Tinnitus: Causes, Symptoms and Treatment

Tinnitus: Causes, Symptoms and Treatment

Edited by Jasmine Richards

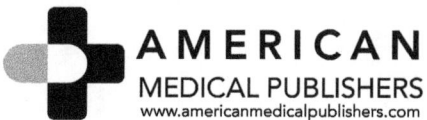

AMERICAN
MEDICAL PUBLISHERS
www.americanmedicalpublishers.com

American Medical Publishers,
41 Flatbush Avenue,
1st Floor, New York,
NY 11217, USA

Visit us on the World Wide Web at:
www.americanmedicalpublishers.com

ISBN: 978-1-63927-415-4

Cataloging-in-Publication Data

Tinnitus : causes, symptoms and treatment / edited by Jasmine Richards.
    p. cm.
Includes bibliographical references and index.
ISBN 978-1-63927-415-4
1. Tinnitus. 2. Hearing disorders. 3. Tinnitus--Etiology. 4. Symptoms.
5. Tinnitus--Treatment. I. Richards, Jasmine.
RF293.8 .T56 2022
617.8--dc23

Table of Contents

Preface

Tinnitus is a hearing disorder in which sound is heard even in the absence of it from any external source. The sound heard is often like a ringing, hissing, roaring, or clicking. It may be loud or soft, high or low pitched. It can affect one ear or both the ears. The persistent sound may cause anxiety, depression and may interfere with concentration. A major cause of tinnitus is noise-induced hearing loss. Ménière's disease, ear infections, brain tumors, exposure to certain medications, head injury and earwax may also cause tinnitus. Tinnitus is determined in a person depending on the description of the audiological abnormalities experienced, and assessment of how the condition is affecting the person's life. The diagnosis may be supported by conducting a neurological examination or an audiogram. Determining the cause of the condition and treating it leads to improvement. Sound therapy, talk therapy and hearing aids can also help the individual in managing the disease. This book elucidates the causes, symptoms and treatment of tinnitus in a comprehensive manner. It strives to provide a fair idea about the modern practices in the management of tinnitus. A number of latest researches have been included to keep the readers up-to-date with the global concepts in this medical condition.

The researches compiled throughout the book are authentic and of high quality, combining several disciplines and from very diverse regions from around the world. Drawing on the contributions of many researchers from diverse countries, the book's objective is to provide the readers with the latest achievements in the area of research. This book will surely be a source of knowledge to all interested and researching the field.

In the end, I would like to express my deep sense of gratitude to all the authors for meeting the set deadlines in completing and submitting their research chapters. I would also like to thank the publisher for the support offered to us throughout the course of the book. Finally, I extend my sincere thanks to my family for being a constant source of inspiration and encouragement.

Editor

Evidence of Key Tinnitus-Related Brain Regions Documented by a Unique Combination of Manganese-Enhanced MRI and Acoustic Startle Reflex Testing

Avril Genene Holt[1]*, David Bissig[1], Najab Mirza[1], Gary Rajah[1], Bruce Berkowitz[1,2]

1 Department of Anatomy and Cell Biology, Wayne State University School of Medicine, Detroit, Michigan, United States of America, **2** Department of Ophthalmology, Wayne State University School of Medicine, Detroit, Michigan, United States of America

Abstract

Animal models continue to improve our understanding of tinnitus pathogenesis and aid in development of new treatments. However, there are no diagnostic biomarkers for tinnitus-related pathophysiology for use in awake, freely moving animals. To address this disparity, two complementary methods were combined to examine reliable tinnitus models (rats repeatedly administered salicylate or exposed to a single noise event): inhibition of acoustic startle and manganese-enhanced MRI. Salicylate-induced tinnitus resulted in wide spread supernormal manganese uptake compared to noise-induced tinnitus. Neither model demonstrated significant differences in the auditory cortex. Only in the dorsal cortex of the inferior colliculus (DCIC) did both models exhibit supernormal uptake. Therefore, abnormal membrane depolarization in the DCIC appears to be important in tinnitus-mediated activity. Our results provide the foundation for future studies correlating the severity and longevity of tinnitus with hearing loss and neuronal activity in specific brain regions and tools for evaluating treatment efficacy across paradigms.

Editor: Jun Yan, Hotchkiss Brain Institute, University of Calgary, Canada

Funding: These studies were supported by the National Institutes of Health [DC007733 to AGH, EY018109 to BAB, P30 Grants (Anatomy and Cell Biology, Wayne State University and Kresge Hearing Research Institute, University of Michigan)], University Medical Student Grant to GR, an unrestricted grant from Research to Prevent Blindness (Kresge Eye Institute) and Wayne State University School of Medicine MD/PhD program for DB. The funders had no role in study design, data collection and analysis, decision to publish, or preparation of the manuscript.

Competing Interests: The authors have declared that no competing interests exist.

* E-mail: agholt@med.wayne.edu

Introduction

Tinnitus, the perception of a ringing, buzzing, or hissing in the absence of an external stimulus due to noise, drugs, or traumatic brain injury, is a rapidly growing major health concern affecting both civilian and military populations [1,2,3,4]. Mounting evidence suggests that tinnitus can be linked with increased spontaneous neuronal activity [5,6,7,8] leading to the use of drugs targeted at reducing spikes of increased activity. However, such approaches have only been partially successful [5,9,10,11,12]. A better understanding of the pathophysiology of tinnitus is needed to improve future treatment efforts.

Animal models of tinnitus (e.g., noise or drug induced) produce increases in spontaneous neuronal activity, which are likely downstream consequences of changes in calcium and calcium channel-dependent neurotransmitter release. Blocking calcium channels with nimodipine has been shown to reduce percepts associated with salicylate-induced tinnitus [13,14,15,16]. Despite such promising results, there is a pressing need to analytically measure calcium ion regulation in auditory-related brain regions to determine whether or not common brain regions and abnormalities exist across tinnitus models.

A recent methodological advance in the tinnitus field involves the use of gap and pre-pulse inhibition of the acoustic startle reflex (ASR) for screening of tinnitus percepts in animal models. The paradigm was designed to assess whether the subject perceives tinnitus by introducing a pre-stimulus "gap" in sound (silence) just prior to the startle stimulus. If the pre-stimulus gap is detected, there is a decreased startle reflex observed when the startle stimulus is presented (Figure 1A–B). If the gap is embedded in a tone that closely matches the animal's tinnitus in frequency and intensity, the result is a full startle reflex that is not blunted [17]. While such psychophysical tests are useful in the assessment of tinnitus percepts, they cannot spatially resolve pathological changes in specific auditory regions and so miss important mechanistic information regarding the initiation and maintenance of tinnitus.

Manganese-enhanced MRI (MEMRI) with systemically administered $MnCl_2$ has been used to examine neuronal activity *in vivo* [18,19,20]. The paramagnetic Mn^{2+} ion (manganese) can enter active neurons through voltage-gated calcium channels, amongst others calcium channels [21,22,23,24,25]. Since manganese efflux from cells is slow [26], activity-dependent accumulation of the ion in brain regions can be measured as a decrease in tissue T_1 at high spatial resolution hours later [27,28,29]. In this manner, MEMRI has been used to measure sound-evoked activity in the midbrain from awake and free moving rodents [20,30]. To-date only one study has used MEMRI to investigate tinnitus, however, analysis was performed in excised tissue [18]. Whether manganese accumulation in auditory-related brain regions will be sensitive enough to detect differences between awake and freely moving animals with and without tinnitus or between groups with tinnitus

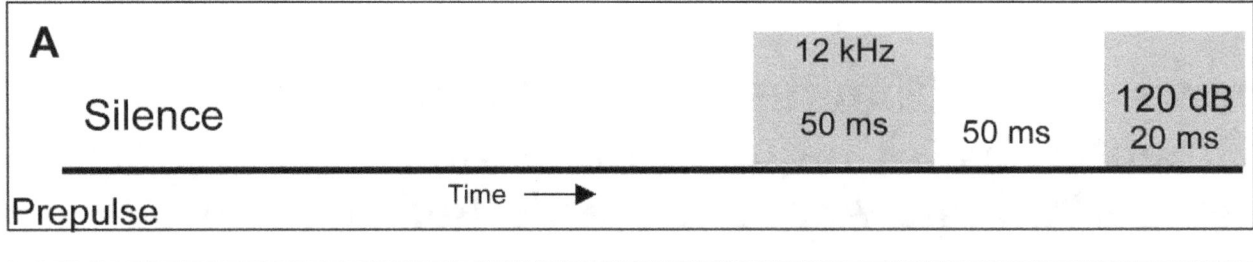

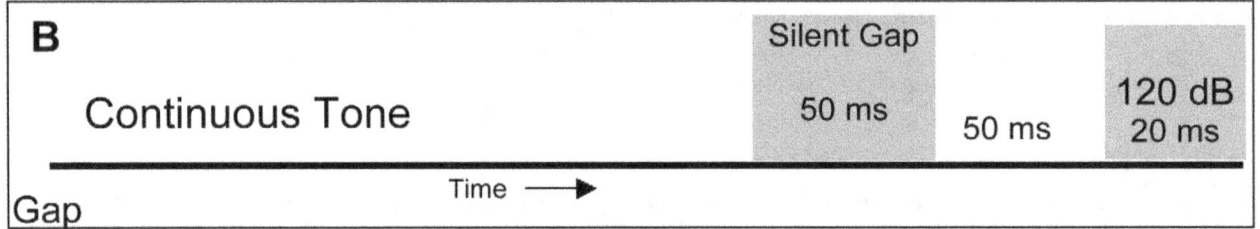

Figure 1. Schematic of acoustic startle reflex (ASR) under conditions of pre-pulse (pASR) or gap (gASR) inhibition. (A) During the pASR test animals are presented with a randomly introduced 120 dB stimulus resulting in a measurable startle response. If a 50 ms tone preceding a 50 ms silent period is introduced and detected just prior to the startle stimulus, usually a decreased startle reflex is observed. **(B)** When a startle stimulus is presented in the presence of a continuous background tone (4,8,12, 16, 20, or 24 kHz) a startle reflex is elicited. If a 50 ms silent gap in the background tone is presented just prior to the startle stimulus then the startle response is decreased. However, if an animal has tinnitus percepts and the tone matches the tinnitus in frequency and loudness then the silent gap is filled in by the animal's tinnitus and the startle response is not significantly blunted.

produced by different means (noise, salicylate, blast wave, etc.) remains to be determined.

In this study, behavioral (ASR) and imaging (MEMRI) assessments were combined to identify and characterize early stages of tinnitus in two different animal models. We have identified a common brain region with increased activity regardless of the method of tinnitus induction, and brain regions in which activation is specific to the method used to induce the tinnitus.

Results

Salicylate and noise exposure result in temporal differences in hearing loss

Relative to that in controls (average of 30 dB across three frequencies), injection of salicylate results in significant changes in hearing thresholds (32 dB; $p = 0.04$) when animals were tested two hours following administration on the second day of treatment (Table 1). After 10 hours with no additional salicylate hearing thresholds returned to normal (Table 2). Therefore, daily administration of salicylate resulted in daily temporary threshold shifts averaging 1–12 dB across frequencies depending upon the time after salicylate administration. In contrast, animals that were exposed to a 10 kHz 118 dB 1/3 octave band noise generally exhibited profound deafness (Table 1) with average thresholds of 98 dB or more in the ear that was not plugged ($p = 6.0 \, E^{-6}$) and elevated thresholds averaging of 51 dB across the three frequencies, tested in the plugged ear, that were not significantly different from control thresholds ($p = 0.09$). Two animals that were noise exposed, but were not imaged had ABR assessment at both 24 and 48 hours with animals tested at 48 hours showing no significant change in hearing thresholds from the 24 hour time point (data not shown). Therefore, in contrast to salicylate-induced changes in hearing threshold, we found no evidence for diminished noise-induced changes in this study. Therefore, changes in hearing, as measured by ABR, were temporary for salicylate-injected animals and permanent (bilaterally, although asymmetrical) for sound

exposed animals (Tables 1 and 2). To determine whether these temporal differences in hearing loss would differentially affect tinnitus percepts we recorded pASR and gASR across both animal models of tinnitus and normal hearing controls.

ASR demonstrates specific tinnitus percepts specific to the animal model

To compare behavioral correlates of salicylate and noise induced tinnitus, the acoustic startle reflex was tested and compared at three time points per group, before salicylate treatment or noise exposure (baseline 2–3 measures), after salicylate administration (after one hour on day two) or noise treatment (after 24 hours) as well as on the day of imaging seven hours after the final administration of salicylate or 55 hours following noise (Figure 2).

For ASR testing animals needed to demonstrate the ability to exhibit a robust startle reflex in response to a brief loud noise as well as the capacity to attenuate the startle reflex in the presence of a pre-pulse or a silent gap in a tone. Of the animals tested for startle reflex under baseline conditions, all of the animals exhibited both a robust sound off startle reflex as well as the ability to inhibit the reflex in approximately 70% of the 120 total trials - - ten trials recorded for each of the six different frequencies tested at two different sound levels (45 and 60 dB for control and salicylate groups, 70 and 95 dB for the noise exposed group).

Control animals showed a robust attenuation of both the pASR and the gASR regardless of the frequency that was tested (Figure 3). However, inhibition of the acoustic startle reflex was less variable at 60 dB when compared to 45 dB (data not shown) suggesting that the higher intensity pre-pulse or background tones increased ASR sensitivity when comparing performance across frequencies. Therefore results are presented for the 60 dB levels.

In pre-drug baseline testing, rats in the salicylate group detected either the prepulse (Figure 3A) or the gap (Figure 3B) and demonstrated the ability to suppress the startle reflex. Across frequencies, pASR testing revealed robust suppression of the

Table 1. Summary of hearing thresholds following salicylate or noise treatment: Auditory brainstem responses.

Frequency	4 kHz		12 kHz		20 kHz		Average		P-value [a]	
Treatment	*Left*	*Right*	*Left*	*Right*	*Left*	*Right*	*Left*	*Right*		
Control [b, c]	31±5.74	29±3.85	29±2.49	28±2.40	30±4.77	30±3.30	30±4.33	29±3.18	-	
Salicylate [b, c]	30±2.50	33±3.50	32±3.95	32±2.38	31±3.11	32±2.22	31±3.01	32±2.62	0.05	
Noise I [b, c]	**33±6.85**	96±9.00	**65±22.81**	100 ↑	**62±19.25**	100 ↑	**53±21.80**	99±5.20	**Noise-Plugged**	**0.16**
									Noise-Unplugged	0.004
Noise II [b, c]	90±14.14	**30±2.12**	100 ↑	**58±14.14**	100 ↑	**51±24.04**	97±8.16	**46±18.25**	**Noise-Plugged**	**0.19**
									Noise-Unplugged	0.001

[a]Significance p≤0.05.
[b]Hearing threshold, expressed in decibels (dB).
[c]Error (±) is expressed as SEM.
100 ↑ More than 100 dB.
Bold indicates the protected (plugged) ear (Noise I left ear protected Noise II had the right ear protected).

startle reflex ($46.5\% \pm 1.69$) prior to treatment. Greater suppression was observed one hour after salicylate treatment on the second day ($69.5\% \pm 1.50$; $p < 0.0001$), and seven hours after salicylate treatment on the third day ($59\% \pm 2.34$; $p < 0.0001$; Figure 3A). Relative to the full startle response amplitude (100%) gASR testing at 12 kHz (Figure 3B) resulted in a robust attenuation of startle ($26\% \pm 2.92$). After salicylate treatment, gASR startle amplitude was significantly increased at 12 kHz ($12\% \pm 3.85$; $p = 0.05$) over baseline, but was not significantly different from baseline 7 hours post treatment (Figure 3B). In addition, salicylate treated animals exerted significantly more force in response to the startle stimulus only when compared to controls both during pASR (Figure 4A) testing (0.90 ± 0.08; $p < 0.0001$ 1 hr after injection; 0.93 ± 0.14; $p < 0.0001$ seven hrs after injection) and gASR (Figure 4B) testing (0.22 ± 0.04; $p = 0.02$ 1 hr after injection; 0.25 ± 0.03; $p \leq 0.05$ seven hrs after injection). Thus, gASR testing demonstrated cyclical salicylate-induced tinnitus as shown by ABR (Table 2), while pASR testing demonstrated a more sustained hyperacusis (Figure 3A) with both tests reflecting increased force following treatment when comparing force exerted in response to startle stimulation only (Figure 4).

Just as with the control and the salicylate groups, the baseline measures in the noise group indicated the ability of the animals to reliably inhibit pASR and gASR (Figure 5). Following exposure to a 10 kHz 118 dB 1/3 octave band sound animals sustained a substantive threshold shift (Table 1). Therefore the intensities for the pre-pulse (pASR) and background tones (gASR) were increased to levels that could be detected by the animals (70 and 95 dB). Despite the noise exposure, animals attenuated pASR

Table 2. Hearing thresholds at two time points following salicylate administration: Auditory brainstem responses.

Frequency	4 kHz	12 kHz	20 kHz
Treatment			
Control [a,b]	30±5.04	28±2.45	30±4.15
6 hrs after injection [a,b]	34±2.99	34±2.50	33±2.89
10 hrs after injection [a,b]	30±2.22	30±1.73	30±1.50

[a]Hearing threshold, expressed in decibels (dB).
[b]Error (±) is expressed as SEM.

responses across all frequencies at each time point tested (baseline – 30%, 24 hrs – 20%, 55 hrs – 24%) confirming that the animals were able to hear the pre-pulse (Figure 5A) with the decrease from 30% to 20 and 24% suggesting hearing loss effects. When tested for inhibition of gASR, there was a significant reduction in the ability to inhibit the acoustic startle reflex at both post-noise time points at the frequencies of 12 (baseline – 28%, 24 hrs – 16% $p = 0.0079$, 55 hrs – 14% $p = .0008$) and 16 kHz (baseline – 33%, 24 hrs – 21% $p = 0.0079$, 55 hrs – 17% $p = 0.0003$), reflecting the capacity of gASR to demonstrate not only the hearing loss but the perception of tinnitus as well. The results suggest that the tinnitus percepts were fairly tonal in nature and were experienced across two (12 kHz and 16 kHz) of the tested frequencies (Figure 5B–C).

In animals that were not exposed to salicylate or noise, (the control group), the ability to inhibit the gASR remained constant (Figure 6). However, the salicylate group showed a decreased ability to inhibit gASR one hour after salicylate treatment, but by seven hours the ability to attenuate gASR had returned to normal levels. For noise-exposed animals, the ability to inhibit the gASR remained decreased at both time points following noise exposure (Figure 6). These results further support the idea that the tinnitus experienced by the salicylate group was transient while the noise-exposed group experienced a more uninterrupted tinnitus.

MEMRI measures tinnitus-dependent differential regional brain activity

Salicylate and noise groups were given manganese 8 hours prior to imaging. This corresponded to a time when animals exhibited behavioral correlates of tinnitus (ASR testing of salicylate and noise groups).

All manganese-injected animals exhibited the expected high signal intensities in the anterior pituitary [31]. Raw signal intensities (before normalization to muscle) were analyzed at this location to verify that control and tinnitus groups experienced similar brain systemic manganese exposure: Between groups, raw signal intensities were similar at the anterior pituitary and adjacent muscle alike (one-way ANOVAs, $P > 0.05$). These raw intensities were correlated ($r = 0.49$; $P = 0.016$), indicating that normalization to muscle would reduce inter-subject variability in brain signal intensities. After normalization to adjacent muscle, no group differences were found at the anterior pituitary (one-way ANOVA, $P > 0.05$).

In non-auditory regions (listed in Table 3), no significant group differences in manganese uptake were found (one-way ANOVAs, $P > 0.05$). For completeness, mean normalized signal intensities for

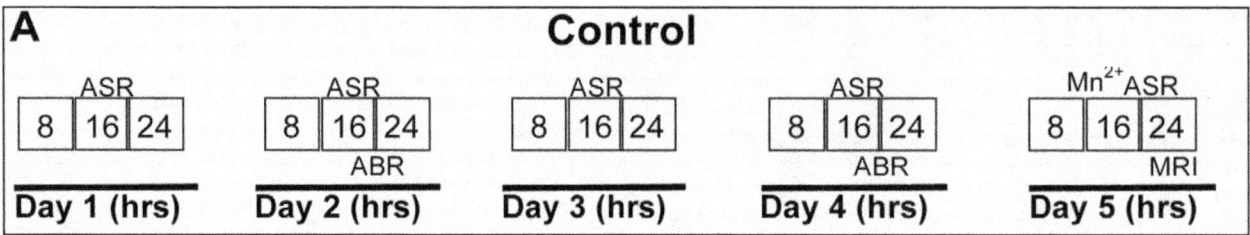

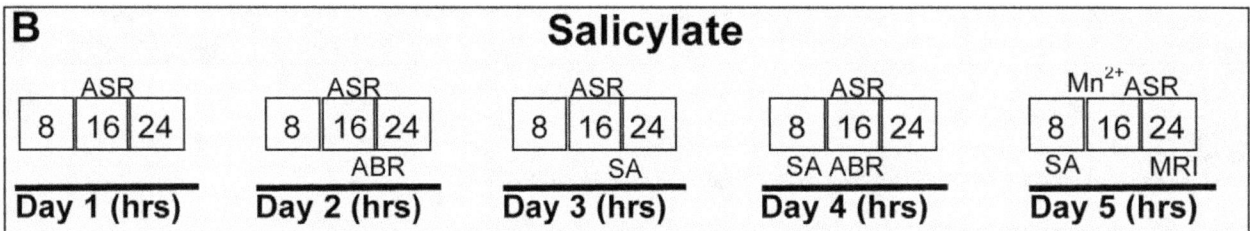

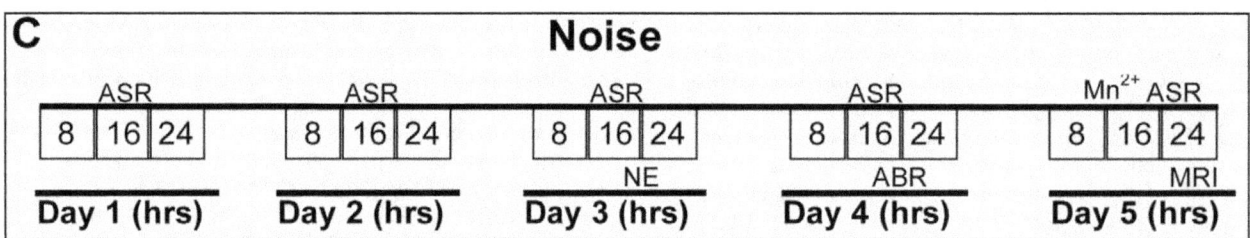

Figure 2. Time line showing day and approximate time of day for each procedure. Acoustic startle reflex testing (ASR) for tinnitus perception, auditory brainstem response testing (ABR) for hearing loss, tinnitus induction, manganese injection and imaging in control (**A**), salicylate (**B**) and noise (**C**) groups during a given day. 8 – first eight hrs of day, 16 – second eight hr period of day, 24 – last eight hr period of day, SA – salicylate injection, NE – noise exposure, Mn^{2+} - manganese injection, MRI – magnetic resonance imaging.

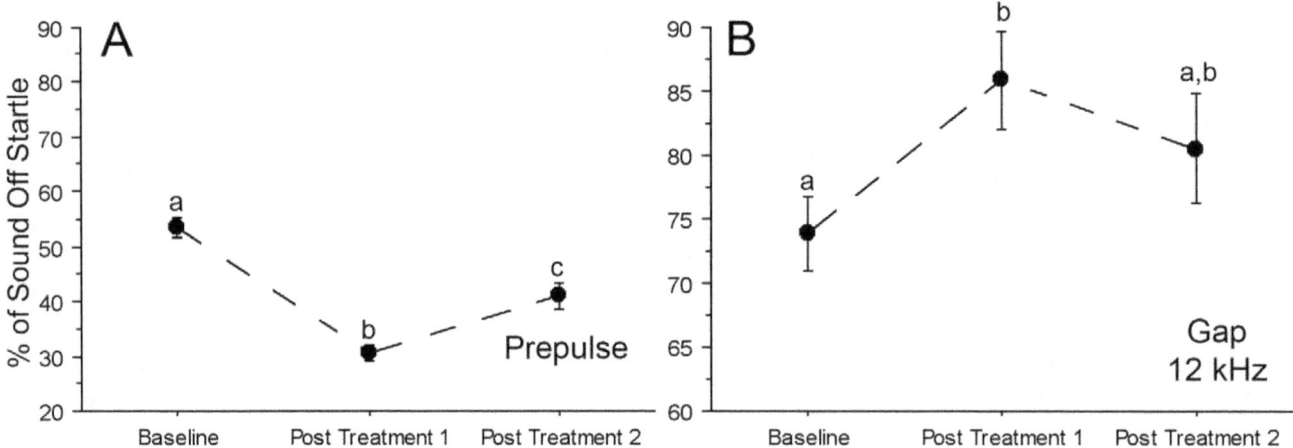

Figure 3. Salicylate results in a decreased ability to blunt the acoustic startle response (ASR) under conditions of gap inhibition. Performance during ASR testing was recorded before treatment (Baseline), 1 hr following the second day of salicylate administration (Post Treatment 1) and seven hrs following the third day of salicylate administration (Post Treatment 2). Relative to a full startle response (100%), untreated rats detected the gap and prepulse and could suppress the startle reflex across all frequencies (baseline in **A**). Across all frequencies significant decreases in pASR were observed relative to baseline both one hour following salicylate administration (Post Treatment 1) and seven hours after treatment (Post Treatment 2) (**A**). When compared to baseline, $p = 0.0001$ for both Post Treatment 1 and 2 (compare a–b and a–c). Post Treatment 1 and 2 were also significantly different from one another (b–c; $p = 0.0004$). At 12 kHz the % sound off startle initially changed by 12% ($p = 0.05$) from Baseline to Post Treatment 1, but was not significantly different from Baseline during Post Treatment 2 testing (**B**). Differing letters denote significance across time points, $p \leq 0.05$ was significant; error bars equal SEM.

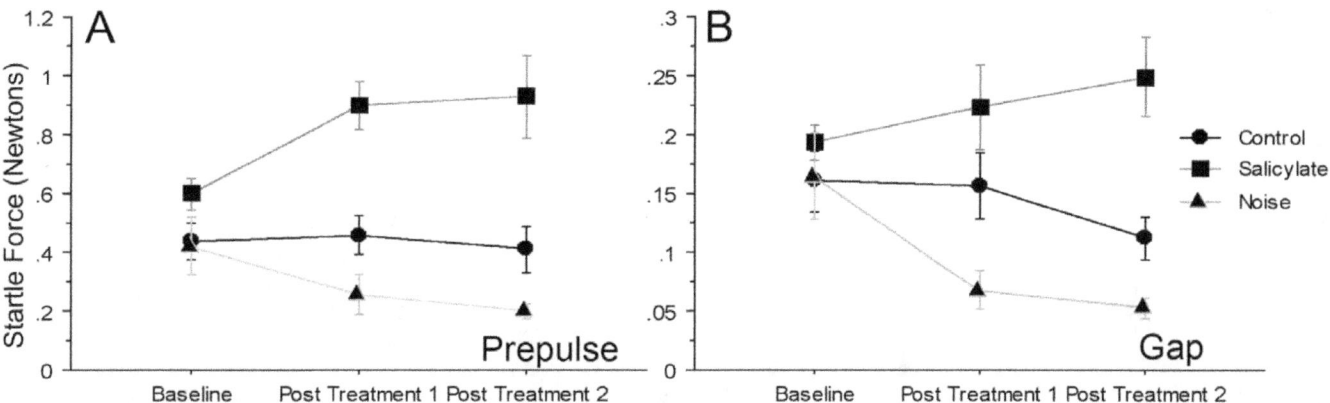

Figure 4. Treatment with salicylate or noise results in changes in startle force elicited by the startle stimulus. There was no significant difference in Baseline acoustic startle response (ASR) values during Prepulse (**A**) or Gap (**B**) tests when comparing control, salicylate and noise groups. Follwing salicylate treatment there were significant differences in startle force when compared to controls during prepulse testing for both Post Treatment 1 and Post Treatment 2 (p≤0.0001 in each case) as well as gap testing (Post Treatment 2 p = 0.002). For the noise treated group there no significant differences in startle force when compared to controls during prepulse testing for Post Treatment 1 or Post Treatment 2 (p = 0.093) nor gap testing for Post Treatment 1 or 2 (p = .09). p≤0.05 was significant; error bars equal SEM.

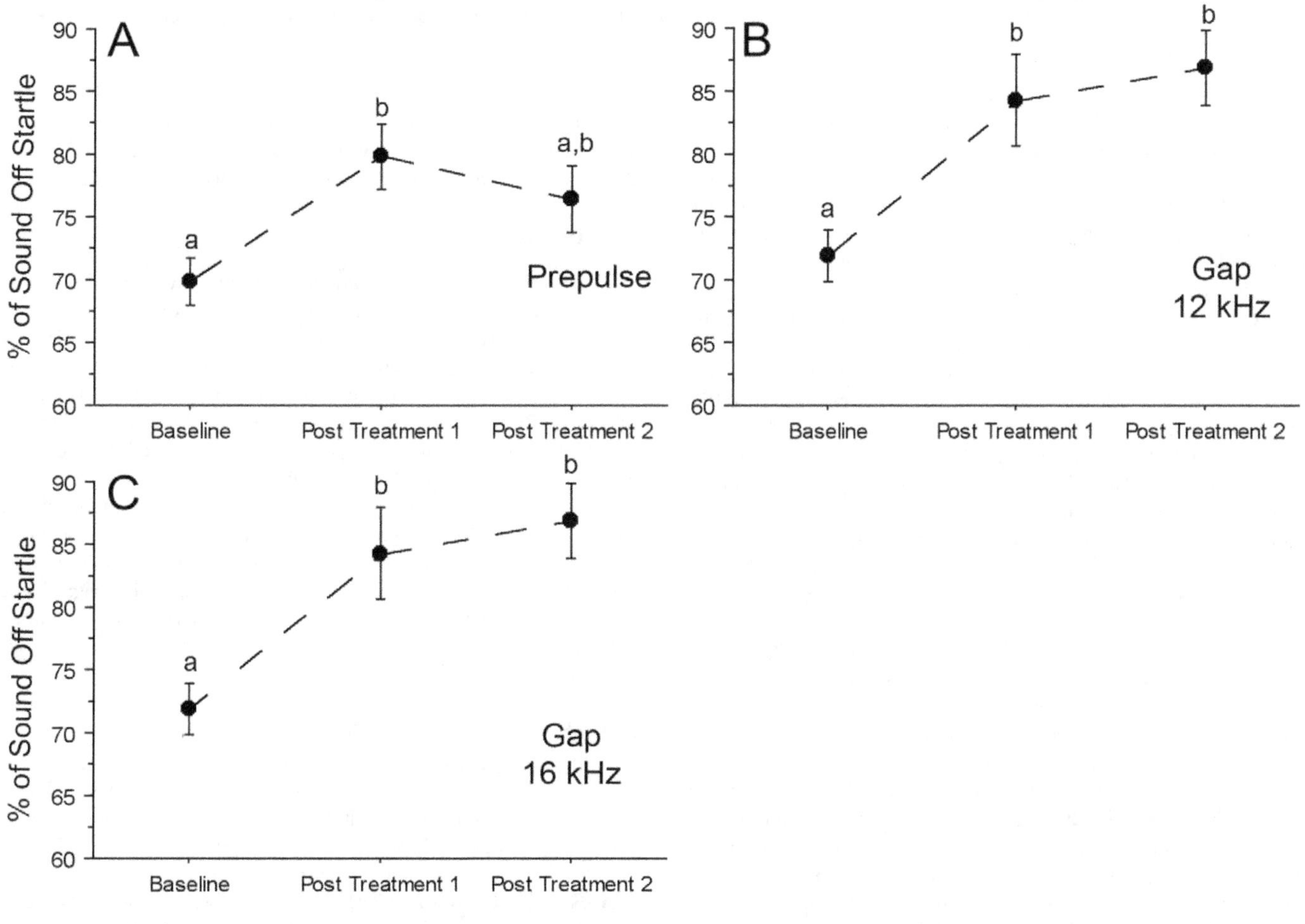

Figure 5. Hearing loss (pre-pulse) and tinnitus (Gap) perception following exposure to loud noise. A decreased ability to blunt the acoustic startle response (ASR) occurred under conditions prepulse inhibition (**A**), but was more pronounced during gap inhibition testing (**B,C**). Performance during ASR testing was recorded before noise exposure (Baseline), on the second day following noise exposure (Post Treatment 1) and on the third day following noise exposure (Post Treatment 2). (**A**) Relative to a full startle response (100%) animals were able to suppress the ASR by 30% during prepulse detection trials (baseline). (**B**) However, during post treatment 1 testing, at 12 kHz suppression was only 16% and by 48 hrs (post treatment 2) only 13%. (**C**) Also, at 16 kHz baseline gASR was 33% but by 24 hrs after noise exposure (post treatment 1) was only 21% of baseline and after 48 hrs (post treatment 2) 17% of baseline. Differing letters denote significance across time points, p≤0.05 was considered significant; error bars equal SEM.

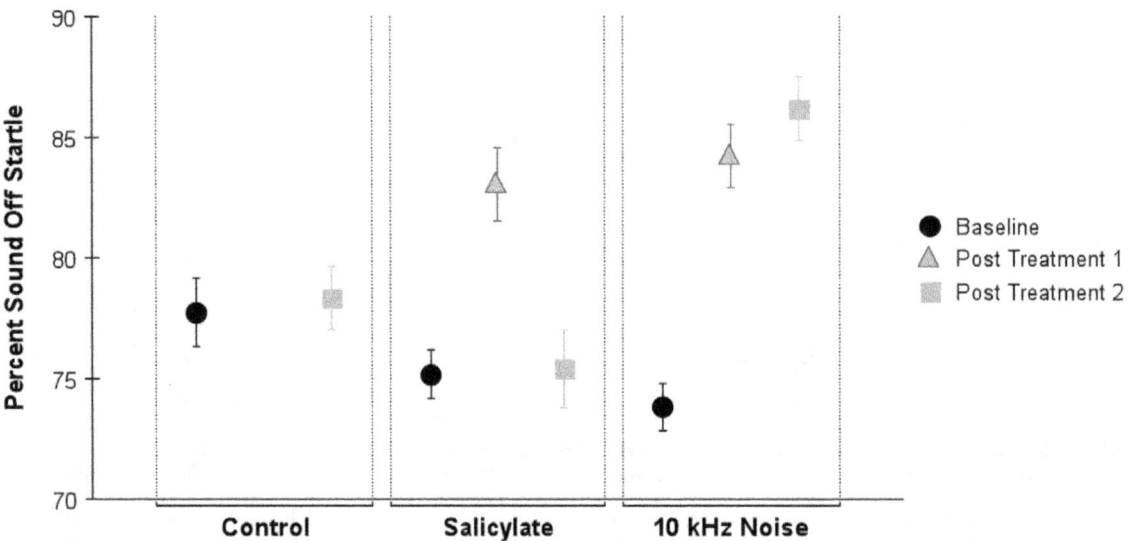

Figure 6. Summary graph of gap ASR comparing experimental groups (control, salicylate, noise) at three different time points (baseline, post treatment 1 and post treatment 2). For control animals the percent inhibition of startle remains constant. For the salicylate group post treatment 1 testing resulted in decreased inhibition of gASR, but by post treatment 2 testing, gASR had returned to normal levels. The 10 kHz noise group demonstrated a decreased ability to inhibit gASR at both time points following noise exposure when compared to baseline. Error bars equal SEM.

these regions, along with specific two-tailed t-test comparisons of the control group to each experimental group, are presented in Table 3. Layer-specific analysis of the cortex revealed no group differences (P>0.05 for all cortical depths tested in all regions). Normalized signal intensities, averaged over cortical depths corresponding to layers II through VI, are similarly provided in Table 3.

Significant group differences were found in the DCN (Figure 7A–B; $F_{[2,17]}$ = 5.22; P = 0.017) and the DCIC (Figure 8A–B; $F_{[2,17]}$ = 7.60; P = 0.004). In post-hoc testing (two-tailed t-tests, uncorrected p-values reported), DCN manganese uptake was similar in noise-exposed and control groups (P>0.05), but elevated in the salicylate-exposed group (vs. noise P = 0.033; vs. control, P = 0.023; Figure 7A–B). In contrast, DCIC manganese uptake was elevated in animals with tinnitus (control vs. noise, P = 0.025; control vs. salicylate, P = 0.005); and there was no significant difference between salicylate- and noise-exposed groups (P>0.05; Figure 8A–B;). Statistical conclusions were identical when Tukey's Honestly Significant Difference test was used for post-hoc analysis (data not shown).

Besides the DCIC and DCN, no group differences in manganese uptake were found for any other sub-cortical structures (Figure 7–8 and Table 3). Sub-divisions of the inferior colliculus besides the DCIC (i.e. the ECIC and CNIC) failed to reach statistical significance (Figure 8), we found no evidence for group-wise regional differences within the inferior colliculus: Tests for both the ECIC and CNIC regions reached marginal significance (for each region, $F_{[2,17]}$>2.73; P<0.10), and showed a similar between-group pattern of manganese uptake (Figure 8 i.e. control<salicylate; noise≈salicylate). In each group, normalized signal intensities trended lower in the ECIC and CNIC than in the DCIC (Table 3), though only for the CNIC was this difference significant in all three groups (paired two-tailed t-tests, P<0.002 for each). In control animals, VCN signal intensities were greater than in the DCIC, though still lower than in the DCN (paired two-tailed t-tests; p = 0.009 and 0.001 respectively, Table 3).

The pattern of regional signal intensities seen in the auditory regions of control animals (DCN>VCN>DCIC>CNIC>Aud) is

intriguing. However, several factors unrelated to baseline neuronal activity may complicate between-region comparisons of MEMRI data (e.g. differences in myelination, proximity to ventricular space).

Discussion

The literature suggests anomalous neural activity within central auditory pathways associated with tinnitus inducing drugs and noise [32,33,34,35]. However, this is the first study in which all subjects undergoing tinnitus assessment also underwent imaging analysis in vivo. Using this approach we found that both salicylate and noise-induced tinnitus result in increased neuronal activity in DCIC neurons. The IC is the point of integration of all ascending and descending projections to the auditory cortex with the DCIC receiving the largest portion of the descending fibers [36,37,38,39,40,41,42]. The DCIC receives ascending projections from the DCN, the anteroventral cochlear nucleus (AVCN) and the dorsal nucleus of the lateral lemniscus (DNLL). Significant changes in activity were not observed in MGN or the auditory cortex. Future work may detect a spread of increased neuronal activity to those regions over time.

ASR characterization of tinnitus percepts

First, we evaluated the tinnitus status of each rat. Using inhibition of startle techniques, pASR and gASR, we were able to correlate a decrease in the ability to inhibit the ASR at specific frequencies with the perception of tinnitus. These data support and extend previous results using this technique to characterize tinnitus.

ASR inhibition discriminates fluctuations in salicylate induced tinnitus. In the salicylate group, relative to a full startle response, all animals exhibited the ability to inhibit their ASR prior to treatment. One hour following salicylate administration, ASR suppression was diminished, though only for pre-startle tones centered on a frequency of 12 kHz (11–13 kHz). These results closely match previous studies, which identify salicylate-induced tinnitus with percepts ranging from ~10–16 kHz [43,44,45,46,47,48,49]. Six hours after the last

Table 3. Effects of salicylate and noise exposure on neuronal activity in different brain regions as measured by manganese enhanced MRI.

Tinnitus Group		Control [bcd]	Salicylate [bcd]	Noise [bcd]
Brain Region				
Amyg [a]	mean	160.8±4.0	158.7±6.8	169.7±6.6
	p-value		0.77	0.23
Au1 [a]	mean	149.9±1.8	145.2±4.7	151.9±4.6
	p-value		0.39	0.69
AuD	mean	148.7±2.1	144.7±4.8	152.5±5.2
	p-value		0.46	0.52
DCN [a]	mean	210.3±6.8	242.4±12.1	209.9±5.2
	p-value		0.02	0.96
VCN	mean	189.0±5.6	189.5 ±3.9	187.4±9.0
	p-value		0.94	0.79
VCPO	mean	195.8±7.4	190.9±3.5	198.8±4.5
	p-value		0.55	0.73
Floc [a]	mean	172.0±5.2	168.3±1.9	169.1±3.4
	p-value		0.52	0.64
Pfloc	mean	162.7±4.1	158.0±2.1	158.0±3.1
	p-value		0.43	0.38
LGN [a]	mean	152.2±3.0	154.6±4.9	164.5±6.0
	p-value		0.94	0.79
MGN	mean	167.3±4.7	170.4±3.5	170.9±5.0
	p-value		0.59	0.59
CNIC [a]	mean	163.1±3.4	174.2±3.6	170.9±4.2
	p-value		0.03	0.15
DCIC	mean	176.7±3.2	195.2±5.0	186.4±2.2
	p-value		0.01	0.03
ECIC	mean	175.7±3.5	186.5±2.3	181.6±3.9
	p-value		0.02	0.25
SC	mean	162.9±4.7	169.8±4.4	169.8±4.8
	p-value		0.28	0.34
TeA [a]	mean	156.2±2.2	153.4±4.2	154.7±2.8
	p-value		0.58	0.69
V1	mean	148.2±2.5	147.0±3.7	154.5±4.3
	p-value		0.80	0.24
V1B	mean	150.0±3.4	156.0±3.3	157.3±2.7
	p-value		0.23	0.12
V1M	mean	147.2±3.4	154.8±3.8	157.9±3.1
	p-value		0.17	0.04
V2L	mean	154.9±2.7	155.8±3.1	153.5±3.2
	p-value		0.73	0.84
V2MM & V2ML	mean	145.9±2.6	149.0±4.3	154.0±4.1
	p-value		0.44	0.12

[a]Bold text indicates beginning of new brain region.
[b]Signal intensity, expressed as the percentage of adjacent muscle; arbitrary units (a.u.).
[c]Significance $p \leq 0.05$.
[d]Error (±) is expressed as SEM.

salicylate injection, gASR inhibition was not significantly different from baseline, likely reflecting the decrease in systemic salicylate and therefore decreased tinnitus perception. These results are consistent with those of other studies demonstrating that salicylate induced tinnitus in the rat is stable in terms of hearing loss and tinnitus perception by the third day of treatment and that the perception of tinnitus is reversible [43,44,45,46,47,48,49].

ASR inhibition suggests salicylate induced tinnitus results in hyperacusis. We also tested the performance of the animals in pASR testing. We typically use pASR to verify that animals can detect tones and thus negate hearing loss as a factor on performance. Prior to treatment animals were able to inhibit their ASR in response to a pre-pulse. Following salicylate treatment the inhibition was more robust. Previous studies as well as the current study have noted a general increase in startle amplitude for animals administered salicylate [49,50,51]. Because each startle event is compared to the full startle response from each session, the ability to suppress the startle response following salicylate administration would be expected to diminish. This was not the case in the present work, suggesting an improvement in auditory perception leading to a heightened suppression of the startle response that has been termed "hyperacusis". This type of sensitivity to loud noise is often observed in human subjects with tinnitus.

ASR inhibition differentiates frequency specific changes in noise-induced tinnitus. In animal models, noise has also been used to induce tinnitus, as defined via behavioral testing, [17,52,53]. In addition to the current study, other reports demonstrate that exposure to the equivalent of a 10 kHz 118 dB 1/3 octave band tone results in tinnitus, but also profound deafness [54]. Since the ASR performance is dependent upon hearing, in the current study one ear in each animal from the noise group was plugged during the noise exposure, leaving that ear capable of detecting the tones for pASR and gASR in addition to resulting in an asymmetric hearing loss. The fact that only one functional ear is necessary for pASR and gASR tinnitus assessment has previously been reported [17]. To compensate for increased hearing thresholds in the plugged ear, intensity levels were raised for ASR testing. To determine whether the animals had the ability to hear well enough to inhibit the ASR, we first tested pASR. Animals were able to consistently decrease their startle amplitude from the full startle response (i.e. 100%). Next, performance on the gASR test was assessed and both 12 kHz and 16 kHz showed evidence of tinnitus-like percepts at both time points (24 and 48) hours following noise exposure.

Thus, a total of two ASR sessions were recorded following treatment with either salicylate or noise. The second post treatment ASR test was given 54 to 56 hours following the initial induction of tinnitus. For the salicylate group this time point corresponded with seven hours following the day three salicylate injection (post treatment 2 ASR) and results from gASR testing showed no significant difference between the post treatment 2 gASR (7 hours following the day three salicylate injection) and baseline measures perhaps indicating a lack or decrease of tinnitus percepts. These results support previous findings showing the diminution of tinnitus percepts within four–six hours following salicylate administration [51]. For the noise group, frequencies associated with tinnitus percepts post-treatment, continued to exhibit gASR measures significantly different from baseline measures even on the second day of assessment following exposure. Our results confirm findings from previous studies showing that gASR is an advantageous and reliable technique for assessment of tinnitus whether induced by salicylate [30] or noise [17,51]. Given our ASR results in both the salicylate and noise groups we concluded that the animals experienced tinnitus-like percepts. However, ASR tests do not provide insight into specific tinnitus-related brain pathophysiology such as altered regulation of ions (i.e., calcium).

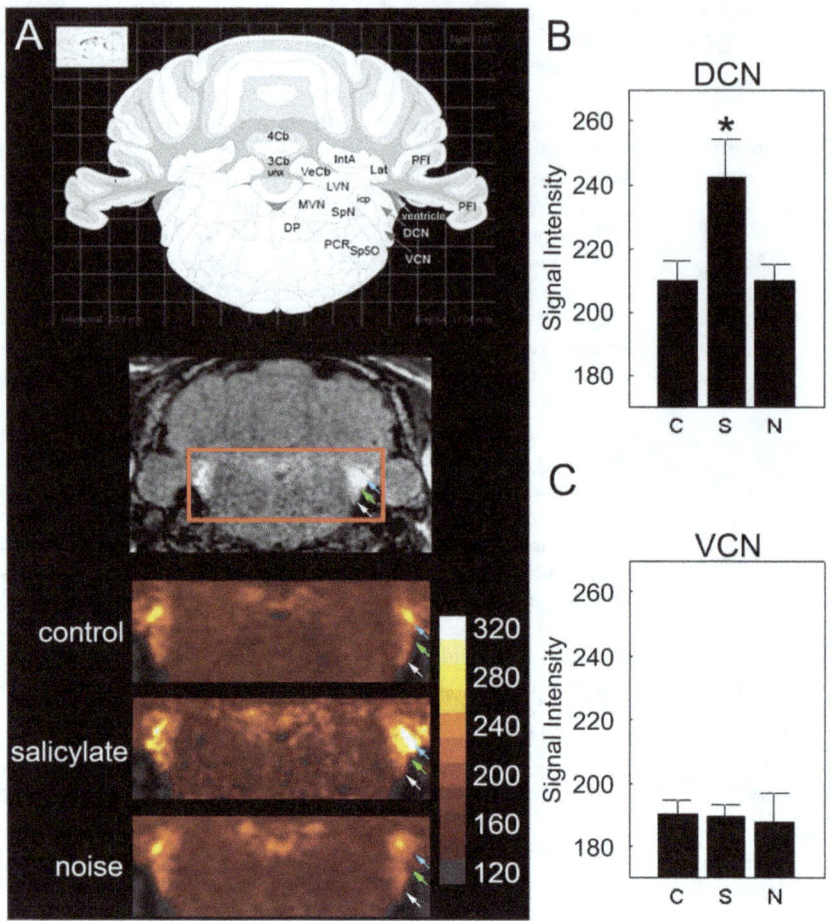

Figure 7. Salicyate increases MEMRI measured signal intensity in the DCN but not the VCN. In the dorsal cochlear nucleus (DCN) a significant increase in signal intensity was observed (**A–B**) in the salicylate treated group (242. 37±12.08; p = 0.02) when compared to controls (210.26±6.76), but no change was observed in the VCN (**A, C**). Noise exposure does not change MEMRI measured signal intensity in the DCN (209. 90±5.22; p = 0.02) or VCN (187. 41±9.02; p = 0.02) 48 hrs post noise exposure (**A–C**). Signal intensity is calculated as a percentage of nearby muscle. Asterisk denotes significance, p≤0.05; error bars equal StDev, C – control, S – salicylate, N - noise exposed In MRI panels white arrows indicate VCN, green arrows indicate DCN, and blue arrows indicate ventricular space.

MEMRI demonstrates differential brain region activation in salicylate and noise induced tinnitus

Manganese, an activity-dependent contrast agent, accumulates in active neurons through, for example, voltage-gated calcium channels. Increased neuronal activity results in increased cellular manganese uptake. For a given region of interest then, differences in manganese accumulation, measured non-invasively with MRI, reflect differences in neuronal activity during the period of manganese accumulation, before anesthesia and MR imaging [55]. The use of MEMRI avoids a major drawback of doing functional studies in MRI scanners for testing of central auditory structures: an extremely noisy scanner environment. Since manganese uptake is activity dependent and loss from the cell is slow, neuronal activity in awake animals can thus be encoded outside of the magnet with activity readout hours later.

In the present study, MRI images with high spatial resolution were needed to analyze the relatively small regions in the auditory brainstem. To this end, brain manganese levels were measured using signal intensities from T_1-weighted images. Normalization to adjacent tissue is a common part of this approach, either to a negative-control brain region [56,57] or to nearby muscle [18,27,55,58]. The tissue used for normalization must be carefully selected, as underlying group differences there may obscure or over-emphasize group differences in regions of experimental interest. The quality of normalization can be gauged by evaluating negative-control regions, where no group differences are expected. In the present work, negative findings at the anterior pituitary and throughout the visual system – covering a broad range of enhancement levels – are consistent with appropriate normalization, as are the heterogeneous results for neighboring and identically-normalized auditory regions (e.g. VCN vs. DCN). Future work may benefit from T_1 mapping of the brain [31] since this will be sensitive to a broader range of tissue manganese concentrations while being unaffected by receive-coil artifacts – the primary motive for normalizing signal intensities in the present study.

Recent studies have suggested that MEMRI can be used to image the auditory brainstem [18,20,59]. For example, MEMRI was used to identify tinnitus related activated brain regions ex vivo [18]. Previous lower-resolution studies have utilized PET and MRI to identify tinnitus associated brain regions that show changes in neuronal activity [60], however the low resolution of these techniques has prevented detailed identification of brain regions involved. Further corroboration of the sensitivity of the MEMRI for use in the auditory system is the interesting correlation of signal intensity and brain regions in normal hearing controls. We found

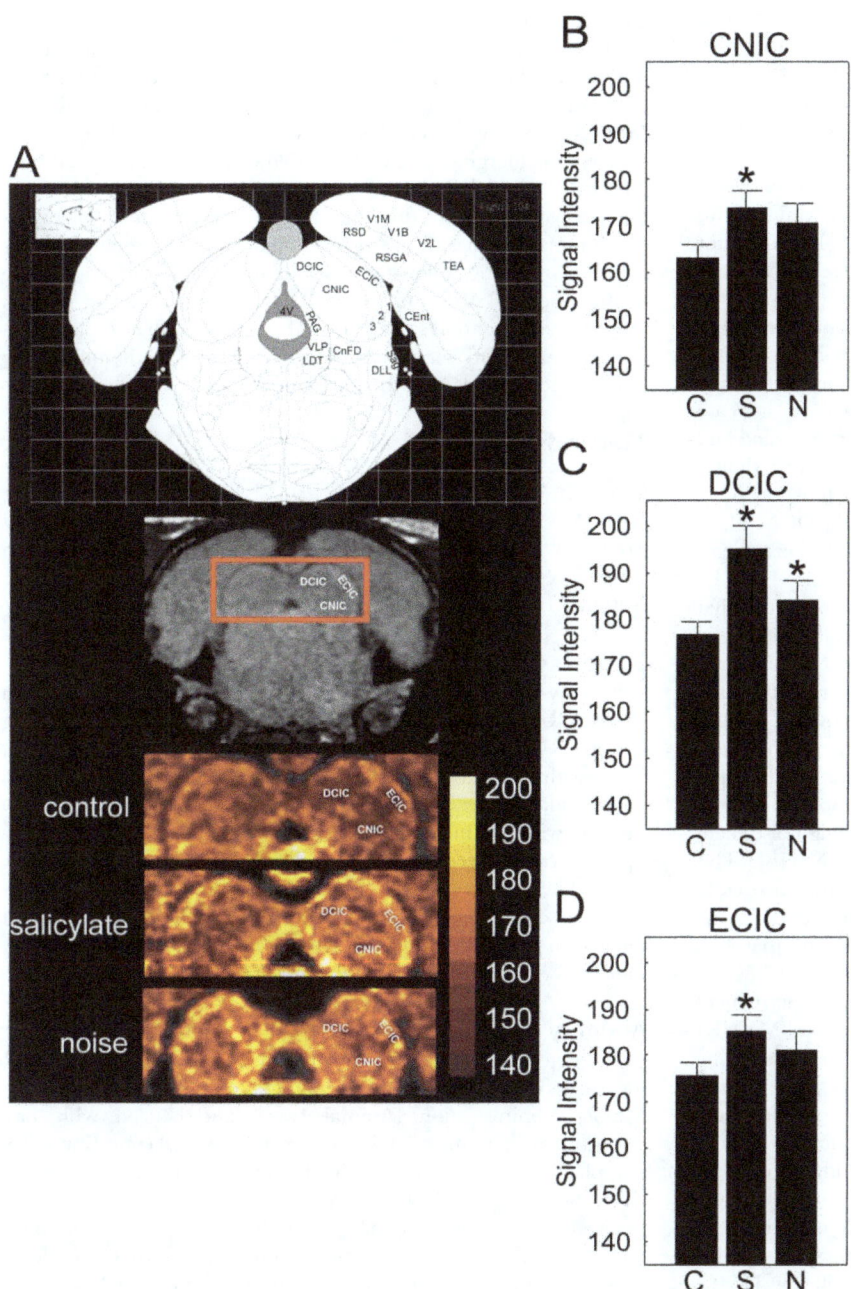

Figure 8. Effects of salicyate and noise exposure on MEMRI measured signal intensity in the inferior colliculus after three days of salicylate administration and 48 hrs post noise exposure. Signal intensity was compared across groups (A–D). In the salicylate group, manganese accumulation was supernormal in the central nucleus of the inferior colliculus (B; CNIC; 174. 20±3.60; p = 0.03), as well as the dorsal cortex (C; DCIC; 195. 21±4.96; p = 0.005) and external cortex (D; ECIC; 186. 52±2.35; p = 0.02) when compared to controls. In the noise exposed group, only the DCIC had increased signal intensity (186. 35±2.17; p = 0.03). Asterisks denote significance, p≤0.05; error bars equal StDev, C – control, S – salicylate, N - noise exposed.

higher signal intensities in the DCN when compared to the VCN. This fits well with other studies in which the VCN is reported to have lower levels of spontaneous neuronal activity as assessed via electrophysiology when compared to the DCN [61,62,63]. Following deafferentation, the DCN continues to show spontaneous activity while the VCN is quieted [64,65,66]. Our results support these findings with the DCN exhibiting significantly more manganese uptake than the VCN in normal hearing animals and with only DCN showing changes in activity following tinnitus induction.

MEMRI associated changes in neuronal activity within auditory pathways occurred bilaterally. In the current study, brains of animals with salicylate and noise induced tinnitus-like percepts were compared during the early stages of tinnitus onset. In the DCN and DCIC, there were no differences observed in manganese uptake in the right and left sides. Since the injections of salicylate were systemic, this result was not surprising. However, in previous studies where a tone was presented directly into a single ear, the changes in neuronal activity were lateralized, [5,18,67] but when the IC was studied there was no difference in hemispheres (Melcher 2009). In the current study, a plug was inserted into one ear for protection against profound hearing loss. This "protection" resulted in an asymmetry in terms of hearing loss in the right versus left ears possibly contributing to lateralized tinnitus percepts. However our imaging studies suggest that the tinnitus that was induced, at least during the early stages we tested, was not hemisphere specific. We surmise that while the plug was sufficient to preserve hearing well enough for animals to successfully perform during ASR testing, the plug did not prevent tinnitus-associated uptake of manganese in central pathways associated with the plugged ear.

Specific tinnitus induction results in differential manganese uptake. In the cochlear nucleus only the DCN showed an increase in manganese uptake in our study, a result only observed in the salicylate group. Salicylate has been shown to increase spontaneous activity in the DCN using extracellular recording and with imaging techniques. Using electrophysiology and a very similar noise exposure to that of our study, another study has previously shown increases in neuronal spontaneous activity in the DCN [8]. In the current study we did not observe changes in the DCN of animals from the noise group. Perhaps the observed differences can be attributed to the time point we used for assessment. In that electrophysiology study DCN activity was initially decreased following exposure with increases in activity observed by five days. We assessed changes in neuronal activity in the noise group two days following the noise exposure. Assessing neuronal activity at a later time point, when increased DCN activity is expected from noise-induced tinnitus may yield significant differences from baseline. In a previous tinnitus related MEMRI study, while no changes in neuronal activity were observed in the DCN following noise there were increases in manganese uptake in the PVCN [18]. This discrepancy between that study and the current one may be due to the difference in noise exposure. The previous study used a noise exposure that resulted in a temporary threshold shift that had returned to normal levels prior to manganese injection, while the acoustic exposure in the current study results in a permanent threshold shift and profound deafness. In the previous MEMRI study, manganese was administered to animals showing psychophysical evidence of tinnitus months after the sound exposure. Therefore results from that study would include changes in neuronal activity reflecting uptake due to chronic tinnitus and not the early stages of tinnitus reported in the current study. More work is now needed to resolve these issues.

In the inferior colliculus, both salicylate- and noise-induced tinnitus resulted in significantly elevations in manganese uptake. These results suggest an important role of IC, specifically DCIC, involvement in tinnitus-related neuronal activity. Consistent with this, tinnitus-associated changes in neuronal activity within the IC have been reported following salicylate [60,67,68,69] and noise alike [18,53,70,71,72].

In the present study, we found no significant activity differences in the auditory cortex. This coincides with recent studies in the rat using electrophysiology where changes in spike amplitude, but not spontaneous activity were observed following salicylate and noise [72]. However, in contrast to our results, PET studies in humans and animals as well as autoradiography have suggested that changes in auditory cortex activity occur in subjects with tinnitus. One possible reason for this differential finding may be use of guinea pigs in these earlier studies instead of rats, and/or use of a different tracer (deoxyglucose), rather than manganese. Although our results are based on linearization of the auditory cortices, which provides a sensitive assessment of changes in individual cortical layers [55], we did not find significant differences in manganese uptake in the auditory cortex.

Conclusion

Our goal was to study in awake rats changes in neuronal activity in tinnitus related brain regions that are common to different types of tinnitus using two complementary approaches (ASR and MEMRI). Since the current study focused on similarities and differences emerging hours – days following tinnitus onset and the mechanisms involving the maintenance of chronic may be very different, in the future this approach can be expanded for use in longitudinal studies and in evaluation of treatment efficacy regardless of time following onset or method of induction. The combination of ASR and MEMRI should prove to be quite a powerful combination since MEMRI has high spatial resolution, is not susceptible to scanner noise artifacts and both manganese uptake and ASR can be measured repeatedly.

Methods

Ethics Statement

All procedures were approved by the Wayne State School of Medicine "Laboratory Animal Care and Use Committee" (PHS Animal Welfare Assurance number A3310-01) and conform to the National Institutes of Health guidelines.

Subjects

Twenty-four male Sprague Dawley rats were obtained from Charles River Laboratory. All rats were 2–3 months old weighing 250 g–270 g. The rats were individually housed and maintained at 25°C with a 12 hour light dark cycle. Three groups of animals were studied. The control group consisted of animals in which tinnitus was not induced (n = 8) while in the other two groups tinnitus was induced with either salicylate (n = 6) or noise (n = 6). Limited testing was also performed in animals imaged without manganese (n = 2), animals tested with ASR without Mn^{2+}, but not imaged (n = 2), animals tested with ABR after manganese (n = 2), and ASR 4–10 days after noise exposure (n = 2).

Auditory Brainstem Response (ABR) Testing

To determine the hearing thresholds for each group, ABR measures were recorded before and after treatment, and after $MnCl_2$ administration. Animals were anesthetized with i.m. injections of ketamine HCL (50 mg/kg) and xylazine (2 mg/kg) and placed in a sound attenuating booth (Kinder Scientific Poway, CA). Sub-dermal electrodes were inserted below the pinna (reference electrode), on the top of the head (active electrode), and below the contralateral pinna (ground electrode). A Beyer speaker (Beyer, Germany) was placed into the external ear canal and thresholds were obtained from tone bursts 5 ms in duration for 340 trials for each of three frequencies (4, 12 and 20 kHz) up to 100 dB. Sound was generated and evoked potentials were recorded amplified and filtered using Daqarta (Data AcQuisition And Real-Time Analysis) digital signal processing software package (v4.51, Interstellar Research, Michigan) and a Grass preamplifier. Hearing thresholds were established by determining the lowest intensity of a tone between 0–100 dB that elicits a response at each frequency.

Control Protocol

Testing of the animals in the control group were interspersed with testing of animals in the tinnitus groups. Each of the animals had 2–3 days of baseline ASR's recorded. Eight hours prior to imaging, most control animals (N = 8) were administered 66 mg $MnCl_2 \cdot H_2O$/kg (i.p.). This manganese dose and timing have been shown adequate for functional brain imaging [55]. Two hours prior to imaging, a post-$MnCl_2$ ASR was recorded (Figure 2A). In addition, two of the control rats were imaged without $MnCl_2$ to verify that appropriate enhancement took place in all regions of interest.

Salicylate Protocol

Baseline ASR tests were recorded in each animal (N = 6) for two to three days. Next, animals received a daily i.p. injection (300 mg/kg) of sodium salicylate (Sigma Aldrich) in physiological saline for three days. One hour following the second day of salicylate administration a post treatment-ASR was recorded followed by ABR testing for hearing thresholds. $MnCl_2$ (Sigma, Aldrich) was administered (i.p.; 66 mg $MnCl_2 \cdot H_2O$/kg) one hour after the third salicylate injection, eight hours prior to imaging. A post $MnCl_2$ ASR was recorded two hours prior to imaging (Figure 2B).

Noise Exposure Protocol

Baseline ASR tests were recorded in each animal (N = 6) for two to three days. For acoustic exposure, animals were first placed into individual cages that were set on racks in a custom built noise exposure booth. We have previously shown that the noise exposure used here results in a permanent shift in hearing threshold [54]. Since hearing is necessary for ASR testing, noise exposure was attenuated for one ear: 30 minutes prior to noise exposure, an ear plug was inserted into either the right or the left ear canal (unilaterally, semi-randomly), and the auricle of the plugged ear was folded and secured with a single stitch. Gauze was taped over the stitched ear and a paper neck collar applied during the noise exposure to prevent the animal from injuring the ear. Noise was generated using DaqGen software (Daqarta, Interstellar Research) channeled through 16 overhead speakers and Grass preamplifiers controlled using an Apple computer. Animals were exposed for 4 hours to a 10 kHz, 118 dB one-third octave band tone. To determine the effects of noise exposure on both the plugged and unplugged ears, ABRs and ASRs (using levels that were detectable by the noise exposed animals − 75 and 90 dB) were recorded 24 hrs following sound exposure. On the second day post sound exposure, $MnCl_2$ (66 mg $MnCl_2 \cdot H_2O$/kg) was administered (i.p.) and imaging was conducted eight hours later, with a post $MnCl_2$ ASR recorded two hours prior to imaging (Figure 2C).

Acoustic Startle Reflex (ASR) Testing

Based on previous studies, the acoustic startle reflex provides a useful and reliable method for detecting salicylate and noise induced tinnitus in rats [17,49]. All tests were performed in a noise attenuation chamber with customized hardware and software (Kinder Scientific, Poway, CA). Inside the chamber, animals were placed inside a plexi-glass box resting on a piezoelectric force transducer in a calibrated sound field. The adjustable ceiling of the box was positioned above the animal to constrict excessive movement. All ASR tests were conducted in the light. The ceiling of the box has slits and sits 15 cm from the speaker located at the top of the chamber. The output of the piezo transducer was amplified, filtered, and the root mean square of the waveform measured to estimate startle amplitude.

For each animal both pre-pulse inhibition (pASR) and gap detection inhibition (gASR) of acoustic startle was conducted. First pASR testing was performed, immediately followed by gASR testing. Testing resulted in animals spending no more than one hour per day in the testing chamber. pASR testing aids in the interpretation of gASR data, providing a control for both hearing loss and temporal processing dysfunction. In our paradigm, deficits in gASR accompanied by normal pASR represent the presence of

tinnitus. For the pASR testing, pre-startle tones were presented at 4, 8, 12, 16, 20, and 24 kHz at levels of 45 and 60 dB in all groups with the exception of the Noise Group: Since those animals experienced hearing loss, levels of 75 and 90 dB were used in ASR conducted post noise exposure. Each pre-startle tone was presented for 20 ms, in a silent background 50 ms before the sound off startle (120 dB broad band noise for 50 ms). For each ASR test (pre-pulse - pASR or gap - gASR) a total of 10 trials were run for each frequency at each intensity as well as in the sound off startle condition for pASR and in both the sound off startle condition and the sound in startle condition for gASR. The trials were presented in a pseudo-randomized order, with inter-trial intervals randomized between 1 and 6 s.

During gASR testing, a background tone of either, 4, 8, 12, 16, 20, or 24 kHz at 45 and 60 dB, (or 75 and 90 dB in post noise exposed animals) was presented. A silent gap lasting 20 ms was embedded in the tone 50 ms prior to the startle (120 dB wide band noise). To determine a maximum startle response, a startle was also elicited without any background tone (sound off startle). For each frequency at each sound level, with 10 trials recorded for each condition as with pASR.

MEMRI Image Acquisition

Eight hours post $MnCl_2$ injection, animals were anesthetized with urethane 3.9 ml/kg i.p. (36% solution, prepared fresh daily; Aldrich) and promptly scanned. The timing between injection and scanning was based on previous work showing that brain manganese accumulation is adequate for functional imaging after eight hours [55], as well as a study outlining a detailed time-course for manganese enhancement in the mouse brain. In this approach, MEMRI data report on brain activity between injection and scanning − while animals are awake and freely-moving − with anesthetic choice or scanning environment having little opportunity to influence results [31]. To specifically check the effects of urethane on manganese uptake, we have performed retinal functional studies with MEMRI in the same animal before and after death. We find no differences in retinal signal intensity (data not shown). Thus, there is little reason to think that urethane influences the manganese signal.

For the duration of the scan, each animal was placed on a heated re-circulating water pad with a rectal thermometer to monitor and maintain core body temperature. Scans were performed on a 4.7 T Bruker Avance System using a whole body transmit-only coil and a 3 cm internal diameter receive-only coil. Individual images were acquired using a 3D RARE sequence (repetition time [TR] 330 ms; echo time [TE] 6.9 ms, with a RARE factor of 8, for an effective echo time of 28 ms; number of acquisitions [NA] 4; matrix size 216×248×120; field of view [FOV] 2.81×3.22×3.12 cm^3; providing a resolution of 130 µm×130 µm×260 µm; 37 min/image). All animals were alive when scanning was complete. As described previously [55], we also scanned a "phantom" roughly the size of a rat's head (containing a 10:1 mixture of water and 0.67 mM $MnCl_2$ in saline) using the same parameters employed in animals for later modeling of signal intensity changes as a function of distance from the surface coil.

ASR Data Analysis

In the pASR paradigm results were calculated as the force of the startle response following the pre-pulse preceded startle noise, divided by the sound off (no background sound) startle multiplied by 100. The results are therefore reported as the percent inhibition of the sound off startle. For the gASR paradigm the data were calculated in the same way except for each trial at each frequency and sound level the maximum startle response was recorded both in the presence of the background tone and in a silent background. Data were analyzed using StatView for between group comparisons and SPSS software v 7.0 for repeated measures analysis of variance (for within group comparisons) to determine significant differences and post hoc comparisons to determine which means contributed to the observed effects.

MEMRI Image Analysis

For these experiments increased manganese uptake was equated to changes in ion regulation and increased neuronal activity. Therefore the terms are used interchangeably throughout the text. Image analysis proceeded, with slight modification, as detailed elsewhere [55]. Briefly, the influence of surface coil position on signal intensity was modeled, then corrected for within each image using R scripts developed in-house (v.2.9.0; R Development Core Team (2009); http://www.R-project.org). Next, average signal intensity was measured from several manually-defined regions of interest (ROIs) using MRIcro v.1.40, [73] with tracings of each structure guided by the Paxinos and Watson (6th Edition; 2007) rat brain atlas including several sub-cortical auditory and non-auditory regions: the medial geniculate nucleus (MGN), the central nucleus, dorsal cortex, and external cortex of the inferior colliculus (CNIC, DCIC and ECIC, respectively), the dorsal cochlear nucleus (DCN) and ventral cochlear nucleus (VCN), the paraflocculus (Pfloc), flocculus (Floc), amygdala (amyg), superior colliculus (sup coll), and lateral geniculate nucleus (LGN). Spherical ROIs were used to characterize the CNIC, MGN, LGN, and sup coll (radius: 520 µm). Hand-drawn ROIs spanning three consecutive coronal slices (each 260 µm thick) were used in all other cases, except for the DCN: Owing to the small size of the DCN, its ROI was drawn in two consecutive slices with the broadest cross-sectional areas. Each anatomical region was identified both by its broad contours, and proximity to prominent adjacent structures: The contours of the paraflocculus and cochlear nuclei, for instance, are clearly visible in several coronal slices (e.g. Figure 7A), simplifying comparisons to the Paxinos and Watson atlas and facilitating fine localization of the DCN and VCN. Hand-drawn ROIs were placed at the rostrocaudal center of each anatomical region, and drawn to occupy the entire coronal profile of each region, excluding a buffer ($\geq$1 voxel wide, depending on the ROI) at borders with neighboring brain regions and tissues (e.g. choroid plexus). Appropriate ROI placement was confirmed in parasagittal views, and the subject-to-subject consistency of ROI placement was checked by at least two of the authors.

Several cortical regions, both traditionally auditory – primary auditory cortex (Au1) and dorsal zone of auditory cortex (AuD), and regions not traditionally associated with auditory pathways - temporal association area (TeA), lateral (V2L) and medial (V2M) secondary visual cortex, and the monocular (V1M), binocular (V1B), and rostral (V1) portions of the primary visual cortex – were analyzed in a manner which preserves cortical layer-specific information as previously described [55]. Briefly, high-order

polynomials were fit to the brain/no-brain border in coronal slices. Lines perpendicular to the polynomials were automatically drawn, and tilted in the rostrocaudal plane to be consistent with the brain surface. Brain signal intensities were evenly sampled along these lines and organized as a linearized image of the cortex. Here, a linearized version of the Paxinos and Watson atlas (6th Edition; 2007) was used to divide the linearized cortex into each ROI. Average profiles of signal intensity as a function of cortical depth were then generated for each ROI, and data at cortical depths corresponding to layers II through IV used for between-subject comparisons.

For all functional comparisons of MEMRI data, brain signal intensities were normalized to adjacent tissue, similar to the approach used elsewhere [27,55,56]. Here, ROI signal intensities (SI) were normalized adjacent muscle (normalized ROI SI = ROI SI/muscle SI * 100). Muscle normalization can compensate for any signal intensity gradients that remain after image processing, as well as potential inter-individual differences in peripheral $MnCl_2$ uptake (e.g. liver sequestration). Normalization to a non-auditory brain region, which might better-provide those benefits, was also considered. However, association with tinnitus for most brain regions remains unclear.

To check the quality of muscle normalization, additional analyses were carried out at the anterior pituitary and adjacent muscle. Because the anterior pituitary sits outside of the blood-brain-barrier, it has been used in previous work to gauge non-specific brain enhancement due to systemic increases in manganese [74]. Here, anterior pituitary SI was analyzed using two spherical ROIs (radius: 390 µm) placed to the left and right of midline in coronal sections. To gauge whether muscle normalization would reduce inter-individual variability in brain data, we tested for a positive correlation between pre-normalization SIs for the pituitary and the adjacent muscle (linear regression). To test whether control and tinnitus groups experienced similar levels of manganese uptake, we use one-way ANOVAs to compare pre-normalization SIs for the pituitary and the adjacent muscle alike, as well as normalized pituitary SIs.

Functional comparisons of MEMRI data from controls to each tinnitus group were carried out by performing one-way ANOVAs at each brain region. Significant ANOVA results were further tested using post-hoc t-tests.

Acknowledgments

We would like to acknowledge the technical assistance of Bozena Fyk-Kolodziej, Takashi Shimano, Robin Roberts. Special thanks to Dr. Larry Hughes for guidance with statistical analysis and R. Afram, P. Griffith, and S. Naidu for their help with manuscript preparation.

Author Contributions

Conceived and designed the experiments: AGH BB. Performed the experiments: NM GR. Analyzed the data: AGH DB NM GR. Contributed reagents/materials/analysis tools: AGH BB. Wrote the paper: AGH DB.

References

1. Cave KM, Cornish EM, Chandler DW (2007) Blast injury of the ear: clinical update from the global war on terror. Mil Med 172: 726–730.
2. Fagelson MA (2007) The association between tinnitus and posttraumatic stress disorder. Am J Audiol 16: 107–117.
3. Lew HL, Jerger JF, Guillory SB, Henry JA (2007) Auditory dysfunction in traumatic brain injury. J Rehabil Res Dev 44: 921–928.
4. Snow JB (2004) Tinnitus: theory and management. Hamilton [Ont.] Lewiston, NY: BC Decker; Sales and distribution, U.S., BC Decker. xv, 368 p.
5. Bauer CA, Turner JG, Caspary DM, Myers KS, Brozoski TJ (2008) Tinnitus and inferior colliculus activity in chinchillas related to three distinct patterns of cochlear trauma. J Neurosci Res 86: 2564–2578.
6. Brozoski TJ, Bauer CA, Caspary DM (2002) Elevated fusiform cell activity in the dorsal cochlear nucleus of chinchillas with psychophysical evidence of tinnitus. J Neurosci 22: 2383–2390.
7. Kaltenbach JA (2007) The dorsal cochlear nucleus as a contributor to tinnitus: mechanisms underlying the induction of hyperactivity. Prog Brain Res 166: 89–106.

8. Kaltenbach JA, Afman CE (2000) Hyperactivity in the dorsal cochlear nucleus after intense sound exposure and its resemblance to tone-evoked activity: a physiological model for tinnitus. Hear Res 140: 165–172.

9. Bahmad FM Jr., Venosa AR, Oliveira CA (2006) Benzodiazepines and GABAergics in treating severe disabling tinnitus of predominantly cochlear origin. Int Tinnitus J 12: 140–144.

10. Denk DM, Heinzl H, Franz P, Ehrenberger K (1997) Caroverine in tinnitus treatment. A placebo-controlled blind study. Acta Otolaryngol 117: 825–830.

11. Salembier L, De Ridder D, Van de Heyning PH (2006) The use of flupirtine in treatment of tinnitus. Acta Otolaryngol Suppl. pp 93–95.

12. Wenzel GI, Warnecke A, Stover T, Lenarz T (2010) Effects of extracochlear gacyclidine perfusion on tinnitus in humans: a case series. Eur Arch Otorhinolaryngol 267: 691–699.

13. Dieler R, Davies C, Shehata-Dieler WE (2002) [The effects of quinine on active motile responses and fine structure of isolated outer hair cells from the Guinea pig cochlea]. Laryngorhinootologie 81: 196–203.

14. Kay IS, Davies WE (1993) The effect of nimodipine on salicylate ototoxicity in the rat as revealed by the auditory evoked brain-stem response. Eur Arch Otorhinolaryngol 250: 51–54.

15. Liu Y, Li X, Ma C, Liu J, Lu H (2005) Salicylate blocks L-type calcium channels in rat inferior colliculus neurons. Hear Res 205: 271–276.

16. Liu Y, Zhang H, Li X, Wang Y, Lu H, et al. (2007) Inhibition of voltage-gated channel currents in rat auditory cortex neurons by salicylate. Neuropharmacology 53: 870–880.

17. Turner JG, Brozoski TJ, Bauer CA, Parrish JL, Myers K, et al. (2006) Gap detection deficits in rats with tinnitus: a potential novel screening tool. Behav Neurosci 120: 188–195.

18. Brozoski TJ, Ciobanu L, Bauer CA (2007) Central neural activity in rats with tinnitus evaluated with manganese-enhanced magnetic resonance imaging (MEMRI). Hear Res 226: 168–179.

19. Berkowitz BA, Roberts R, Goebel DJ, Luan H (2006) Noninvasive and simultaneous imaging of layer-specific retinal functional adaptation by manganese-enhanced MRI. Invest Ophthalmol Vis Sci 47: 2668–2674.

20. Yu X, Wadghiri YZ, Sanes DH, Turnbull DH (2005) In vivo auditory brain mapping in mice with Mn-enhanced MRI. Nat Neurosci 8: 961–968.

21. Drapeau P, Nachshen DA (1984) Manganese fluxes and manganese-dependent neurotransmitter release in presynaptic nerve endings isolated from rat brain. J Physiol 348: 493–510.

22. Cross DJ, Flexman JA, Anzai Y, Sasaki T, Treuting PM, et al. (2007) In vivo manganese MR imaging of calcium influx in spontaneous rat pituitary adenoma. AJNR Am J Neuroradiol 28: 1865–1871.

23. Gadjanski I, Boretius S, Williams SK, Lingor P, Knoferle J, et al. (2009) Role of n-type voltage-dependent calcium channels in autoimmune optic neuritis. Ann Neurol 66: 81–93.

24. Itoh K, Sakata M, Watanabe M, Aikawa Y, Fujii H (2008) The entry of manganese ions into the brain is accelerated by the activation of N-methyl-D-aspartate receptors. Neuroscience 154: 732–740.

25. Berkowitz BA, Roberts R, Penn JS, Gradianu M (2007) High-resolution manganese-enhanced MRI of experimental retinopathy of prematurity. Invest Ophthalmol Vis Sci 48: 4733–4740.

26. Aoki I, Naruse S, Tanaka C (2004) Manganese-enhanced magnetic resonance imaging (MEMRI) of brain activity and applications to early detection of brain ischemia. NMR Biomed 17: 569–580.

27. Alvestad S, Goa PE, Qu H, Risa O, Brekken C, et al. (2007) In vivo mapping of temporospatial changes in manganese enhancement in rat brain during epileptogenesis. Neuroimage 38: 57–66.

28. Chuang KH, Koretsky A (2006) Improved neuronal tract tracing using manganese enhanced magnetic resonance imaging with fast T(1) mapping. Magn Reson Med 55: 604–611.

29. Sun N, Li Y, Tian S, Lei Y, Zheng J, et al. (2006) Dynamic changes in orbitofrontal neuronal activity in rats during opiate administration and withdrawal. Neuroscience 138: 77–82.

30. Yu X, Zou J, Babb JS, Johnson G, Sanes DH, et al. (2008) Statistical mapping of sound-evoked activity in the mouse auditory midbrain using Mn-enhanced MRI. Neuroimage 39: 223–230.

31. Lee JH, Silva AC, Merkle H, Koretsky AP (2005) Manganese-enhanced magnetic resonance imaging of mouse brain after systemic administration of MnCl2: dose-dependent and temporal evolution of T1 contrast. Magn Reson Med 53: 640–648.

32. Cacace AT, Lovely TJ, McFarland DJ, Parnes SM, Winter DF (1994) Anomalous cross-modal plasticity following posterior fossa surgery: some speculations on gaze-evoked tinnitus. Hear Res 81: 22–32.

33. Cacace AT, Lovely TJ, Winter DF, Parnes SM, McFarland DJ (1994) Auditory perceptual and visual-spatial characteristics of gaze-evoked tinnitus. Audiology 33: 291–303.

34. Lockwood AH, Salvi RJ, Coad ML, Towsley ML, Wack DS, et al. (1998) The functional neuroanatomy of tinnitus: evidence for limbic system links and neural plasticity. Neurology 50: 114–120.

35. Moody DB (2004) Animal Models of Tinnitus. In: Snow JB, ed. Tinnitus: Theory and Management. Hamilton [Ont.] Lewiston, NY: BC Decker; Sales and distribution, U.S., BC Decker. pp 80–95.

36. Andersen RA, Snyder RL, Merzenich MM (1980) The topographic organization of corticocollicular projections from physiologically identified loci in the AI, AII, and anterior auditory cortical fields of the cat. J Comp Neurol 191: 479–494.

37. Diamond IT, Jones EG, Powell TP (1969) The projection of the auditory cortex upon the diencephalon and brain stem in the cat. Brain Res 15: 305–340.

38. Druga R, Syka J (1984) Ascending and descending projections to the inferior colliculus in the rat. Physiol Bohemoslov 33: 31–42.

39. Druga R, Syka J, Rajkowska G (1997) Projections of auditory cortex onto the inferior colliculus in the rat. Physiol Res 46: 215–222.

40. Faye-Lund H (1985) The neocortical projection to the inferior colliculus in the albino rat. Anat Embryol (Berl) 173: 53–70.

41. Syka J, Masterton RB (1988) Auditory pathway: structure and function. New York: Plenum Press, xi, 363 p. [361] leaf of plates p.

42. Winer JA, Larue DT, Diehl JJ, Hefti BJ (1998) Auditory cortical projections to the cat inferior colliculus. J Comp Neurol 400: 147–174.

43. Bauer CA, Brozoski TJ, Rojas R, Boley J, Wyder M (1999) Behavioral model of chronic tinnitus in rats. Otolaryngol Head Neck Surg 121: 457–462.

44. Guitton MJ, Caston J, Ruel J, Johnson RM, Pujol R, et al. (2003) Salicylate induces tinnitus through activation of cochlear NMDA receptors. J Neurosci 23: 3944–3952.

45. Jastreboff PJ, Brennan JF, Coleman JK, Sasaki CT (1988) Phantom auditory sensation in rats: an animal model for tinnitus. Behav Neurosci 102: 811–822.

46. Jastreboff PJ, Sasaki CT (1994) An animal model of tinnitus: a decade of development. Am J Otol 15: 19–27.

47. Lobarinas E, Sun W, Cushing R, Salvi R (2004) A novel behavioral paradigm for assessing tinnitus using schedule-induced polydipsia avoidance conditioning (SIP-AC). Hear Res 190: 109–114.

48. Ruttiger L, Ciuffani J, Zenner HP, Knipper M (2003) A behavioral paradigm to judge acute sodium salicylate-induced sound experience in rats: a new approach for an animal model on tinnitus. Hear Res 180: 39–50.

49. Yang G, Lobarinas E, Zhang L, Turner J, Stolzberg D, et al. (2007) Salicylate induced tinnitus: behavioral measures and neural activity in auditory cortex of awake rats. Hear Res 226: 244–253.

50. Sun W, Lu J, Stolzberg D, Gray L, Deng A, et al. (2009) Salicylate increases the gain of the central auditory system. Neuroscience 159: 325–334.

51. Turner JG, Parrish J (2008) Gap detection methods for assessing salicylate-induced tinnitus and hyperacusis in rats. Am J Audiol 17: S185–192.

52. Bauer CA, Brozoski TJ (2001) Assessing tinnitus and prospective tinnitus therapeutics using a psychophysical animal model. J Assoc Res Otolaryngol 2: 54–64.

53. Heffner HE, Harrington IA (2002) Tinnitus in hamsters following exposure to intense sound. Hear Res 170: 83–95.

54. Holt A, Lomax L, Lomax M, Altschuler R (2005) Differential Gene Expression in Two Models of Tinnitus The Association for Research in Otolaryngology. New Orleans, LA. pp 329.

55. Bissig D, Berkowitz BA (2009) Manganese-enhanced MRI of layer-specific activity in the visual cortex from awake and free-moving rats. Neuroimage 44: 627–635.

56. Angenstein F, Niessen HG, Goldschmidt J, Lison H, Altrock WD, et al. (2007) Manganese-enhanced MRI reveals structural and functional changes in the cortex of Bassoon mutant mice. Cereb Cortex 17: 28–36.

57. Berkowitz BA, Roberts R, Bissig D (2010) Light-dependant intraretinal ion regulation by melanopsin in young awake and free moving mice evaluated with manganese-enhanced MRI. Mol Vis 16: 1776–1780.

58. Fa Z, Zhang P, Huang F, Li P, Zhang R, et al. (2010) Activity-induced manganese-dependent functional MRI of the rat visual cortex following intranasal manganese chloride administration. Neurosci Lett 481: 110–114.

59. Yu X, Sanes DH, Aristizabal O, Wadghiri YZ, Turnbull DH (2007) Large-scale reorganization of the tonotopic map in mouse auditory midbrain revealed by MRI. Proc Natl Acad Sci U S A 104: 12193–12198.

60. Paul AK, Lobarinas E, Simmons R, Wack D, Luisi JC, et al. (2009) Metabolic imaging of rat brain during pharmacologically-induced tinnitus. Neuroimage 44: 312–318.

61. Francis HW, Manis PB (2000) Effects of deafferentation on the electrophysiology of ventral cochlear nucleus neurons. Hear Res 149: 91–105.

62. Hirsch JA, Oertel D (1988) Intrinsic properties of neurones in the dorsal cochlear nucleus of mice, in vitro. J Physiol 396: 535–548.

63. Oertel D (1991) The role of intrinsic neuronal properties in the encoding of auditory information in the cochlear nuclei. Curr Opin Neurobiol 1: 221–228.

64. Evans EF, Nelson PG (1973) On the functional relationship between the dorsal and ventral divisions of the cochlear nucleus of the cat. Exp Brain Res 17: 428–442.

65. Koerber KC, Pfeiffer RR, Warr WB, Kiang NY (1966) Spontaneous spike discharges from single units in the cochlear nucleus after destruction of the cochlea. Exp Neurol 16: 119–130.

66. Pfeiffer RR (1966) Classification of response patterns of spike discharges for units in the cochlear nucleus: tone-burst stimulation. Exp Brain Res 1: 220–235.

67. Heffner HE, Koay G (2005) Tinnitus and hearing loss in hamsters (Mesocricetus auratus) exposed to loud sound. Behav Neurosci 119: 734–742.

68. Chen GD, Jastreboff PJ (1995) Salicylate-induced abnormal activity in the inferior colliculus of rats. Hear Res 82: 158–178.

69. Jastreboff PJ, Sasaki CT (1986) Salicylate-induced changes in spontaneous activity of single units in the inferior colliculus of the guinea pig. J Acoust Soc Am 80: 1384–1391.

70. Melcher JR, Levine RA, Bergevin C, Norris B (2009) The auditory midbrain of people with tinnitus: abnormal sound-evoked activity revisited. Hear Res 257: 63–74.

71. Ma WL, Hidaka H, May BJ (2006) Spontaneous activity in the inferior colliculus of CBA/J mice after manipulations that induce tinnitus. Hear Res 212: 9–21.

72. Norena AJ, Moffat G, Blanc JL, Pezard L, Cazals Y (2010) Neural changes in the auditory cortex of awake guinea pigs after two tinnitus inducers: salicylate and acoustic trauma. Neuroscience.

73. Rorden C, Brett M (2000) Stereotaxic display of brain lesions. Behav Neurol 12: 191–200.

74. Chuang KH, Koretsky AP (2009) Accounting for nonspecific enhancement in neuronal tract tracing using manganese enhanced magnetic resonance imaging. Magn Reson Imaging 27: 594–600.

2

Long-Term Tinnitus Suppression with Linear Octave Frequency Transposition Hearing Aids

Elisabeth Peltier[1], Cedric Peltier[1], Stephanie Tahar[1], Evelyne Alliot-Lugaz[1], Yves Cazals[2]*

1 Laboratoire Chelles surdité, Chelles, France, 2 Laboratoire de Neurosciences Intégratives et Adaptatives, Aix-Marseille Université, CNRS UMR 7260, Féderation de Recherche 3C (Cerveau, Comportement, Cognition), Marseille, France

Abstract

Over the last three years of hearing aid dispensing, it was observed that among 74 subjects fitted with a linear octave frequency transposition (LOFT) hearing aid, 60 reported partial or complete tinnitus suppression during day and night, an effect still lasting after several months or years of daily use. We report in more details on 38 subjects from whom we obtained quantified measures of tinnitus suppression through visual analog scaling and several additional psychoacoustic and audiometric measures. The long-term suppression seems independent of subject age, and of duration and subjective localization of tinnitus. A small but significant correlation was found with audiogram losses but not with high frequency loss slope. Long-term tinnitus suppression was observed for different etiologies, but with a low success rate for sudden deafness. It should be noted that a majority of subjects (23) had a history of noise exposure. Tinnitus suppression started after a few days of LOFT hearing aid use and reached a maximum after a few weeks of daily use. For nine subjects different amounts of frequency shifting were tried and found more or less successful for long-term tinnitus suppression, no correlation was found with tinnitus pitch. When the use of the LOFT hearing aid was stopped tinnitus reappeared within a day, and after re-using the LOFT aid it disappeared again within a day. For about one third of the 38 subjects a classical amplification or a non linear frequency compression aid was also tried, and no such tinnitus suppression was observed. Besides improvements in audiometric sensitivity to high frequencies and in speech discrimination scores, LOFT can be considered as a remarkable opportunity to suppress tinnitus over a long time scale. From a pathophysiological viewpoint these observations seem to fit with a possible re-attribution of activity to previously deprived cerebral areas corresponding to high frequency coding.

Editor: Xi (Erick) Lin, Emory Univ. School of Medicine, United States of America

Funding: These authors have no support or funding to report. The work is simply the result of research based upon observations from daily work of hearing aid dispensers. The corresponding author who wrote the manuscript is a profesional research worker belonging to the Institut National de la Santé et de la Recheche Médicale (the French Medical Research Council).

Competing Interests: The authors have declared that no competing interests exist.

* E-mail: yves.cazals@univ-amu.fr

Introduction

Tinnitus, the perception of a sound without an external stimulus, often occurs together with hearing loss. It is a pathology which affects approximately 10% of the population worldwide [1]. It has long been observed that tinnitus sounds most loud and annoying in a quiet environment [2,3] whereas noisy surroundings can produce a partial to complete suppression of tinnitus. Thus for many hearing-impaired people the use of a hearing aid besides providing improved perception of external sounds, can be beneficial against tinnitus [4,5,6]. Most often the tinnitus suppressing effects provided by external sounds do not last much after returning to a quiet environment, and if any, the long term suppressive effects are weak [7]. In addition, hyperacusis often associated with tinnitus [8,9] can limit the use of amplification of external sounds which may exacerbate tinnitus perception.

Special hearing aids delivering a noise as tinnitus masker were developed several decades ago; dedicated studies report some success but overall do not bring strong evidence of benefit [10]. Masking of tinnitus is obtained for about half of the subjects [11], but the constant noise may become too bothersome [12], or can adversely interfere with the hearing of other sounds. In addition to tinnitus masking during the masker sound, many subjects report that at cessation of masking, tinnitus can remain attenuated for seconds up to a few minutes, a phenomenon called residual inhibition [13,14].

The perceived pitch of tinnitus is very often associated with audiometric losses at the corresponding frequencies [15,16,17]. This association strongly suggests the hearing loss as a first source of tinnitus although it remains unknown why people with similar hearing losses are or are not affected by tinnitus. For a majority of hearing-impaired people the hearing loss affects the high frequencies and, as a correlate, tinnitus sufferers also most often report high frequency tinnitus pitches [12,16].

When the degree of hearing loss at some frequencies is moderate or severe the quality and discriminability of sounds at these frequencies can be so deteriorated that providing amplified sounds at these frequencies do not bring benefit and may even be detrimental [18]. As information given by high frequencies can be a decisive help for sound identification and for speech intelligibility, transposition of high to lower frequencies has been tried in hearing aids for decades [19]. Up to now frequency lowering techniques continue to be a matter of studies [20,21] and hearing aid manufacturers presently offer some algorithms. A

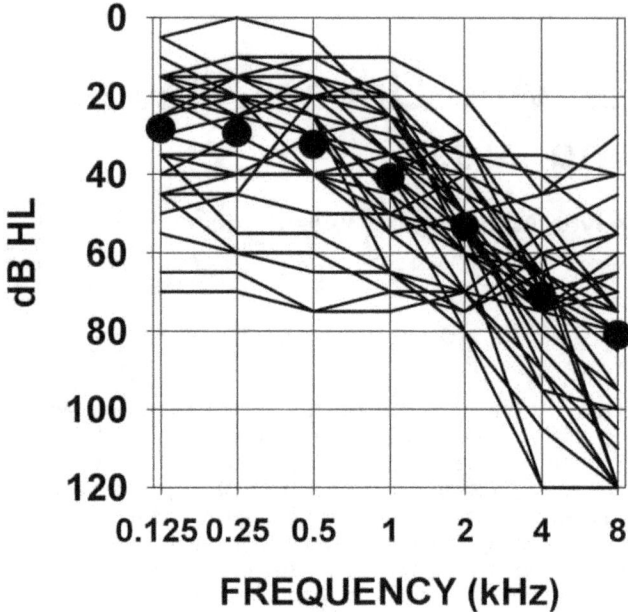

Figure 1. Audiograms of all the studied subjects. Abscissa : frequencies in kHz, ordinate : sound level in audiometric dB. Black circles : mean values.

recent study provides details upon technical differences between the two main hearing aids using frequency lowering algorithms : the Phonak SR using a non linear frequency compression, and the Widex AE using a linear frequency transposition [22]. It indicates that both provide improved audibility of high frequencies together with some signal distortion, but also result in considerably different percepts of the same original sounds.

The present study reports on tinnitus suppression over day and night for months to years, observed from hearing impaired subjects after several days or weeks of using daily the linear octave frequency transposition hearing aid.

Materials and Methods

The data presented in this article were obtained over the last three years from two hearing aid dispensing centers. The selection of subjects for whom to try fitting with a linear octave frequency transposition (LOFT) hearing aid was based on the presence of a considerable hearing loss at high frequencies. About one third of these subjects had previous experience with another hearing aid but complained about it, for the other two thirds the LOFT aid was a first choice. Over the years the presence of invalidating tinnitus was also considered as a criterion for this choice. The patients were followed weekly during trials of different settings. Generally patients were given two settings of frequency transposition and were asked to alternate uses and appreciate their satisfaction over a period of at least two weeks. Although data logs in these hearing aids provided numbers of hours of use for the different settings which were collected into computer data bases, this large amount of data were not retrieved for analysis.

For each subject, basic medical informations were obtained at the first patient visit. In subsequent visits classical audiometric gains and speech intelligibility curves were measured and a brief description of patient satisfaction was also taken. For 38 subjects more precisely considered in this report, several tinnitus assessments were performed. The subjective level of tinnitus was obtained by using a visual analog scale (VAS) ranging from 0 to 10 in twenty steps. Localization of tinnitus was noted and approximations of its pitch and loudness were obtained by comparison with audiometer tones using reference frequencies of 2,3,4,6 and 8 kHz. For 31 subjects, estimates of tinnitus masking were also performed using the best tone-match frequency; for 12 of them masking was obtained at levels of 70 dB HL or more and for 13 of them hyperacusis prevented masking success.

The results presented here above were also examined exclusively for the 23 subjects with a history of noise exposure, all results were found similar.

All statistical tests and plots were performed using the SigmaStat SigmaPlot software version 12. In agreement with French legislation, data in this study were obtained by professional health workers on their own patients and were not transmitted to anyone else (monocentric study), in addition data were treated anonymously.

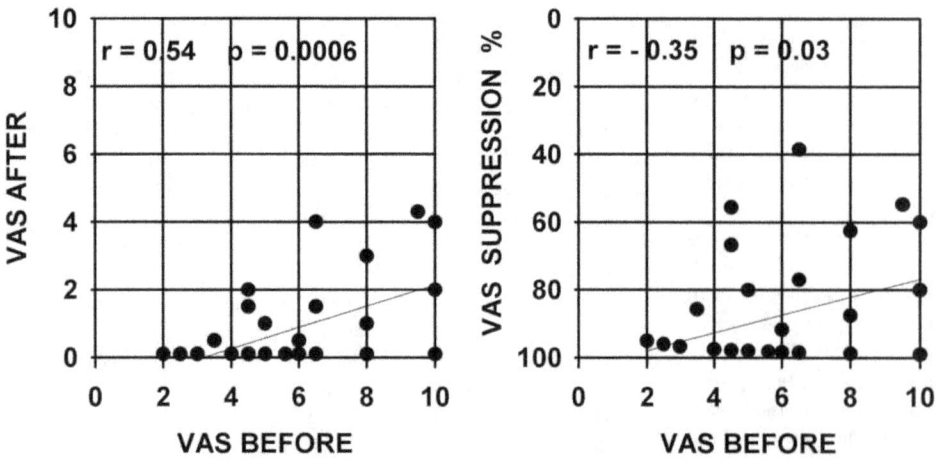

Figure 2. Subjective level of tinnitus before and after LOFT aid use. VAS : visual analog scale, values represent quantified subjective level of tinnitus. Abscissa : VAS score before LOFT aid use. Left graph : ordinate is VAS score after LOFT aid use. Right graph : same data but expressed as percent of suppression. Text in each graph indicates value of correlation coefficient (r) and statistical significance level (p).

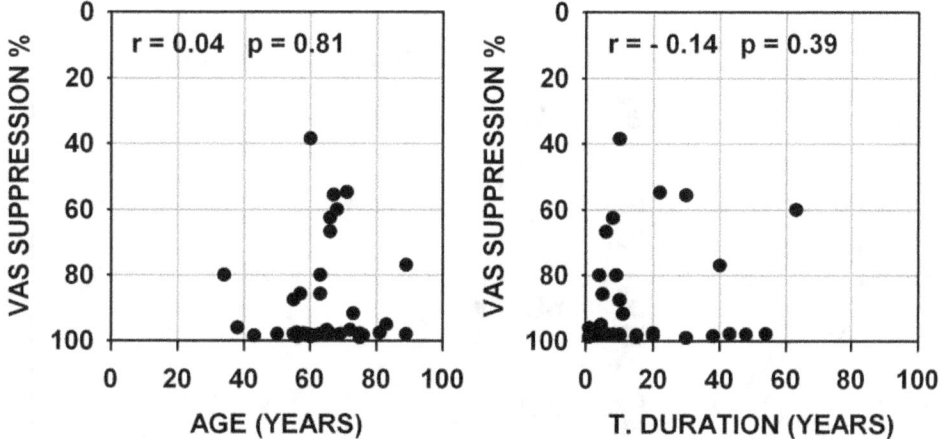

Figure 3. Percent of tinnitus suppression versus subject age or duration of tinnitus. Ratios of tinnitus suppression versus subjects age (left graph) and duration of tinnitus (right graph). Text in each graph indicates value of correlation coefficient (r) and statistical significance level (p).

Results

Among 74 subjects tested with LOFT amplification, long-term tinnitus suppression was obtained for 60 of them (81%). At present, long-term tinnitus suppression for day and night has been reported as permanent by all 60 subjects who use the LOFT aid daily; for our group of subjects this suppression spreads from some weeks to about two years and a half. As for etiologies of hearing impairment, subjects could be classified in six categories presenting different success rates, these success rates were statistically tested using the X-square and Fischer tests. For three subjects the etiology was chimiotherapy (antibiotic or anticancer drugs), among these all underwent tinnitus suppression (not statistically significant). Deafness occurred after surgery for 3 subjects, tinnitus suppression was successful for all 3 (not statistically significant). For 8 cases suffering from sudden deafness, tinnitus suppression was obtained in 2 cases only, this low rate was not found statistically significant likely due to the small number of observations but still suggests a real trend. For 8 subjects head trauma was identified as the cause of hearing impairment, for all of them tinnitus suppression was successful (p<0.001). Hereditary deafness was diagnosed for 15 subjects, long-term tinnitus suppression was

successful for 12 of them a statistically significant proportion (p<0.003). Finally 37 subjects had a history of noise exposure and tinnitus suppression was obtained for 32 of them (p<0.001). As for subjects for whom tinnitus was not suppressed, we did not find any etiologic or audiometric special feature.

The more detailed data presented hereafter are restrained to 38 subjects for whom quantified measures of subjective tinnitus strength were obtained using a visual analog scale, and for whom several additional psychoacoustic and audiometric data could be collected. These 38 subjects presented somewhat similar audiograms with most often a rather steep hearing loss slope at high frequencies, all audiograms are presented in figure 1. The values of tinnitus strength as given by the subjects using a visual analog scale score before and after using a LOFT hearing aid are presented in figure 2 (left graph). The right graph shows the same data but in the form of percent of suppression obtained by the ratio : (VAS before minus VAS after)/VAS before which was then multiplied by 100. It can be seen from this figure that, over all individuals, tinnitus was subjectively evaluated as about half-suppressed to totally suppressed in the long-term. There is a significant correlation (Pearson product-moment correlation coefficient)

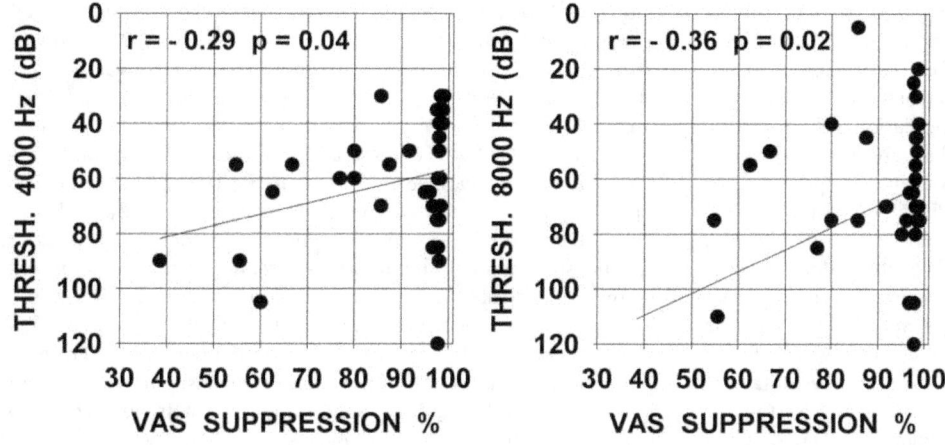

Figure 4. Percent of tinnitus suppression versus audiometric threshold at 4000 Hz and 8000 Hz. Abscissa : tinnitus suppression ratio (%) Ordinate : audiometric threshold in dB -left graph at 4000 Hz, -right graph at 8000 Hz. Text in each graph indicates value of correlation coefficient (r and statistical significance level (p).

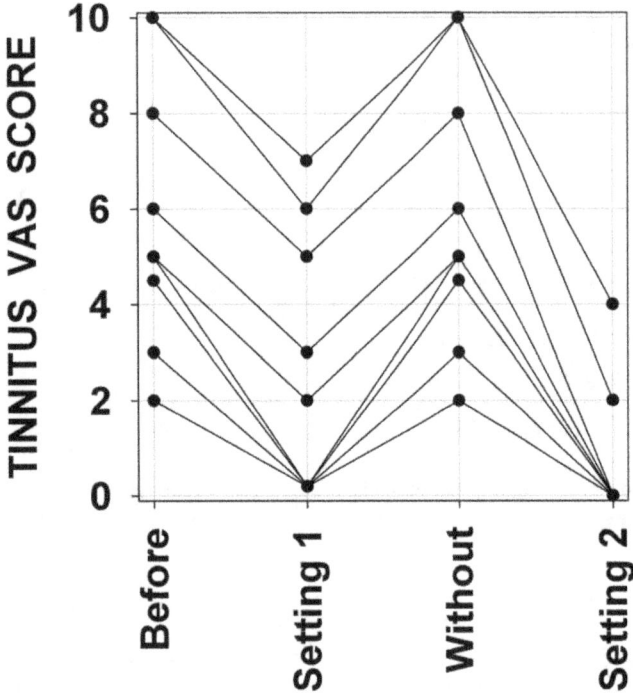

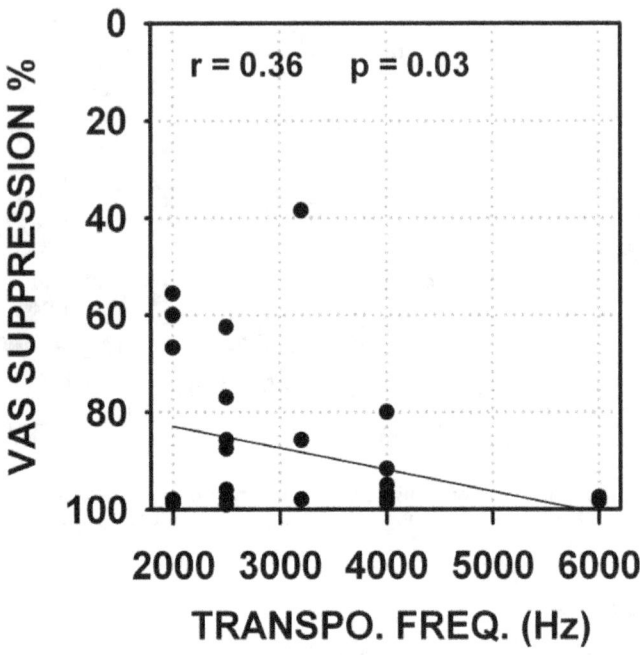

Figure 5. Variations of tinnitus subjective levels for 9 subjects in four conditions. Abscissa : subjective level of tinnitus. Ordinate : before LOFT aid use (Before), with a first frequency transposition setting (Setting 1), during a period without LOFT aid (Without) and with a second frequency transposition setting (Setting 2).

Figure 6. Percent of tinnitus suppression versus value of transposition frequency. Abscissa : value of transposition frequency, ordinate : tinnitus suppression ratio (%).Text in each graph indicates value of correlation coefficient (r) and statistical significance level (p).

between the subjective strength of tinnitus before LOFT use and the level of tinnitus suppression after LOFT use. The stronger the tinnitus was originally judged, the proportionally smaller was the percent of LOFT induced suppression. The correlation values are statistically significant but are not of high value and correspond approximately to 29–12% of the observed variability in the data. There was no correlation between the amount of tinnitus suppression and the age of the patient or the duration of tinnitus (figure 3); even for quasi life-long tinnitus complete suppression could be obtained. No correlation was observed between the level for tinnitus masking and/or the presence of hyperacusis and the amount of tinnitus suppression. Significant correlations were found between audiogram thresholds and subjective amount of tinnitus suppression. In figure 4 are presented graphs of threshold level versus amount of tinnitus suppression for frequencies of 4 and 8 kHz, frequencies to which tinnitus pitches were most often approximated. As seen in the figure, correlation values can be considered statistically significant but values are low; no correlation was found for 1 and 2 kHz thresholds but, unexpectedly, for 125, 250 and 500 Hz thresholds significant correlations were found but still with low values (respectively −0.44, −0.38 and −0.36). For each subject the high frequency slope of the audiogram was computed using a linear regression line approximation based on threshold values at 1,2,4 and 8 kHz, the slope value was expressed in dB per octave. No correlation was found between these slope values and the tinnitus VAS scores obtained. For all subjects an approximate pitch estimation of their tinnitus was obtained by comparison with audiometer tones, pitch estimates were matched by the subjects to frequencies of 2,3,4,6 or 8 kHz tones with a predominance for 4 kHz. No correlation was found between the amount of long-term tinnitus suppression

and the frequency of the tinnitus pitch approximation. Tinnitus localization (right ear, left ear, bilateral or central) was also documented, suppression was found independent of tinnitus localization. Clearly tinnitus suppression was obtained in the LOFT aided ear but could also affect tinnitus in the opposite ear to various degrees but this point remains poorly documented in our data.

The precise time course for the setting of long-term tinnitus suppression is generally poorly documented in our data because most subjects were not monitored on a fine time-base. However several subjects offered to provide a follow-up self-report. These subjects reported a long-term tinnitus suppression increasing over several days or weeks of LOFT aid use. For various reasons some subjects stopped using their aid for days to weeks, they all reported a reappraisal of their tinnitus within a day; when a LOFT aid was reused, the tinnitus suppression became effective again within a day of use. For several subjects two different amounts of frequency transposition trials were separated by a period of no aid use. Figure 5 presents VAS scores obtained in these different conditions for 9 subjects, it can be seen that in the period of no aid use subjective tinnitus strength returned to original values and that a different amount of frequency transposition could provide more tinnitus suppression. The amount of frequency transposition was empirically adjusted for each individual upon examination of the audiogram and mostly upon week trials and subject's choice. The subjects reported their choice to be based upon best hearing as sounding most natural, and not upon tinnitus suppression. There is a weak correlation between the amount of frequency transposition and the strength of tinnitus suppression as can be seen in figure 6. We found no correlation between tinnitus pitch and most efficient amount of frequency transposition for tinnitus suppression.

Discussion

It seems quite reasonable to think that tinnitus is often associated with auditory deprivation. Indeed for hearing-impaired persons complaining about tinnitus, an association with the audiometric loss seems to be most frequently observed [15,16,17]. Furthermore, normally-hearing subjects after some minutes in a silent cabin report tinnitus which resembles very much tinnitus described from complaints of hearing-impaired persons [3]. Tinnitus may then correspond to an abnormal neural activity associated with brain areas deprived of sound activation, hypothetically through alteration of lateral inhibition and/or synchrony and setting of hyper-reactivity presumably in link with hyperacusis often associated with tinnitus [23].

It also seems quite clear that reactivation of deprived sensorineural areas can be associated with tinnitus suppression. Indeed there are many reports of tinnitus and temporary hearing loss from exposures to excessive sound levels showing that tinnitus disappears together with recovery of hearing loss [24], similar concomitances were made in many other pathological conditions such as Meniere's disease, sudden deafness and drug ototoxicity. In cases of permanent hearing loss, there are suggestions that a reactivation of deprived areas can attenuate tinnitus [25].

In line with the two propositions above, we speculate that the tinnitus suppression reported in the present study could correspond to a perceptive re-attribution of transposed frequencies to auditory brain areas deprived by deafness. It might not be necessarily a re-excitation of deprived channels but it could act as a sort of gate mechanism. Because usual amplification and non linear frequency transposition did not provide similar tinnitus suppression for subjects of this study, both characteristics of linearity and of octave transposition may be of importance. Linearity allows conservation of harmonic relation – as spectral peaks remain at integer (although not necessarily successive) multiples-, which is well known as a strong factor for unifying components into a single auditory perception, preserving sound naturalness, a feature indicated by subjects in their choice of LOFT setting. In addition octave transposed components blend much better than components transposed at non octave ratios [26]. Remarkably in this line is the octave confusion often observed in tinnitus pitch matching [27] which may be an illustration of the perceptive strength of octave transposition. These two aspects may be critical for frequency transposed information to be perceptually fused with the un-transposed parts. Hypothetically once perceptually fused the transposed components might fit internal patterns used for recognition which would consequently re-attribute activity to deprived areas.

Author Contributions

Conceived and designed the experiments: EP. Performed the experiments: EP CP ST EA-L. Analyzed the data: EP YC. Contributed reagents/materials/analysis tools: YC. Wrote the paper: YC.

References

1. Holmes S, Padgham ND (2009) Review paper : more than ringing in the ears: a review of tinnitus and its psychosocial impact. Journal of Clinical Nursing, 18: 2927–2937.
2. Tucker DA, Phillips SL, Ruth RA, Clayton WA, Royster E, et al. (2005) The effect of silence on tinnitus perception. Otolaryngol Head Neck Surg. 132: 20–24.
3. Del Bo L, Forti S, Ambrosetti U, Costanzo S, Mauro D, et al. (2008) Tinnitus aurium in persons with normal hearing: 55 years later. Otolaryngol Head Neck Surg. 139: 391–394.
4. Dutt SN, McDermott AL, Irving RM, Donaldson I, Pahor AL, et al. (2002) Prescription of binaural hearing aids in the United Kingdom: a knowledge, attitude and practice (KAP) study. J Laryngol Otol Suppl. 28: 2–6.
5. Trotter MI, Donaldson I (2008) Hearing aids and tinnitus therapy: a 25-year experience. J Laryngol Otol. 122: 1052–1056.
6. Del Bo L, Ambrosetti U (2007) Hearing aids for the treatment of tinnitus. Prog Brain Res. 166: 341–345.
7. Moffat G, Adjout K, Gallego S, Thai-Van H, Collet L, et al. (2009) Effects of hearing aid fitting on the perceptual characteristics of tinnitus. Hearing Res 254: 82–91.
8. Jastreboff PJ, Gray WC, Gold SL (1996) Neurophysiological approach to tinnitus patients. Am J Otol. 17: 236–240.
9. Anari M, Axelsson A, Eliasson A, Magnusson L (1999) Hypersensitivity to sound. Scan. Audiol. 28: 219–230.
10. Hobson J, Chisholm E, El Refaie A (2010) Sound therapy (masking) in the management of tinnitus in adults. Cochrane Database Syst Rev. 12:CD006371.
11. Vernon J, Griest S, Press L (1990) Attributes of tinnitus and the acceptance of masking. Am J Otolaryngol 11: 44–50.
12. Cazals Y, Bourdin M (1983) Etude acoustique des acouphènes. Revue de Laryngologie 104 : 433–438.
13. Terry AM, Jones DM, Davis BR, Slater R (1983) Parametric studies of tinnitus masking and residual inhibition. Br J Audiol. 17: 245–256.
14. Roberts LE, Moffat G, Baumann M, Ward LM, Bosnyak DJ (2008) Residual inhibition functions overlap tinnitus spectra and the region of auditory threshold shift. JARO 9: 417–435

15. Wegel Rl (1931) A study of tinnitus. Arch Otolaryngol. 14: 158–165.
16. Henry J.A., Meikle M., Gilbert A (1999) Audiometric correlates of tinnitus pitch: insights from the Tinnitus data registry. In: Hazell, J. (Ed.), Proceedings of the Sixth International Tinnitus Seminar. The Tinnitus and Hyperacusis Centre, London, 51–57.
17. Norena A, Micheyl C, Chéry-Croze S, Collet L (2002) Psychoacoustic characterization of the tinnitus spectrum: implications for the underlying mechanisms of tinnitus. Audiol Neurootol. 7: 358–369.
18. Vickers DA, Moore BCJ, Baer T (2001) Effects of low-pass filtering on the intelligibility of speech in quiet for people with and without dead regions at high frequencies. J. Acoust. Soc. Am. 110, 1164–1175.
19. Simpson A (2009) Frequency lowering devices for managing high frequency hearing loss : a review. Trends in Amplification, 13: 87–106.
20. Robinson JD, Stainsby TH, Baer T, Moore BC (2009) Evaluation of a frequency transposition algorithm using wearable hearing aids. Int J Audiol. 48: 384–393.
21. Füllgrabe C, Baer T, Moore BC (2010) Effect of linear and warped spectral transposition on consonant identification by normal-hearing listeners with a simulated dead region. Int J Audiol. 49: 420–433.
22. McDermott HJ (2011) A technical comparison of digital frequency-lowering algorithms available in two current hearing aids. PLoS One. 6: e22358.
23. Eggermont JJ (2012) Hearing loss, hyperacusis, or tinnitus: What is modeled in animal research? Hear Res. 2012 Feb 7. [Epub ahead of print].
24. Atherley GRC, Hempstock TI, Noble WG (1968) Study of tinnitus induced temporarily by noise. J Acoust Soc Am, 44: 1503–1506.
25. Diesch E, Andermann M, Flor H, Rupp A (2010) Functional and structural aspects of tinnitus-related enhancement and suppression of auditory cortex activity. Neuroimage. 50: 1545–59.
26. Bergman AS (1990) Auditory scene analysis.The perceptual organization of sound. MIT Press, 773 p.
27. Henry JA, Dennis KC, Schechter MA (2005) General review of tinnitus: prevalence, mechanisms, effects and management. J Speech Lang Hear Res 48: 1204–1235.

3

Tinnitus: Distinguishing between Subjectively Perceived Loudness and Tinnitus-Related Distress

Elisabeth Wallhäusser-Franke[1]*, Joachim Brade[2], Tobias Balkenhol[1], Roberto D'Amelio[1,3], Andrea Seegmüller[1], Wolfgang Delb[1]

1 Department of Phoniatrics and Audiology, Medical Faculty Mannheim, Heidelberg University, Mannheim, Germany, 2 Department of Medical Statistics and Biomathematics, Medical Faculty Mannheim, Heidelberg University, Mannheim, Germany, 3 Department of Internal Medicine IV and Neurocenter, University Clinic, Saarland University, Homburg/Saar, Germany

Abstract

Objectives: Overall success of current tinnitus therapies is low, which may be due to the heterogeneity of tinnitus patients. Therefore, subclassification of tinnitus patients is expected to improve therapeutic allocation, which, in turn, is hoped to improve therapeutic success for the individual patient. The present study aims to define factors that differentially influence subjectively perceived tinnitus loudness and tinnitus-related distress.

Methods: In a questionnaire-based cross-sectional survey, the data of 4705 individuals with tinnitus were analyzed. The self-report questionnaire contained items about subjective tinnitus loudness, type of onset, awareness and localization of the tinnitus, hearing impairment, chronic comorbidities, sleep quality, and psychometrically validated questionnaires addressing tinnitus-related distress, depressivity, anxiety, and somatic symptom severity. In a binary step-wise logistic regression model, we tested the predictive power of these variables on subjective tinnitus loudness and tinnitus-related distress.

Results: The present data contribute to the distinction between subjective tinnitus loudness and tinnitus-related distress. Whereas subjective loudness was associated with permanent awareness and binaural localization of the tinnitus, tinnitus-related distress was associated with depressivity, anxiety, and somatic symptom severity.

Conclusions: Subjective tinnitus loudness and the potential presence of severe depressivity, anxiety, and somatic symptom severity should be assessed separately from tinnitus-related distress. If loud tinnitus is the major complaint together with mild or moderate tinnitus-related distress, therapies should focus on auditory perception. If levels of depressivity, anxiety or somatic symptom severity are severe, therapies and further diagnosis should focus on these symptoms at first.

Editor: Berthold Langguth, University of Regensburg, Germany

Funding: This work was partly supported by auric Hörsysteme and Schaaf und Maier Hörgeräte. The funders had no role in study design, data collection and analysis, decision to publish, or preparation of the manuscript.

Competing Interests: This work was partly supported by auric Hörsysteme and Schaaf und Maier Hörgeräte.

* E-mail: elisabeth.wallhaeusser@medma.uni-heidelberg.de

Introduction

Subjective tinnitus is a sound that does not originate from an external or body sound source and that is heard only by those affected. Tinnitus is a widespread symptom with 30–40% of the adult population experiencing tinnitus during their life, and 0.5–2.5% being severely affected by a tinnitus that interferes with life quality [1–4]. The majority of tinnitus patients are hearing impaired [4], and many additionally express hypersensitivity to environmental sounds [5]. Treatment of hearing loss by hearing aids or cochlear implants may reduce the tinnitus perception [6–8] suggesting interplay between tinnitus and hearing impairment. In addition, a patient's reaction to tinnitus determines the degree of tinnitus-related distress which is largely independent from psychoacoustic measures [9,10]. Besides that, especially those patients with high tinnitus-related distress show a high prevalence of depressivity, anxiety and somatic symptoms [11–14]. Depressivity and anxiety tend to worsen tinnitus-related distress and vice

versa, but the relation between tinnitus and these psychopathologies is not undisputed [15].

Most therapeutic interventions focus on the reduction of tinnitus-related distress without primarily trying to reduce tinnitus loudness [16–18], partly reflecting the lack of successful approaches to reduce loudness. It should not be ignored, however, that the subjectively perceived loudness may be the major complaint, and that it may be associated with low tinnitus-related distress [19]. This together with the finding, that severe tinnitus-related distress may be associated with low subjective loudness [19] suggests that these measures represent separate tinnitus parameters that are both relevant to the affected individuals. They may independently become incapacitating and then demand specific therapeutic interventions.

The subjectively perceived loudness of tinnitus can be recorded by numeric rating scales which typically range from 0 or 1 (low loudness) to 10 (high loudness) and which have been used in several studies on tinnitus (e.g. [20,21]). Numeric rating scales provide high measurement resolution and are easy to score [22], they reflect the subjective impression of tinnitus loudness experienced by the patients which may deviate from the tinnitus loudness that is measured by psychoacoustic matching procedures [23]. Tinnitus-related distress on the other hand is measured with psychometrically validated questionnaires (e.g. [24,25]).

Aim of the present questionnaire-based study was to determine factors that differentially affect subjectively perceived tinnitus loudness and tinnitus-related distress. Data were collected from 4705 persons affected by tinnitus. The questionnaire included items about tinnitus characteristics such as localization and type of sound, tinnitus duration, subjectively perceived tinnitus loudness, and hearing impairment. Strength of tinnitus-related distress was recorded with the psychometrically validated short version of the Tinnitus Questionnaire (MTQ, [26]). Depressive symptoms, anxiety and somatic symptom severity were addressed with modules of the psychometrically validated Patient Health Questionnaire (PHQ, [27,28]).

Methods

Data collection and sample

During September of 2010 a questionnaire with a total of 256 items was distributed by mail to all of the 13,349 registered patient members of the German Tinnitus Association (Deutsche Tinnitus-Liga, DTL). The questionnaire was accompanied by a letter in which the participants were informed, that by filling out and sending in the questionnaire they agreed to the use of their data for research purposes. 4752 questionnaires were received, and the data of 4705 questionnaires were entered into the data base. The rest was omitted mainly because of invalid membership numbers. The questionnaires were pseudonymized in that they contained the membership code but not the participants' names. The study protocol was approved by the local ethics committee (Ethikkommission II) of the Medical Faculty Mannheim of Heidelberg University and by the data safety commissioner of the Medical Faculty Mannheim of Heidelberg University according to the principles expressed in the Declaration of Helsinki.

Besides information about age and gender the following information included in the questionnaire was used for the present study:

Tinnitus characteristics and hearing loss

In the questionnaire type of tinnitus sound, type of tinnitus onset (slowly/suddenly), its duration and localization as well as the time of daily tinnitus awareness was assessed. Subjectively perceived loudness was recorded on a numeric rating scale (T-NRS) from 0 (tinnitus audible only during silence) to 10 (louder than all external sounds). To asses the potential presence of hearing impairments it was asked, if an audiogram was taken, if hearing impairment had been diagnosed by an otolaryngologist, and if hearing aids were used. Response options were 'yes' or 'no'. This did not accurately reflect the amount of hearing loss, but did tell whether hearing impairments were uni- or bilateral and which side was affected.

Tinnitus-related distress

Tinnitus-related distress was addressed by the psychometrically validated brief version of the tinnitus questionnaire (MTQ: [26]) with sum scores from 0 (no distress) to 24 (maximum distress). Sum scores were derived only from cases with complete MTQ-scales. In line with Hiller and Goebel [26] sum scores below 8 were classified as mild tinnitus-related distress, while sum scores above 18 were seen as indicator of severe tinnitus-related distress.

Psychological factors

Three psychometrically validated modules of the Patient Health Questionnaire (PHQ) were used to address depressivity (PHQ-9), anxiety (GAD-7), and somatic symptom severity (PHQ-15) [27,28]. Response options for PHQ-9 and GAD-7 were 0 (not bothered at all) to 3 (bothered almost every day). Response options for PHQ-15 were 0 (not bothered at all) to 2 (bothered a lot). Higher scores indicated greater symptom severity in all scales, and a cut point at 15 distinguished between mild/moderate and severe/most severe symptom levels [28,29]. A case was eliminated for classification in a module, if a single item in that module was missing. Since in the PHQ-15 one item addressed pre-menopausal women and one item addressed sexually active persons exclusively, these items were scored 0 if left blank producing a slight underestimation of somatic symptom severity in theses cases.

Finally, one question each asked about difficulties to initiate and to maintain sleep, and the presence of chronic somatic morbidities as well as chronic pain and dizziness were recorded.

Data analysis

Data management and data analysis were performed with the Statistical Package for the Social Sciences (SPSS) 18.0 for Windows (Chicago, Illinois) and SAS for Windows 9.2 (SAS Institute Inc., Cary, NC, USA). Percentages are reported for categorical variables (% in table 1) and means ± standard deviations (mean [standard deviation]) for sum score and NRS variables. A correlation analysis for tinnitus-related distress (MTQ) and subjective loudness (T-NRS) showed a moderate correlation between them (Spearman's rho for non-parametric data: 0.524). Therefore, further analyses were performed separately for both tinnitus measures.

To identify the variables with the strongest association with MTQ and T-NRS respectively, groups with mild (MTQ-score≤7) versus severe (MTQ-score≥19) tinnitus-related distress, and with low (T-NRS≤2) versus high loudness (T-NRS≥8) were compared. Conceivably loudness and distress clusters do partially overlap. Data were categorized into major (problematic) versus minor with a cut-off score of ≥15 (major) for the variables PHQ-9, GAD-7 and PHQ-15 distinguishing severe levels of depressivity, anxiety and somatic symptom severity [28,29]. Based on this grouping odds ratios were computed. The presence (major) of hearing impairment, dizziness, chronic pain, somatic comorbidities, and sleep problems were contrasted to their absence (minor). In addition, the tinnitus characteristics sudden onset, constant awareness of the tinnitus, and localization were included. An odds ratio (OR) of 2 and above respectively of 0.5 and below, indicating a 2 (or more)-fold likelihood respectively a 0.5 (or less)-fold likelihood of a characteristic were considered relevant. In addition to the point estimates, 95% confidence intervals were calculated for the odds ratios to quantify the range of the effect size. The predictive power on T-NRS or MTQ of variables with an OR≥2 or ≤0.5 in the univariate analyses was assessed in a binary stepwise logistic regression model.

Results

Data were derived from 4705 questionnaires. The age range was 18 to 94 years (58.63 [11.76] years; females: 57.44 [12.22]; males: 59.47 [11.39]), and the overall female proportion was 40.9%. Mild tinnitus-related distress (MTQ-score≤7) was reported by 37.6%, whereas distress related to the tinnitus was judged as being intermediate (8≤MTQ-score≤18) by 49.0%, and 13.4% of the participants felt severely distressed by their tinnitus (MTQ-score≥19). Low subjective loudness was commonly associated with

Table 1. Influence of Tinnitus characteristics, hearing impairments, and psychopathological factors on subjectively perceived tinnitus loudness and on tinnitus-related distress.

Characteristic %	Total	Subjective Tinnitus Loudness (T-NRS)			Tinnitus-Related Distress (MTQ)		
		Low	High	OR (95% CI)	Mild	Severe	OR (95% CI)
		(T-NRS≤2)	(T-NRS≥8)		(MTQ≤7)	(MTQ≥19)	
	N = 4705	N = 379	N = 1338		N = 1754	N = 623	
Age>50 years	74.9	**59.8**	**82.0**	**3.1 [2.4–3.9]**	73.0	75.6	1.1 [0.9–1.4]
Female	40.9	43.0	38.4	1.2 [1.0–1. 5]	39.7	36.8	1.1 [0.9–1.4]
Time since tinnitus onset							
< = 12 months	1.3	1.3	1.1	0.8 [0.3–2.2]	1.2	1.5	1.3 [0.6–2.9]
<12 months and < = 5 years	14.7	20.6	10.9	**0.5 [0.4–0.6]**	11.7	19.1	1.8 [1.4–2.3]
>5 years	84.0	78.1	88.0	**2.1 [1.5–2.8]**	87.1	79.4	0.6 [0.5–0.7]
Tinnitus onset							
sudden	66.2	69.9	67.1	0.9 [0.7–1.1]	65.8	66.9	1.1 [0.9–1.3]
slowly progressive	41.4	31.7	43.0	1.6 [1.3–2.1]	39.4	39.8	1.0 [0.8–1.2]
Permanent awareness	79.2	**49.3**	**92.3**	**13.6 [10.2–18.3]**	70.9	91.6	**5.4 [3.8–7.5]**
Localization of the tinnitus							
left	19.6	27.2	14.6	**0.5 [0.4–0.6]**	22.0	14.0	0.6 [0.5–0.7]
right	14.4	16.6	12.3	0.7 [0.5–1.0]	15.6	11.1	0.9 [0.7–1.2
binaural/central	74.2	**61.5**	**82.4**	**2.9 [2.3–3. 8]**	68.5	84.1	**2.4 [1.9–3.1]**
Hearing impairment							
unilateral left	18.3	20.8	17.4	0.8 [0.6–1.1]	18.2	18.2	1.0 [0.8–1.3]
unilateral right	13.6	11.1	12.0	1.1 [0.8–1.6]	13.7	12.8	0.9 [0.7–1.2]
bilateral	44.5	**26.6**	**56.7**	**3.6 [2.8–4.6]**	39.8	54.3	1.8 [1.5–2.2]
Influence of Hearing aid							
tinnitus lower	29.9	**36.5**	**22.2**	**0.5 [0.3–0.8]**	**39.6**	**16.0**	**0.3 [0.2–0.4]**
tinnitus louder	5.1	6.8	6.4	1.0 [0.4–2.5]	**2.6**	**10.8**	**4.6 [2.3–9.2]**
Dizziness	27.6	**17.9**	**33.0**	**2.3 [1.7–3.0]**	21.3	41.6	**2.6 [2.2–3.2]**
Chronic pain	66.2	**50.9**	**73.5**	**2.7 [2.1–3.4]**	52.4	81.9	**3.9 [3.1–4.9]**
Somatic comorbidities	53.7	**42.0**	**59.9**	**2.1 [1.6 –2.7]**	56.1	60.3	1.6 [1.3–2.0]
Sleep Problems	76.5	**60.4**	**83.9**	**3.4 [2.7–4.4]**	60.9	94.8	**11.6 [8.1–16.8]**
Psychopathologies							
Depressivity (PHQ-9≥15)	10.6	**5.3**	**20.0**	**4.5 [2.8–7.2]**	1.5	42.6	**48.0 [31.3–73.7]**
Anxiety (GAD-7≥15)	7.3	**3.0**	**14.0**	**5.3 [2.8–9.8**	0.8	32.1	**61.6 [34.8–109.2]**
Somatic Symptom Severity (PHQ-15≥15)	13.1	**3.5**	**22.5**	**8.0 [4.4–14.4]**	2.9	39.8	**22.1 [15.8–31.1]**

In this table, population percentages (%) as well as characteristics (%) of subgroups with low (< = 2) and high (≥8) subjectively perceived tinnitus loudness measured on a numeric rating scale (T-NRS) from 0 (tinnitus audible only during silence) to 10 (louder than all external sounds), and mild (MTQ score≤7) and severe (MTQ score≥19) tinnitus-related distress are shown. Absolute numbers deviate because of missing data in single items. Percentages for type of tinnitus onset and tinnitus localization exceed 100%, because participants with two distinguishable tinnitus tones coded multiple categories. Variables with values marked in bold because of odds ratios (OR) of 2 and above or 0.5 or below were included in the regression analysis.
CI – confidence interval of OR, MTQ – short version of the tinnitus questionnaire, N – number.

mild distress, whereas high subjective loudness tended to be associated with severe distress. These categories were not congruent, however. In 13 participants (0.3%) a subjective loudness score (T-NRS) of two and lower combined with severe tinnitus–related distress, whereas 209 participants (4.4%) reported a combination of loud (T-NRS≥8) but only mildly distressing tinnitus. Overall, the correlation between T-NRS and MTQ was found to be moderate (r = 0.524 Spearman's rho based on MTQ sum scores). Gender effects were not apparent, whereas older age and tinnitus duration of more than 5 years were associated with louder but not with a more distressing tinnitus. Sudden onset was prevalent, and of the 50% that named a possible cause, the majority (n = 1716) suspected stress followed by sudden hearing loss (1389) and noise trauma (354) as putative reasons. Ringing, continuous, binaural-central tinnitus prevailed, and unilateral tinnitus was more frequently located on the left ear which coincided with a higher incidence of left unilateral hearing impairment (table 1). The subjectively perceived loudness had increased since tinnitus onset in 34.9% of the participants while a decrease was reported by 7.7%. In contrast, decreases in tinnitus-related distress (28.4%) were as common as increases (25.4%).

Auditory-related factors

Altogether 78.1% reported a hearing impairment that had been diagnosed audiometrically by an otolaryngologist. This percentage rose with age (56.2% below age 40; 84.1% above age 70). Percentages of bilateral hearing impairment, binaural-central localization and permanent awareness of the tinnitus differed substantially when comparing low and high subjective tinnitus loudness (table 1).

42% of the individuals indicating hearing impairments used hearing aids. 29.9% of them experienced a decrease while 5.1% experienced an increase in the subjective loudness of the tinnitus when using hearing aids. Participants with low subjective loudness (T-NRS≤2) as well as participants with mild distress (MTQ≤7) benefitted most from the use of hearing aids, whereas those with severe tinnitus-related distress (MTQ≥19) reported loudness increases most often and decreases least often (table 1).

Psychological factors

Correlations between depressivity, anxiety, somatic symptom severity and T-NRS were low (Spearman's Rho: PHQ-9: 0.351; GAD-7: 0.301; PHQ-15: 0.312). Correlations between MTQ and the PHQ-scales (PHQ-9: 0.663; GAD-7: 0.610; PHQ-15: 0.535) exceeded those between MTQ and T-NRS (0.524). Most noteworthy was the high incidence of elevated PHQ scores in the group with severe tinnitus-related distress (table 1). Correlations between the three PHQ scales exceeded all other correlations (PHQ-9/GAD7: 0.805; PHQ-9/PHQ-15: 0.762; GAD-7/PHQ-15: 0.654). Altogether 726 participants, equalling 18.6% of the whole sample, reached a score of 15 and above in at least one of the PHQ scales. Severe somatic symptom severity was most common (13.1% of whole sample) followed by depressivity (10.4%) and anxiety (7.3%), and 3.6% expressed severe levels in all PHQ-scales. Based on the population with a severe level in at least one of the PHQ scales (726 = 100%), the percentage with comorbid severe depressivity, anxiety and somatic symptom severity was highest in the subgroup with severe tinnitus-related distress (39.8%), and lowest in the subgroup with mild tinnitus-related distress (2.9%; Fig. 1).

Influence of somatic comorbidities and sleep quality

More than 50% of the sample reported somatic comorbidities. Percentages were lower only in the group with low subjective loudness. Reports of sleep disturbances, chronic pain and dizziness peaked in the group with severe tinnitus-related distress. Analysis of OR revealed that sleep disturbances, chronic pain and dizziness were associated with tinnitus-related distress, and that all variables were associated with subjective loudness although to a lesser extent (table 1).

Differentiation between subjective tinnitus loudness and tinnitus-related distress

Univariate analyses showed that groups with low and high subjective tinnitus loudness differed substantially (OR≥2 or ≤0.5) with respect to the percentage of subjects that was permanently aware of the tinnitus, somatic symptom severity, binaural/central localization of the tinnitus, anxiety and depressivity, binaural hearing impairment, tinnitus duration, and in the variables sleep problems, age, chronic pain, dizziness, and somatic comorbidities. Dominance of loudness over distress was most obvious for those with loud but only mildly distressing tinnitus (n = 209). In this group the low sum scores in the PHQ scales (PHQ-9: 4.0 [3.6], GAD-7: 3.2 [2.9]; PHQ-15: 5.7 [4.0]) were most notable.

In contrast, groups with mild respectively severe tinnitus-related distress differed most in the percentage of elevated depressivity, anxiety, somatic symptom severity, and sleep disturbances. Permanent awareness and localization of the tinnitus as well as chronic pain and dizziness were less influential, whereas bilateral hearing impairment age and tinnitus duration had no substantial influence.

The predominant characteristic in the group with severe tinnitus-related distress was the high prevalence of psychologically relevant symptoms as indicated by elevated scores in the PHQ scales. Conspicuous were also the high percentages of those with comorbid chronic pain and dizziness. Moreover, the majority had difficulties in initiating or maintaining sleep, and overall benefit from hearing aids was lower than average. Influence of the psychopathological variables was most obvious in a small cluster of 13 subjects who reported low subjective tinnitus loudness but severe tinnitus-related distress. Mean sum scores of PHQ-9 (13.3 [5.0]), GAD-7 (12.2 [6.5]) and PHQ-15 (15.2 [9.0] were high, whereas hearing impairments (69.2%; bilateral: 46.2%) were less frequent than average.

In a step-wise regression analysis the predictive power of auditory and non-auditory variables on tinnitus-related distress respectively subjective tinnitus loudness with the factors showing OR of 2 and above or of 0.5 and below was calculated. Factors found to be relevant for subjective tinnitus loudness was above all the factor "permanent awareness" of the tinnitus followed by "binaural/central localization", sleep problems and pain. In contrast, most influential variables on tinnitus-related distress were depressivity and anxiety followed by sleep problems and permanent awareness of the tinnitus. In addition the variables binaural/central tinnitus localization as well as somatic symptom severity and pain had significant influence (table 2). Noteworthy was also that decreases of subjective tinnitus loudness while using a hearing aid were significantly more likely for those with mild tinnitus-related distress than for those with severe tinnitus-related distress as indicated by an OR below 0.5 (table 1, 2).

Discussion

The results of the present study are based on data obtained from 4705 participants with tinnitus. The observed distribution of tinnitus characteristics is in accordance with those found in epidemiological tinnitus studies [21,26,30]. The results show that subjective tinnitus loudness and tinnitus-related distress are only moderately correlated, and that the variables that exert a major influence on either tinnitus measure differ substantially. Bilateral hearing impairment rather increases the risk for a tinnitus that is perceived as being loud, whereas variables associated with psychopathologies rather increase the risk for severe tinnitus-related distress. Therefore subjective tinnitus loudness should be treated as a separate characteristic of the tinnitus in addition to tinnitus-related distress. These findings are in line with earlier reports [19,26,31], and with imaging studies that suggest involvement of different brain areas in the processing of the tinnitus percept compared to tinnitus-related distress, i.e. the reaction on this percept (rev. in [13]). Moreover they can be seen as an explanation for the finding that therapies like cognitive behavioural therapy which aim at the reaction on the tinnitus, do not influence its perception, i.e. the subjectively perceived loudness [16–18]. In addition, there is evidence that the subjectively perceived loudness can be diminished temporarily while not influencing tinnitus-related distress by electrically stimulating dorsolateral prefrontal cortex [20].

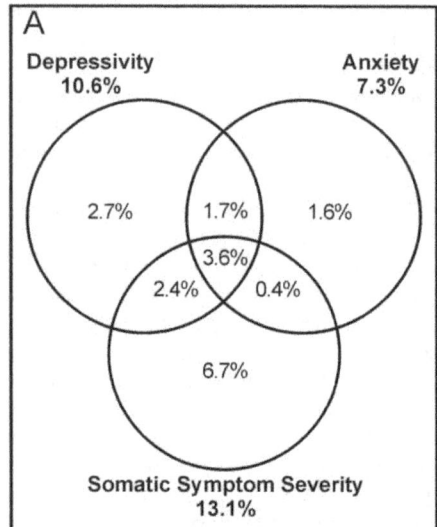
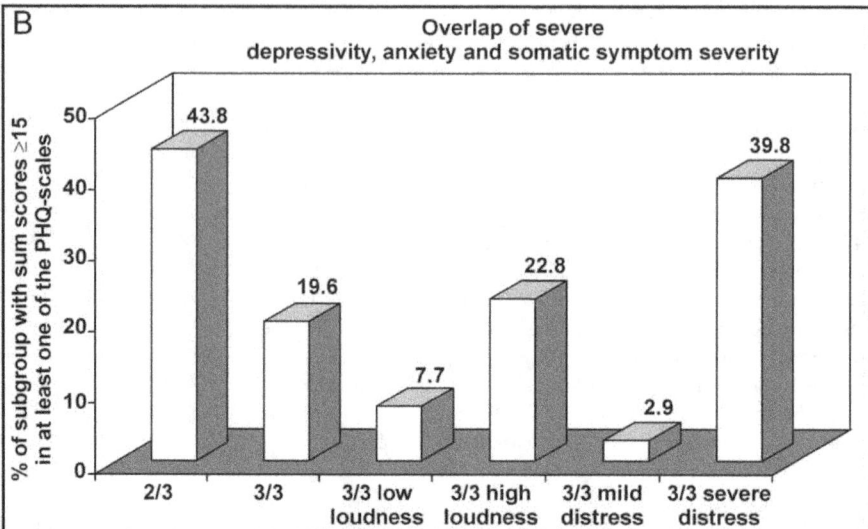

Figure 1. Comorbidity of depressivity, anxiety, and somatic symptom severity derived from scores of the Patient Health Questionnaire (PHQ). A: Somatic symptom severity was most common (13.1% of whole sample) followed by depressivity (10.6%) and anxiety (7.3%). 3.6% of the whole sample were affected by elevated levels of depressivity, anxiety and somatic symptom severity at the same time, and an additional 4.5% showed elevated levels in two scales. **B**: The 726 participants with scores of 15 or above in at least one of the three PHQ scales (1/3) were set to 100%. Of these, 318 (43.8%) exhibited severe levels in at least 2 PHQ-scales (2/3), while 142 (19.6%) had severe levels in all scales (3/3). The percentage of participants with scores of 15 and above in all three scales (3/3) was least common in the subgroup with mild tinnitus-related distress (2.9%), while it was most common in the subgroup with severe tinnitus-related distress with 39.8%. Differences between subgroups with low and high subjective loudness had the same direction, but were less pronounced. PHQ scales: PHQ-9 – depressivity, GAD-7 – anxiety, PHQ-15 – somatic symptom severity.

Tinnitus related distress: the influence of psychopathologic variables

To our knowledge this study analyzes the largest sample of subjects with tinnitus that has ever been evaluated with psychometrically validated questionnaires addressing depressivity, anxiety and somatic symptom severity in conjunction with subjective tinnitus loudness and tinnitus-related distress. The observed percentages of severe depressivity and anxiety are slightly higher than in the general population [32]. In the subgroup with severely distressing tinnitus (MTQ>18), however, this percentage

is multiplied, which is in accordance with reports on a close association of a severely distressing tinnitus with depressive symptoms and anxiety [2,12,14,33,34].

In addition, severe somatic symptom severity is increased in the group with severe tinnitus-related distress compared to the study population in general. The threshold we used for the distinction between moderate and severe cases requires the presence of at least seven bothering somatic symptoms, and is seen as a reliable distinction between presence of somatoform disorders in comparison to their absence [28]. The present finding also is in line with

Table 2. Results of the stepwise regression analysis.

Tinnitus-related distress (MTQ)	OR [95% CI]	Subjective tinnitus loudness (T-NRS)	OR [95% CI]
Depressivity (PHQ-9)****	19.67 [5.29–73.12]	Permanent awareness of tinnitus****	24.04 [9.25–62.45]
Anxiety (GAD-7)*	14.19 [1.52–132.42]	Binaural tinnitus localization***	4.77 [2.00–11.37]
Sleep problems****	11.99 [3.46–41.51]	Sleep Problems**	3.23 [1.40–7.49]
Permanent awareness of tinnitus***	10.61 [2.43–46.29]	Pain*	2.84 [1.20–6.73]
Binaural tinnitus localization**	4.14 [1.62–10.57]		
Somatic Symptom Severity (PHQ-15)*	4.75 [2.43–46.29]		
Pain*	2.23 [1.14–4.38]		
Tinnitus lower with hearing aid*	0.32 [0.15–0.7]		

Variables with significant impact on tinnitus-related distress and subjectively perceived tinnitus loudness were determined in a stepwise regression analysis comparing mild versus severe distress and low versus high loudness, respectively. Concordance of the model was 89.7 for tinnitus-related distress and 81.3 for subjective tinnitus loudness. Odds ratios (ORs) and 95% confidence intervals (95% CI) are shown.
*$p<0.05$,
**$p<0.01$,
***$p<0.001$,
****$p<0.0001$.
MTQ – short version of the tinnitus questionnaire, T-NRS – numeric rating scale for subjectively perceived tinnitus loudness.

observations that tinnitus patients with high levels of self- and somatic attention express greater emotional and tinnitus-related distress [35–37], and that depressed tinnitus patients display strong somatic focus resulting in a tendency to report large numbers of medically unexplained symptoms [36].

In agreement with former tinnitus studies [14,35,36], somatic symptom severity as a determining factor for tinnitus-related distress is most frequent followed by depressivity, while anxiety is least frequent in the present sample. Although depressivity, anxiety, and somatic symptom severity are often coexistant, there is no complete overlap in the study sample. Moreover relative frequencies deviate between the subgroups with low and high subjective loudness as well as between subgroups with mild and severe tinnitus-related distress, and they deviate from those seen in a large primary care population [28].

An important issue that cannot be settled with this cross-sectional survey is whether these comorbidities are primary or secondary to the tinnitus. Longitudinal studies with a small number of acute tinnitus patients suggest that psychopathological conditions exist beforehand and constitute risk factors for the development of a distressing tinnitus or that they arise together with the tinnitus [33,37]. This does not exclude the possibility, however, that tinnitus promotes the progression of psychopathologies and it appears likely that both developments exist.

Variables that predominantly influence the subjectively perceived tinnitus loudness and the effect of hearing aids

The rate of hearing impairment in the present study is high. Its incidence increases with age, and bilateral hearing impairment is more frequent in the group that experiences loud tinnitus. These findings agree with those of others [3,38–40]. A relation between the amount of hearing loss and subjective tinnitus loudness was reported by two studies comprising together about 1000 audiometrically screened tinnitus patients indicating that tinnitus loudness correlates with the presence and the degree of threshold shifts [39,40].

Hearing impairment is thought to be the permissive condition for the development of the tinnitus perception. Therefore restoring auditory input is expected to reduce the subjectively perceived tinnitus loudness. Though, results of such interventions are variable and the overall success rate is low [6,41]. The results of the present study indicate that recovery of auditory input reduces subjective tinnitus loudness while using the hearing aid in about 30% of all hearing aid users. Most important, however, the results suggest that hearing aids are more effective in individuals that have a non-distressing tinnitus, whereas the risk to increase the perceived tinnitus loudness when using hearing aids is disproportionately high in individuals with severe tinnitus-related distress.

Limitations

Some limitations apply to the present analysis. Our tinnitus population may not represent the tinnitus population as a whole,

but may be dominated by individuals that are concerned by their tinnitus and became active by joining a patient organization. Therefore the reported characteristics may not be entirely representative for the general tinnitus population. Furthermore the evidence relies on self-report questionnaires and therefore may be influenced by misconceptions. However, characteristics of the investigated tinnitus population are in line with the published literature [11,14,21,30,34].

Conclusion

Subjectively perceived tinnitus loudness as measured here represents a distinctive quality of tinnitus which needs to be assessed separately and in addition to tinnitus-related distress and to psychoacoustic tinnitus characteristics. This can be done effectively by numeric rating scales. Study participants with a severely distressing tinnitus expressed elevated levels of depressivity, anxiety, and somatic symptom severity, and the high incidence of sleep problems, chronic pain and dizziness in the highly distressed tinnitus patients appears to be associated foremost with these factors. Therefore, especially in subjects with high tinnitus-related distress, the potential presence of severe depressivity, anxiety and somatic symptom severity should be assessed separately from tinnitus-related distress by validated psychopathology questionnaires.

A combination of the MTQ questionnaire with established questionnaires addressing psychopathologies such as PHQ-9, GAD-7, and PHQ-15 in conjunction with audiological examination and recording of the subjectively perceived tinnitus loudness represents a powerful and easy to handle tool to characterize tinnitus patients. While these parameters are already assessed in specialized tinnitus centres, they also need to be evaluated during routine otolaryngologic examination of tinnitus patients. As suggested by the differential effect of hearing aids in distressed and non-distressed participants, a comprehensive characterization may optimize patient allocation and consequently the therapeutic outcome of existing tinnitus therapies.

Acknowledgments

The authors want to thank the German Tinnitus Association (DTL), the DTL members who participated and the past president of the DTL, Elke Knör, for enabling this study. The authors also wish to acknowledge the help of the medical students Alexander Eiffler, Tobias Hofbauer and Herve Nguewoun who inscribed the data into the database.

Author Contributions

Conceived and designed the experiments: EWF WD RD TB. Performed the experiments: EWF. Analyzed the data: EWF JB WD. Wrote the paper: EWF WD. Organized the study: EWF AS.

References

1. Krog NH, Engdahl B, Tambs K (2010) The association between tinnitus and mental health in a general population sample: results from the HUNT Study. J Psychosom Res 69: 289–298.
2. Nondahl DM, Cruickshanks KJ, Huang GH, Klein BE, Klein R, et al. (2011) Tinnitus and its risk factors in the Beaver Dam offspring study. Int I Audiol 50: 313–320.
3. Shargorodsky J, Curhan GC, Farwell WR (2010) Prevalence and characteristics of tinnitus among US adults. Am J Med 123: 711–718.
4. Sindhusake D, Golding M, Newall P, Rubin G, Jakobsen K, et al. (2003) Risk factors for tinnitus in a population of older adults: the blue mountains hearing study. Ear Hear 24: 501–507.
5. Jastreboff PJ, Jastreboff MM (2006) Tinnitus retraining therapy: a different view on tinnitus. ORL 68: 23–30.
6. Del Bo L, Ambrosetti U (2007) Hearing aids for the treatment of tinnitus. Prog Brain Res 166: 341–345.
7. Henry JA, Zaugg TL, Myers PJ, Schechter MA (2008) Using therapeutic sound with progressive audiologic tinnitus management. Trends in Amplification 12: 188–207.
8. Olze H, Szczepek AJ, Haupt H, Zirke N, Graebel S, et al. (2011) The impact of cochlear implantation on tinnitus, stress and quality of life in postlingually deafened patients. Audiol Neurootol 17: 2–11.
9. Dauman R, Tyler RS (1992) Some considerations on the classification of tinnitus. In: Aran JM, Dauman R, eds. Tinnitus 91 – Proceedings of the Fourth

International Tinnitus Seminar. Bordeaux: Kugler Publications, Amsterdam. pp 225–229.

10. Jastreboff PJ, Gray WC, Gold SL (1996) Neurophysiological approach to tinnitus patients. Am J Otol 17: 236–240.

11. Delb W, D'Amelio R, Schonecke OW, Iro H (1999) Are there psychological or audiological parameters determining tinnitus impact? In: Hazell JWP, ed. Proceedings of the Sixth International Tinnitus Seminar. Cambridge: Oxford University Press. pp 446–451.

12. Dobie RA (2003) Depression and tinnitus. Otolaryngol Clin North Am 36: 383–388.

13. Langguth B, Landgrebe M, Kleinjung T, Sand GP, Hajak G (2011) Tinnitus and depression.World J Biol Psychiatry. Early Online. pp 1–12.

14. Zöger S, Svedlund J, Holgers KM (2006) Relationship between tinnitus severity and psychiatric disorders. Psychosomatics 47: 282–288.

15. Ooms E, Meganck R, Vanheule S, Vinck B, Watelet JB, et al. (2011) Tinnitus Severity and the Relation to Depressive Symptoms: A Critical Study. Otolaryngol Head Neck Surg 145: 276–281.

16. Delb W, D'Amelio R, Boisten CJ, Plinkert PK (2002) Evaluation of the tinnitus retraining therapy as combined with a cognitive behavioral group therapy. HNO 50: 997–1004.

17. Martinez-Devesa P, Perera R, Theodoulou M, Waddell A (2010) Cognitive behavioural therapy for tinnitus. Cochrane Database Syst Rev 9: CD005233.

18. McKenna L (1998) Psychological treatments for tinnitus. In Vernon JA, ed. Tinnitus treatment and relief. Needham Heights, MA: Allyn & Bacon. pp 140–155.

19. Hiller W, Goebel G (2007) When tinnitus loudness and annoyance are discrepant: audiological characteristics and psychological profile. Audiol Neurootol 12: 391–400.

20. Frank E, Schecklmann M, Landgrebe M, Burger J, Kreuzer P, et al. (2012) Treatment of chronic tinnitus with repeated sessions of prefrontal transcranial direct current stimulation: outcomes from an open-label pilot study. J Neurol 259: 327–33.

21. Stouffer JL, Tyler RS (1990) Characterization of tinnitus by tinnitus patients. J Speech Hear Disord 55(3): 439–453.

22. Meikle MB, Stewart BJ, Griest SE, Henry JA (2008) Tinnitus outcomes assessment. Trends Amplif 12: 223–235.

23. Henry JA, Meikle MB (2000) Psychoacoustic measures of tinnitus. J Am Acad Audiol 1: 138–155.

24. Hallam RS, Jakes SC, Hinchcliffe R (1998) Cognitive variables in tinnitus annoyance. British J Clin Psychol 27: 213–222.

25. Hiller W, Haerkötter C (2005) Does sound stimulation have additive effects on cognitive-behavioral treatment of chronic tinnitus? Behav Res Ther 43: 595–612.

26. Hiller W, Goebel G (2006) Factors influencing tinnitus loudness and annoyance. Arch Otolaryngol Head Neck Surg 132: 1323–1330.

27. Kroenke K, Spitzer RL, Williams JB, Löwe B (2010) The Patient Health Questionnaire Somatic, Anxiety, and Depressive Symptom Scales: a systematic review. Gen Hosp Psychiatry 32: 345–359.

28. Löwe B, Spitzer RL, Williams JBW, Mussell DSWM, Schellberg D, et al. (2008) Depression, anxiety and somatisation in primary care: syndrome overlap and functional impairment. Gen Hosp Psychiatry 30: 191–199.

29. Kroenke K, Spitzer RL, Williams JBW (2002) The PHQ-15: validity of a new measure for evaluating the severity of somatic symptoms. Psychosom Med 64: 258–266.

30. Axelsson A, Ringdahl A (1989) Tinnitus - a study of its prevalence and characteristics. Br J Audiol 23: 53–62.

31. Stouffer JL, Tyler RS (1990) Subjective tinnitus loudness. Hear Instr 41: 17–19.

32. Wiltink J, Beutel ME, Till Y, Ojeda FM, Wild PS, et al. (2011) Prevalence of distress, comorbid conditions and well being in the general population. J Affect Disord 130: 429–437.

33. Langenbach M, Olderog M, Michel O, Albus C, Köhle K (2005) Psychosocial and personality predictors of tinnitus-related distress. Gen Hosp Psychiatry 27: 73–77.

34. Holgers KM, Zöger S, Svedlund K (2005) Predictive factors for development of severe tinnitus suffering – further characterisation. Int J Audiol 44: 584–592.

35. Newman CW, Wharton JA, Jacobson GP (1997) Self-focused and somatic attention in patients with tinnitus. J Am Acad Audiol 8: 143–149.

36. Hiller W, Janca A, Burke KC (1997) Association between tinnitus and somatoform disorders. J Psychosom Res 43: 613–624.

37. D'Amelio R, Archonti C, Scholz S, Falkai P, Plinkert PK, et al. (2004) Psychological distress associated with acute tinnitus. HNO 52: 599–603.

38. Schlee W, Kleinjung T, Hiller W, Goebel G, Kolassa IT, et al. (2011) Does tinnitus distress depend on age of onset? PLoS One 2011;6(11): e27379.

39. Savastano M (2008) Tinnitus with or without hearing loss: are its characteristics different? Eur Arch Otorhinolaryngol 265: 1295–1300.

40. Mazurek B, Olze H, Haupt H, Szczepek AJ (2010) The more the worse: the grade of noise-induced hearing loss associates with the severity of tinnitus. Int J Environ Res Public Health 7: 3071–3079.

41. Wedel vH, Strahlmann U, Zorowka P (1989) Effectiveness of various non-medicinal therapeutic measures in tinnitus. A long-term study. Laryngorhinootologie 68: 259–266.

4

Temporomandibular Joint Disorder Complaints in Tinnitus: Further Hints for a Putative Tinnitus Subtype

Veronika Vielsmeier[1]*, **Jürgen Strutz**[1], **Tobias Kleinjung**[2], **Martin Schecklmann**[3], **Peter Michael Kreuzer**[3], **Michael Landgrebe**[3], **Berthold Langguth**[3]

1 Department of Otorhinolaryngology, University of Regensburg, Regensburg, Germany, 2 Department of Otorhinolaryngology, University of Zurich, Zurich, Switzerland, 3 Department of Psychiatry and Psychotherapy, University of Regensburg, Regensburg, Germany

Abstract

Objective: Tinnitus is considered to be highly heterogeneous with respect to its etiology, its comorbidities and the response to specific interventions. Subtyping is recommended, but it remains to be determined which criteria are useful, since it has not yet been clearly demonstrated whether and to which extent etiologic factors, comorbid states and interventional response are related to each other and are thus applicable for subtyping tinnitus. Analyzing the Tinnitus Research Initiative Database we differentiated patients according to presence or absence of comorbid temporomandibular joint (TMJ) disorder complaints and compared the two groups with respect to etiologic factors.

Methods: 1204 Tinnitus patients from the Tinnitus Research Initiative (TRI) Database with and without subjective TMJ complaints were compared with respect to demographic, tinnitus and audiological characteristics, questionnaires, and numeric ratings. Data were analysed according to a predefined statistical analysis plan.

Results: Tinnitus patients with TMJ complaints (22% of the whole group) were significantly younger, had a lower age at tinnitus onset, and were more frequently female. They could modulate or mask their tinnitus more frequently by somatic maneuvers and by music or sound stimulation. Groups did not significantly differ for tinnitus duration, type of onset (gradual/abrupt), onset related events (whiplash etc.), character (pulsatile or not), hyperacusis, hearing impairment, tinnitus distress, depression, quality of life and subjective ratings (loudness etc.).

Conclusion: Replicating previous work in tinnitus patients with TMJ complaints, classical risk factors for tinnitus like older age and male gender are less relevant in tinnitus patients with TMJ complaints. By demonstrating group differences for modulation of tinnitus by movements and sounds our data further support the notion that tinnitus with TMJ complaints represents a subgroup of tinnitus with clinical features that are highly relevant for specific therapeutic management.

Editor: Ulrich Thiem, Marienhospital Herne - University of Bochum, Germany

Funding: The study was funded by the Tinnitus Research Initiative. The funders had no role in study design, data collection and analysis, decision to publish, or preparation of the manuscript.

Competing Interests: The authors have declared that no competing interests exist.

* E-mail: veronika.vielsmeier@klinik.uni-regensburg.de

Introduction

Tinnitus is the perception of sound in the absence of any external sound source and it is considered to be a very heterogeneous condition [1]. A large variety of different etiologic factors can cause tinnitus. On a phenotypic level, tinnitus can be perceived unilaterally, bilaterally or centrally in the head, the perceived sound can be tone-like or noise-like and tinnitus can be accompanied by many comorbidities such as hyperacusis, insomnia, anxiety or depression [2,3,4]. In face of such heterogeneity, subtyping of different forms of tinnitus has been proposed as a strategy to facilitate both diagnosis and therapy of tinnitus [5]. In order to be clinically useful the different subtypes should be pathophysiologically different, easily distinguishable and predictive for the outcome of specific interventions. The condition of tinnitus consisting of a "typewriter" like sound may serve as a rare but useful example for a subtype which is caused by vascular-nerve conflict and which has been shown to be responsive to

carbamazepine treatment [6]. Successful classification criteria would improve both research and clinical management. Thus there is an important need to identify clinical criteria for useful subtyping of tinnitus patients.

Here we investigated whether comorbid temporomandibular joint complaints may constitute such a discriminating criterion. Since the first description by Costen in 1934 [7] the association of tinnitus with temporomandibular joint (TMJ) dysfunction has been confirmed in many studies [8,9,10,11]. In a recent pilot study we found that tinnitus patients with TMJ problems tend to be younger, more frequently female and to have better hearing function in contrast to those with tinnitus but without TMJ symptoms [12].

Moreover, in many cases tinnitus can be modulated by jaw movements [13,14]. Actually, an improvement of tinnitus symptoms mediated by a specific therapy of TMJ disorders has been reported [8,15].

Table 1. Assessment instruments.

Assessed characteristics	Assessment instrument
clinical and demographic characteristics	Tinnitus Sample Case History Questionnaire (TSCHQ) (Langguth et al. 2007)
tinnitus handicap	Tinnitus Handicap Inventory (THI) (Newman et al)
tinnitus severity	Tinnitus Questionnaire (TQ) (Goebel and Hiller)
depressive symptoms	Beck Depression Inventory (BDI) (Beck et al. 1961)
quality of life	World Health Organisation Quality of Life Scale (WHOQoL)
tinnitus loudness	Numeric Rating Scale (0–10): Loudness
tinnitus discomfort	Numeric Rating Scale (0–10): Discomfort
Tinnitus annoyance	Numeric Rating Scale (0–10): Annoyance
Tinnitus ignorability	Numeric Rating Scale (0–10): Ignorability
Tinnitus unpleasentness	Numeric Rating Scale (0–10): Unpleasentness

Neuronal pathways, by which the trigeminal afferents can interact with the central auditory system, have been identified in animal studies [16–17]. Trigeminal input propagates via the trigeminal ganglia and the trigeminal nucleus to the dorsal cochlear nucleus [18,19] and can influence activity in central auditory pathways [20], especially in case of cochlear damage [21]. Moreover an interaction of somatosensory stimulation with tinnitus loudness has been reported in people with tinnitus [22] and has been interpreted as a hint for the activation of the non-modality specific extralemniscal pathways in tinnitus [23,24]. Based on (i) the observation that tinnitus is frequently related with TMJ disorders or neck problems, (ii) the finding that many patients can manipulate their tinnitus by jaw, neck or head movements and (iii) the identification of neuronal pathways mediating somatosensory input to the dorsal cochlear nucleus, the concept of "somatosensoric tinnitus" has been proposed [25]. Since then "somatosensoric tinnitus" has been considered as a potentially useful subtype of tinnitus [26,27,28,29,30] even if data about an association between the comorbidity "TMJ disorder" and the ability to manipulate the tinnitus by jaw or head movements are scarce [14].

Here, we used the Tinnitus Research Initative Database [31] to compare tinnitus patients with and without self-reported TMJ complaints with respect to their clinical characteristics. Special emphasis was set on differences in the ability to modulate the tinnitus by somatosensoric maneuvers in order to test the association between TMJ comorbidity and somatic modulation claimed by the concept of somatosensoric tinnitus.

Materials and Methods

The data analysis was based on data of the Tinnitus Research Initiative Database. Data management was conducted according to the Data Handling Plan (TRI-DHP V07, May 9th, 2011). Data analysis was conducted according to the Standard Operating Procedure (TRI-SA V01, May 9th, 2011), thereby following a study-specific Statistical Analysis Plan (SAP-004, June 27th, 2011) that was written according to the SAP template (TRI-SAP, May 12th, 2011). Statistical details can be found below. All documents are to be found under http://database.tinnitusresearch.org/. 1204 patients from the Tinnitus Research Initiative (TRI) Database were investigated. Patients presented

between 2005 and 2011 at different tinnitus centers worldwide (Regensburg, Aachen, Germany; Antwerp, Belgium; Volta Redonda, Belo Horizonte, and Porto Alegre, Brazil; Buenos Aires, Argentina). Patients completed the self-measurement questionnaires (see table 1) before their first presentation at the clinic. The diagnosis of tinnitus was confirmed by clinical specialists (medical doctors and/or audiologists with experience in the diagnosis and management of tinnitus). Patients with complete information with respect to the question "Do you suffer from temporomandibular disorder?" (answer: yes or no) in the Tinnitus sample case history questionnaire of the TRI case report form were included. Patients gave written informed consent to record their data in the database and to perform analyses with the data. The project has been approved by the local ethics committee (Ethikkommission der Fakultät für Medizin der Universität Regensburg). There was no overlap with an earlier study [12] as data of this former sample were not included in the data analysis.

Assessment was performed before the first consultation in the tinnitus clinics and included the Tinnitus Sample Case History Questionnaire (TSCHQ), the Tinnitus Handicap Inventory, the Tinnitus Questionnaire, the Beck Depression Inventory, the World Health Organisation Quality of Life Scale (WHOQoL), and several tinnitus numeric rating scales (loudness, discomfort, annoyance, ignorability and unpleasantness) (see table 1).

Among these variables, we were interested in demographic characteristics like age, gender and age at tinnitus onset. Furthermore, we investigated the possible masking of the tinnitus by music or sounds and the ability of modulating the tinnitus by somatic maneuvers. In addition, we analyzed tinnitus duration, pulsatile character, onset related events, the self-reported suffering from hyperacusis, and the mean hearing level (dB HL over all measured frequencies (0.125–8 kHz) of both ears).

If no data were available at the screening visit (first consultation), we used data from the baseline visit of a clinical intervention. If both screening and baseline data were available we used the mean of both time points. For continuous variables (e.g., age) we contrasted both groups (with and without TMJ complaints) with Student t-tests. For categorical variables (e.g., gender), we used χ^2-tests of independence to investigate differences in the proportion of these variables in both groups. We calculated 23 contrasts; to avoid false positive results we declare only contrasts with a Bonferroni corrected significance threshold of 0.0022 as significant ($p = 5\% / 23 = 0.0022$).

Results

261 patients complained about problems of the TMJ (22%), whereas 943 (78%) reported that they have no symptoms of the temporomandibular joint. Tinnitus patients with TMJ disorders complaints were more frequently female (with TMJ disorder: 54%; without: 33%), significantly younger and had an earlier tinnitus onset compared to those without TMJ disorder. Moreover patients with tinnitus and temporomandibular joint disorder were more frequently able to mask their tinnitus by sounds or music (with TMJ disorder: 85%; without: 74%) and they could more frequently modulate their tinnitus by somatic maneuvers (with TMJ disorder: 48%; without: 30%).

Other tinnitus related aspects such as tinnitus duration, character of onset, pulsatile character, onset related events, hyperacusis, and hearing function did not show any significant differences between the two groups. In addition, scores of the THI, BDI and quality of life scales as well as numeric ratings with respect to tinnitus did not show group differences.

An overview of the results can be found in table 2. Figure 1 depicts results for gender, maskability of tinnitus with acoustic stimuli, and ability to modulate tinnitus by somatic maneuvers. Figure 1 depicts the relative frequencies of significant categorical variables as can be seen in table 2.

Discussion

In order to further substantiate the findings of a pilot study [12] we analyzed a large sample (1204 patients) from the TRI database to investigate the clinical characteristics of tinnitus patients with TMJ complaints in comparison to tinnitus patients without any TMJ complaints. In contrast to the former pilot study, in which the TMJ disorder was diagnosed by a specialized dentist, here information about TMJ complaints was obtained from patients' self-report in the Tinnitus Case History Questionnaire [32]. We abstained from further differentiating the underlying pathology of the TMJ complaints, since the putative neurobiological mechanism for the interaction between TMJ complaints and tinnitus is abnormal trigeminal input to the dorsal cochlear nucleus [20,21].

About one out of five tinnitus patients affirmed TMJ problems. Patients with comorbid TMJ complaints were more frequently female and of a younger age and had also experienced an earlier onset of tinnitus. All these findings are exactly in line with the results from the pilot study [12], suggesting that self-reported TMJ complaints are considered to be a reliable piece of information that proves diagnostic value in the assessment of tinnitus. However, we could not confirm a difference in hearing function between tinnitus patients with and without TMJ complaints. In the pilot study the difference in hearing function was driven primarily by patients with TMJ complaints as the primary complaint and such patients were not included in this study. Only patients presenting in a tinnitus clinic with the primary complaint of tinnitus were included in this study. Thus these findings further underscore that the sample recruitment strategy is of high relevance in the investigation of comorbidities of tinnitus [33].

In addition, we found that tinnitus patients with TMJ complaints can modulate their tinnitus by somatic maneuvers or by music and sound more frequently than tinnitus patients without TMJ problems. A possible association between TMJ complaints and somatic modulation has been postulated before [25], but to our knowledge our data are the first that empirically confirm this association. One earlier study with a substantial smaller sample size did not find such an association [14]. Since our study involved almost ten times more patients, this discrepancy may be related to study power. Whereas an association between TMJ comorbidity

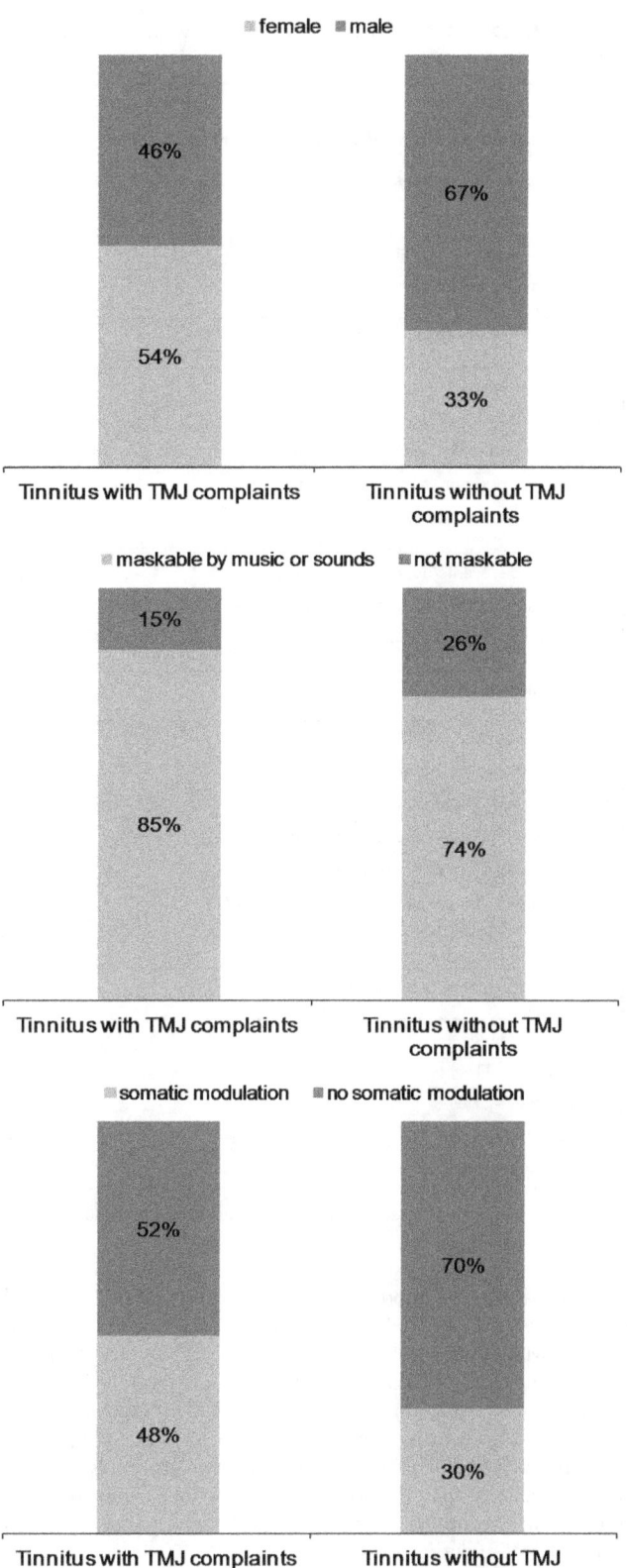

Figure 1. Relative proportion of gender, tinnitus maskability, and somatic modulation of tinnitus in dependence from complaints about temporomandibular joint disorder (categorical variables with significant contrasts between groups) (see separate documents).

Table 2. Comparison of tinnitus patients with and without complaints about temporomandibular joint disorder (see separate documents).

Temporomandibular joint disorder complaints (n=1204)	Yes (n=261, 22%)	No (n=943, 78%)	Statistics
demographic characteristics			
age (years) (n=1181)	50.7±13.9	53.6±13.1	T=3.141; df=1179; p=0.002*
age at tinnitus onset (years) (n=1088)	41.5±14.5	45.2±14.4	T=3.570; df=1086; p<0.001*
gender (female/male) (n=1204)	140/121	311/632	χ^2=37.245; df=1; p<0.001*
tinnitus and audiologic characteristics			
duration (n=1089)	8.9±9.5	8.2±9.5	T=0.947; df=1087; p=0.344
onset (gradual/abrupt) (n=1139)	114/136	442/447	χ^2=1.325; df=1; p=0.250
pulsatile (no/yes with heartbeat/yes other than heartbeat) (n=1180)	196/34/27	758/90/75	χ^2=4.486; df=2; p=0.106
maskable by music or sounds (no/yes) (n=1027)	33/190	213/591	χ^2=13.107; df=1; p<0.001*
somatic modulation (no/yes) (n=1183)	134/123	648/278	χ^2=28.568; df=1; p<0.001*
onset related event (sound/whiplash/hearingloss/stress/headtrauma/others/multiple events/no event) (n=1204)	17/11/25/61/5/62/44/36	54/12/95/219/6/253/154/150	χ^2=14.556; df=7; p=0.042
hyperacousis (never/rarely/some-times/usually/always) (n=1181)	27/28/97/46/59	113/138/361/147/165	χ^2=6.175; df=4; p=0.186
mean hearing level (dB HL over all frequencies of both ears) (n=849)	22.7±15.8	23.6±14.1	T=0.767; df=847; p=0.443
questionnaires			
tinnitus questionnaire (n=981)	41.7±18.1	40.7±17.8	T=0.709; df=979; p=0.479
tinnitus handicap inventory (n=1160)	50.4±22.2	47.2±23.3	T=1.927; df=1158; p=0.054
Beck depression inventory (n=1117)	12.3±8.8	10.6±8.3	T=2.722; df=1115; p=0.007
WHO quality of life questionnaire domain 1 (n=729)	13.9±3.2	14.5±2.9	T=2.359; df=727; p=0.019
WHO quality of life questionnaire domain 2 (n=730)	13.7±2.8	14.1±2.7	T=1.595; df=728; p=0.111
WHO quality of life questionnaire domain 3 (n=728)	14.2±3.5	14.5±3.1	T=1.235; df=726; p=0.217
WHO quality of life questionnaire domain 4 (n=730)	15.4±2.7	15.9±2.3	T=1.986; df=728; p=0.047
numeric rating scales (scale: 1–10)			
loudness (n=1138)	6.3±2.4	6.4±2.2	T=0.682; df=1136; p=0.495
discomfort (n=1136)	7.0±2.3	7.0±2.4	T=0.076; df=1134; p=0.939
annoyance (n=1139)	6.6±2.5	6.7±2.4	T=0.806; df=1137; p=0.420
ignorability (n=1137)	6.6±2.8	6.8±2.7	T=1.289; df=1135; p=0.198
unpleasantness (n=1140)	6.5±2.6	6.7±2.4	T=1.110; df=1138; p=0.267

*p<0.0022 (Bonferroni corrected significance threshold: 5% divided by 23 single contrasts).

and the ability to modulate tinnitus by jaw, head or neck movements was expected, the significant difference in the rate of patients who could mask their tinnitus by environmental sounds, was an unexpected finding. Notably, this observation of higher masking rates in the tinnitus group with TMJ complaints is not confounded by hearing function, since there was no significant difference in audiometric data between the two groups. Rather this finding suggests that abnormal trigeminal input influences the interaction of tinnitus related neuronal abnormalities and the processing of auditory stimuli.

We are aware of the limitations of our study. First audiometric data were not available for the whole sample but only for 849 patients (66%). Moreover the criterion of TMJ complaints was based on self-report and we have no information about the exact underlying pathology and the laterality of the TMJ complaints. Thus further studies are needed to confirm our findings, to explore the relevance of the underlying TMJ pathology and to address the relation between TMJ laterality and tinnitus laterality.

Trigeminal somatosensoric input and auditory input converge at the dorsal cochlear nucleus (DCN) [34,35]. This convergence at the DCN is generally considered to represent the neuronal correlate for the clinically observed interactions between the somatosensory system and tinnitus [16,26]. Thus, one could speculate that abnormal auditory and trigeminal input to the DCN in patients with TMJ complaints leads to plastic changes of multisensoric processing in the DCN [25,36,37] which may provide an explanation for the observed higher rates of tinnitus modulation by both auditory and somatic modulation in this tinnitus subgroup. Support for this theory derives from recent animal experiments, which demonstrated plastic changes in the auditory-somatosensory integration in the DCN in noise-exposed animals, especially those that developed tinnitus [20]. Functional neuroimaging studies in tinnitus patients confirmed this interaction by demonstrating an enhanced response to jaw protrusion in cochlear nucleus and inferior colliculus in tinnitus patients as compared to controls [38].

The activation of the extralemniscal pathways has been proposed as an alternative explanation for the interaction between the somatosensory and the auditory system in tinnitus patients [23,24]. This theory is based on the observation that electrical stimulation of the median nerve can modulate tinnitus loudness [39]. Finally TMJ disorders may influence tinnitus by modifying perceived hearing level at the middle ear. This theory could be further explored by investigating the relationship between the exact TMJ pathology and tinnitus.

The findings of this study are considered highly relevant in the quest for relevant clinical criteria for tinnitus subtyping, since it is clearly demonstrated that comorbid TMJ complaints exert an impact on the ability to modulate tinnitus by somatic maneuvers and sound. This difference in symptom modulation is likely to be relevant for the success of specific therapeutic interventions that involve auditory stimulation [40] or somatosensoric interventions [41]. Thus, based on our findings we propose TMJ complaints as a criterion for tinnitus subtyping and invite further studies to investigate its relevance in clinical practice.

In summary, our findings of reduced relevance of the risk factors "older age" and "male gender" together with higher rates of modulation by somatic or auditory stimuli in tinnitus patients with comorbid TMJ complaints suggest, that "comorbid TMJ complaints" represents a valuable criterion for defining a subgroup of tinnitus that exhibits clinical features that could be highly relevant, in future clinical research, for the evaluation of specific therapeutic interventions.

Acknowledgments

We want to thank Andreia Aazevedo, Ricardo Figueiredo, Claudia Coelho, Marcello Rates and Carolina Binetti for contributing data to the database. We also want to thank Susanne Staudinger, Konstantin Martin and Sandra Pfluegl for assistance with data management.

Author Contributions

Conceived and designed the experiments: VV JS MS BL. Performed the experiments: VV MS PMK BL. Analyzed the data: VV MS ML. Contributed reagents/materials/analysis tools: VV MS. Wrote the paper: VV TK PMK BL.

References

1. Langguth B, Kleinjung T, Landgrebe M (2011) Tinnitus: The Complexity of Standardization. Eval Health Prof.
2. Langguth B, Kleinjung T, Landgrebe M (2011) Severe tinnitus and depressive symptoms: a complex interaction. Otolaryngol Head Neck Surg 145: 519; author reply 520.
3. Langguth B, Landgrebe M, Kleinjung T, Sand GP, Hajak G (2011) Tinnitus and depression. World J Biol Psychiatry.
4. Chandra RK, Epstein VA, Fishman AJ (2009) Prevalence of depression and antidepressant use in an otolaryngology patient population. Otolaryngol Head Neck Surg 141: 136–138.
5. Tyler R, Coelho C, Tao P, Ji H, Noble W, et al. (2008) Identifying tinnitus subgroups with cluster analysis. Am J Audiol 17: S176–184.
6. Nam EC, Handzel O, Levine RA (2010) Carbamazepine responsive typewriter tinnitus from basilar invagination. J Neurol Neurosurg Psychiatry 81: 456–458.
7. Costen JB (1997) A syndrome of ear and sinus symptoms dependent upon disturbed function of the temporomandibular joint. 1934. Ann Otol Rhinol Laryngol 106: 805–819.
8. Wright EF, Bifano SL (1997) Tinnitus improvement through TMD therapy. J Am Dent Assoc 128: 1424–1432.
9. Dolowitz DA, Ward JW, Fingerle CO, Smith CC (1964) The Role of Muscular Incoordination in the Pathogenesis of the Temporomandibular Joint Syndrome. Laryngoscope 74: 790–801.
10. Chole RA, Parker WS (1992) Tinnitus and vertigo in patients with temporomandibular disorder. Arch Otolaryngol Head Neck Surg 118: 817–821.
11. Bernhardt O, Mundt T, Welk A, Koppl N, Kocher T, et al. (2011) Signs and symptoms of temporomandibular disorders and the incidence of tinnitus. J Oral Rehabil.
12. Vielsmeier V, Kleinjung T, Strutz J, Burgers R, Kreuzer PM, et al. (2011) Tinnitus with Temporomandibular Joint Disorders: A Specific Entity of Tinnitus Patients? Otolaryngol Head Neck Surg.
13. Pinchoff RJ, Burkard RF, Salvi RJ, Coad ML, Lockwood AH (1998) Modulation of tinnitus by voluntary jaw movements. Am J Otol 19: 785–789.
14. Sanchez TG, Guerra GC, Lorenzi MC, Brandao AL, Bento RF (2002) The influence of voluntary muscle contractions upon the onset and modulation of tinnitus. Audiol Neurootol 7: 370–375.
15. Wright EF (2007) Otologic symptom improvement through TMD therapy. Quintessence Int 38: e564–571.
16. Roberts LE, Eggermont JJ, Caspary DM, Shore SE, Melcher JR, et al. (2010) Ringing ears: the neuroscience of tinnitus. J Neurosci 30: 14972–14979.
17. Dehmel S, Cui YL, Shore SE (2008) Cross-modal interactions of auditory and somatic inputs in the brainstem and midbrain and their imbalance in tinnitus and deafness. Am J Audiol 17: S193–209.
18. Shore S, Zhou J, Koehler S (2007) Neural mechanisms underlying somatic tinnitus. Prog Brain Res 166: 107–123.
19. Zhou J, Shore S (2004) Projections from the trigeminal nuclear complex to the cochlear nuclei: a retrograde and anterograde tracing study in the guinea pig. J Neurosci Res 78: 901–907.
20. Dehmel S, Pradhan S, Koehler S, Bledsoe S, Shore S (2012) Noise overexposure alters long-term somatosensory-auditory processing in the dorsal cochlear nucleus–possible basis for tinnitus-related hyperactivity? J Neurosci 32: 1660–1671.
21. Shore SE (2011) Plasticity of somatosensory inputs to the cochlear nucleus–implications for tinnitus. Hear Res 281: 38–46.
22. Moller AR, Moller MB, Yokota M (1992) Some forms of tinnitus may involve the extralemniscal auditory pathway. Laryngoscope 102: 1165–1171.
23. Moller AR (2003) Pathophysiology of tinnitus. Otolaryngol Clin North Am 36: 249–266, v–vi.
24. Moller AR (2007) The role of neural plasticity in tinnitus. Prog Brain Res 166: 37–45.
25. Levine RA (1999) Somatic (craniocervical) tinnitus and the dorsal cochlear nucleus hypothesis. Am J Otolaryngol 20: 351–362.
26. Levine RA, Nam EC, Oron Y, Melcher JR (2007) Evidence for a tinnitus subgroup responsive to somatosensory based treatment modalities. Prog Brain Res 166: 195–207.
27. Latifpour DH, Grenner J, Sjodahl C (2009) The effect of a new treatment based on somatosensory stimulation in a group of patients with somatically related tinnitus. Int Tinnitus J 15: 94–99.
28. Biesinger E, Reisshauer A, Mazurek B (2008) [The role of the cervical spine and the craniomandibular system in the pathogenesis of tinnitus. Somatosensory tinnitus]. HNO 56: 673–677.
29. Vanneste S, Plazier M, der Loo E, de Heyning PV, Congedo M, et al. (2010) The neural correlates of tinnitus-related distress. Neuroimage 52: 470–480.
30. Kapoula Z, Yang Q, Le TT, Vernet M, Berbey N, et al. (2011) Medio-lateral postural instability in subjects with tinnitus. Front Neurol 2: 35.
31. Landgrebe M, Zeman F, Koller M, Eberl Y, Mohr M, et al. (2010) The Tinnitus Research Initiative (TRI) database: a new approach for delineation of tinnitus subtypes and generation of predictors for treatment outcome. BMC Med Inform Decis Mak 10: 42.
32. Langguth B, Goodey R, Azevedo A, Bjorne A, Cacace A, et al. (2007) Consensus for tinnitus patient assessment and treatment outcome measurement: Tinnitus Research Initiative meeting, Regensburg, July 2006. Prog Brain Res 166: 525–536.
33. Langguth B, Landgrebe M, Kleinjung T, Sand GP, Hajak G (2011) Tinnitus and depression. World J Biol Psychiatry 12: 489–500.
34. Shore SE (2011) Plasticity of somatosensory inputs to the cochlear nucleus - Implications for tinnitus. Hear Res.
35. Kaltenbach JA (2007) The dorsal cochlear nucleus as a contributor to tinnitus: mechanisms underlying the induction of hyperactivity. Prog Brain Res 166: 89–106.
36. Kaltenbach JA (2006) Summary of evidence pointing to a role of the dorsal cochlear nucleus in the etiology of tinnitus. Acta Otolaryngol Suppl: 20–26.
37. Tzounopoulos T (2008) Mechanisms of synaptic plasticity in the dorsal cochlear nucleus: plasticity-induced changes that could underlie tinnitus. Am J Audiol 17: S170–175.
38. Lanting CP, de Kleine E, Eppinga RN, van Dijk P (2010) Neural correlates of human somatosensory integration in tinnitus. Hear Res 267: 78–88.
39. Moller AR, Moller MB, Jannetta PJ, Jho HD (1992) Compound action potentials recorded from the exposed eighth nerve in patients with intractable tinnitus. Laryngoscope 102: 187–197.
40. Vernon JA, Meikle MB (2003) Masking devices and alprazolam treatment for tinnitus. Otolaryngol Clin North Am 36: 307–320, vii.
41. Biesinger E, Kipman U, Schatz S, Langguth B (2010) Qigong for the treatment of tinnitus: a prospective randomized controlled study. J Psychosom Res 69: 299–304.

5

Predisposition for and Prevention of Subjective Tinnitus Development

Sönke Ahlf[9], Konstantin Tziridis*[9], Sabine Korn, Ilona Strohmeyer, Holger Schulze

Experimental Otolaryngology, University of Erlangen-Nuremberg, Erlangen, Germany

Abstract

Dysfunction of the inner ear as caused by presbyacusis, injuries or noise traumata may result in subjective tinnitus, but not everyone suffering from one of these diseases develops a tinnitus percept and vice versa. The reasons for these individual differences are still unclear and may explain why different treatments of the disease are beneficial for some patients but not for others. Here we for the first time compare behavioral and neurophysiological data from hearing impaired Mongolian gerbils with (T) and without (NT) a tinnitus percept that may elucidate why some specimen do develop subjective tinnitus after noise trauma while others do not. Although noise trauma induced a similar permanent hearing loss in all animals, tinnitus did develop only in about three quarters of these animals. NT animals showed higher overall cortical and auditory brainstem activity *before* noise trauma compared to T animals; that is, animals with low overall neuronal activity in the auditory system seem to be prone to develop tinnitus after noise trauma. Furthermore, T animals showed increased activity of cortical neurons representing the tinnitus frequencies *after* acoustic trauma, whereas NT animals exhibited an activity decrease at moderate sound intensities by that time. Spontaneous activity was generally increased in T but decreased in NT animals. Plastic changes of tonotopic organization were transient, only seen in T animals and vanished by the time the tinnitus percept became chronic. We propose a model for tinnitus prevention that points to a global inhibitory mechanism in auditory cortex that may prevent tinnitus genesis in animals with high overall activity in the auditory system, whereas this mechanism seems not potent enough for tinnitus prevention in animals with low overall activity.

Editor: Iris Schrijver, Stanford University School of Medicine, United States of America

Funding: This work was supported by the Interdisciplinary Center for Clinical Research (IZKF, project E7) at the University Hospital Erlangen. The funders had no role in study design, data collection and analysis, decision to publish, or preparation of the manuscript.

Competing Interests: The authors have declared that no competing interests exist.

* E-mail: konstantin.tziridis@uk-erlangen.de

[9] These authors contributed equally to this work.

Introduction

Diseases of the inner ear leading to hearing loss (HL) may result in subjective tinnitus [1]. Enigmatically, not everyone suffering from HL develops a tinnitus percept and conversely not in everyone who suffers from tinnitus a permanent hearing impairment can be detected [2]. The reasons for these individual differences are still unclear and may explain why different treatments of the disease are beneficial for some patients but not for others [3].

The development of a tinnitus percept is often related to neuronal plasticity on multiple levels of the central auditory system including the auditory cortex ([4,5,6,7] for review see [8]). Current models of tinnitus genesis usually consider damage of cochlear hair cells that induce an imbalance in lateral inhibition on subsequent neuronal levels as causal for such central plasticity [9], but even if the inducing event is identical not every animal or human subsequently suffers from tinnitus. In this report we follow the hypothesis that there must be some predisposition in the central auditory system of some but not all individuals that protects them from the development of subjective tinnitus. In search of this predisposition we recorded neuronal activity from the auditory brainstem and cortex of the same individuals of Mongolian gerbils before and after an acoustic trauma and compared the data obtained from animals that showed an acute tinnitus percept in

behavioral testing (group T) with data from those that did not (group NT). Possible differences in these two groups of animals may further elucidate the neuronal mechanisms that lead to subjective tinnitus and thereby may help to find a prophylaxis against tinnitus development and improve actual treatments for tinnitus patients (e.g. [10]).

Materials and Methods

Ethics Statement

For the welfare of the animals the researchers were responsible. The gerbils were housed in a standard animal rack (Bio A.S. Vent Light, Ehret Labor- und Pharmatechnik, Emmendingen, Germany) in groups of 2 to 3 animals per cage with free access to water and food at 20 to 24°C room temperature. The use and care of animals was approved by the state of Bavaria (Regierungspräsidium Mittelfranken, Ansbach, Germany).

Behavioral Measurements

A total of thirty five 8 to 10 weeks old male Mongolian gerbils (*Meriones unguiculatus*) purchased by Charles River (Charles River GmbH, Sulzfeld, Germany) were used in this study. Animals were handled before the beginning of the experiments and accustomed to the setup environment to minimize stress. Behavioral testing of animals was performed in an IAC (Industrial Acoustics Company GmbH, Niederkrüchten, Germany) acoustic chamber on a TMC (Technical Manufacturing Corporation, Peabody, MA, USA) low-vibration table. The behavioral setup consisted of a 15 cm long transparent acrylic tube (inner diameter 4.0 to 4.3 cm, depending on the body size of the animal) placed 10 cm in front of a speaker (Canton Plus X Series 2; Canton, Weilrod, Germany) onto a Honeywell FSG15N1A piezo sensor (Honeywell AG, Offenbach, Germany). The tube's front end was closed with a stainless steel grate (wire mesh width 0.5 mm) allowing acoustic stimulation with no detectable distortion (signal to noise ratio at least 70 dB, checked via HP spectrum analyzer: 3563A Control Systems Analyzer; Hewlett-Packard GmbH, Böblingen, Germany). Sound pressure level was controlled via a B&K Type 2610 measuring amplifier fed with a B&K Type 2669 preamplifier/B&K Type 4190 condensor microphone combination (Brüel & Kjaer GmbH, Bremen, Germany). Stimulus generation and data acquisition was controlled using custom-made Matlab 2008 programs (Math-Works, Natick, MA, USA; stimulation/recording sampling rate 20 kHz). For sound generation the frequency response function of the speaker was calibrated to produce an output spectrum that was flat within +/−1 dB.

Animals were placed in the tube, in which it fits well and is able to move back and forth roughly 2 cm. We allowed 15 min habituation time before 3 different types of prepulse inhibition (PPI) modulated auditory startle response (ASR) paradigms (Figure 1) were performed, usually in a single 4 h block before and 5 to 11 days (median 7 days) after the acoustic trauma. Between different stimulus sets a break of 5 minutes was used to prevent behavioral adaptation. Interstimulus intervals were varied randomly (mean 10±2.5 sec SD) and each stimulus was repeated 15 times. Stimulation paradigms were: first, an hearing threshold estimation paradigm to obtain behavioral audiograms (set 1) [11] consisting of a 90 dB SPL pure tone startle stimulus (duration: 6 ms, with 2 ms cosine-squared rise and fall ramps; 0.5 to 8.0 kHz in octave steps) preceded by 100 ms by a 0 to 50 dB SPL prestimulus of the same frequency and length. Stimuli with different frequencies were presented pseudorandomized in blocks of different prestimulus intensities starting from 0 dB SPL and rising to 50 dB SPL (cf. Figure 1, upper panel). Second, two different forms of gap-noise paradigms were used to demonstrate the existence of possible tinnitus percepts and to give a rough estimate of the perceived tinnitus frequencies [12]. The first of these used a gap-noise paradigm with a white noise background of 50 dB SPL and 90 dB SPL pure tone startle stimuli of 1 to 8 kHz in octave steps with or without a 15 ms prestimulus-gap in the noise 100 ms before the stimulus (stimulus set 2, Figure 1, center panel) with the rationale of utilizing tinnitus related anxiety as frequency specific factor that induces freezing behavior (cf. [13,14,15]). Each frequency was presented separately with and without gap, starting from 1 kHz in ascending steps to 8 kHz. The last paradigm (stimulus set 3) had an identical timing and presentation regime as stimulus set 2 with the startle-stimulus being a click and the noise being bandpass filtered to mean frequencies ranging from 1 to 16 kHz in octave steps and a width of ±0.5 octave (Figure 1, lower panel) with the rationale of the tinnitus frequency masking the gap in the noise band that fits its spectrum best [12]. Both gap-noise paradigms for the detection of tinnitus percepts yielded similar results (cf. below).

Data of all PPI paradigms were checked by eye: Trials in which the animals moved within 100 ms before the startle stimulus were discarded; only responses within the first 50 ms after startle stimulus onset were used for further analysis. Response data in the threshold paradigm (stimulus set 1) were fitted with a sigmoidal

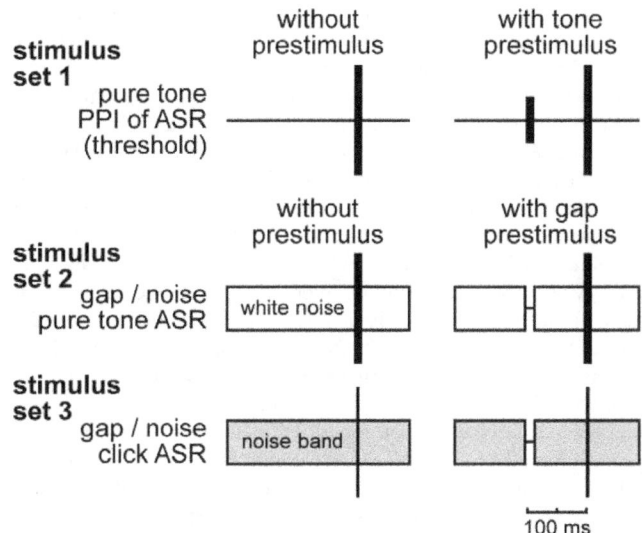

Figure 1. Behavioral paradigms using prepulse inhibition (PPI) of the acoustic startle response (ASR). Upper panel: Hearing threshold estimation paradigm in silence, with 90 dB pure tone startle stimuli ranging from 0.5 to 16 kHz in octave steps and prestimuli of the same frequency with intensities ranging from 0 to 50 dB SPL in 10 dB steps (=stimulus set 1). **Center panel:** Behavioral tinnitus test (stimulus set 2, [12]) with white noise background and pure tone startle stimuli ranging from 1 to 8 kHz (in octave steps) utilizing a silent gap of 15 ms as prestimulus. **Lower panel:** Behavioral tinnitus test (stimulus set 3, [15]) with bandpass noise (width of 1 octave) of different center frequencies (1 to 16 kHz in octave steps), a click as startle stimulus and a gap as prestimulus.

Boltzmann function; hearing thresholds were defined as the sound level at the inflection point of the function at each frequency before and after trauma (cf. [16]). The data in the two gap-noise paradigms (sets 2 and 3) were normalized to minimize variance of the response amplitudes and to avoid possible effects of the acoustic trauma on different stimulation frequencies. In other words, we tried to control for differences in the startle amplitudes resulting from the hearing loss at the trauma frequency. This normalization also guarantees that the reduced ASR response after acoustic trauma is not due to hearing loss rather than a tinnitus percept. The normalization was performed by dividing the actual amplitude by the median amplitude of the startle stimulus alone (set 1 pure tone startle stimulus without prestimulus). This was done for pre and post trauma conditions and all frequencies separately; then the effect of the PPI relative to pre trauma values was calculated in percent.

Acoustic Trauma and Auditory Brainstem Recordings

An acoustic trauma at 2 kHz (115 dB SPL, 75 min) in deep ketamine-xylazine-anesthesia (mixture of ketamine, xylazine, NaCl and atropine at a mixing ratio of 9:1:8:2, initial dose: 0.3 ml s.c.) was used to induce a frequency specific HL in all animals and possibly the subsequent development of a tinnitus percept. The tone was generated by a HP 33120A waveform generator, amplified and presented free-field to both ears by a speaker placed 5 cm in front of the animal's head (Canton Plus X Series 2). Anesthesia during trauma was maintained via subcutaneous infusion of the anesthetic solution supported by a syringe pump at a rate of 0.2 to 0.3 ml/h. The animal's body temperature was kept constant by a warming pad.

Auditory brainstem responses (ABR) were measured after the pre trauma ASR experiments but before surgery (cf. below) and again directly after the acoustic trauma to measure the acute trauma effect. Data were obtained via subcutaneously placed thin silver wire electrodes (0.25 mm diameter) using a Plexon Multichannel Acquisition Processor (Plexon system with HLK2-card; Plexon Inc., Dallas, TX, USA) after amplification by a JHM NeuroAmp 401 (J. Helbig Messtechnik, Mainaschaff, Germany) and stored with a custom-made Matlab program (10 kHz sampling rate). Auditory stimuli were generated by a custom-made Matlab program and presented free field to one ear at a time via a frequency response function corrected speaker (SinusLive neo 25S, pro hifi, Kaltenkirchen, Germany) at circa 0.5 cm distance from the animal's pinna while the contralateral ear was tamped with an ear plug (e.g. [17]). Stimuli presented were clicks (0.1 ms duration) and pure tones (4 ms duration including 1 ms cosine-squared rise and fall times) ranging from 0.5 to 16.0 kHz in half-octave steps. 120 stimuli were presented in pairs of two phase inverted stimuli (intrastimulus interval 100 ms) and an interstimulus interval of 500 ms between stimulus pairs. Stimulation was pseudo-randomized using a fixed list of all combinations of stimulus frequencies and sound pressure levels (0 to 90 dB SPL in 5 dB steps). To obtain ABR-based audiograms the mean ABR waves were compared to the mean amplitude 200 to 100 ms before the stimulus (baseline). Thresholds were defined automatically by a custom-made Matlab program at the highest attenuation at which the evoked amplitude raised over 2 standard deviations of the baseline; data were discarded at frequencies where this procedure was not possible, e.g., at low signal to noise ratios. For additional analysis the root mean square (RMS) value of the ABR signal was calculated from 1 ms to 5 ms after stimulus onset.

Electrophysiological Unit Recordings in Primary Auditory Cortex (AI)

Recording in AI was chosen, as it is the first and – at least for the gerbil – most important cortical representation of perceived sounds. Two to five days after obtaining baseline ASR and ABR data, i.e., before the acoustic trauma, the skull of the anesthetized animals was trepanned to expose the left auditory cortex. A 2.5 cm aluminum head-post and recording chamber was implanted. Recording began two to four days after surgery. Animals were again ketamine-xylazine anesthetized, placed on a warming pad and fixated via the aluminum head-post. Over 2 to 3 sessions every second day, single and multi-unit responses to tones in 5 to 7 tracks with 2 to 4 recording locations each in AI were recorded using tungsten microelectrodes (1 MΩ impedance, 1–2 μm tip diameter, Plexon microelectrodes PLX-ME-W-3-PC-3-1.0-A-254). Verification of recording sites was done using neuronal response characteristics (latency, tuning sharpness (Q30), temporal response patterns (phasic/tonic), tonotopic organization (cf. [18])).

Stimulation consisted of pure tones (200 ms including 1 ms cosine-squared rise and fall times) ranging from 0.25 to 16.0 kHz in quarter-octave or half-octave steps presented at 70 dB SPL with 500 ms interstimulus intervals. Additionally to these iso-intensity measurements, tuning curves were recorded using pure tones in the mentioned frequency range but at different intensities ranging from 0 to 90 dB SPL. The recorded unit activity was analyzed with custom-made Matlab and IDL programs. Best frequency (BF; frequency with highest discharge rate at 70 dB SPL) as well as spontaneous rate (mean activity within a time window from 50 ms before to stimulus onset), evoked rate at BF and evoked rates at all tested stimulation intensities and frequencies were calculated for each unit individually.

Results

Assessment of Noise Trauma Induced Hearing Loss and Tinnitus Development

Under deep ketamine-xylazine anesthesia a total of 35 animals received a noise trauma (2 kHz pure tone, cf. Methods) that produced a spectrally defined acute HL in all animals that could be detected at least until the end of our experiments (4 animals exemplarily retested up to 16 weeks after the trauma). HL was quantified by both ABR and behavioral audiograms before and after the trauma (cf. below). Animals were also tested for tinnitus with behavioral tests (cf. Methods and [19,20]). We determined whether an animal developed a tinnitus percept and if so approximated the individually perceived frequency. It turned out that about three quarters (26 out of 35) of the animals developed a tinnitus percept while the remaining 9 animals did not. This percept was usually strongest at frequencies at and/or 1 octave above the trauma frequency in one or both gap-noise paradigms. Figure 2A depicts the behavioral responses to stimulus set 3 of two exemplary animals with a spectrally narrow (left) or wide (right) tinnitus percept, respectively. Narrow tinnitus percepts (16/26, 61.5%) were defined as having only one or two neighboring frequencies affected, while wide tinnitus percepts had at least three frequencies affected. The example of an animal with a spectrally narrow tinnitus percept shown in the left panel of Figure 2A had a significant PPI impairment (as reflected in increased ASR) at 4 and 8 kHz only (Tukey post-hoc tests after one-factorial ANOVA). In contrast, for the animal with a spectrally wide tinnitus percept shown on the right we detected significantly impaired PPI at 4 frequencies. Figure 2B gives an overview across the frequency distributions of the tinnitus percepts in both groups. The two distributions are not significantly different from each other (Kolmogorov-Smirnov test, p = 0.12) with both showing the peak of the distributions around 2 to 4 kHz. For all further analysis we therefore combined the data of these two groups again.

Figure 3 compares the results of the two behavioral paradigms for tinnitus detection. The top panel shows the behavioral data for stimulus set 2 across all animals, the bottom panel depicts data for stimulus set 3. Grey bars show post trauma PPI changes in animals that developed a tinnitus percept (group T), white bars those for animals that did not develop a tinnitus (group NT). For group T (narrow and wide tinnitus percept) and stimulation set 2 (Figure 3, top panel) a significant impairment of PPI as a sign of tinnitus could be detected at all tested frequencies after the trauma (single sample t-tests vs. 0 all $p<0.001$; mean $\pm$ SD at 1 kHz: $25.7\pm95.0\%$; 2 kHz: $45.7\pm114.7\%$; 4 kHz: $48.1\pm98.3\%$; 8 kHz: $25.9\pm49.1\%$) but was strongest at 2 and 4 kHz (Tukey-tests after significant one-factorial ANOVA). NT animals on the other hand showed no impairment or even a significant improvement of PPI (1 kHz: $6.5\pm93.0\%$; 2 kHz: $-8.2\pm72.0\%$; 4 kHz: $-17.6\pm35.4\%$, $p<0.001$; 8 kHz: $-2.2\pm32.8\%$). In stimulation set 3 (Figure 3, bottom panel) T animals showed a significant impairment of PPI at all tested frequencies after the trauma (single sample t-tests vs. 0 all $p<0.001$ except 2 kHz where p = 0.002; 1 kHz: $24.5\pm126.9\%$; 2 kHz: $23.2\pm158.1\%$; 4 kHz: $19.6\pm86.4\%$; 8 kHz: $16.3\pm24.8\%$; 16 kHz: $13.4\pm19.8\%$) while the distribution – without any clear peak as indicated by the non-significant one-factorial ANOVA – was not identical to the one shown above (Kolmogorov-Smirnov test, $p<0.05$). NT animals again showed no impairment or even improved their PPI responses significantly (1 kHz: $-9.1\pm23.8\%$, $p<0.001$; 2 kHz: $-21.9\pm28.7\%$, $p<0.001$; 4 kHz: $-8.9\pm33.5\%$, p = 0.002; 8 kHz: $-1.5\pm14.9\%$; 16 kHz: $3.7\pm13.3\%$). In other words, whereas group T developed significantly impaired PPI as a sign of tinnitus

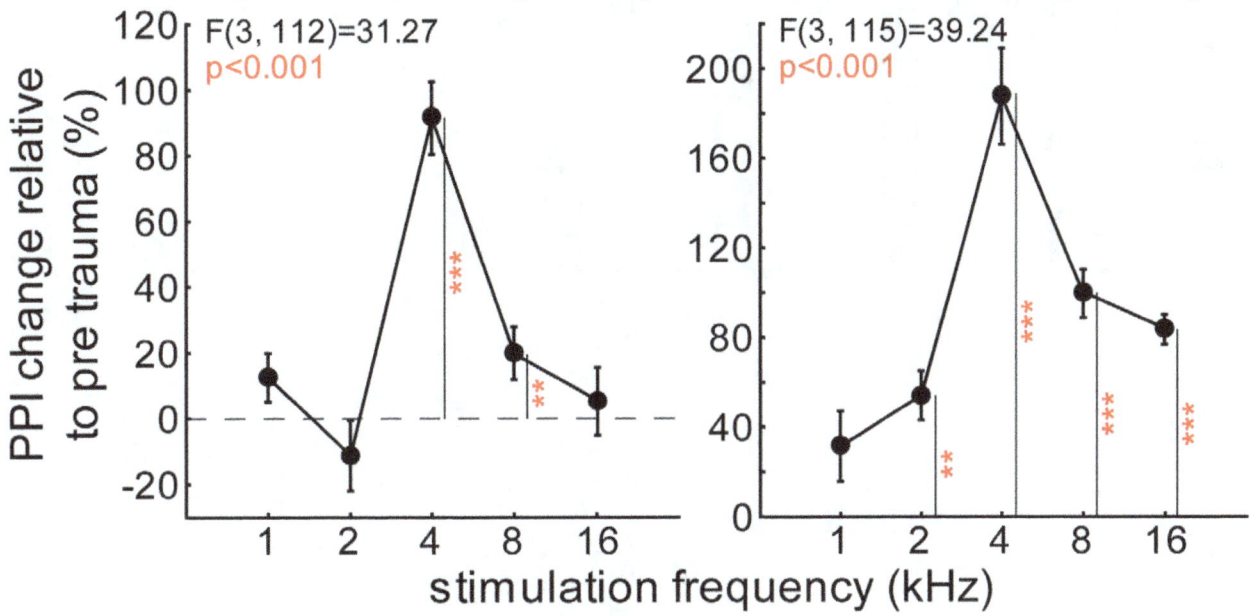

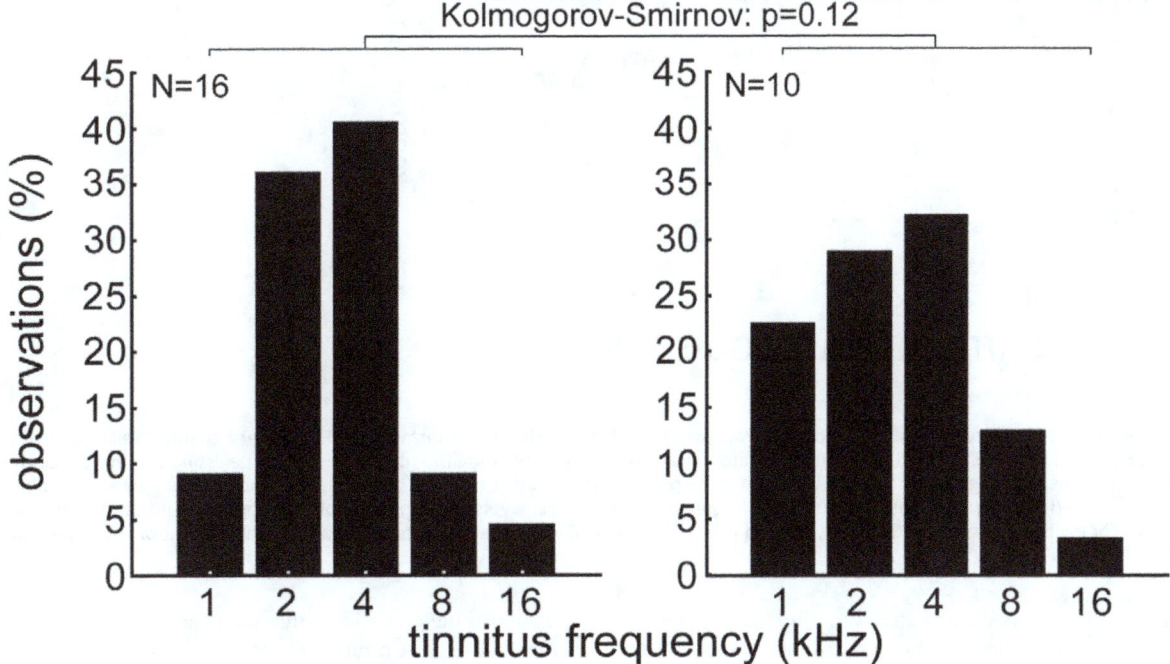

Figure 2. Frequency distributions of perceived tinnitus frequencies. A Data from two exemplary animals tested with stimulus set 3 with narrow (left panel) and wide tinnitus percepts (right panel), respectively. In both cases the one-factorial ANOVAs indicated frequency dependency of the PPI changes relative to pre trauma but in the first case only for two and in the second case for four frequencies. Whiskers indicate standard error of the mean (SEM) **B** Frequency distributions for narrow (16 animals) and wide tinnitus percepts (10 animals) with observation frequency given in percent. Both distributions are not significantly different from each other.

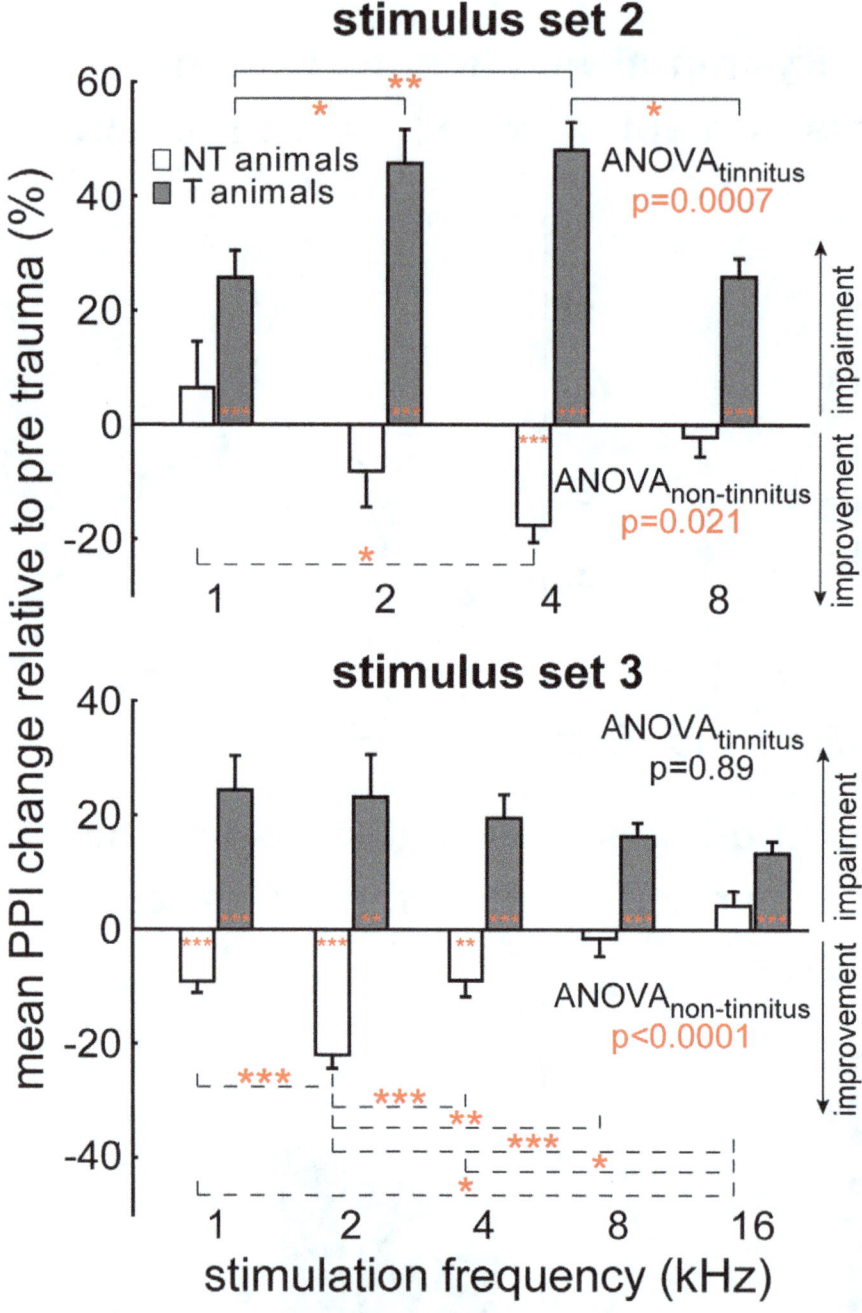

Figure 3. Behavioral tinnitus tests (gap-noise paradigms) in 35 animals. Mean normalized PPI response changes relative to pre trauma (in percent ± SEM) of group T (black) and NT (white); upward deviations indicate PPI impairment indicative for an existing tinnitus percept, downward gives PPI improvement. Upper panel: stimulus set 2, the responses are sorted for startle stimulus frequency. Lower panel: stimulus set 3, the responses are sorted for the bandpass noise center frequency. Significance levels of single sample t-tests vs. 0 indicating an impairment or improvement for each frequency and the Tukey-tests of the 1-factorial ANOVA indicating frequency specific impairment or improvement: * p<0.05, ** p<0.01, *** p<0.001.

in both paradigms, NT animals even showed significantly improved PPI at frequencies from one octave below to one octave above the trauma frequency compared to pre trauma conditions.

In Figure 4 the development of the tinnitus percept is exemplarily assessed over time in 4 T animals by 1-factorial ANOVAs in tinnitus and non-tinnitus frequencies (defined at day 2 post trauma) separately. The impairment of PPI, as indicative of a tinnitus percept in these T animals increased over time and reached a peak after 3 to 4 weeks post trauma. The data

demonstrate (t-tests vs. 0) that the acute tinnitus percept is evident from day 2 post trauma on. At 3 weeks post trauma we also find the non-tinnitus frequencies to be affected; this may point to a peak tinnitus percept around that time which than becomes chronic (tested up to 16 weeks) and the non-tinnitus frequencies become unaffected again. Therefore, the neuro-plastic processes that lead to the development of a chronic subjective tinnitus seem to be finished after about 3 weeks post trauma in this animal model.

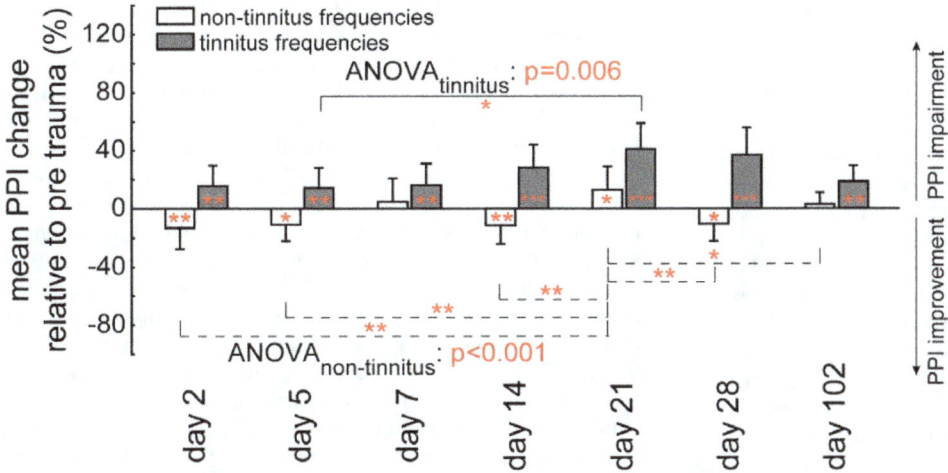

Figure 4. Development of tinnitus percept over time (stimulation set 2). Mean prepulse inhibition change relative to pre trauma response (in percent ± SEM) for non-tinnitus frequencies (open bars) and all tinnitus frequencies (black bars) obtained up to 102 days after trauma, exemplary in four T animals. An impairment of PPI is plotted upward, an improvement downward; significant difference of data to pre trauma is depicted by asterisks in each bar (one sample t-tests vs. 0). Connecting lines indicate significant Tukey post-hoc tests. Significance levels: * p<0.05, ** p<0.01, *** p<0.001.

All animals showed a significant hearing loss (HL) which was similar in their ABR and behavioral audiograms (Figure 5). The ABR thresholds averaged over all animals and frequencies increased significantly: mean ABR after the trauma pre 44.2±11.2 dB SPL, post 52.9±11.6 dB SPL (F (1, 732) = 153.51, p<0.001). As can be seen in Figure 5A this HL was frequency dependent, as indicated by the significant one-factorial ANOVA for the HL over all stimuli (click and pure tones of different frequencies; F(11, 179) = 3.27; p<0.001) with a maximal HL around the trauma frequency and half an octave above. The HL assessed by the behavioral audiogram is depicted in Figure 5B. We also find a general threshold increase (single sample t-tests HL for each frequency vs. 0, always p<0.001) but the one-factorial ANOVA only shows a tendency for frequency-specificity (F(5, 202) = 2.07, p = 0.08).

We also analyzed the HL of both tinnitus animal groups (T and NT) dependent on the stimulation frequency by 2-factorial ANOVAs and found neither in the ABR nor in the behaviorally determined thresholds any frequency specific differences between the animal groups. This was true for the interactions as well as for the mean HL over all frequencies which in ABR measurements of the NT animals amounted 23.2±23.8% and in the T animals 24.0±30.5% (2-factorial ANOVA, F(1, 167) = 0.03; p = 0.87) and 70.4±49.2% and 82.8±51.9% (2-factorial ANOVA, F(1, 162) = 1.76, p = 0.19) in the behavioral audiograms for NT and T animals, respectively. In other words, the existence or non-existence of a tinnitus percept in our animal groups cannot be explained by differences in the induced trauma as determined with these physiological or behavioral measures. Nevertheless, as the variance between the different specimens was quite high in both

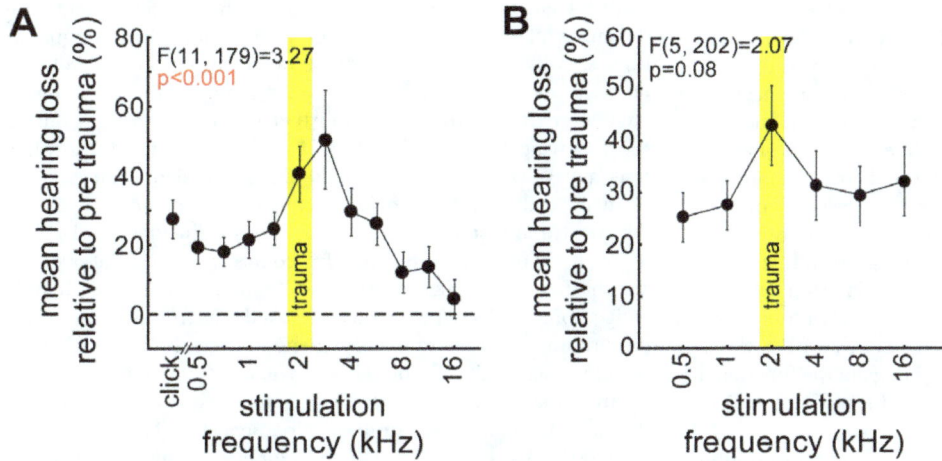

Figure 5. ABR and behaviorally determined hearing loss. A Significant one-factorial ANOVA (mean ± SEM) of the hearing loss (in percent relative to pre trauma) over the different stimulation frequencies as obtained by ABR measurements of all investigated animals. The yellow area indicates the trauma frequency. **B** One-factorial ANOVA of the hearing loss obtained by behavioral threshold paradigm (stimulus set 1). The statistics indicate only a tendency for frequency specific hearing loss around the trauma frequency. In both methods of HL determination the trauma frequency is affected most.

groups (large standard deviations) an effect on the individual HL level cannot completely be ruled out.

Neurophysiological Correlates of HL and Tinnitus in Primary Auditory Cortex Field AI

The behavioral differences in T and NT animals were paralleled by different plastic changes of neuronal responses in primary auditory cortex field AI: We recorded pure tone responses from a total of 627 single and multi-units (490 units in T and 137 units in NT group). Out of these, 331 units were recorded before (278 in T, 53 in NT group) and 296 units after the acoustic trauma (212 in T, 84 in NT group) over several recording sessions, usually 2 sessions before and 3 after the trauma.

Figure 6A shows the mean evoked response rates as a function of pure tone frequency across all units in NT animals before and after trauma (left panel). The same data were replotted in the right panel but now aligned to the BF of each unit. With a 2-factorial ANOVA we found an overall decrease of evoked rate in NT animals after the trauma (pre: 11.50 ± 1.07 spikes/sec, post: 6.14 ± 0.53 spikes/sec, $F(1, 1410) = 43.98$, $p < 0.001$) that was not uniformly distributed across all frequencies (2-factorial ANOVA; $p = 0.009$) but most prominent below the trauma frequency (significant Tukey-tests at 0.5, 0.7 and 1 kHz). Figure 6B depicts the respective mean evoked rates recorded in the T animals. No significant change of mean rate averaged over all frequencies (pre: 7.11 ± 0.37 spikes/sec, post: 7.88 ± 0.61 spikes/sec, $F(1, 4285) = 2.04$, n.s.) nor any interaction between frequency and trauma status could be found. Interestingly, comparing the data from Figure 6A and 6B, it is obvious that the mean evoked rates in T and NT animals were different before the trauma (mean over all frequencies for NT: 10.88 ± 15.14, T: 6.75 ± 10.59; $F(1, 4260) = 83.43$, $p < 0.001$; interaction: $F(21, 4260) = 2.49$, $p < 0.001$, Tukey-tests significant at 0.5, 0.7 and 1 kHz) but reached similar levels after the trauma (no significant difference over all frequencies for NT: 6.82 ± 8.21 and T: 7.49 ± 14.78, $F(1, 3526) = 1.17$ or in interaction of frequency and group $F(21, 3526) = 0.40$; $p > 0.05$ for both). The mean evoked response rates in group T showed a significant increase only when aligning the data to the individually perceived lowest tinnitus frequency (Figure 6C). Tukey post-hoc tests indicated these differences to be exactly at this tinnitus frequency and one octave above and therefore this may be a neuronal correlate of the tinnitus percept.

Further changes or predispositions of neuronal response properties were observed as summarized in Figure 7. First of all, the described changes in evoked discharge rates were "anti-paralleled" by changes in the spontaneous rate that significantly increased in the T group whereas it did not change in the NT group (Figure 7A) after the trauma. These changes or non-changes in spontaneous rate may also represent neuronal correlates for the existence or non-existence of a tinnitus percept in group T or NT, respectively. Figure 7B demonstrates that the pure tone evoked response rate at the BF was different between groups T and NT already *before* the trauma, which could already be inferred from the analyses described in Figure 6. Furthermore, in line with previous reports [5,7] we observed a significant change in mean BF in the T group that is indicative for a neuro-plastic change in the functional topography of the tonotopic organization of AI that is not seen in the NT group (Figure 7C).

This trauma-induced plasticity of the tonotopic organization in AI of T animals was further analyzed and compared to NT animals in Figure 8: There, the spatio-temporal dynamics of the changes are plotted as a function of time and BF for both T and NT animals (right and left column, respectively)., We separated the data for the day of recording into four groups, first, the pre trauma

data (blue) and second the recordings performed at three different time ranges post trauma (reddish colors), namely the day of the trauma, i.e., immediately after obtaining the ABR (top panels), day 2 to 3 post trauma and finally days 5 to 7 post trauma. The BFs of units in these groups were binned in octave bands and the frequency distributions of the BFs of T and NT animals at the three post trauma time points were compared to the pre trauma condition (tested with Kolmogorov-Smirnov tests, corrected for multiple testing). As can be seen in Figure 8, the BF distributions of NT animals (Figure 8A) did not show any significant changes over time. On the other hand, the BF distributions of the T animals (Figure 8B) – while not different from NT animals before the trauma – did show strong and significant shifts over time: On the day of the trauma we found a strong shift to an over-representation of frequencies below the acoustic trauma, on day 2 and 3 the whole distribution shifted to an over-representation of frequencies above the trauma frequency, and finally after one week the distribution changed back to pre trauma conditions. In other words, after dramatic disturbances of the tonotopic organization immediately post trauma, the animals showing a tinnitus percept, seem to be completely normal again in their tonotopic organization of AI by one week post trauma, although the tinnitus percept was still present at that time (cf. Figures 3 and 4).

Because of this finding of these temporal dynamics of the noise-trauma induced plasticity of the tonotopic organization, we also analyzed the temporal dynamics of the rate changes shown in Figure 7A and B: While the T animals showed an almost linear increase of the spontaneous rate over time, no changes of spontaneous rate over time were seen in the NT group (not shown). In contrast, changes in evoked discharge rate showed complex temporal dynamics over time: Figure 9A to F give the interactions in the 2-factorial ANOVAs of the mean evoked rates for the same 4 time ranges depicted above (cf. Figure 8) relative to trauma induction (pre trauma, immediately after trauma, 2 to 3 days post trauma and 5 to 7 days post trauma) in both animal groups; all interactions are significant at a p-level below 0.001 allowing Tukey post-hoc tests. Shown are mean evoked rates across all units in AI stimulated with frequencies below the trauma frequency (Figure 9A), at the trauma affected frequencies (2 to 4 kHz; Figure 9B, cf. Figure 5A) and frequencies above the trauma (Figure 9C). As can be seen, the different animal groups show different temporal dynamics of evoked rate changes within these three frequency ranges: Whereas NT animals show a strong and significant decrease of evoked rate below the trauma frequency immediately after the trauma with no further significant changes during the following week (NT_{pre} vs. NT_0 to NT_{4-7}: Tukey post-hoc tests always $p < 0.001$), T animals display no significant changes of mean evoked rate with low frequency stimulation relative to the pre trauma status with only one minor fluctuation (T_{2-3} vs. T_{4-7}: $p = 0.003$, Figure 9A). In contrast, at and above the trauma frequency (Figure 9B, C), NT animals show less changes with strongest decrease of mean evoked rate towards one week post trauma at the trauma frequency range (NT_{pre} vs. NT_{4-7}: $p = 0.04$), while the T animals show a significant increase of the mean evoked rate by that time at the frequencies where the tinnitus is perceived (trauma frequencies: T_{pre} vs. T_{4-7}: $p = 0.001$, T_0 vs. T_{4-7}: $p < 0.001$; above trauma frequencies: T_{pre} vs. T_{2-3}: $p < 0.001$, T_0 vs. T_{2-3}: $p = 0.005$).

Interestingly, when mean evoked rate changes are plotted only for responses at the BFs of the individual units, a different picture was found (Figure 9E): There, no significant changes could be detected for the NT group while within the T group there was a

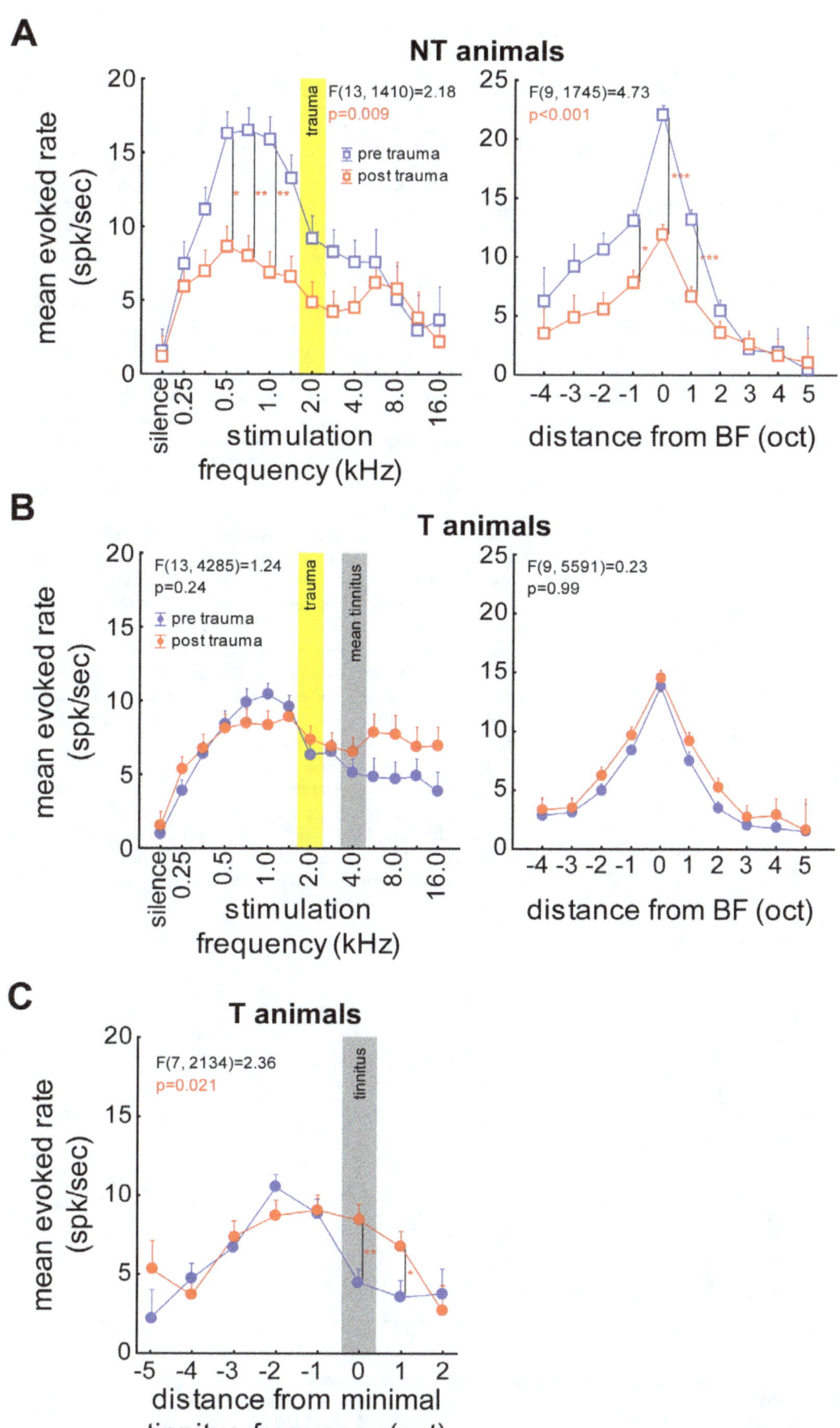

Figure 6. Neuronal evoked response to iso-intensity pure tone stimulation. Mean response (+SEM) of all recorded neurons of groups NT and T during 70 dB SPL stimulation. **A left panel** Shown is the interaction of the 2-factorial ANOVA of trauma status (blue: before; red: after) over frequencies (trauma: yellow area) of the pure tone evoked response rates in group NT. **right panel** Interaction of the 2-factorial ANOVA of trauma status and frequencies (octaves) of mean response rates aligned to the BF of each individual unit. NT animals show a strong decrease in evoked rate below 2 kHz and around the BF after the trauma. **B left panel** Same display as in A for group T with the mean minimal tinnitus frequency (grey bar). **right panel** Same display as in A, data aligned to the BF of each unit. Note that in this group the BF shifts after the trauma towards higher frequencies (cf. panel C). T animals do not show this reduction of evoked rate that NT animals exhibit. **C** Interaction of frequency (octaves) and trauma status of data from group T aligned to individual minimal tinnitus frequency now becomes significant with increased mean evoked rate after the trauma at the tinnitus frequency and one octave above. T animals show a frequency specific increase of evoked response after the trauma with aligning the recorded data to the behaviorally determined tinnitus frequency. Tukey post-hoc test significance level: * p<0.05, ** p<0.01, *** p<0.001.

strong significant increase of mean BF-evoked rate immediately after the trauma that returned back to normal on day 2 to 3 post trauma (T_0 vs. T_{pre} and T_{2-3}: p<0.001, T_0 vs. T_{4-7}: p = 0.02). For stimulation frequencies at least one octave below BF, no significant changes were seen for T animals while there was a decrease in response rate for NT animals (NT_{pre} vs. NT_0: p = 0.03, NT_{pre} vs. NT_{4-7}: p = 0.01, Figure 9D), and for frequencies at least one octave above BF (Figure 9F) there was a significant increase in mean response rate in T animals, but this change was only seen after the changes at BF had vanished again, i.e., from day 2–3 on (T_{pre} vs. T_{2-3}: p = 0.01, T_{pre} vs. T_{4-7}: p = 0.002, T_0 vs. T_{2-3}: p = 0.04). For the NT animals, again a decrease in response rate over time was seen at this frequency range (NT_{pre} vs. NT_0: p = 0.006, NT_{pre} vs. NT_{4-7}: p = 0.001).

Figure 10 finally depicts mean ABR strength (root-mean-square (RMS) values of ABR amplitudes; A, C) and evoked rate (rate-intensity functions; B, D) as a function of sound intensity in T (C, D) and NT animals (A, B). We compared data measured before and directly after the trauma by 2-factorial ANOVAs for three frequency bands, namely below the trauma frequency (left column), the frequencies most affected by the trauma (2 to 4 kHz; middle column, cf. Figure 5A) and the frequencies above this affected range (right column).

Interestingly, the significant decrease in mean response rate of AI neurons of the NT group that was shown in Figure 6A could only be detected for moderate sound pressure levels (grey area in Figure 10B) and was only significant for frequencies below the trauma frequency (Figure 10B, left panel inset). For high sound pressure levels of 90 dB SPL, we found the inverse effect in group NT, namely a general increase in mean response

rate after the trauma across all tested frequency ranges (Figure 10B). In contrast, no such changes were seen in the T group: There, we observed only minor changes in mean response rate in the rate-intensity functions for frequencies up to 4 kHz (Figure 10D, left and middle panels), but a strong and general increase of almost 50% across all intensities for frequencies above 4 kHz with a parallel shift of the whole mean rate-intensity function. In general, there was no such shift but rather a change in the shape of the rate-intensity functions in the NT animals (from a sigmoidal to an exponential curve progression; Figure 10B).

Comparing these changes of cortical rate-intensity functions to the ABR data we found that the observed changes of cortical response rates were in general paralleled by similar changes in ABR strength, with the exception that significantly strengthened responses in the T animals after trauma were seen in all frequency ranges and not only above 4 kHz (Figure 10C). Therefore it may be concluded that at least some of the changes we observed in AI simply reflect changes that occur already at levels of the auditory pathway downstream of the auditory cortex, although top-down influences are also conceivable (cf. [21,22]).

Finally, comparing the overall level of mean ABR strength and evoked discharge rate between T and NT animals (Fig. 10 A vs. C and B vs. D, respectively), we found generally smaller ABR amplitudes (F(1, 14888) = 1296.7, p<0.001) and the lower spike rates in AI (F(1, 32637) = 65.57, p<0.001) before and after trauma in the T compared to the NT animals.

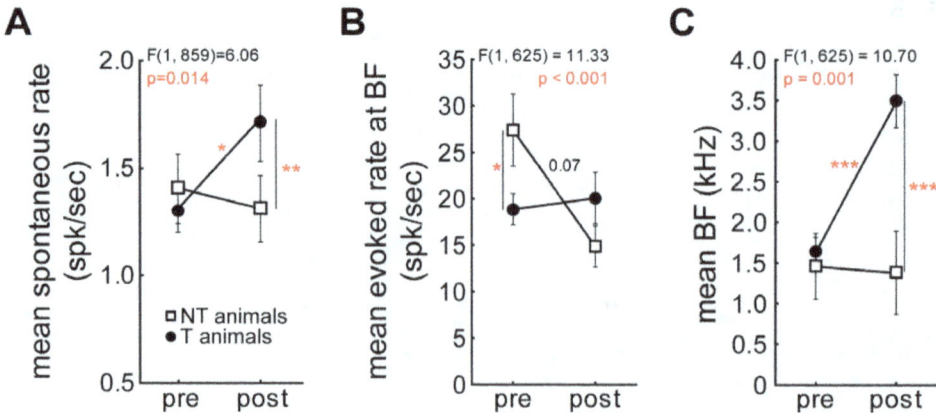

Figure 7. Trauma induced changes of neuronal response parameters. Interactions of the ANOVAs of the mean values (± SEM) of neuronal response parameters in groups T (filled circles) and NT (open squares) before and after acoustic trauma. **A** Significant interaction of trauma status and animal group in the spontaneous rate with an increase in activity after the trauma in T animals only. **B** Evoked rate at BF is different before but not after the trauma between both groups. **C** BF of all recorded units changes only in T animals after the trauma indicating a reorganization of tonotopic maps. Tukey post-hoc test significance levels: * p<0.05, *** p<0.001.

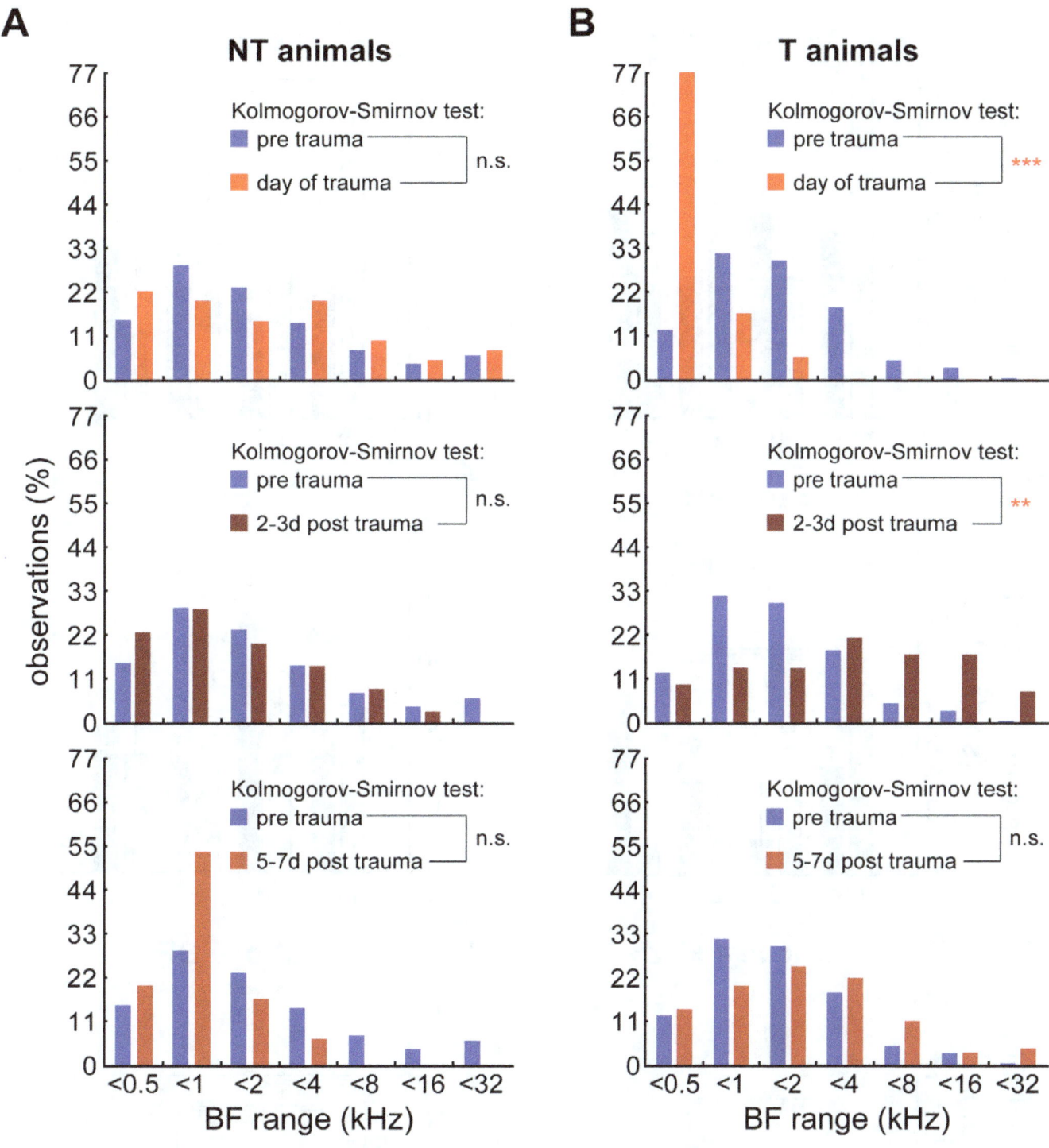

Figure 8. Changes in BF frequency distributions over time. A Comparison of the frequency distribution of BF (observations in %) binned in one octave steps of NT animals before the trauma (blue) with the data obtained on 3 different time points post trauma, from top to bottom: day of trauma, 2 to 3 days after trauma, 5 to 7 days after trauma. Distributions are tested by Kolmogorov-Smirnov tests corrected for multiple comparisons. The distributions do not change over time. **B** Comparison of the BF distributions of T animals on the same three time points. The distributions show strong shifts over time. Kolmogorov-Smirnov significance levels: ** p<0.01, *** p<0.001.

Discussion

Methodological Considerations

In this report we aimed to understand why different individuals suffering from similar peripheral auditory impairment often but not always do develop a tinnitus percept. Therefore it is crucial to this study to undoubtedly identify those animals that did develop a tinnitus percept after noise trauma and distinguish them from those who did not. To achieve this goal we employed a multistep procedure: First, we quantified the noise trauma induced hearing

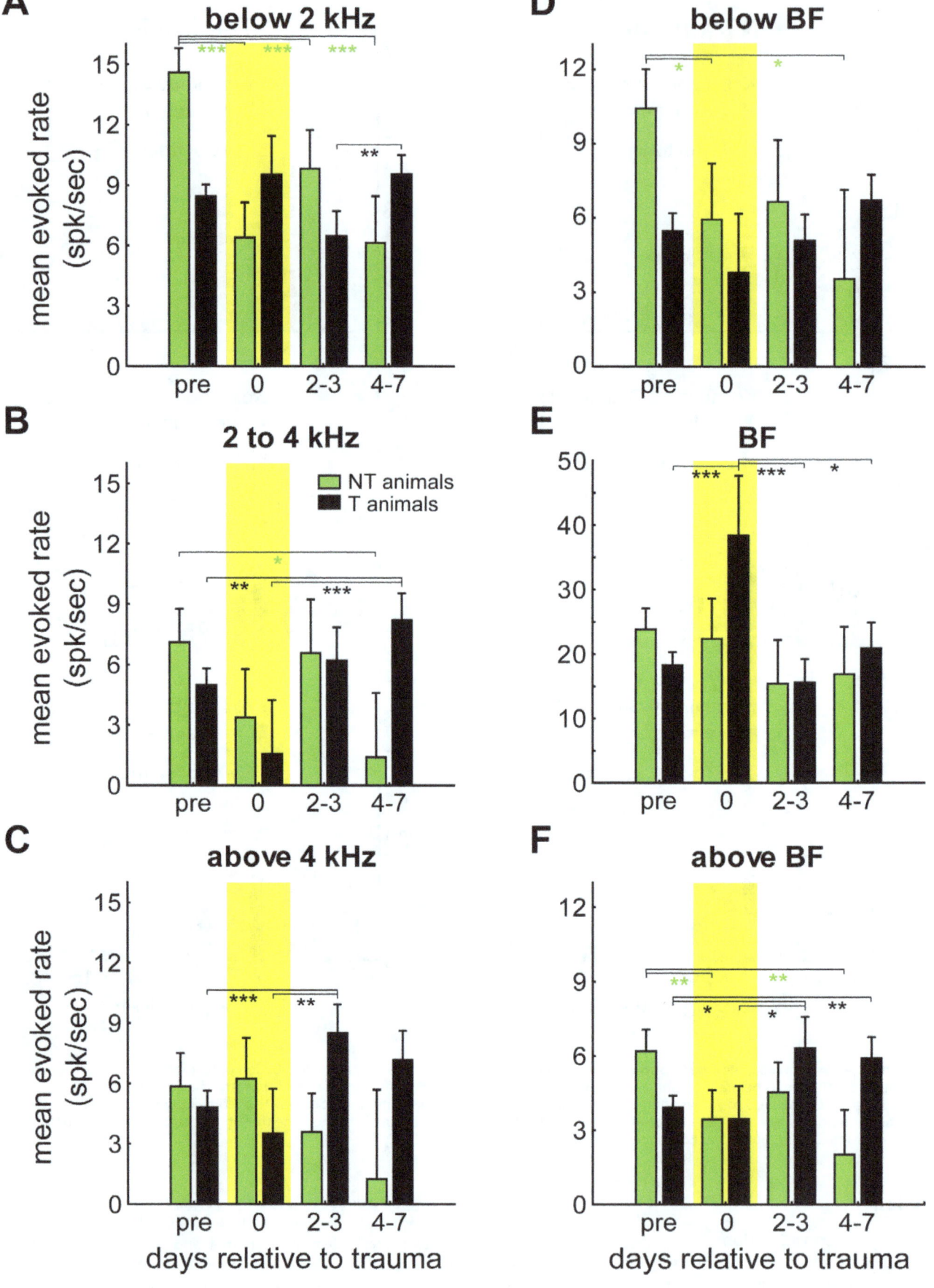

Figure 9. Changes in mean evoked rate over time. Results of the 2-factorial ANOVAs of mean evoked rates of all recorded units as a function of recording time and animal group (green = NT, black = T) separately for different frequency ranges; all interactions are significant with $p < 0.001$, asterisks indicate significant Tukey post-hoc tests, whiskers give the SEM. **A** Mean evoked rate of all units stimulated with frequencies below the trauma; only NT animals show a decrease in responses relative to pre trauma. **B** Mean evoked rate at trauma affected frequencies; increase of response over time only in T animals. **C** Mean evoked rate above the trauma frequencies; again, only T animals show increase of response rates over time. **D** Mean evoked rate of frequencies at least 1 octave below the individual BF of every unit; only NT animals show decrease of activity relative to pre trauma. **E** BF responses of all recorded units; in T animals a significant increase of response strength can be found only at the day of the trauma, immediately post trauma. **F** Mean evoked rates at least one octave above BF; in T animals an increase of response can be found only from day 2–3 on, while in NT animals the responses decrease already at the day of the trauma. Tukey post-hoc test significance levels: * $p < 0.05$, ** $p < 0.01$, *** $p < 0.001$.

loss using both electrophysiological (ABR) and behavioral approaches (PPI of ASR) which led to similar estimates of hearing loss (cf. Figure 5; [16]). Only those animals were included in the study that showed a hearing impairment of at least 15 dB at the trauma frequency of 2 kHz to prevent any effect of hidden hearing loss [23]. Thereby, the paradigm we used to induce this hearing loss was relatively mild, which in recent studies turned out to be ideal to induce the development of tinnitus in rodent models compared to severe acoustic traumata, probably because in the latter case the hearing loss is less restricted to a certain frequency range and therefore the effect on decreased lateral inhibition is spectrally less focused. [24,25]. Second, we used two different behavioral approaches to detect a tinnitus percept in our animals, namely the gap-noise modulated PPI paradigm adapted from Turner and colleagues [12,20,26] and fear-potentiation modulated PPI paradigms, e.g., inspired from Guitton and colleagues [15]. Although the two methods yield slightly different estimates of tinnitus frequency (cf. Figure 3), the outcome was highly comparable with respect to the question if there was a tinnitus percept at all or not as all animals displayed a tinnitus percept in both paradigms with at least one overlapping frequency. We normalized all PPI responses individually for all frequencies tested to counteract the effects of the different perception thresholds and of the trauma. We then grouped the animals according to their behavior into individuals with and without tinnitus and investigated the pure tone responses of neurons within AI. Finally, we correlated the neurophysiological data (ABR and AI recordings) with the behavioral data. The fact that we could describe a number of highly significant differences in the neuronal responses pre and post trauma between animals classified behaviorally as having a tinnitus percept (group T) or not (group NT) further strengthens the results of the behavioral tinnitus detection procedures employed here (cf. Figures 6 to 10). Therefore, based on this combination of behavioral and electrophysiological parameters collected in this report it is very likely that the individual specimen tested here were correctly grouped into T and NT animals.

Predisposition for Subjective Tinnitus Development

The most prominent pre trauma differences in T and NT animals were the higher sound-evoked activities within the auditory system (as apparent in both ABR and AI recordings) of the NT group compared to the T group (cf. Figures 6; 7B; 9 and 10). Obviously this higher neuronal activity allows the auditory system of animals in the NT group to differently react to noise-induced peripheral damage compared to the T animals. One might speculate on the different neuronal mechanisms that lead, after a noise trauma, to the development or prevention of tinnitus in T and NT animals, respectively:

In T animals the trauma-induced damage to the receptor epithelium of the cochlea obviously triggers a number of neuroplastic changes throughout the auditory system that may be either transient or permanent (cf. [27,28]). In our model, the

plastic reorganization of the tonotopic organization of the primary auditory cortex that has already been described by a number of studies [29,30,31,32,33,34] turned out to be only transient, but showed complex temporal dynamics: A shift of the BF-representation to lower frequencies immediately after trauma was followed by a shift to higher frequencies a few days later and back to normal after about one week post trauma (cf. Figure 8). Intriguingly, these changes in tonotopic organization in AI were accompanied by significantly but also transiently increased response rates at the BF of the units (Figure 9E). As changes at off-BF frequencies appeared later and were permanent rather that transient (Figure 9F), this points to a mechanism of plastic changes that affect the tonotopic organization and which are active within the receptive field of the units during a short, transient post trauma period. During this temporal disturbance of the tonotopic organization in AI obviously some further plastic changes take place that stay permanent even after the tonotopic order is back to pre trauma conditions. These seem to be most prominent at frequencies above BF, i.e. above the center of the spectral receptive field. In our data, these plastic changes are represented by a number of increased (spontaneous and evoked) neuronal response rates that are in part stimulation frequency specific and correlated to the behaviorally estimated perceived tinnitus frequencies (cf. Figures 6C; 7A; 9C, F; 10C, D). We believe that these neurophysiological changes described during the first week post trauma reflect the transition from an acute to a chronic state of subjective tinnitus in the T group, as the tinnitus percept is still present after the plastic reorganizations are finished (cf. Figure 4). Finally, as the changes of the tonotopic representation in AI and evoked rates at BF were transient in the T animals whereas the increases in neuronal discharge rate – spontaneous and at high, tinnitus-related frequencies – persisted beyond one week post trauma, we believe that the latter are the neurophysiological correlates of the tinnitus percept rather than the former.

Tinnitus Prevention

In NT animals we saw a different picture, as the noise-trauma induced neuroplastic changes were completely different compared to the T group: In the NT group, coming from a higher overall level of sound induced activity in the auditory system, we measured a significant decrease in evoked response rates both in AI and ABR recordings (cf. Figures 6A; 7B) but no change in spontaneous rate (cf. Figure 7A) or tonotopic organization (cf. Figures 7C; 8A). Interestingly it turned out that this reducing effect on evoked response rate could only be seen at moderate sound intensities, while there were no changes for low intensities and even increased evoked responses for the highest intensity testes (90 dB SPL; cf. Figure 10A, B). Based on these observations we propose the following model of tinnitus prevention in NT animals:

We believe that there is an active neuronal process that is able to prevent the development of a tinnitus percept in the NT group, whereas it is not in the T group. Based on our data the main predisposition for this ability to prevent tinnitus development seems to be the higher overall neuronal activity – both

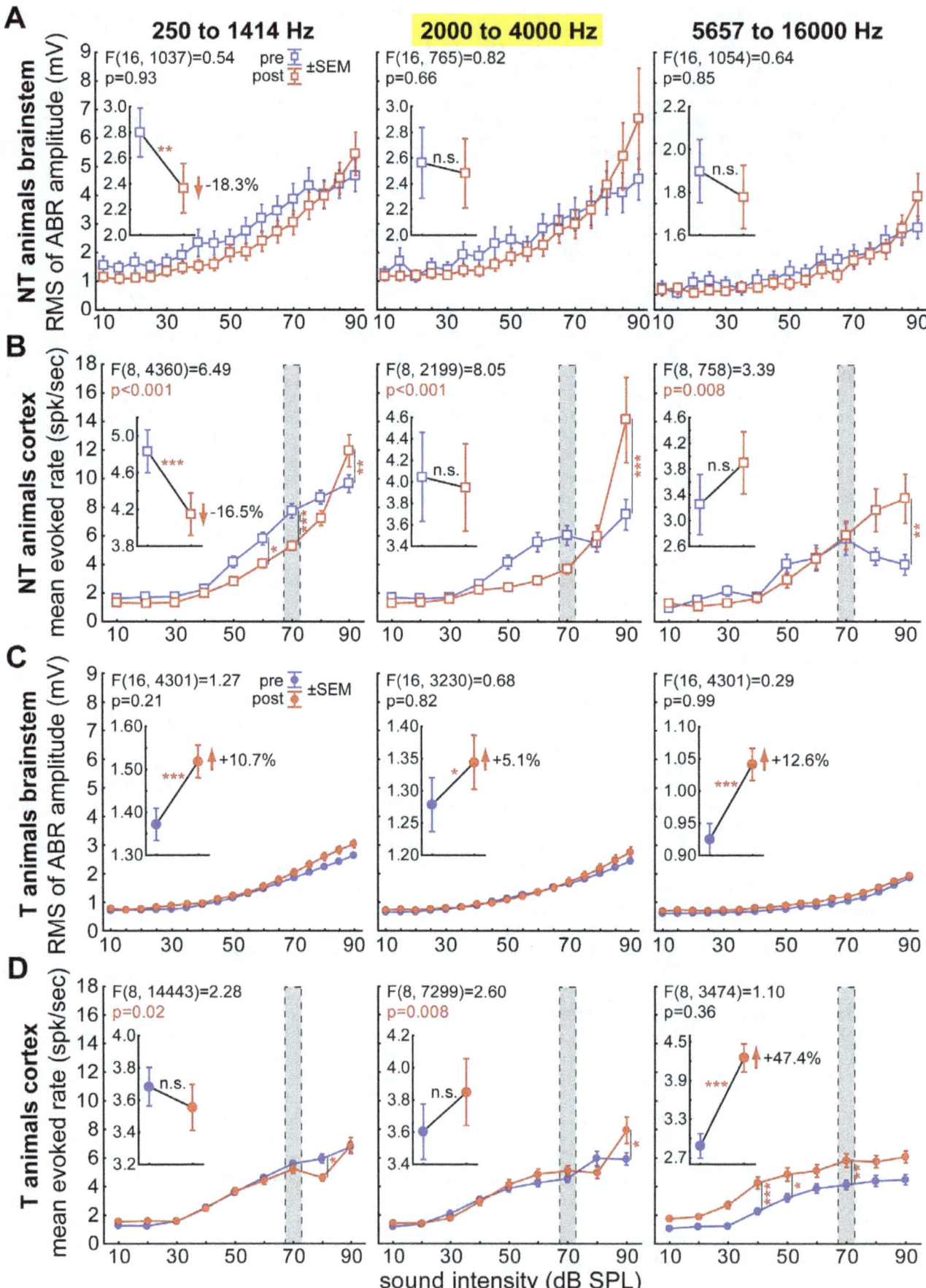

Figure 10. Intensity functions of brainstem and cortical responses in NT and T animals. A Brainstem responses (RMS of ABR amplitudes) of NT animals over the different stimulation intensities grouped for frequencies below the trauma, frequencies affected most by the trauma and frequencies above the trauma affected range. Given is the interaction of the 2-factorial ANOVA of measurement time (pre or post trauma) and intensities, Whiskers give the SEM, asterisks indicate significant Tukey post-hoc tests. No interaction is found here while the mean over all intensities (insets) indicates a significant decrease of ABR response after the trauma for frequencies below 2 kHz. **B** Mean rate-intensity functions of the evoked responses of the neurons in AI in NT animals plotted the same way as in A, the gray area indicates the iso-intensity measurement range shown, e.g., in Figure 6. The interaction is significant in all three cases indicating intensity specific changes while over all intensities only the activity below the trauma drops significantly. **C** ABR of T animals, no significant interaction could be found, but mean over all intensities the ABR amplitudes increase in all frequency ranges. **D** Mean rate-intensity functions of neurons in AI of T animals, the interaction is significant for the lower two frequency ranges indicating intensity specific changes without a general increase of activity. This can only be found above the trauma in the range of the tinnitus frequencies. Tukey post-hoc test significance level: * $p < 0.05$, ** $p < 0.01$, *** $p < 0.001$.

spontaneous and evoked – in the auditory system of the NT compared to the T animals. Obviously this neuronal process is able to reduce evoked activity, thereby preventing changes in spontaneous activity, evoked activity at high stimulation frequencies and tonotopic organization. A candidate for a transmitter system that may mediate this effect is the $GABA_A$-system, as it allows for a fast and global inhibition of the whole auditory cortex in response to sound [35,36,37,38,39,40,41]. We believe that the inhibition relevant here is global rather than frequency specific, as the reduction in response rate is rather focused on frequencies below the trauma frequency (cf. Figures 6A; 9A, D; 10A, B), whereas the tinnitus percept seems to be related to increased response rates at frequencies above the trauma frequency (cf. Figure 6B; 9C, F; 10D). Our hypothesis is that a global inhibitory mechanism that counteracts the development of increased rates at high frequencies is able to prevent tinnitus development, but at the same time, as it acts in a non-frequency specific manner, reduces the response rates at lower frequencies. This mechanism seems to work only for moderate sound intensities that are in the range of the normal auditory surround of the animals, possibly because the stimulation of the auditory system in this intensity range is needed to further trigger the malfunctional development of tinnitus during a critical period post trauma. At lower intensities it may not be necessary to activate this global inhibitory mechanism to prevent the tinnitus development, and at high intensities, were we observed increased response rates even in the NT group, it may be overstrained so that tinnitus would still develop. As the latter possibility would be a situation of permanent ongoing noise exposure for the animals, it may well be that our NT animals would have developed a tinnitus if the loud stimulation would have continued permanently (continuous noise pollution) rather than only during short, 200 ms stimuli during recording. Both scenarios, noise reduced environments for T animals and noise-intense environments for NT animals after the trauma may be used to test these hypotheses in future studies.

We propose that the high pre trauma neuronal activity in the NT group allows for its described significant reduction, whereas the low pre trauma activity in the T group is not sufficient to trigger this mechanism or, alternatively, global cortical inhibition is already at its limits, causal for the lower neuronal activity in these animals and cannot be increased further. In this case, the plastic recalibrations of neuronal response rates that take place in the T animals in the course of tinnitus chronification also trigger disturbances of the tonotopic organization in AI that remain transient, probably because they merely reflect the response rate recalibration process itself [28,42] and are again dominated by the tonotopic organization of the thalamic input after the rate recalibration is finished.

Finally, our view of an insufficient additional inhibitory capacity in T compared to NT animals is supported by recently published results from Yang and colleagues [43] reporting an abolishment of the tinnitus percept in rats after injection of GABAergic enhancers but not after applying excitation reducing pharmaceutics.

In summary we believe that an overall high neuronal activity in the auditory system opens the possibility to activate a global inhibitory mechanism that is able to prevent the development of a subjective tinnitus after a trauma-induced damage to the peripheral receptor epithelium of the cochlea. A closer understanding of this mechanism might open the possibility to develop a prophylaxis strategy to prevent the development of a subjective tinnitus in hearing impaired patients, e.g. after acute noise trauma. In this context, GABAergic enhancers [43] or other therapeutical interventions [10,44] that are able to reduce overall neuronal activity may be a promising strategy to follow.

Acknowledgments

We are grateful to Dr. Christo Pantev for valuable comments on an earlier version of the manuscript, and Julia C. Stepper for skillful assistance in the experiments as well as for animal caretaking.

Author Contributions

Conceived and designed the experiments: KT HS. Performed the experiments: SA SK IS. Analyzed the data: SA KT. Wrote the paper: KT HS.

References

1. Hoffman HJ, Reed GW (2004) Epidemiology of Tinnitus. In: Snow JB, editor. Tinnitus: theory and management: BC Decker Inc. 16–41.
2. Kim DK, Park SN, Park KH, Choi HG, Jeon EJ, et al. (2010) Clinical characteristics and audiological significance of spontaneous otoacoustic emissions in tinnitus patients with normal hearing. J Laryngol Otol 125: 246–250.
3. Langguth B, Salvi R, Elgoyhen AB (2009) Emerging pharmacotherapy of tinnitus. Expert Opin Emerg Drugs 14: 687–702.
4. Bauer CA, Turner JG, Caspary DM, Myers KS, Brozoski TJ (2008) Tinnitus and inferior colliculus activity in chinchillas related to three distinct patterns of cochlear trauma. J Neurosci Res 86: 2564–2578.
5. Engineer ND, Riley JR, Seale JD, Vrana WA, Shetake JA, et al. (2011) Reversing pathological neural activity using targeted plasticity. Nature 470: 101–104.
6. Gerken GM (1996) Central tinnitus and lateral inhibition: an auditory brainstem model. Hear Res 97: 75–83.
7. Mühlnickel W, Elbert T, Taub E, Flor H (1998) Reorganization of auditory cortex in tinnitus. Proc Natl Acad Sci U S A 95: 10340–10343.
8. Guitton MJ (2012) Tinnitus: pathology of synaptic plasticity at the cellular and system levels. Front Syst Neurosci 6: 12.
9. Eggermont JJ (2003) Central tinnitus. Auris Nasus Larynx 30 Suppl: S7–12.
10. Okamoto H, Stracke H, Stoll W, Pantev C (2010) Listening to tailor-made notched music reduces tinnitus loudness and tinnitus-related auditory cortex activity. Proc Natl Acad Sci U S A 107: 1207–1210.
11. Young JS, Fechter LD (1983) Reflex inhibition procedures for animal audiometry: a technique for assessing ototoxicity. J Acoust Soc Am 73: 1686–1693.
12. Turner JG, Parrish J (2008) Gap detection methods for assessing salicylate-induced tinnitus and hyperacusis in rats. Am J Audiol 17: S185–192.
13. Apergis-Schoute AM, Debiec J, Doyere V, LeDoux JE, Schafe GE (2005) Auditory fear conditioning and long-term potentiation in the lateral amygdala

require ERK/MAP kinase signaling in the auditory thalamus: a role for presynaptic plasticity in the fear system. J Neurosci 25: 5730–5739.

14. Ben Mamou C, Gamache K, Nader K (2006) NMDA receptors are critical for unleashing consolidated auditory fear memories. Nat Neurosci 9: 1237–1239.

15. Guitton MJ, Pujol R, Puel JL (2005) m-Chlorophenylpiperazine exacerbates perception of salicylate-induced tinnitus in rats. Eur J Neurosci 22: 2675–2678.

16. Walter M, Tziridis K, Ahlf S, Schulze H (2012) Context Dependent Auditory Threshold Determined by Brainstem Audiometry and Prepulse Inhibition in Mongolian Gerbils. Open Journal of Acoustics 2: 34–49.

17. Stuermer IW, Scheich H (2000) Early unilateral auditory deprivation increases 2-deoxyglucose uptake in contralateral auditory cortex of juvenile Mongolian gerbils. Hear Res 146: 185–199.

18. Thomas H, Tillein J, Heil P, Scheich H (1993) Functional organization of auditory cortex in the mongolian gerbil (Meriones unguiculatus). I. Electrophysiological mapping of frequency representation and distinction of fields. Eur J Neurosci 5: 882–897.

19. Campeau S, Davis M (1992) Fear potentiation of the acoustic startle reflex using noises of various spectral frequencies as conditioned stimuli. Animal Learning & Behavior 20: 177–186.

20. Turner JG, Brozoski TJ, Bauer CA, Parrish JL, Myers K, et al. (2006) Gap detection deficits in rats with tinnitus: a potential novel screening tool. Behav Neurosci 120: 188–195.

21. Bajo VM, Moore DR (2005) Descending projections from the auditory cortex to the inferior colliculus in the gerbil, Meriones unguiculatus. J Comp Neurol 486: 101–116.

22. Budinger E, Heil P, Scheich H (2000) Functional organization of auditory cortex in the Mongolian gerbil (Meriones unguiculatus). IV. Connections with anatomically characterized subcortical structures. Eur J Neurosci 12: 2452–2474.

23. Schaette R, McAlpine D (2011) Tinnitus with a normal audiogram: physiological evidence for hidden hearing loss and computational model. J Neurosci 31: 13452–13457.

24. Devarajan K, Gassner D, Durham D, Staecker H (2012) Effect of Noise Exposure Duration and Intensity on the Development of Tinnitus. ARO. Abs. 593.

25. Turner J, Larsen D (2012) Relationship Between Noise Exposure Stimulus Properties and Tinnitus in Rats: Results of a 12-Month Longitudinal Study. ARO. Abs. 594.

26. Turner JG (2007) Behavioral measures of tinnitus in laboratory animals. Prog Brain Res 166: 147–156.

27. Norena AJ, Tomita M, Eggermont JJ (2003) Neural changes in cat auditory cortex after a transient pure-tone trauma. J Neurophysiol 90: 2387–2401.

28. Kotak VC, Fujisawa S, Lee FA, Karthikeyan O, Aoki C, et al. (2005) Hearing loss raises excitability in the auditory cortex. J Neurosci 25: 3908–3918.

29. Dietrich V, Nieschalk M, Stoll W, Rajan R, Pantev C (2001) Cortical reorganization in patients with high frequency cochlear hearing loss. Hear Res 158: 95–101.

30. Eggermont JJ (2006) Cortical tonotopic map reorganization and its implications for treatment of tinnitus. Acta Otolaryngol Suppl: 9–12.

31. Eggermont JJ, Roberts LE (2004) The neuroscience of tinnitus. Trends Neurosci 27: 676–682.

32. Norena AJ, Eggermont JJ (2003) Changes in spontaneous neural activity immediately after an acoustic trauma: implications for neural correlates of tinnitus. Hear Res 183: 137–153.

33. Norena AJ, Moffat G, Blanc JL, Pezard L, Cazals Y (2010) Neural changes in the auditory cortex of awake guinea pigs after two tinnitus inducers: salicylate and acoustic trauma. Neuroscience 166: 1194–1209.

34. Weisz N, Muller S, Schlee W, Dohrmann K, Hartmann T, et al. (2007) The neural code of auditory phantom perception. J Neurosci 27: 1479–1484.

35. Foeller E, Vater M, Kossl M (2001) Laminar analysis of inhibition in the gerbil primary auditory cortex. J Assoc Res Otolaryngol 2: 279–296.

36. Horikawa J, Hosokawa Y, Kubota M, Nasu M, Taniguchi I (1996) Optical imaging of spatiotemporal patterns of glutamatergic excitation and GABAergic inhibition in the guinea-pig auditory cortex in vivo. J Physiol 497 (Pt 3): 629–638.

37. Middleton JW, Kiritani T, Pedersen C, Turner JG, Shepherd GM, et al. (2011) Mice with behavioral evidence of tinnitus exhibit dorsal cochlear nucleus hyperactivity because of decreased GABAergic inhibition. Proc Natl Acad Sci U S A 108: 7601–7606.

38. Kurt S, Moeller CK, Jeschke M, Schulze H (2008) Differential effects of iontophoretic application of the GABAA-antagonists bicuculline and gabazine on tone-evoked local field potentials in primary auditory cortex: interaction with ketamine anesthesia. Brain Res 1220: 58–69.

39. Browne CJ, Morley JJ, Parsons CH (2012) Tracking the Expression of Excitatory and Inhibitory Neurotransmission-Related Proteins and Neuroplasticity Markers after Noise Induced Hearing Loss. PLoS One 7: 11.

40. Kurt S, Deutscher A, Crook JM, Ohl FW, Budinger E, et al. (2008) Auditory cortical contrast enhancing by global winner-take-all inhibitory interactions. PLoS One 3: e1735.

41. Moeller CK, Kurt S, Happel MF, Schulze H (2010) Long-range effects of GABAergic inhibition in gerbil primary auditory cortex. Eur J Neurosci 31: 49–59.

42. Pinto DJ, Hartings JA, Brumberg JC, Simons DJ (2003) Cortical damping: analysis of thalamocortical response transformations in rodent barrel cortex. Cereb Cortex 13: 33–44.

43. Yang S, Weiner BD, Zhang LS, Cho S, Bao S (2011) Homeostatic plasticity drives tinnitus perception in an animal model. Proc Natl Acad Sci U S A 108: 14974–14979.

44. Flor H, Hoffmann D, Struve M, Diesch E (2004) Auditory discrimination training for the treatment of tinnitus. Appl Psychophysiol Biofeedback 29: 113–120.

6

Short and Intense Tailor-Made Notched Music Training against Tinnitus: The Tinnitus Frequency Matters

Henning Teismann[1]*, Hidehiko Okamoto[1,2], Christo Pantev[1]

1 Institute for Biomagnetism and Biosignalanalysis, University of Muenster, Muenster, Germany, 2 Department of Integrative Physiology, National Institute for Physiological Sciences, Okazaki, Japan

Abstract

Tinnitus is one of the most common diseases in industrialized countries. Here, we developed and evaluated a short-term (5 subsequent days) and intensive (6 hours/day) tailor-made notched music training (TMNMT) for patients suffering from chronic, tonal tinnitus. We evaluated (i) the TMNMT efficacy in terms of behavioral and magnetoencephalographic outcome measures for two matched patient groups with either low ($\leq$8 kHz, N = 10) or high ($>$8 kHz, N = 10) tinnitus frequencies, and the (ii) persistency of the TMNMT effects over the course of a four weeks post-training phase. The results indicated that the short-term intensive TMNMT took effect in patients with tinnitus frequencies $\leq$8 kHz: subjective tinnitus loudness, tinnitus-related distress, and tinnitus-related auditory cortex evoked activity were significantly reduced after TMNMT completion. However, in the patients with tinnitus frequencies $>$8 kHz, significant changes were not observed. Interpreted in their entirety, the results also indicated that the induced changes in auditory cortex evoked neuronal activity and tinnitus loudness were not persistent, encouraging the application of the TMNMT as a longer-term training. The findings are essential in guiding the intended transfer of this neuro-scientific treatment approach into routine clinical practice.

Editor: Michael A. Fox, Virginia Commonwealth University Medical Center, United States of America

Funding: This work was supported by grants from the Deutsche Forschungsgemeinschaft (Pa 392/10-3, Pa 392/13-1), the Tinnitus Research Initiative, the Japan Society for the Promotion of Science for Young Scientists, and the Strategic Research Program for Brain Sciences (Development of Biomarker Candidates for Social Behavior). The funders had no role in study design, data collection and analysis, decision to publish, or preparation of the manuscript.

Competing Interests: The authors have declared that no competing interests exist.

* E-mail: h.teismann@uni-muenster.de

Introduction

Chronic tinnitus is a disease that deserves attention and study, because to this date there is no standard cure. Chronic tinnitus is one of the most common auditory disorders, currently affecting 10 to 15% of the adult general population [1]. Unfortunately, patients often fail to cope with or compensate their tinnitus, and then their quality of life can be considerably limited. Many patients even exhibit severe co-morbid disorders like insomnia or depression [2].

Tinnitus is likely a result of maladaptive plasticity in the central auditory pathway [3]. The original tinnitus signal is most often triggered by hearing loss. Based on auditory neural input deprivation, the excitation-inhibition balance in the central auditory pathway is disturbed, most probably by the weakening of inhibitory networks. Consequently, maladaptive brain changes lead to neuronal hyperactivity, increased neuronal synchrony, and possibly burst firing. All these neuronal phenomena have been shown to be associated with the tinnitus perception [4].

In order to effectively cure tinnitus, the neurons that underlie this auditory phantom perception need to be identified and targeted. It has been argued that the target neurons are those coding frequencies affected by hearing loss, for instance because tinnitus spectra and the spectra of the most effective tinnitus maskers resemble frequency regions affected by hearing loss [5,6]. However, even though most tinnitus patients indeed have hearing loss as detectable by a standard audiometric examination, there also are tinnitus patients who have normal standard hearing thresholds [7], or patients with hearing loss in whom there is no

clear relationship between tinnitus pitch and audiogram profile [8]. Furthermore, many people with hearing loss do not have tinnitus.

An essential supplement to measuring the hearing threshold is the determination of the perceived tinnitus pitch. In patients with *tonal* tinnitus, usually the "tinnitus frequency" (i.e. the frequency that sounds most similar to the tinnitus [9]) can be matched, and it has been demonstrated that auditory cortex neurons coding the tinnitus frequency are involved into tinnitus perception [10,11,12]. Thus, these neurons are a potential treatment target. However, it should be noted that the reliable determination of the tinnitus frequency is not at all trivial: a high-frequency audiometer covering the frequency range up to 16 kHz [13] should be utilized, pitfalls like octave confusions need to be considered, and the reliability of matching increases when patients are trained [14].

As mentioned before, there is no standard cure for tinnitus [4]. One major problem is that there are several different treatment target candidates in the brain (e.g. auditory cortex, thalamus, dorsal/ventral cochlear nuclei, inferior colliculus, cochlear nerve, or the limbic system [15]). Another problem is to hit potential targets with the necessary precision (e.g. using tools like transcranial magnetic stimulation, or transcranial direct current stimulation [16]). However, it appears plausible to assume that the auditory cortex would principally be a treatment target, because the tinnitus percept arises here, and changes in auditory cortex must exist when tinnitus is present [17].

The seemingly most obvious avenue to target tinnitus is via the auditory modality, using for instance broadband noise to mask and

Table 1. Patient characteristics and baseline values of outcome measures broken by patient group.

Patient groups	Patient characteristics	Values [mean ± sd]
Tinnitus frequency ≤8 kHz	Age [years]	32.2±8.2
	Tinnitus duration [years]	5.1±6.4
	Tinnitus-related distress [0 – 40 points]	8.5±6.8
	General psychopathological distress [0 – 90 points]	21.7±13.7
	Subjective tinnitus loudness [0 – 100 points]	61.2±11.8
Tinnitus frequency >8 kHz	Age [years]	34.4±9.1
	Tinnitus duration [years]	5.8±4.9
	Tinnitus-related distress [0 – 40 points]	6.7±5.9
	General psychopathological distress [0 – 90 points]	33.0±30.0
	Subjective tinnitus loudness [0 – 100 points]	51.7±18.8

habituate the tinnitus perception [18]. However, auditory stimulation treatments might often be too unspecific, i.e. they do not take into account parameters of the individual patient profile, such as the tinnitus sound quality, the tinnitus frequency, or the hearing threshold.

In a previous study [12,19], assuming that maladaptive plastic changes generally are reversible [20,21,22], we developed and evaluated a customized auditory stimulation treatment strategy (tailor-made notched music training (TMNMT)), which individually targets auditory cortical areas coding the tinnitus frequency. We succeeded to reverse maladaptive plasticity processes associated with the tinnitus perception to a certain degree, probably by reducing the excitability of auditory neurons that coded the tinnitus frequency, resulting in subjective tinnitus loudness reduction. Similar findings were also reported by [13].

However, our previous study raised several critical questions. The answers to these questions would have implications for the application of this neuro-scientific treatment approach during routine clinical practice. For instance, an important query is whether the TMNMT effects remain persistent over time after training cessation. Another relevant issue concerns patient profile variables that may influence TMNMT efficacy. Eventually, it remains to be investigated how long the TMNMT has to last until effects become measurable and noticeable.

In the present study, employing behavioral and magnetoencephalographic (MEG) outcome measures, we investigated (i) the efficacy of a short and more intensive variant of the TMNMT (i.e. 24 hours of notched music distributed over 5 subsequent days), (ii) the durability of the induced TMNMT effects (by employing a follow-up observation phase of 31 days), and crucially, (iii) the relevancy of the tinnitus frequency for TMNMT efficacy in two groups of matched tinnitus patients with chronic tonal tinnitus and either low (i.e. ≤8 kHz) or high (i.e. >8 kHz) tinnitus frequencies.

Results

The two patient groups that were compared in terms of TMNMT efficacy (tinnitus frequency ≤8 kHz (N = 10) vs. tinnitus frequency >8 kHz (N = 10)) did not significantly differ in age (t(18) = −0.57, p = 0.58), tinnitus duration (t(18) = −0.27, p = 0.79), general psychopathological distress (as assessed with the SCL-90-R inventory [23]) (t(18) = −1.4, p = 0.162), and hearing loss (there was neither a significant main effect of group (F(1,18) = 0.1, p = 0.76), nor were there significant interactions of group with ear (F(1,18) = 0.21, p = 0.65), frequency (F(12,216) = 1.13, p = 0.34), or

ear *and* frequency (F(12,216) = 0.52, p = 0.90)). Furthermore, before TMNMT onset (i.e. at baseline) tinnitus-related distress (as assessed with the Tinnitus Questionnaire [24]) (t(18) = 0.63, p = 0.54) and tinnitus loudness diary values (t(18) = 1.35, p = 0.19) did not significantly differ between groups (Table 1). Therefore, the two groups were comparable regarding both relevant tinnitus-related characteristics as well as baseline values of the dependent variables. Retrospectively, neither total music listening times (t(18) = 1.07, p = 0.299) nor subjective music enjoyment (t(18) = −0.28, p = 0.785) did significantly differ between the two patient groups.

To assess effects of the TMNMT on tinnitus perception and tinnitus-related evoked auditory cortex activity, as well as to study the persistency of such potential effects, we normalized the values of the dependent variables obtained at the points in time **(i)** shortly after TMNMT completion, **(ii)** 3 days after TMNMT completion, **(iii)** 17 days after TMNMT completion, and **(iv)** 31 days after TMNMT completion relative to the baseline values (formula: (values at **(i)**, **(ii)**, **(iii)**, and **(iv)**/values at baseline)-1) separately for the two patient groups, and tested whether the normalized values at the different points in time were significantly different from zero (if so, there would be a significant change relative to baseline) by means of planned comparisons. To account for multiple comparisons, we controlled the false discovery rate at 5 % [25]. t-values and corresponding p-values are summarized in Table 2.

As shown in Figure 1, for the patients with tinnitus frequencies ≤8 kHz, **(i)** shortly after TMNMT completion normalized tinnitus loudness was significantly reduced (t = −2.3, p<0.03). There were no significant changes in tinnitus-related distress (Figure 2), normalized N1m ratio, and normalized auditory steady-state response (ASSR) ratio (Figure 3). Moreover, there was no significant difference in normalized loudness diary values before vs. after TMNMT units (t(9) = 0.58, p = 0.29). **(ii)** 3 days after TMNMT completion, there was a significant reduction in normalized N1m ratio (t = −2.14, p<.02) (Figure 3). There were no significant changes in normalized tinnitus loudness, normalized tinnitus-related distress, and normalized ASSR ratio (Figures 1, 2, and 3). **(iii)** 17 days after TMNMT completion, normalized tinnitus-related distress (t = −2.11, p<0.02) (Figure 2), normalized tinnitus loudness (t = −2.15, p<0.02) (Figure 1), and normalized N1m ratio (t = −1.97, p<0.03) (Figure 3) were significantly reduced. There was no significant change in normalized ASSR ratio (Figure 3). **(iv)** 31 days after TMNMT completion, normalized tinnitus-related distress was significantly reduced (t = −2.38, p<0.01) (Figure 2). There was no significant change in normalized tinnitus loudness (Figure 1).

Table 2. Statistical t- (df = 9) and (unilateral) p-values of the calculated planned comparisons broken by patient group and as functions of outcome measure and time point.

Patient groups	Outcome measures	Shortly after TMNMT[a]	3 days after TMNMT	17 days after TMNMT	31 days after TMNMT
Tinnitus frequency ≤8 kHz	Tinntus-related distress [t (p)]	−1.99 (0.0385)	−1.52 (0.065)	−2.11 (0.0175)*	−2.38 (0.0085)*
	Tinnitus loudness [t (p)]	−2.3 (0.0235)*	−0.96 (0.1805)	−2.15 (0.016)*	−1.12 (0.132)
	N1m [t (p)]	−0.34 (0.372)	−2.14 (0.0165)*	−1.97 (0.0245)*	n.m.[1]
	ASSR [t (p)]	−0.03 (0.488)	0.43 (0.332)	0.39 (0.349)	n.m.
Tinnitus frequency >8 kHz	Tinntus−related distress [t (p)]	−0.06 (0.4775)	0.48 (0.3225)	0.47 (0.317)	0.99 (0.161)
	Tinnitus loudness [t (p)]	−0.69 (0.2535)	0.2 (0.42)	1.12 (0.1325)	−0.67 (0.252)
	N1m	n.a.[2]	n.a.	n.a.	n.a.
	ASSR	n.a.	n.a.	n.a.	n.a.

[a] Tailor-made notched music training.
*Significant; false discovery rate controlled at 5 %. [1] Not measured. [2] Not analyzable.

For the patients with tinnitus frequencies >8 kHz, there were no significant changes in normalized tinnitus loudness or normalized tinnitus-related distress at any of the four points in time (Figures 1 and 2). Due to technical limitations (see methods section), N1m and ASSR data are not available for this group.

Discussion

For the first time, we succeeded to demonstrate that short and intensive TMNMT could effectively reduce subjective tinnitus loudness and tinnitus-related distress. Crucially, we found this effect only in patients with tinnitus frequencies ≤8 kHz. While the loudness reduction effect was already significant shortly after TMNMT completion, then fluctuated and vanished, the distress

reduction was only a trend at this point in time, which then however manifested and stabilized circa two weeks after TMNMT completion. Moreover, in patients with tinnitus frequencies ≤8 kHz, there was a significant N1m source strength reduction three days after TMNMT completion, which seems to have slowly decayed, yet which still outlasted until the next MEG measurement two weeks later.

The loudness reduction effect observed here in tinnitus patients with tinnitus frequencies ≤8 kHz replicates the effect seen in our previous study [12,19], however on a different, much shorter time scale. Thus, it seems to be possible to significantly alleviate subjective tinnitus loudness by listening to tailor-made notched music over the course of only a few days, when the daily listening time is considerable. Therefore, the TMNMT becomes potentially feasible for many tinnitus patients.

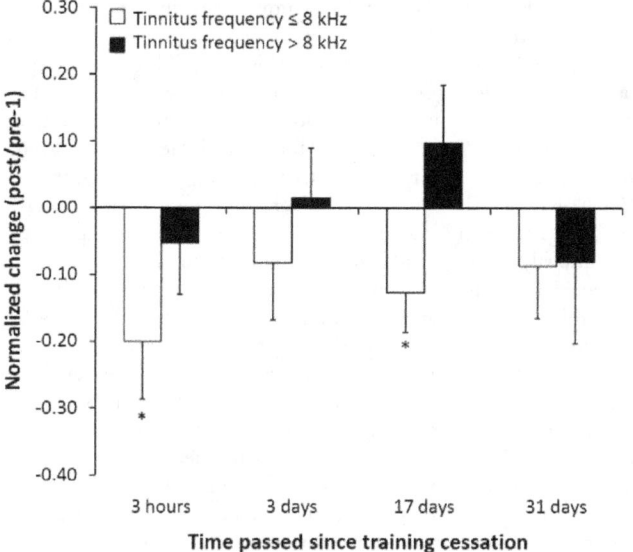

Figure 1. Tinnitus loudness ratios. Normalized tinnitus loudness changes relative to baseline at four time points after training completion for both patient groups. White bars represent the low tinnitus frequency (≤8 kHz) group, black bars represent the high tinnitus frequency (>8 kHz) group. Asterisks denote significant changes, the error bars denote standard errors of the mean. Positive values indicate aggravation, and negative values indicate alleviation.

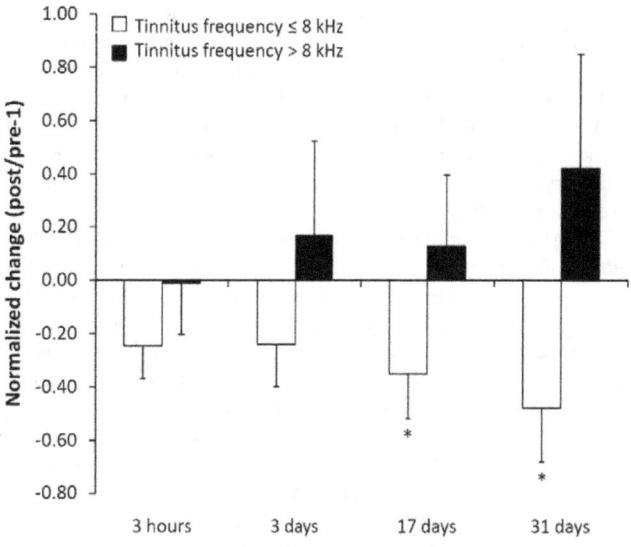

Figure 2. Tinnitus-related distress ratios. Normalized tinnitus-related distress changes relative to baseline at four time points after training completion for both patient groups (arrangement according to Figure 1).

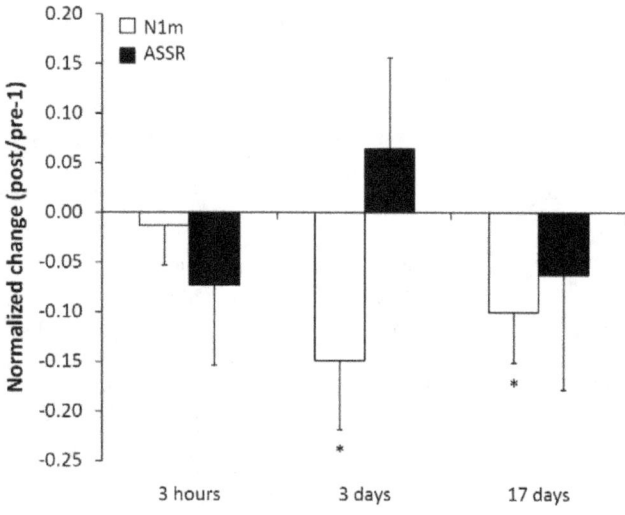

Figure 3. N1m and ASSR source strength ratios. Normalized N1m and auditory steady-state response (ASSR) changes relative to baseline at three time points after training completion for the patient group characterized by tinnitus frequencies ≤8 kHz. White bars represent N1m source strength, black bars represent ASSR source strength. Asterisks denote significant changes, the error bars denote standard errors of the mean. Positive values indicate increment, and negative values indicate decrement. Please note that for the patient group characterized by tinnitus frequencies >8 kHz auditory evoked fields are not available due to technical limitations of the MEG sound delivery system (limit =8 kHz).

It arises the question what are the neuronal mechanisms that could underlie the observed tinnitus loudness reduction effect. We suggest that TMNMT would have induced a circumscribed auditory functional deafferentation [26] or transient sensory input deprivation, respectively. This deprivation may have rather rapidly led to a reduction of excitability of auditory cortex neurons coding the notched frequencies, among them the tinnitus frequency. The excitability reduction might have been caused by the (transient) strengthening of locally weakened inhibitory impact [27] in the auditory cortex of the patients [12]. For instance, there is evidence in adult rat barrel cortex that inhibitory synapse density could be dominantly and proportionally (relative to excitatory synapse density) increased within 24 hours of sensory stimulation [28,29].

The neurons coding the tinnitus frequency are likely involved into tinnitus perception [11,12,19,27]. However, given that the patients studied here did not exhibit severe hearing loss (and therefore vast tonotopic reorganization would not be expected), these neurons could probably still be excited via their original thalamo-cortical tuning (in this case by auditory input corresponding to the tinnitus frequency, which was used as test stimulus during the MEG measurements). At the same time, it would be possible to inhibit these neurons via their neighbors in frequency space. Thus, when the patients were listening to their notched music, due to the notch the neurons coding the tinnitus frequency would have been hardly excited. Their neighbors, however, would have been excited strongly, and they could have projected lateral or co-tuned inhibition [30] to the target neurons coding the tinnitus frequency. Over time, this type of stimulation could have led to reduction in the excitability of auditory cortex neurons coding the tinnitus frequency, and eventually to changes in tinnitus perception.

Importantly, the loudness reduction effect did not seem to be persistent: already 3 days after TMNMT completion, it was no longer measurable. We interpret this only short-lasting effect duration as indication that the induced plastic changes were merely functional and therefore transient in their nature – to elicit more stable and persistent effects, i.e. large-scale structural changes [31], the training needs to be performed over a longer period of time, presumably at least several weeks or even months. This assumption is also strongly supported by studies investigating rehabilitative training approaches for different diseases thought to be associated with maladaptive brain plasticity, for instance focal hand dystonia [20], and phantom limb pain [21,32].

The tinnitus-related distress reduction effect observed here in tinnitus patients with frequencies ≤8 kHz exhibits a rather different time course than the loudness reduction effect. While there is merely a reduction trend directly after the TMNMT, the effect becomes significantly larger and more stable over time. At first glance, this development appears somewhat surprising. However, it should be considered that the tinnitus questionnaire measured emotional and cognitive distress. The questionnaire items target tinnitus-related cognitions, thoughts, and feelings, whose alteration may need some time to reach the conscious level. Hence, from a psychological point of view, the delayed distress reduction effect may reflect the subjects' awakening that (i) the TMNMT indeed had been effective (e.g. given that the tinnitus became louder again sometime after TMNMT completion), that (ii) the TMNMT could be repeated anytime, and that (iii) it could be performed over a longer period of time, potentially increasing its effectiveness.

An additional crucial finding was that the TMNMT efficacy depended on the tinnitus frequency. Even though we had relatively amplified high frequency music energy during the filtering process (Figure 4), and despite having utilized a headphone that reliably transduced very high frequencies, the TMNMT was on average only effective for patients with tinnitus frequencies ≤8 kHz, but not for patients with frequencies above this value. From a theoretical viewpoint, this finding is plausible for several reasons: (i) the sensitivity of the human cochlea is comparably low for very high frequencies [33]. Thus, much larger sound pressure levels must be used to make very high frequencies audible. (ii) Age-related hearing loss progresses from the highest to the lower frequencies [33]. Hence, this factor adds to the cochlea's general relative insensitivity for very high frequencies. (iii) Music usually contains relatively little very high frequency energy. (iv) Eventually, during listening the patients might involuntarily have paid most attention to the rather low frequencies (for instance to the voices of the singers), which are more relevant for music perception and enjoyment than the rather high frequencies. Taken together, these arguments demonstrate that it would be challenging to effectively suppress the activity of target neurons coding very high tinnitus frequencies, and it remains to be investigated whether the TMNMT could principally work for tinnitus patients with tinnitus frequencies >8 kHz. On the one hand, it appears reasonable to assume that for such cases the treatment stimulus should contain a sufficient amount of high frequency energy. On the other hand, we presume that it would be important that the treatment stimulus and strategy remained interesting or motivating enough to activate attention- and reward-related networks of the brain thought to promote plastic change. One possibility would be to further enrich the music spectrum in the high frequency range, for instance by adding high-pass noise.

The results showed a significant reduction in N1m source strength for tinnitus patients with tinnitus frequencies ≤8 kHz

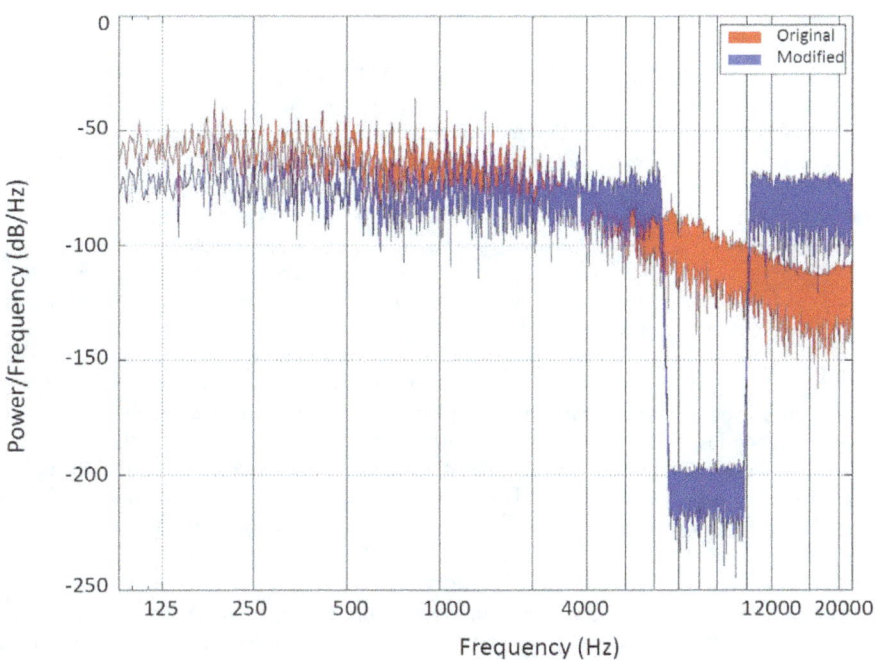

Figure 4. Music spectra. Exemplary frequency spectra of original (red) and modified (i.e. flattened and notched) (blue) music pieces. Here, the notch is centered at 7100 Hz.

(Figure 3). Notably, this effect was not significant shortly after TMNMT completion, but three days later, with effect size becoming lesser 2 weeks later. Basically, this reduction effect replicates an effect seen in our previous study [12,19]. The observed decay of the effect over the course of the two weeks following TMNMT completion suggests that the short-term training-induced changes were not persistent.

Based on our previous findings [12,19], we presumed that tinnitus frequency-evoked N1m amplitude change and tinnitus loudness change were associated. Yet, in the present study, the N1m amplitude change did not correspond as well to the tinnitus loudness change as in the previous study, possibly because subjective tinnitus loudness does not only depend on neural activity in auditory cortex [3,4]. Nonetheless, there is evidence that listening to notched music can reduce notch center-frequency evoked (here: tinnitus frequency-evoked) N1m amplitude on very short [26] and rather long time scales [12,19]. Further, listening to music (or noise) that is notched around the tinnitus frequency can alleviate tinnitus loudness and annoyance [12,13,19]. Still, the relationship between tinnitus frequency-evoked N1m amplitude change and tinnitus loudness change (or changes in other aspects of tinnitus perception) may be rather complex. For instance, it is known that both N1m amplitude [34] and tinnitus perception [35] are sensitive to parameters such as alertness, attention focus, or mood, and the impact of these parameters on N1m amplitude and tinnitus loudness may not necessarily be equivalent. Moreover, tinnitus perception is multifaceted, and the *variability of changes between different aspects of tinnitus perception* (e.g. loudness, awareness, annoyance, or distress) is presumably higher on rather short compared to rather long time scales. Thus, it is less likely to find a simple correlation between change in tinnitus perception and change in auditory cortex neural activity on a rather short time scale. However, regarding these arguments and our previous findings [12,19], and considering the present observation that the overall time courses of tinnitus frequency-evoked N1m amplitude

change and tinnitus loudness change (i.e. reduction and return to baseline) are in line, we suggest that the reduction of neural activity in auditory cortex could be closely related to subjective tinnitus loudness alleviation.

In our previous study [12,19], in addition to the N1m effect, we had observed a significant ASSR source strength reduction induced by the long-term TMNMT, which was positively correlated with the tinnitus loudness reduction. Yet, a significant ASSR change was not found in the present study. However, the arguments presented above regarding the N1m basically apply to the ASSR as well. Moreover, it may be that plastic changes in the primary auditory cortex (as reflected by ASSR) would need longer to develop than corresponding changes in non-primary auditory cortex (as reflected by N1m), particularly if top-down modulation is expected to play a critical role. During the present study, the patients had been instructed to listen to their training music with as much pleasure as possible, and therefore top-down modulation probably has taken place. Furthermore, while primary auditory cortex activity is most strongly modulated by bottom-up input, non-primary auditory cortex activity is strongly shaped by both bottom-up *and* top-down input [36]. Moreover, there is evidence indicating that non-primary auditory cortex may be more plastic than primary auditory cortex [37,38]. Eventually, it has been argued [37] that attention-related modulations in primary auditory cortex may be *driven* by non-primary auditory cortex attention-related changes, given that the alterations are more robust here [38,39].

In conclusion, this study demonstrates that it was possible to (i) transiently alleviate subjective tinnitus loudness, and to (ii) more steadily reduce perceived tinnitus-related distress in patients with chronic tonal tinnitus, not more than moderate hearing loss, and tinnitus frequencies ≤8 kHz by means of short and intensive TMNMT. Neurophysiological TMNMT effects were measurable in non-primary auditory cortical areas. The direction (i.e. reduction) and the time course (i.e. build-up and decay) of neuronal activity change induced by the training imply that the short-term TMNMT could partly and transiently reverse mal-adaptive plastic changes contributing to the tinnitus perception. Taken together, towards the goal of transferring the TMNMT approach into routine clinical practice, the findings motivate (i) the administration of the TMNMT as a long-term treatment, (ii) the targeted advancement of the TMNMT for patients with tinnitus frequencies >8 kHz, and (iii) the systematic utilization of attention-, emotion-, and motivation-related brain networks for the purpose of TMNMT efficacy.

Materials and Methods

Participants

We recruited 24 adult patients with chronic (≥3 months) tonal (i.e. peep- or whistle-like) tinnitus, and without severe hearing loss (≤50 dB HL between 125 and 16000 Hz, measured in octave steps for frequencies up to 1 kHz, and in ½ octave steps for frequencies above 1 kHz, utilizing the Orbiter 922DH clinical audiometer (GN Otometrics, Denmark)). 20 patients completed the 5 days TMNMT. 4 patients (2 patients per group) dropped out during the TMNMT due to underestimation of participation effort. The completers were divided into two groups based on their tinnitus frequencies: (1) patients with tinnitus frequencies ≤8 kHz (N = 10),

and (2) patients with tinnitus frequencies >8 kHz (N = 10). The value 8 kHz was chosen in order to achieve comparability to our previous long-term TMNMT study [12], where we had included only patients with tinnitus frequencies ≤8 kHz.

In order to reduce possible placebo effects, the patients were explained before study onset that they would randomly receive one out of two treatments: either (1) the target music training, or (2) the alternative music training. In fact, all patients received the target music training (i.e. training (1)). The alternative music training (training (2)) was not administered. The patients were informed that in case of both trainings the music would be modified in an individual (and audible) way based on the tinnitus frequency. However, patients were not told how exactly the music would be modified in any of the two training versions to guarantee complete blinding. After completion of the study, the patients were debriefed. Patients gave written informed consent for the participation in the study. The study was performed in accordance with the Declaration of Helsinki. The study was approved by the Ethics Commission of the Medical Faculty, University of Muenster, Germany.

Music modification

The patients provided 6 hours of their most enjoyable music in CD audio quality (sampling rate 44100 Hz, 16 bit, stereo). In a first processing step, the music energy spectrum was digitally

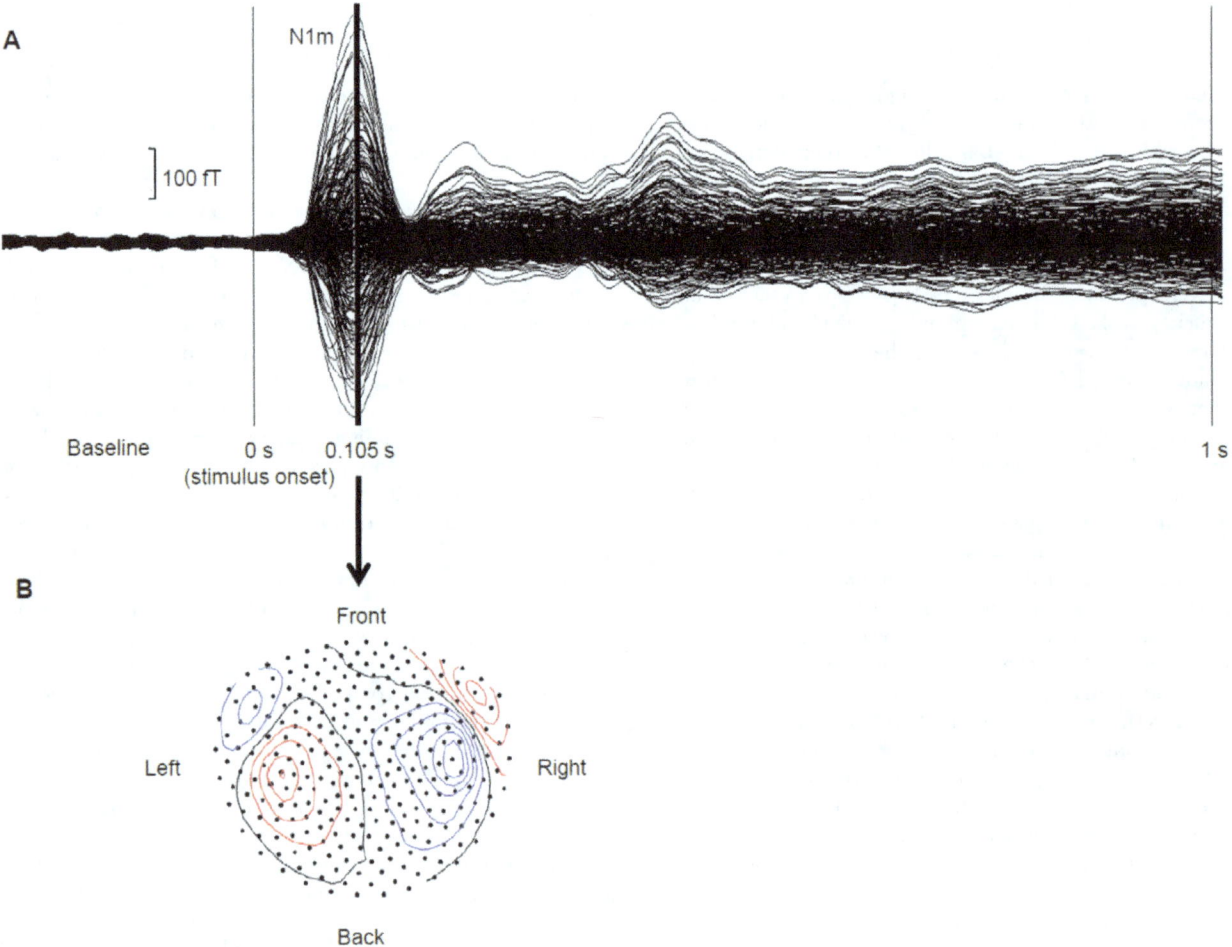

Figure 5. Auditory evoked field. A Example of a 30 Hz low-pass filtered auditory evoked field exhibiting a clear N1m response peaking 0.1 s after stimulus onset. **B** Example of a contour plot corresponding to the 0.01 s time interval prior to the N1m peak shown in A. The plot displays clear dipolar patterns over left and right hemispheres.

"flattened" by redistributing energy from lower to very high frequency ranges. In a second processing step, the frequency band of one octave width centered at the individual tinnitus frequency was digitally removed from the music energy spectrum by means of a Butterworth notch filter (bandwidth: (tinnitus frequency/$\sqrt{2}$) to (tinnitus frequency $\times \sqrt{2}$); order: 150) (Figure 4).

Music training

The TMNMT was performed over the course of 5 subsequent days. The patients were instructed to listen to their training music for 3 hours on days 1 and 5, and for 6 hours (2 times 3 hours) on days 2, 3, and 4. Patients listened to the notched music via supplied closed headphones (Beyerdynamic DT-770, 32 Ohm Edition) and with comfortable loudness (patient-driven). Listening times had to be documented on a daily basis.

Behavior measurements

Tinnitus-related distress was measured with the E+C subscale of the German version of the Tinnitus Questionnaire [24] (i) shortly before TMNMT onset, (ii) shortly after TMNMT completion, and (iii) 3 days, (iii) 17 days, and (iv) 31 days after TMNMT completion.

Moreover, the subjective tinnitus loudness status was measured by means of a visual analogue scale (VAS) throughout the study on a daily basis, beginning 14 days prior to TMNMT onset (familiarization phase), and ending 31 days after TMNMT completion (tinnitus loudness diary). During (i) the TMNMT, (ii) the 7 days prior to TMNMT onset, and (iii) the 9 days following TMNMT offset, subjective tinnitus loudness was measured 4 times per day at times of day that corresponded to the times before and after music listening during the training phase (e.g. at 8:00, 11:15, 14:00 and 17:15). At the remaining days, the loudness was measured once per day (always at the same time of day, e.g. always at 8:00). Subjects were instructed to perform the loudness estimation always at one and the same quiet location. Moreover, during the training phase subjects were supposed to wait for 15 minutes after finishing a music listening unit before they made the loudness measurement.

MEG measurements

Auditory evoked fields (AEF) were measured by means of a 275 channel MEG system (Omega 275, CTF, VSM MedTech Ltd.) in a silent magnetically shielded room. However, for patients with tinnitus frequencies >8 kHz, the AEFs could not be measured with sufficient quality, which was a consequence of the spectral sound transmission properties of the tubal system utilized to deliver the sound stimuli to the patients' ears (frequencies >8 kHz are strongly attenuated). Therefore, for this group AEFs are not available. The baseline MEG measurement took place directly before training onset. Course measurements were performed (i) shortly (approx. 3 hours) after training completion, (ii) 3 days after training completion, and (iii) 17 days after training completion. To evoke auditory fields, two different sound stimuli were delivered

randomly to either the left or the right ears of the patients. The carrier frequency of one stimulus corresponded to a patient's individual tinnitus frequency. The carrier frequency of the other stimulus was 500 Hz (control stimulus), which was distinctly separate from the tinnitus frequencies of all included subjects. The tinnitus frequency stimulus evoked activity from a cortical region contributing to the tinnitus perception, while the control stimulus evoked activity from a cortical area not involved in the tinnitus perception.

The stimuli had duration of 1.0 s. The initial 0.3 s were sinusoidal, whereas the remaining 0.7 s were amplitude-modulated with a modulation frequency of 40 Hz and a modulation depth of 100 %. The utilization of such stimuli allows the recording of both clean transient N1m and sustained auditory steady-state responses (ASSR) simultaneously [40]. The loudness of the control stimulus was set to 45 dB above individual hearing threshold. The tinnitus frequency stimulus was matched in loudness to the control stimulus prior to the baseline measurement. The power difference between the two test stimuli was kept identical across all course measurements. The sound onset asynchrony was randomized between 2.0 and 3.0 s.

The contour maps of both N1m (Figure 5) and ASSR responses displayed clear dipolar patterns over both hemispheres, motivating the use of a single dipole model for source analysis. For N1m analysis, the grand-averaged magnetic fields were baseline corrected and 30 Hz low-pass filtered. The 0.01 s time window prior to the N1m peak was used for equivalent current dipole estimations (one dipole per hemisphere), and the maximal N1m source strength for each condition (tinnitus frequency vs. control frequency) and each hemisphere was calculated by using the source space projection technique [41]. For ASSR analysis, the grand-averaged magnetic fields were baseline corrected and 32 to 48 Hz band-pass filtered. The source space projection technique (based on N1m sources) was used to calculate the average ASSR source strengths across the time interval from 0.7 to 1.0 s for each condition (tinnitus frequency vs. control frequency) and each hemisphere.

In order to eliminate effects of head position differences on source strength within subjects between course measurements, we calculated ratios between the source strengths evoked by the tinnitus frequency stimulus and the source strengths evoked by the control stimulus.

Acknowledgments

We are grateful to Andreas Wollbrink, Karin Berning, Ute Trompeter, and Hildegard Deitermann for technical assistance.

Author Contributions

Conceived and designed the experiments: HT HO CP. Performed the experiments: HT. Analyzed the data: HT. Contributed reagents/materials/analysis tools: HO. Wrote the paper: HT HO CP.

References

1. Heller AJ (2003) Classification and epidemiology of tinnitus. Otolaryngol Clin North Am 36: 239–248.
2. Dobie RA (2003) Depression and tinnitus. Otolaryngol Clin North Am 36: 383–388.
3. Eggermont JJ, Roberts LE (2004) The neuroscience of tinnitus. Trends Neurosci 27: 676–682.
4. Rauschecker JP, Leaver AM, Muhlau M (2010) Tuning out the noise: limbic-auditory interactions in tinnitus. Neuron 66: 819–826.
5. Norena AJ (2010) An integrative model of tinnitus based on a central gain controlling neural sensitivity. Neurosci Biobehav Rev 35: 1089–1109.
6. Roberts LE, Eggermont JJ, Caspary DM, Shore SE, Melcher JR, et al. (2010) Ringing ears: the neuroscience of tinnitus. J Neurosci 30: 14972–14979.
7. Kim DK, Park SN, Park KH, Choi HG, Jeon EJ, et al. (2010) Clinical characteristics and audiological significance of spontaneous otoacoustic emissions in tinnitus patients with normal hearing. J Laryngol Otol 125: 246–250.
8. Pan T, Tyler RS, Ji H, Coelho C, Gehringer AK, et al. (2009) The relationship between tinnitus pitch and the audiogram. Int J Audiol 48: 277–294.
9. Henry JA, Meikle MB (2000) Psychoacoustic measures of tinnitus. J Am Acad Audiol 11: 138–155.

10. Diesch E, Struve M, Rupp A, Ritter S, Hulse M, et al. (2004) Enhancement of steady-state auditory evoked magnetic fields in tinnitus. Eur J Neurosci 19: 1093–1104.

11. Muhlnickel W, Elbert T, Taub E, Flor H (1998) Reorganization of auditory cortex in tinnitus. Proc Natl Acad Sci U S A 95: 10340–10343.

12. Okamoto H, Stracke H, Stoll W, Pantev C (2010) Listening to tailor-made notched music reduces tinnitus loudness and tinnitus-related auditory cortex activity. Proc Natl Acad Sci U S A 107: 1207–1210.

13. Lugli M, Romani R, Ponzi S, Bacciu S, Parmigiani S (2009) The windowed sound therapy: a new empirical approach for an effectiv personalized treatment of tinnitus. Int Tinnitus J 15: 51–61.

14. Moore BC, Vinay, Sandhya (2010) The relationship between tinnitus pitch and the edge frequency of the audiogram in individuals with hearing impairment and tonal tinnitus. Hear Res 261: 51–56.

15. Langguth B, Salvi R, Elgoyhen AB (2009) Emerging pharmacotherapy of tinnitus. Expert Opin Emerg Drugs 14: 687–702.

16. Lefaucheur JP (2009) Methods of therapeutic cortical stimulation. Neurophysiol Clin 39: 1–14.

17. Eggermont JJ (2006) Cortical tonotopic map reorganization and its implications for treatment of tinnitus. Acta Otolaryngol Suppl. pp 9–12.

18. Jastreboff PJ (1990) Phantom auditory perception (tinnitus): mechanisms of generation and perception. Neurosci Res 8: 221–254.

19. Stracke H, Okamoto H, Pantev C (2010) Customized notched music training reduces tinnitus loudness. Commun Integr Biol 3: 274–277.

20. Candia V, Elbert T, Altenmuller E, Rau H, Schafer T, et al. (1999) Constraint-induced movement therapy for focal hand dystonia in musicians. Lancet 353: 42.

21. Flor H, Elbert T, Knecht S, Wienbruch C, Pantev C, et al. (1995) Phantom-limb pain as a perceptual correlate of cortical reorganization following arm amputation. Nature 375: 482–484.

22. Giraux P, Sirigu A, Schneider F, Dubernard JM (2001) Cortical reorganization in motor cortex after graft of both hands. Nat Neurosci 4: 691–692.

23. Hardt J, Gerbershagen HU, Franke P (2000) The symptom check-list, SCL-90-R: its use and characteristics in chronic pain patients. Eur J Pain 4: 137–148.

24. Goebel G, Hiller W (1994) [The tinnitus questionnaire. A standard instrument for grading the degree of tinnitus. Results of a multicenter study with the tinnitus questionnaire]. HNO 42: 166–172.

25. Benjamini Y, Hochberg Y (1995) Controlling the False Discovery Rate - a Practical and Powerful Approach to Multiple Testing. Journal of the Royal Statistical Society Series B-Methodological 57: 289–300.

26. Pantev C, Wollbrink A, Roberts LE, Engelien A, Lutkenhoner B (1999) Short-term plasticity of the human auditory cortex. Brain Res 842: 192–199.

27. Diesch E, Andermann M, Flor H, Rupp A (2010) Functional and structural aspects of tinnitus-related enhancement and suppression of auditory cortex activity. Neuroimage 50: 1545–1559.

28. Knott GW, Quairiaux C, Genoud C, Welker E (2002) Formation of dendritic spines with GABAergic synapses induced by whisker stimulation in adult mice. Neuron 34: 265–273.

29. Zito K, Svoboda K (2002) Activity-dependent synaptogenesis in the adult Mammalian cortex. Neuron 35: 1015–1017.

30. Oswald AM, Schiff ML, Reyes AD (2006) Synaptic mechanisms underlying auditory processing. Curr Opin Neurobiol 16: 371–376.

31. Feldman DE (2009) Synaptic mechanisms for plasticity in neocortex. Annu Rev Neurosci 32: 33–55.

32. Flor H, Elbert T, Muhlnickel W, Pantev C, Wienbruch C, et al. (1998) Cortical reorganization and phantom phenomena in congenital and traumatic upper-extremity amputees. Exp Brain Res 119: 205–212.

33. Fastl H, Zwicker E (2007) Psychoacoustics. Facts and models. Berlin Heidelberg: Springer.

34. Naatanen R, Picton T (1987) The N1 wave of the human electric and magnetic response to sound: a review and an analysis of the component structure. Psychophysiology 24: 375–425.

35. Møller A, Langguth B, DeRidder D, Kleinjung T, eds (2010) Textbook of tinnitus. New York: Springer.

36. Okamoto H, Stracke H, Bermudez P, Pantev C (2010) Sound Processing Hierarchy within Human Auditory Cortex. J Cogn Neurosci.

37. Jaaskelainen IP, Ahveninen J, Belliveau JW, Raij T, Sams M (2007) Short-term plasticity in auditory cognition. Trends Neurosci 30: 653–661.

38. Petkov CI, Kang X, Alho K, Bertrand O, Yund EW, et al. (2004) Attentional modulation of human auditory cortex. Nat Neurosci 7: 658–663.

39. Ahveninen J, Jaaskelainen IP, Raij T, Bonmassar G, Devore S, et al. (2006) Task-modulated "what" and "where" pathways in human auditory cortex. Proc Natl Acad Sci U S A 103: 14608–14613.

40. Engelien A, Schulz M, Ross B, Arolt V, Pantev C (2000) A combined functional in vivo measure for primary and secondary auditory cortices. Hear Res 148: 153–160.

41. Tesche CD, Uusitalo MA, Ilmoniemi RJ, Huotilainen M, Kajola M, et al. (1995) Signal-space projections of MEG data characterize both distributed and well-localized neuronal sources. Electroencephalogr Clin Neurophysiol 95: 189–200.

7

Psychoacoustic Tinnitus Loudness and Tinnitus-Related Distress Show Different Associations with Oscillatory Brain Activity

Tobias Balkenhol, Elisabeth Wallhäusser-Franke, Wolfgang Delb*

Department of Phoniatrics and Audiology, Medical Faculty Mannheim, Heidelberg University, Mannheim, Germany

Abstract

Background: The phantom auditory perception of subjective tinnitus is associated with aberrant brain activity as evidenced by magneto- and electroencephalographic studies. We tested the hypotheses (1) that psychoacoustically measured tinnitus loudness is related to gamma oscillatory band power, and (2) that tinnitus loudness and tinnitus-related distress are related to distinct brain activity patterns as suggested by the distinction between loudness and distress experienced by tinnitus patients. Furthermore, we explored (3) how hearing impairment, minimum masking level, and (4) psychological comorbidities are related to spontaneous oscillatory brain activity in tinnitus patients.

Methods and Findings: Resting state oscillatory brain activity recorded electroencephalographically from 46 male tinnitus patients showed a positive correlation between gamma band oscillations and psychoacoustic tinnitus loudness determined with the reconstructed tinnitus sound, but not with the other psychoacoustic loudness measures that were used. Tinnitus-related distress did also correlate with delta band activity, but at electrode positions different from those associated with tinnitus loudness. Furthermore, highly distressed tinnitus patients exhibited a higher level of theta band activity. Moreover, mean hearing loss between 0.125 kHz and 16 kHz was associated with a decrease in gamma activity, whereas minimum masking levels correlated positively with delta band power. In contrast, psychological comorbidities did not express significant correlations with oscillatory brain activity.

Conclusion: Different clinically relevant tinnitus characteristics show distinctive associations with spontaneous brain oscillatory power. Results support hypothesis (1), but exclusively for the tinnitus loudness derived from matching to the reconstructed tinnitus sound. This suggests to preferably use the reconstructed tinnitus spectrum to determine psychoacoustic tinnitus loudness. Results also support hypothesis (2). Moreover, hearing loss and minimum masking level correlate with oscillatory power in distinctive frequency bands. The lack of an association between psychological comorbidities and oscillatory power may be attributed to the overall low level of mental health problems in the present sample.

Editor: Berthold Langguth, University of Regensburg, Germany

Funding: The authors have no funding or support to report.

Competing Interests: The authors have declared that no competing interests exist.

* E-mail: wolfgang.delb@medma.uni-heidelberg.de

Introduction

Tinnitus is an auditory percept that does not originate from a physical sound source but is generated within the auditory system. Therefore, a subjective tinnitus is heard only by the affected individual. Cochlear hearing impairment is seen as a permissive if not a necessary condition for tinnitus [1–3]. As hearing impairments become more common with advancing age, it is not surprising that the prevalence of tinnitus increases with age [3,4]. Although tolerated well by many, tinnitus may be the cause for substantial deterioration of life quality [5]. Concerning the impact of tinnitus on an individual, a perceptive component reflected by the subjectively perceived tinnitus loudness and an affective component reflected by the amount of tinnitus-related distress are distinguished [6,7]. In particular, severely distressing tinnitus tends to be associated with increased levels of depressivity, anxiety, and somatic symptom severity [6,8,9].

As a consciously experienced, often continuous, and prominent signal tinnitus should be represented in the spontaneous activation pattern of the cortex. In line with this assumption, magnetoencephalographic (MEG) studies showed that the presence of tinnitus is associated with increased gamma band activity in the auditory cortex (AC) [10–12]. This finding is corroborated by electroencephalographic (EEG) studies that demonstrate the emergence of elevated gamma activity in persons who experience acute tinnitus [13]. Furthermore, gamma band activity in the AC shows some correlation with tinnitus intensity [14], and enhanced gamma activity is localized contralateral to the tinnitus ear in individuals with unilateral tinnitus (MEG: [12], EEG: [15]). Synchronization of fast oscillatory responses in the beta and gamma range is increased during demanding tasks that involve cooperation of widespread cortical regions. This is seen in a variety of cognitive tasks that require routing of signals across distributed cortical networks, perceptual grouping, attention-dependent stimulus selection, sensory-motor integration, working memory, and perceptual awareness [16]. Both synchronization and strength of neuronal oscillations in the gamma frequency range influence the amount and speed of information transfer [17].

At the same time alpha oscillatory activity is decreased in subjects with tinnitus compared to non-tinnitus controls [11,12,18]. Sensory systems exhibit pronounced alpha-like oscillatory activity during resting conditions. Therefore, low levels of alpha activity are thought to reflect a state of excitation while high levels are linked to reduced excitatory drive [19]. Weisz and coworkers [2,20] proposed that the dominant alpha activity at rest is functionally related to ongoing inhibitory activity that prevents spontaneous synchronization of cell assemblies. In line with this interpretation, auditory alpha activity, which also is referred to as tau activity [21], desynchronizes during presentation of auditory stimuli [20]. Thus, reduced alpha oscillatory power as seen in tinnitus patients suggest that tinnitus is associated with loss of cortical inhibition, a notion that is corroborated by findings of a down regulation of inhibition in deafferented regions of the AC in animal models of tinnitus [22], and the finding that functional deafferentation of central auditory areas by hearing loss leads to a significant reduction of alpha power in humans [23].

In the clinical setting a variety of audiological tinnitus characteristics are measured of which tinnitus loudness and tinnitus maskability are particularly important for the patient and the therapist. Tinnitus loudness is determined by different matching procedures, but the results of these measurements are not always satisfactory because they do not necessarily represent the patient's subjectively perceived tinnitus loudness. Minimum masking level on the other hand describes the minimal noise level that is necessary to eliminate the tinnitus perception, and represents a patient's ability to effectively use environmental sound to control the tinnitus perception. While there have been reports on correlates of tinnitus loudness in oscillatory brain activity, electrophysiological correlates of tinnitus maskability and the underlying mechanism remain unclear. In our study we set out to test the following hypotheses on tinnitus and spontaneous oscillatory brain activity:

Hypothesis (1): Loudness of the tinnitus sound correlates with gamma band oscillatory power during absence of external auditory stimulation. Conventionally, tinnitus loudness is measured by a variety of audiological matching procedures (see [24] for a review) or by subjective rating scales [25]. Both methods have limitations. Whereas loudness estimates derived by subjective rating scales are likely to be influenced by the distress attributed to the tinnitus, matching to pure tones at the tinnitus frequency or at 1 kHz might underestimate its loudness, since even if patients describe their tinnitus as extremely loud, measurements are usually found to be only a few dB above threshold [24]. Therefore we developed a new method to reconstruct the tinnitus sound, resulting in sounds that closely matched the individual tinnitus percept of a patient. We hypothesized, that tinnitus loudness estimates derived by comparison to sound synthesized in that way show a better correlation with brain activity than tinnitus loudness estimates derived by comparison to pure tones that are less similar to the tinnitus.

While many of the publications including those cited above compare tinnitus subjects with non-tinnitus subjects, the relation between the subjectively perceived tinnitus loudness and brain oscillatory activity has only been addressed by van der Loo and coworkers [14], and up to now there is no report on the association of tinnitus loudness determined by matching with an external auditory stimulus and oscillatory brain activity.

Hypothesis (2): Tinnitus loudness and tinnitus-related distress are associated with distinct spontaneous brain oscillations. From patient reports it is evident that tinnitus loudness and tinnitus-related distress are distinct characteristics of the tinnitus [6,26], therefore we hypothesized that tinnitus loudness and tinnitus-related distress correlate with distinct aspects of brain activity. Estimates of tinnitus-related distress were derived from a self-report questionnaire.

In the exploratory part of the present study we focused on the following aspects:

(3) We explored the association between oscillatory band power and hearing loss as well as minimum masking level, which are both highly relevant for patients. The relevance of MML has been outlined above and hearing impairment is seen as a permissive, although not sufficient condition for the establishment of tinnitus [1–3]. According to the model originally proposed by Llinas et al. [10] hearing impairment should be related to oscillatory brain activity. To the best of our knowledge, this is the first study that addresses this aspect.

(4) Finally, we explored how psychological comorbidities that often accompany tinnitus [6], and that are known to influence oscillatory brain activity, have distinct influence on oscillatory brain activity in tinnitus patients. Even though the relation between tinnitus-related distress and oscillatory brain activity has been addressed repeatedly [11,27,28], comorbidities such as depressivity and anxiety [6] have not been taken into account.

Since gender differences and oversensitivity to external sounds (hyperacusis) might influence resting state EEG power distribution [29], tinnitus and non-tinnitus participants were restricted to males with normal sound sensitivity.

Methods

The present study was approved by the ethics committee of the Medical Faculty Mannheim (Ethikkommission II) of Heidelberg University according to the principles expressed in the Declaration of Helsinki. Subjects were acquired by newspaper advertisements and consecutively enrolled in the study. All subjects of the patient and the control group were informed about aim and scope of the study and gave written consent. All participants were males and right handed.

Tinnitus patient group

Mean age of the 46 tinnitus patients included in the study was 54.8 years (range 22 to 68 years) and it did not differ from that of the control group (ANOVA: $p = 0.21$). Tinnitus was present bilaterally in 27 and unilaterally in 19 (left: 12; right: 7). Pure tone tinnitus was experienced by 40 participants while 6 had noise-like tinnitus. Mean hearing level (MHL) in the frequency range from 0.125 kHz to 16 kHz was 32.0 dBHL ± 10.0 dBHL (Fig. 1). Only 4 subjects had a highly distressing tinnitus according to the Tinnitus Questionnaire (TQ Hallam et al. [30], German version [31]) with a main score above 47. Average uncomfortable loudness thresholds (UCL) between 0.125 kHz and 10 kHz of all tinnitus patients in the study were normal with 85 dBHL or above.

Control group

None of the 10 participants included in the control group had a history of tinnitus or any other type of ear-related pathology, and all had scores of 60 or below in any of the Symptom Ckecklist-90-R (SCL-90-R) subscales indicating unproblematic psychological conditions. Mean age was 50.4 years (range 25 to 62 years), and hearing loss between 0.125 kHz and 16 kHz averaged to 19.1 dBHL ± 11.7 dBHL (Fig. 1, Table 1).

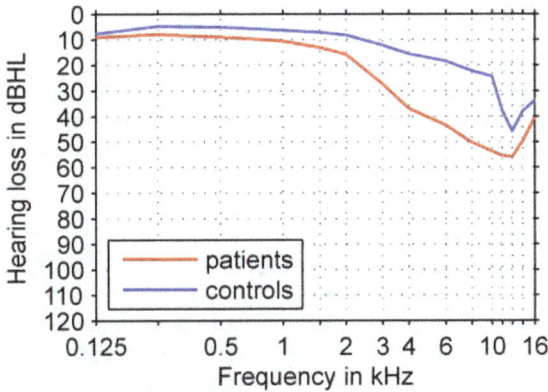

Figure 1. Averaged audiograms of the patient and control groups. Hearing ability was determined between 0.125 kHz and 16 kHz. Group means are shown. Tinnitus patients exhibit more pronounced hearing loss than controls above 2 kHz. Note that the controls as a group exhibit noticeable hearing impairment above 10 kHz.

Psychoacoustic measurements

Thresholds were measured in 1 dB steps with pure tones at the standard frequencies of the audiogram (range from 0.125 kHz to 10 kHz) and in addition at 11.2 kHz, 12.5 kHz, 14 kHz, and 16 kHz (audiometer: Auritec AT900; headphones: Sennheiser HDA200). Mean hearing loss (MHL) was calculated by averaging across all frequencies f_i.

Uncomfortable loudness thresholds (UCL) were recorded at the standard frequencies. For this purpose the sound pressure level of each pure tone was presented at hearing threshold and its level was increased continuously until the sound became uncomfortable. Subjects indicated UCL by pressing a button.

Minimum masking levels (MML) were determined with white noise at the tinnitus ear. In cases of bilateral tinnitus MML was determined for each ear. White noise was presented at hearing threshold and increased in 1 dB step sizes until it masked a subject's tinnitus, which the subject indicated by pressing a button.

Tinnitus reconstruction. Tinnitus reconstruction was based on psychoacoustic tinnitus spectra as described earlier [32] and expanded to a novel heuristic, easy to handle method. Reconstructions were performed with $M = 15$ pure tones at the standard frequencies and with the additional high frequencies f_i of the audiogram (see above). Pure tones were presented to the tinnitus ear or to the ear with less hearing loss in cases of bilateral tinnitus. First, a given pure tone was adjusted to the perceived tinnitus loudness, then the patient rated its contribution to his tinnitus on a numeric rating scale (0: no contribution, 10: perfect match). This was repeated three times and ratings were averaged for each frequency f_i. Thereupon average scores were processed with a custom MATLAB script (The Mathworks, Natick, Massachusetts, USA) to synthesize the tinnitus sound which was played back monaurally at a sampling rate of $F_S = 44.1$ kHz. Pure tone tinnitus $y(n)$ was synthesized by processing the averaged scores A_i as follows:

$$y(n) = \sum_{i=1}^{M} \frac{4^{A_i}}{4^{10}} \sin(2\pi f_i n / F_S) \qquad (1)$$

During play back of the generated sound to the patients via headphone (Sennheiser HDA200), loudness of each frequency component (parameter A_i) was fine-tuned by the examiner on a

Table 1. Participant characteristics.

Parameter	Tinnitus group	Control group	p-value
N	46	10	-
Age (years)	54.8 ± 9.5	50.4 ± 12.6	0.21
UCL (dBHL)	98.9 ± 6.8	96.7 ± 7.3	0.37
MHL (dBHL)	32.0 ± 10.0	19.1 ± 11.7	0.0008
GSI	52.9 ± 7.8	45.7 ± 8.9	0.02
PSDI	49.8 ± 8.3	47.3 ± 7.3	0.38
PST	53.2 ± 6.6	45.8 ± 9.0	0.005
DEP	52.9 ± 9.4	44.4 ± 10.2	0.04
SOM	49.5 ± 9.9	47.4 ± 8.5	0.69
ANX	51.3 ± 9.0	42.6 ± 6.2	0.009
TinDur (years)	10.0 ± 9.4	-	-
TinDis	24.7 ± 14.7	-	-
TL_{dBSL} (dBSL)	18.7 ± 10.2	-	-
TL_{sones} (sones)	4.2 ± 4.3	-	-
TL_{1kHz} (dBHL)	36.2 ± 15.2	-	-
TL_P (dBHL)	66.4 ± 16.3	-	-
TL_{P-HL} (dBSL)	15.9 ± 10.1	-	-
f_{tin} (kHz)	8.8 ± 3.8	-	-
MML (dBHL)	55.4 ± 15.8	-	-
MML − MHL (dBSL)	23.4 ± 17.1	-	-
RTS	9.3 ± 0.4	-	-

Group means and standard deviations are reported. Auditory measures: mean hearing loss (MHL, left and right ear averaged for the frequency range 0.125 kHz to 16 kHz); mean threshold of uncomfortable loudness (UCL, left and right ear averaged for the frequency range 0.125 kHz to 10 kHz). Psychological measures derived from the SCL-90-R: global severity index (GSI), positive symptom total (PST), positive symptom distress index (PSDI), depressiveness subscale (DEP), somatization subscale (SOM), anxiety subscale (ANX). Tinnitus characteristics: tinnitus duration (TinDur), tinnitus-related distress (TinDis) derived from the Tinnitus Questionnaire (scores <47: low tinnitus-related distress, scores ≥47: high tinnitus-related distress). Tinnitus loudness measures (TL, see section "Psychoacoustic measurements" and Table 2); frequency of the major peak in tinnitus spectrum (f_{tin}); minimum masking level when masking with white noise (MML) as well as minimum masking level above mean hearing threshold (MML − MHL); rating of similarity of reconstructed tinnitus sound to own tinnitus (RTS, 0: no match, 10: perfect match).

graphical user interface. The procedure was stopped if no further improvements of the matching score were achieved.

Amplitude modulated tinnitus was approximated by

$$y_{AM}(n) = 1 - \frac{1}{2} A_{AM}[1 - \sin(2\pi df_{AM} n / F_S)] \qquad (2)$$

with the parameters A_{AM} and df_{AM} representing modulation amplitude and frequency. If tinnitus contained a noise component the corresponding tinnitus spectrum was reconstructed in a last step by:

$$y_{tin}(n) = [y_{noise}(n) + y(n)] y_{AM}(n) \qquad (3)$$

For adjusting $y_{noise}(n)$, white noise was band-pass filtered and the cutoff frequencies were selected according to the noise spectrum in a patient's tinnitus. Note that the reconstructed tinnitus covered all frequency components up to 16 kHz.

Averaged across all tinnitus participants, similarity of the reconstructed tinnitus sound to a patient's own tinnitus reached an average similarity index of 9.3 ± 0.4 when rated on a numeric rating scale (0: no contribution, 10: perfect match), indicating a very good fit of the reconstructed tinnitus sound. Averaged across all tinnitus participants, the major peak of the reconstructed tinnitus spectrum was located at $8.8\ \text{kHz} \pm 3.8\ \text{kHz}$ (Table 1 for details).

Tinnitus loudness. Overall five different tinnitus loudness estimates were determined (Table 2). The first tinnitus estimate was obtained in a monaural matching procedure using the reconstructed tinnitus sound as described above and MHL was subtracted from the whole tinnitus spectrum. The largest peak in the spectrum was defined as the tinnitus loudness estimate TL_{dBSL}. In addition, tinnitus loudness was calculated in sone as

$$\text{TL}_{\text{sones}} = k \left[10^{\text{MHL}/20} \left[10^{\text{TL}_{\text{dBSL}}/20} - 1 \right] \right]^{0.6} \quad (4)$$

with $k = 0.1$ (see [24,33]).

Third, in order to account for recruitment phenomena [33], a 1 kHz pure tone was presented via headphone and its loudness was adjusted in 1 dB steps until it was perceived by the patient as loud as his own tinnitus (TL_{1kHz}). A further loudness measure TL_{P} was generated by matching the loudness of the pure tone which corresponded to the major peak of the tinnitus spectrum to the tinnitus loudness experienced by the patient. Finally, the loudness measure $\text{TL}_{\text{P-HL}}$ was obtained by subtracting hearing loss at the major peak of the tinnitus spectrum from TL_{P}.

Tinnitus-related distress and psychometric testing

Tinnitus-related distress was evaluated with the Tinnitus Questionnaire (TQ Hallam et al. [30], German version [31]). This 52 item questionnaire yields a sum-score between 0 to 84 and estimates separate subscores for emotional distress, cognitive distress, intrusiveness, auditory perceptual difficulties, sleep disturbance, and somatic complaints. Sum-scores below 47 indicate low to moderate tinnitus-related distress, whereas values of 47 and above indicate high to very high tinnitus-related distress.

In addition, the German version of the Symptom Checklist-90-R (SCL-90-R [34,35]) was completed by all participants. The SCL-90-R contains subscales for somatization, obsessive-compulsive behavior, interpersonal sensitivity, depression, anxiety, hostility, phobic anxiety, paranoid ideation, and psychoticism. Beyond that, the following global scores were derived: The global severity index (GSI) sets the intensity of perceived distress in reference to all items of the SCL-90-R and is the best single predictor for the

current level or depth of mental distress. The positive symptom total (PST) score is a measure for the quantity of items indicating distress. The positive symptom distress index (PSDI) reflects the average level of distress reported for individual symptoms and it is interpreted as a measure of symptom intensity. Combination of the subscores GSI, PSDI, and PST yields a general psychological distress estimate (GPD).

EEG recording

EEG recordings took place in a dimly lit sound booth shielded against electromagnetic interference (EMI) and connected with the recording room via a glass window. Participants were seated comfortably with uncrossed arms and legs in an armchair that had a head-rest. They were instructed to relax and to avoid any movements.

Eyes were closed during EEG recording, and analysis was confined to resting EEG recorded for 120 s. A cap (g.GAMMA-cap, g.tec Medical Engineering GmbH, Austria) with 22 sintered Ag/AgCl surface electrodes was placed at the standard positions of the extended 10–20 system (Fp1, Fp2, F7, F3, F1, Fz, F2, F4, F8, T7, C3, Cz, C4, T8, P7, P3, Pz, POz, P4, P8, O1, O2) and referenced to linked ear lobes. The electrooculogram (EOG) was monitored with 4 sintered Ag/AgCl surface electrodes (LO1, LO2, IO1, IO2). Impedances were checked to be below 5 kOhm and the sampling rate was set to 512 Hz. EEG signals were acquired by two cascaded 24 bit biosignal amplification units (g.USBamp, g.tec Medical Engineering GmbH, Austria). EEGs were inspected for indicators of sleep such as spindles, enhanced theta oscillations or a slowed alpha rhythm, and only subjects who stayed awake were included.

Data preprocessing and editing

EEG data were pre-processed and analyzed offline with MATLAB. Slow fluctuations were removed by local linear regression (see http://chronux.org/ for details). Length of the moving window and step size were set to $l_w = 1$ s and $l_s = 0.5$ s, respectively. Artifacts at 50 Hz and multiples due to power line interferences were removed by adaptive filter techniques using a separate adaptive filter with two filter coefficients for each interference frequency [36].

Episodic artifacts including muscle artifacts, eye blinks, teeth clenching, or body movement were removed by visual inspection using the MATLAB scripts of EEGLAB [37]. EOG artifacts were removed automatically with a custom MATLAB script by applying the following steps: Low-pass filtering of EOG channels with 5 Hz cutoff frequency, decomposing EEG and EOG signals into independent components with a second order blind identi-

Table 2. Psychoacoustic measures for tinnitus loudness.

Loudness measure	Stimulus for matching procedure	Measure calculated as
TL_{dBSL}	reconstructed tinnitus sound	MHL is subtracted from the level of the major peak in the psychoacoustic tinnitus spectrum after loudness matching
TL_{sones}	reconstructed tinnitus sound	see equation (4)
TL_{1kHz}	sine tone at 1 kHz	-
TL_{P}	sine tone at the major peak of the psychoacoustic tinnitus spectrum	-
$\text{TL}_{\text{P-HL}}$	sine tone at the major peak of the psychoacoustic tinnitus spectrum	hearing loss at the major peak of tinnitus spectrum is subtracted from TL_{P}

Overview on the types of stimuli generated for psychoacoustic tinnitus loudness matching (see section "Psychoacoustic measurements").

fication algorithm [37,38], selection of the EOG components according to their correlation with the recorded EOG channels, high-pass filtering of the selected EOG components with 5 Hz cutoff frequency to remove identified EOG artifacts, and reconstruction of the EEG signal. Subsequent high-pass filtering of the EOG components ensured that automatic artifact removal was restricted to frequencies below 5 Hz where EOG artifacts were expected. After visual artifact removal mean length of the recording was 89.8 s ± 22.6 s.

Power spectral estimation and analysis was done with a multi-taper method (see http://chronux.org/ and [39,40] for details) that tapers the time series by an optimal set of orthogonal tapers (Slepian functions) and applies a Fourier transformation. With the chosen time-bandwidth-product $TW = 3$ and the relation $K = 2TW - 1$ a total number of $K = 5$ tapers were used for power spectral estimation. Mean power spectra were determined by averaging the log-transformed power density spectra of all scalp electrodes for each subject and calculated separately for delta (0.5 Hz to 3 Hz), theta (4 Hz to 7 Hz), alpha (8 Hz to 13 Hz), beta (14 Hz to 30 Hz), and gamma (31 Hz to 64 Hz) band frequencies. Frequencies near the power line artifacts $49\,\text{Hz} < f < 51\,\text{Hz}$ were excluded before averaging results in the gamma frequency range. Because of the relatively low number of 22 electrodes which results in low localization precision [41] we did not apply source localization algorithms.

Statistics

Spearman's rank correlation coefficient ρ was computed for spectral power in the different frequency bands and the psychoacoustic and psychometric factors following a custom MATLAB script [42]. A false discovery rate (FDR) correction was applied to correct for multiple comparisons [43].

Results

Power spectra

An initial ANOVA did not show significant differences for any frequency band between the tinnitus and the control group when averaging power across all 22 electrodes (delta $p = 0.89$, theta $p = 0.34$, alpha $p = 0.59$, beta $p = 0.77$, gamma $p = 0.95$), whereas more detailed correlation analyses revealed significant interactions between tinnitus loudness, tinnitus-related distress, hearing loss and oscillatory band power depending on type of tinnitus loudness measure, oscillation frequency, and control for confounding factors.

Correlation analyses

Mean hearing loss (MHL). MHL did not correlate significantly with oscillatory power averaged over all electrodes in any frequency band, no matter whether controlled for age, general psychological distress (GPD), and tinnitus loudness in dBSL (TL_{dBSL}) or not. When performing the same analysis with tinnitus loudness estimates in the sone scale (TL_{sones}), however, a significant decrease of gamma band power with increasing MHL became apparent ($\rho = -0.35$, $p < 0.03$). Restricting the analysis to patients with pure tone tinnitus and controlling for age, GPD, and TL_{dBSL}, a weakly significant correlation between MHL and alpha band power ($\rho = -0.31$, $p = 0.07$) became apparent, while correlations of MHL and band power averaged over all electrodes in this group reached significance in the alpha, beta, and gamma band when using the tinnitus loudness estimate TL_{sones} (Table 3). For controls, the correlation between MHL and theta band power reached significance ($\rho = -0.71$, $p < 0.03$).

Tinnitus loudness. The correlations of all tinnitus loudness measures (Table 2) with tinnitus-related distress, MHL, and MML are summarized in Table 4. Statistical significance of correlations between these factors depended on the type of loudness measure that was used.

Similarly, statistical significance of correlations between tinnitus loudness and oscillatory brain activity depended on the type of tinnitus loudness that was used (Table 3 and 5). Tinnitus loudness TL_{dBSL} showed a weakly significant correlation with band power averaged over all electrodes in the gamma ($\rho = 0.29$, $p = 0.06$) band. Significance of this correlation improved ($\rho = 0.32$, $p < 0.04$) when controlling for age, GPD, and MHL, and it improved even more when controlling for these factors and tinnitus-related distress in addition ($\rho = 0.39$, $p < 0.02$, Table 5).

When restricting the analysis to patients with pure tone tinnitus (Table 3), the partial correlation between band power averaged over all electrodes and TL_{dBSL} controlled for age, GPD, and MHL became highly significant for the gamma ($\rho = 0.46$, $p < 0.006$) band. Fig. 2 shows that correlation strength across the 22 electrode positions was more uniform for the correlation with gamma (Fig. 2C) than with delta band power (Fig. 2B). These correlations remained significant after correction for multiple comparison (FDR 0.05: $p < 0.002$) in the delta range at the fronto-central electrode positions Fp2, F1, Fz, F2, F4, F8, C3, Cz, and P7, and in the gamma range at all but the T8 and P8 electrode positions. Similar results were seen for delta and gamma band when performing a partial correlation between tinnitus loudness in sone (TL_{sones}) and band power controlled for age, GPD, and MHL in patients with pure tone tinnitus (Table 3).

Analysis of correlation strength at individual electrode positions revealed differential distribution patterns between oscillatory brain activity and the tinnitus loudness TL_{dBSL} in patients with unilateral tinnitus (Fig. 3). For this analysis electrode positions of left and right hemisphere were mirrored to the contralateral hemisphere in patients with right-sided tinnitus. Using the loudness measure TL_{dBSL} and controlling for age, GPD, and MHL demonstrated an asymmetric distribution of correlation strength between tinnitus loudness and oscillatory band power. Relatively high correlations were observed in the delta (Fig. 3A) and gamma (Fig. 3B) band at frontal electrode positions contralateral to the tinnitus ear. However, none of the correlations remained significant after FDR correction (FDR 0.05).

On the contrary, the loudness measure TL_{1kHz}, derived from matching the amplitude of a 1 kHz pure tone to the tinnitus loudness, showed no significant correlation with band power averaged over all electrodes in any frequency range. This did not change when controlling for age, GPD, and MHL (Table 3 and 5). Likewise correlating the loudness measure TL_P, which was derived by adjusting the pure tone corresponding to the major peak in the psychoacoustic tinnitus spectrum to the perceived tinnitus loudness [32], with band power averaged over all electrodes did not show any significant correlation in this analysis. The same was true when TL_{P-HL} was used instead of TL_P.

Minimum masking level (MML). Increase in delta band power averaged over all electrodes correlated significantly with increasing MML ($\rho = 0.40$, $p < 0.007$). This correlation remained highly significant when controlling for age, GPD, and MHL ($\rho = 0.45$, $p < 0.003$), or when controlling for TL_{dBSL} ($\rho = 0.45$, $p < 0.004$), or tinnitus-related distress ($\rho = 0.44$, $p < 0.005$) in addition (Table 3 and 5). A detailed analysis (Fig. 4) localized significant correlations at the right fronto-temporal F8 and T8 electrode positions (FDR 0.05: $p < 10^{-5}$).

When subtracting MHL from MML, correlations became significant for all but the theta frequency band, but remained

Table 3. Partial correlation of band power averaged over all electrodes with audiological parameters for the subgroup with pure tone tinnitus.

Parameter	controlled for (partial correlation)	delta ρ	p	theta ρ	p	alpha ρ	p	beta ρ	p	gamma ρ	p
MHL	age, GPD, TL$_{dBSL}$	−0.11	0.53	−0.16	0.35	−0.31	0.07	−0.21	0.23	−0.12	0.49
MHL	age, GPD, TL$_{sones}$	−0.28	0.10	−0.32	0.06	−0.35	0.04	−0.34	0.04	−0.38	0.02
TL$_{dBSL}$	age, GPD, MHL	0.30	0.09	0.29	0.09	0.11	0.54	0.31	0.07	0.46	0.006
TL$_{sones}$	age, GPD, MHL	0.30	0.08	0.28	0.11	0.10	0.57	0.23	0.18	0.43	0.02
TL$_{1kHz}$	age, GPD, MHL	−0.17	0.34	−0.19	0.28	−0.28	0.10	−0.16	0.37	0.64	0.71
TL$_P$	age, GPD, MHL	−0.05	0.78	0.03	0.87	−0.09	0.62	0.07	0.69	0.13	0.45
TL$_{P-HL}$	age, GPD, MHL	−0.26	0.13	−0.27	0.12	−0.25	0.15	<−0.01	0.98	−0.14	0.42
MML	age, GPD, MHL	0.55	0.0007*	0.25	0.14	0.30	0.08	0.14	0.42	0.15	0.40
MML−MHL	age, GPD, MHL	0.54	0.0008*	0.30	0.08	0.32	0.06	0.25	0.14	0.23	0.19

Correlation coefficients (Spearman's ρ) and corresponding significance levels (p) for tinnitus loudness (TL), minimum masking level (MML), mean hearing loss (MHL) with oscillatory band power in the delta to gamma range are reported. MHL: mean hearing loss averaged for left and right ears and for the frequencies between 0.125 kHz and 16 kHz; TL: tinnitus loudness measures (see section "Psychoacoustic measurements" and Table 2); MML: minimum masking level with white noise; MML−MHL: minimum masking level with white noise above mean hearing threshold. Significant correlations ($p < 0.05$) are indicated by bold letters. Correlations which remained significant after FDR correction (FDR 0.05) are denoted by * at the corresponding p-value.

significant only for the delta band when controlling for age, GPD, and MHL ($\rho = 0.43$, $p < 0.005$) (Table 3, 4, and 5).

Tinnitus-related distress and psychometric parameters. An ANOVA revealed significant differences in theta band power ($p < 0.03$) between patients with low and high tinnitus-related distress when averaging power over all electrodes with more theta band power present in the highly distressed patients. A subsequent correlation analysis of band power averaged over all electrodes and tinnitus-related distress showed a significant correlation in the delta band ($\rho = 0.30$, $p < 0.05$), which did not reach significance anymore when controlled for GPD ($\rho = 0.21$, $p = 0.18$). Similarly, correlations between tinnitus-related distress and power in the delta band averaged over all electrodes did not reach significance when controlling for either the depressivity ($\rho = 0.26$, $p = 0.08$), somatization ($\rho = 0.22$, $p = 0.15$), or the anxiety ($\rho = 0.23$, $p = 0.13$) symptom scale of the SCL-90-R, or when controlling for the tinnitus loudness TL$_{dBSL}$ ($\rho = 0.28$, $p = 0.07$). Results of the correlation analyses are given in Tables 3 and 5. When analyzing correlations of tinnitus-

related distress and band power at individual electrodes (Fig. 5) correlation strength was highest at frontal and temporal parts of the left hemisphere.

General psychological distress scores (GSI, PSDI, and PST) did not correlate significantly with band power averaged over all electrodes in any frequency band. Likewise, none of the correlations between oscillatory band power and the depression, anxiety or somatization symptom scale scores reached significance (Table 5).

Discussion

Results of the present study support hypothesis (1) that increasing tinnitus loudness is associated with increasing gamma oscillatory power. This was found to be the case for the tinnitus loudness estimate derived by adjusting the reconstructed tinnitus sound (TL$_{dBSL}$) to the perceived tinnitus loudness, but not for the psychoacoustically determined tinnitus loudness estimates determined with other types of sound. In addition, delta band power

Table 4. Correlations of tinnitus loudness and distress with auditory parameters.

Parameter	TinDis ρ	p	MHL ρ	p	MML ρ	p	MML−MHL ρ	p
TL$_{dBSL}$ (dBSL)	0.32	0.03	−0.36	0.01	−0.09	0.55	0.14	0.35
TL$_{sones}$ (sones)	0.31	0.03	0.31	0.04	−0.02	0.87	−0.22	0.15
TL$_{1kHz}$ (dBHL)	−0.05	0.73	0.30	0.04	0.34	0.02	0.11	0.46
TL$_P$ (dBHL)	0.06	0.69	0.35	0.02	0.36	0.02	0.04	0.79
TL$_{P-HL}$ (dBSL)	−0.02	0.92	−0.30	0.04	0.09	0.57	0.20	0.17

For the patient group, correlation coefficients (Spearman's ρ) and corresponding significance levels (p) for each of the five different measures for tinnitus loudness (TL, see section "Psychoacoustic measurements" and Table 2) with tinnitus-related distress (TinDis), mean hearing loss (MHL), minimum masking level (MML), as well as minimum masking level above mean hearing threshold (MML−MHL). Mean hearing loss (MHL) was averaged for left and right ears and for the frequency range between 0.125 kHz and 16 kHz. Minimum masking level (MML) was measured with white noise. Significant correlations ($p < 0.05$) are indicated by bold letters. Correlations did not remain significant after FDR correction (FDR 0.05).

Table 5. Correlation of band power averaged over all electrodes with audiological and psychological parameters of the patient group.

Parameter	controlled for (partial correlation)	delta ρ	delta p	theta ρ	theta p	alpha ρ	alpha p	beta ρ	beta p	gamma ρ	gamma p
Age	-	−0.20	0.17	−0.10	0.51	−0.11	0.48	−0.11	0.45	−0.05	0.74
MHL	-	−0.12	0.44	−0.15	0.32	−0.22	0.15	−0.25	0.09	−0.25	0.10
	age, GPD, TL_{dBSL}	−0.02	0.89	−0.09	0.57	−0.22	0.17	−0.17	0.29	−0.19	0.24
	age, GPD, TL_{sones}	−0.09	0.56	−0.14	0.38	−0.19	0.23	−0.26	0.11	−0.35	0.03
TL_{dBSL}	-	0.11	0.45	0.14	0.34	0.05	0.74	0.27	0.07	0.29	0.06
	age, GPD, MHL	0.13	0.41	0.09	0.56	−0.04	0.79	0.20	0.22	0.32	0.04
	age, GPD, MHL, TinDis	0.07	0.67	0.03	0.87	−0.06	0.72	0.23	0.15	0.39	0.02
TL_{sones}	-	0.03	0.85	0.03	0.85	−0.13	0.41	0.04	0.80	0.11	0.48
	age, GPD, MHL	0.11	0.50	0.07	0.68	−0.08	0.64	0.11	0.49	0.28	0.08
	age, GPD, MHL, TinDis	0.03	0.84	−0.01	0.94	−0.10	0.54	0.15	0.37	0.35	0.03
TL_{1kHz}	-	−0.12	0.44	−0.13	0.39	−0.17	0.27	−0.22	0.14	0.05	0.74
	age, GPD, MHL	−0.11	0.50	−0.12	0.44	−0.25	0.11	−0.20	0.21	0.08	0.61
TL_P	-	−0.02	0.91	0.03	0.86	<0.01	0.99	0.09	0.56	0.11	0.45
	age, GPD, MHL	<0.01	0.98	0.08	0.61	0.05	0.75	0.20	0.20	0.21	0.19
$TL_{P−HL}$	-	−0.15	0.32	−0.14	0.34	−0.08	0.60	0.01	0.93	−0.04	0.77
	age, GPD, MHL	−0.18	0.26	−0.20	0.20	−0.21	0.20	−0.07	0.69	−0.14	0.37
MML	-	0.40	0.007*	0.15	0.31	0.25	0.09	0.10	0.52	0.13	0.38
	age, GPD, MHL	0.45	0.003*	0.20	0.20	0.30	0.06	0.17	0.28	0.13	0.41
	age, GPD, MHL, TL_{dBSL}	0.45	0.004*	0.20	0.21	0.30	0.06	0.17	0.31	0.12	0.45
	age, GPD, MHL, TinDis	0.44	0.005*	0.19	0.25	0.30	0.06	0.18	0.27	0.15	0.37
MML−MHL	-	0.43	0.004*	0.25	0.10	0.34	0.03	0.30	0.05	0.32	0.03
	age, GPD, MHL	0.43	0.005*	0.23	0.14	0.30	0.06	0.26	0.11	0.20	0.20
TinDur	-	−0.06	0.71	−0.16	0.29	−0.09	0.54	<0.01	0.97	<−0.01	0.96
TinDis	-	0.30	0.05	0.24	0.11	0.08	0.61	0.05	0.74	−0.10	0.52
	GPD	0.21	0.18	0.21	0.19	0.05	0.73	−0.03	0.84	−0.08	0.63
	DEP	0.26	0.08	0.16	0.30	0.01	0.94	<−0.01	0.95	−0.05	0.72
	SOM	0.22	0.15	0.23	0.13	0.04	0.80	0.03	0.85	−0.10	0.51
	ANX	0.23	0.13	0.16	0.29	−0.05	0.76	<0.01	0.98	−0.06	0.70
	TL_{dBSL}	0.28	0.07	0.21	0.17	0.06	0.68	−0.04	0.79	−0.21	0.17
GSI	-	0.12	0.43	0.13	0.38	0.10	0.50	0.14	0.37	−0.15	0.31
PSDI	-	0.28	0.06	0.13	0.40	0.09	0.57	0.12	0.44	0.03	0.85
PST	-	0.04	0.79	0.14	0.35	0.18	0.24	0.15	0.32	−0.17	0.26
DEP	-	0.15	0.31	0.25	0.10	0.16	0.28	0.14	0.34	−0.12	0.43
SOM	-	0.23	0.12	0.09	0.56	0.09	0.56	0.05	0.74	−0.02	0.89
ANX	-	0.20	0.18	0.21	0.17	0.23	0.12	0.10	0.53	−0.10	0.53

Correlation coefficients (Spearman's ρ) and corresponding significance levels (p) between tinnitus characteristics, minimum masking level (MML), mean hearing loss (MHL), tinnitus-related distress (TinDis), psychometric testing scores and oscillatory band power in the delta to gamma range are reported for the whole tinnitus group. MHL: mean hearing loss averaged for left and right ears between 0.125 kHz and 16 kHz; TL: tinnitus loudness measures (see section "Psychoacoustic measurements" and Table 2); MML: minimum masking level with white noise; MML−MHL: minimum masking level with white noise above mean hearing threshold; TinDur: tinnitus duration in years; TinDis: tinnitus-related distress; DEP: depression subscale of the SCL-90-R; SOM: somatization subscale of the SCL-90-R; ANX: anxiety subscale of the SCL-90-R. Significant correlations ($p < 0.05$) are indicated by bold letters. Correlations which remained significant after FDR correction (FDR 0.05) are denoted by * at the corresponding p-value.

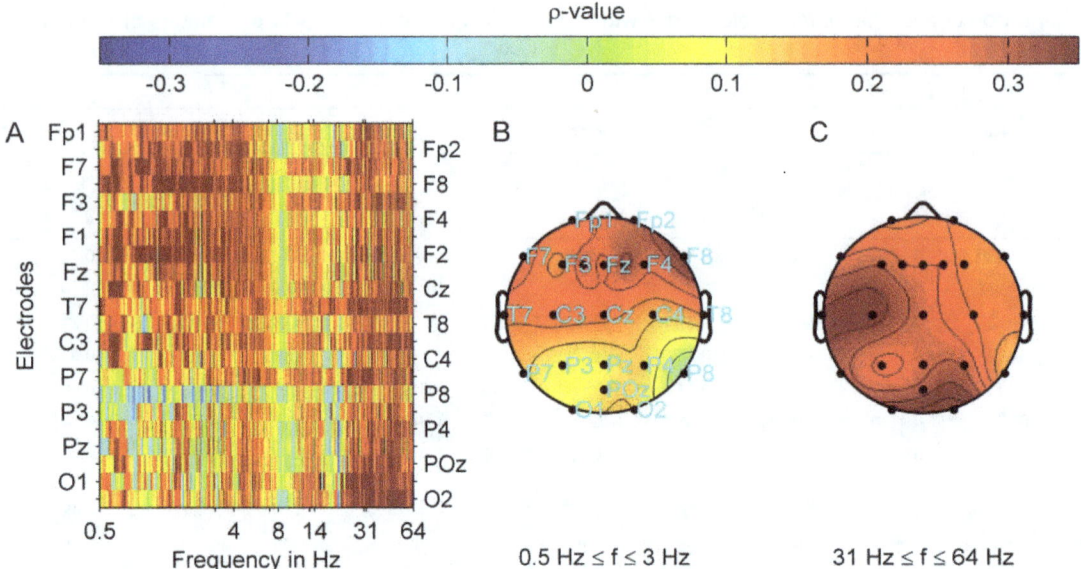

Figure 2. Spatio-spectral distribution of correlation strength between tinnitus loudness and oscillatory band power for the subgroup with pure tone tinnitus. Group averages are shown. Power spectra were interpolated with a resolution of 40 points per 1 Hz. Tinnitus loudness was determined by adjusting the contribution of each frequency component and the loudness of such a reconstructed tinnitus spectrum to the perceived tinnitus. Correlations were controlled for age, global psychological distress (GPD), and mean hearing loss (MHL) between 0.125 kHz and 16 kHz. (A) Correlation strength (Spearman's ρ) at each electrode and frequency point is shown. Plots (B) and (C) show correlation maps corresponding to (A) with averaged correlation strength (ρ) topographies for the tinnitus loudness TL_{dBSL} and delta (B) or gamma (C) oscillatory power. Correlation strength for delta band power and tinnitus loudness was highest in the frontal half of the brain and lowest at posterior locations. For the correlation between gamma band power and tinnitus loudness the distribution of correlation strength across electrode positions was more uniform. Highest correlation strength was reached at the left temporal and right occipital electrode positions. After FDR correction (FDR 0.05: $p < 0.002$) correlations remained significant at all electrode positions except for T8 and P8 locations for the gamma band, whereas significant correlations in the delta band were attained at the fronto-central locations Fp2, F1, Fz, F2, F4, F8, C3, Cz, and at P7.

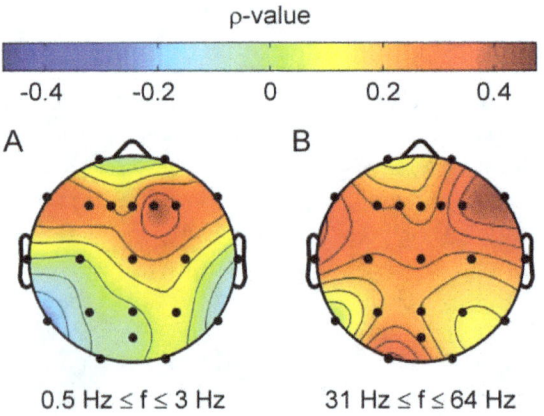

Figure 3. Correlation strength between tinnitus loudness and oscillatory band power for the subgroup with unilateral pure tone tinnitus. Group averages are shown. Electrode positions of left and right hemisphere were interchanged for right-sided tinnitus. Left ear in the plots is the tinnitus ear. Power spectra were interpolated with a resolution of 40 points per 1 Hz. Tinnitus loudness was determined by matching the contribution of each frequency component and the loudness of such a reconstructed tinnitus spectrum to the perceived tinnitus. Correlations with oscillatory band power were controlled for age, global psychological distress (GPD), and mean hearing loss (MHL) between 0.125 kHz and 16 kHz. Note that correlation strength for tinnitus loudness and delta band power is highest at the fronto-central electrodes contralateral to the tinnitus ear (A), whereas it is highest at the contralateral fronto-temporal electrodes for tinnitus loudness and gamma band power (B). Correlation strengths did not remain significant after FDR correction (FDR 0.05).

did significantly increase with the TL_{dBSL} tinnitus loudness estimate. Moreover, increases of loudness-associated gamma and delta activity were localized at the frontal electrodes contralateral to the tinnitus ear for unilateral tinnitus.

Hypothesis (2) that tinnitus loudness and tinnitus-related distress are associated with distinct brain activity patterns was also corroborated by the results of the present study. Tinnitus-related distress does not correlate with gamma band power, and significantly correlates with delta band power at locations which differ from those that correlate with tinnitus loudness. Beyond that high-distress tinnitus was associated with significantly higher theta band power compared to low-distress tinnitus.

The exploratory analysis (3) and (4) revealed that gamma band power decreases with increasing MHL, and that increasing MML correlates with increasing delta band power. In contrast, psychological symptoms such as depressivity and anxiety did not significantly correlate with oscillatory band power.

Tinnitus loudness and tinnitus-related distress

Recording of spontaneous brain activity revealed increases in oscillatory power in the gamma and delta band related to psychoacoustically determined tinnitus loudness. This increase was significant only when determining tinnitus loudness with the reconstructed tinnitus sound (TL_{dBSL}), and when controlling for hearing loss, because MHL shows an inverse correlation with gamma band power. In contrast, increases of tinnitus-related distress assessed with the TQ correlated with increases of activity in the delta band only, and highly distressed tinnitus patients exhibited higher theta band power compared to mildly distressed ones. These findings support the distinction between tinnitus

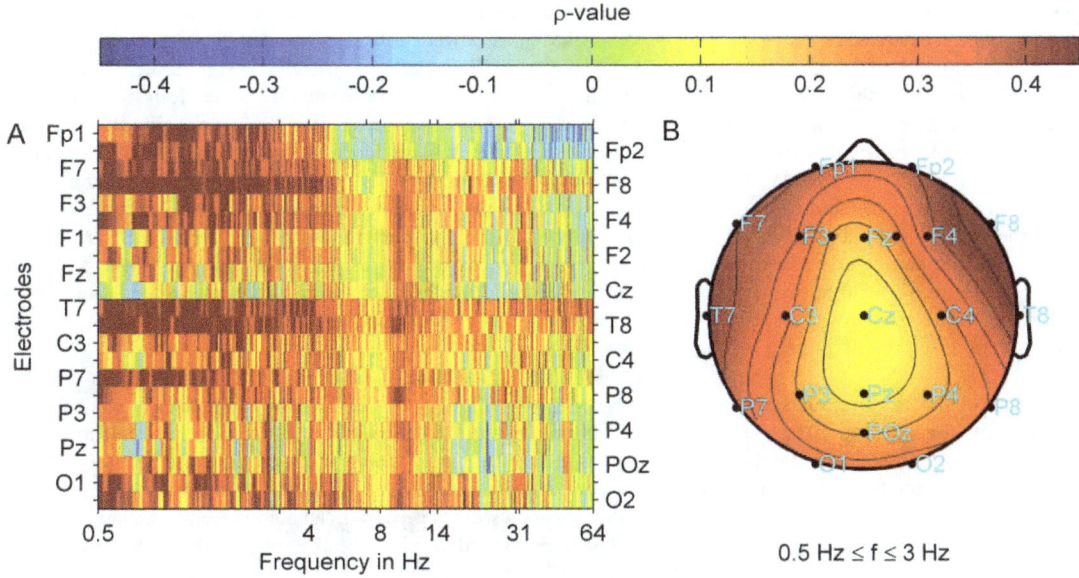

Figure 4. Correlation strength between MML and oscillatory band power. Group average for all tinnitus patients is shown. Power spectra were interpolated with a resolution of 40 points per 1 Hz. Correlations were controlled for age, global psychological distress (GPD) and mean hearing loss (MHL) between 0.125 kHz and 16 kHz. (A) Correlation strength (Spearman's ρ) at each electrode and frequency point is shown. Plot (B) shows the correlation map with averaged correlation strength (ρ) topographies between MML and delta oscillatory power. After FDR correction, correlations at the F8 and T8 electrode position remained significant (FDR 0.05: $p < 10^{-5}$).

loudness and tinnitus-related distress as partly separate aspects of the tinnitus syndrome which was suggested earlier based on questionnaire studies in large tinnitus populations [6,26]. Most importantly, the present findings extent this distinction to physiological differences suggesting that tinnitus loudness and tinnitus-related distress are related to different pathophysiological mechanisms. A distinction between physiological mechanisms related to tinnitus loudness and distress, respectively, is in line with

the results reported by Leaver et al. [7]. These authors observed that neural systems associated with chronic tinnitus differ from those involved in aversive or distressed reactions to the tinnitus. Such a distinction was initially proposed by Jastreboff [44], and it is suggested by the findings of Schlee et al. [27]. As the mean tinnitus-related distress level was rather low in the present study (see Table 1), it is not surprising that the correlation between delta

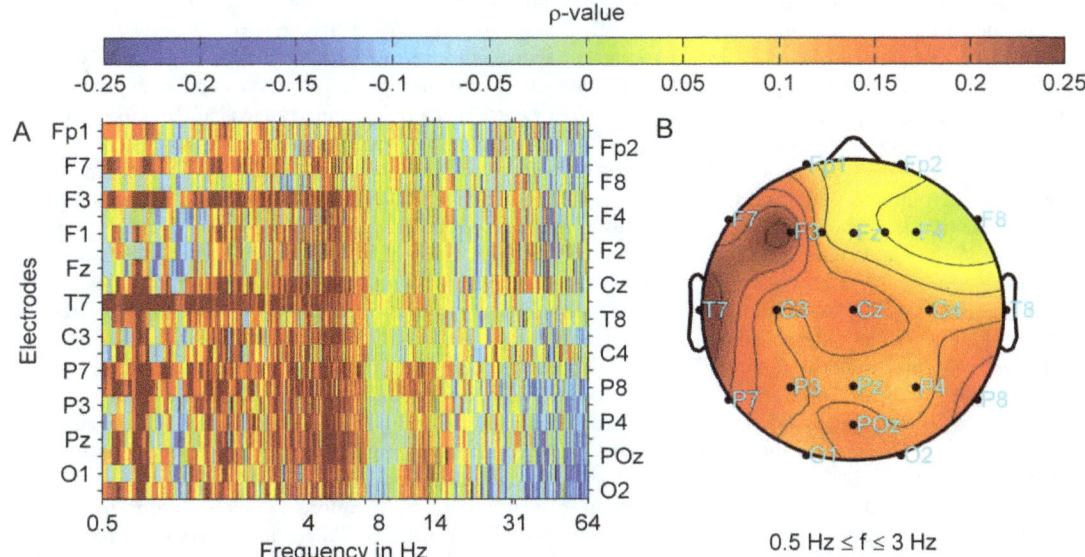

Figure 5. Correlation strength between tinnitus-related distress and oscillatory band power. Group average for all tinnitus patients is shown. Power spectra were interpolated with a resolution of 40 points per 1 Hz. (A) Correlation strength (Spearman's ρ) at each electrode and frequency point is shown. Plot (B) shows the correlation map with averaged correlation strength (ρ) topographies between tinnitus-related distress and delta band power. Irrespective of tinnitus laterality, correlation strength is most pronounced at frontal and temporal locations of the left hemisphere. After FDR correction (FDR 0.05) correlations did not remain significant.

oscillatory power and tinnitus-related distress attains only marginal significance and at this point has to be treated with caution.

In the past, the majority of EEG studies focused on differences between tinnitus and non-tinnitus subjects and did not account for psychological comorbidities although many tinnitus patients suffer from comorbid depressivity or anxiety [45,46], which themselves might cause changes in oscillatory brain activity [47,48]. We tested this in the present study and were unable to demonstrate an association between scores in the depressivity, somatization, or anxiety scales of the SCL-90-R questionnaire and band power. This might be due to the circumstance, however, that mean SCL-90-R scores were rather low even though depressivity and anxiety scores were significantly elevated in the present patient group compared to the control group.

Taken together, the results suggest that the tinnitus syndrome can at least be sub-classified into an intensity/loudness category which represents the strength of the tinnitus-related signal, and into a tinnitus-related distress category. In the following, these two aspects will be discussed separately.

Tinnitus loudness

Tinnitus loudness estimates largely depend on the type of measurement used and it is a matter of controversy which loudness measure represents a valuable estimate. Tinnitus loudness can be assessed in a psychophysical matching procedure in which the loudness of an external auditory signal is matched to the perceived tinnitus loudness [33]. Alternatively, tinnitus loudness can be determined subjectively by ratings on visual analogue scales (VAS) [25]. Fowler [49,50] report that for most tinnitus patients the psychophysically determined tinnitus loudness was only a few dB above threshold, a statement which was frequently confirmed in subsequent studies [24]. This often contrasts to the high tinnitus loudness that is reported by the patients or that is found with VAS ratings. Fowler called this "the illusion of loudness" [49,50]. Interestingly in that respect, VAS loudness ratings typically correlate with tinnitus-related distress [6], whereas the psycho-physically determined tinnitus loudness does not [24,33]. Tyler and Conrad-Armes [33] suggested that the discrepancy between psychophysically determined and subjectively experienced tinnitus loudness can be resolved by calculating the psychophysical loudness estimate in the sone scale (see "Psychoacoustic measurements").

Alternatively, it is possible that the discrepancy between objective and subjective tinnitus loudness estimates originates from recruitment. If a pure tone in a frequency range with significant hearing loss – which is common for the tinnitus frequencies – is used for matching, recruitment phenomena may lead to substantial divergence from the tinnitus loudness estimate derived from matching with a pure tone that corresponds to a frequency region without major hearing loss [33]. An additional factor that influences the perceived loudness of an external sound is its frequency composition since loudness-intensity-functions differ between complex sounds and pure tones [51]. Because the tinnitus spectrum is often complex it appears likely, that the loudness-intensity characteristic of a tinnitus resembles that of a complex sound rather than that of a pure tone.

In the present study, a complex sound, the reconstructed tinnitus spectrum was used for loudness matching in addition to the pure tone corresponding to the major peak of the tinnitus spectrum, and to a 1 kHz pure tone. Because of the reasons outlined above, matching to the complex tinnitus spectrum was expected to achieve better loudness estimates. Logically consistent, only the loudness estimate (TL_{dBSL}) derived from matching with the tinnitus spectrum exhibited a significant correlation with gamma oscillatory activity and at many electrode positions also with delta band power. Correlative strength was not improved by converting this loudness measure to the sone scale (TL_{sones}). In contrast, tinnitus loudness determined by matching with the pure tone that corresponded to the major peak of the tinnitus spectrum did not show a significant correlation with any frequency band, nor did loudness derived by matching with a 1 kHz pure tone (TL_{1kHz}). Taken together, tinnitus loudness determined by matching with the complex reconstructed tinnitus spectrum may represent a better loudness estimate than those derived from the commonly used pure tone matching procedures and therefore is recommended for the psychoacoustic determination of tinnitus loudness.

Significant correlations between the tinnitus loudness estimate measured with TL_{dBSL} and brain oscillatory activity were seen in the gamma and the delta band. It has repeatedly been shown that gamma band activity ($f > 30$ Hz) is elevated in tinnitus subjects compared to controls [13–15,18,20,52], and similar to the present study previous studies reported elevated gamma oscillations in the hemisphere contralateral to the tinnitus ear for unilateral tinnitus [14,15,52] but see [53].

In addition to increases in spontaneous gamma oscillatory activity, increases in delta activity correlated with the TL_{dBSL} tinnitus loudness measure. This finding is in line with previous MEG studies that reported enhanced delta activity in tinnitus subjects with hearing impairment [11,12,54]. Following the thalamocortical dysrhythmia hypothesis originally proposed by Llinas et al. [10], slow wave activity in the delta and theta frequency range is a consequence of input deafferentation, while gamma activity is seen as the tinnitus correlate. Delta activity in tinnitus patients was attenuated by masking [54], as well as during residual inhibition [55], and auditory cortex could be pinpointed as its source [54]. Adjamian et al. [54] did not see a significant correlation between tinnitus loudness and delta band power, which the authors explained by the fact that they correlated subjective loudness rating on a VAS to MEG activity. In contrast, psychoacoustic loudness rating to the reconstructed tinnitus spectrum TL_{dBSL} put forth a significant correlation between tinnitus loudness and delta oscillatory activity. Adjamian et al. [54] speculate that increased slow wave activity during wakening may represent synchronized slowing of activity in large populations of neurons with altered thalamic input due to neural deprivation.

Oscillatory activity in the gamma range is furthermore inversely correlated to hearing impairment. This association has not been reported before, and may be owed to the fact that in contrast to other studies (e.g. [13]) hearing impairment was determined for a wider frequency spectrum in the present study which in particular included the high frequency spectrum. In the rodent auditory system, gamma oscillations occur spontaneously and they remain after lesioning the auditory thalamus. This and intracortical recordings suggest that the observed gamma oscillations are generated intrinsically in auditory cortex [56]. Also in a rodent, it was found that age-related hearing impairment is associated with changes in central processing in addition to cochlear impairments [57]. Reduced gamma oscillatory activity during absence of auditory stimulation in a sound-proof environment as seen in the present recordings might therefore be an indicator of reduced auditory cortical functioning in the tinnitus group. In the control group with less hearing impairment between 2 kHz and 10 kHz, no correlation for MHL and gamma band power could be detected.

Although distinct, because it is generated within the auditory system, tinnitus is an auditory percept. Therefore, processing of this signal should in some aspects resemble the processing of external sounds. External sounds evoke event related potentials (ERP), and gamma oscillations are a component of ERP occurring about 100 ms and 300 ms after sound onset in cat hippocampus, reticular formation and cortex [58]. Gamma oscillations have been associated with attention [59,60] and with emotional content of the sound [61]. This suggests that tinnitus-associated gamma oscillations are influenced by attention and emotion through top-down mechanisms. It is therefore possible that gamma oscillations in tinnitus patients, which were shown to be related to psychophysically determined tinnitus loudness in the present study and to VAS-evaluated tinnitus loudness previously [14], represent activity that is already modified by top-down influences on a primary tinnitus-related signal. Tinnitus loudness obtained by VAS rating shows higher correlations with tinnitus distress than the psychophysiologically determined tinnitus loudness [6]. This in turn might explain the higher correlation between gamma activity and VAS-determined tinnitus loudness [14] as compared to the psychophysiological tinnitus loudness derived by matching with the reconstructed tinnitus spectrum.

In addition, the tinnitus loudness TL_{dBSL} showed significant correlations with delta power at individual electrode positions. In addition to the suggestion that this may be related to auditory deafferentation [54], this can be seen as an expression of the circumstance that tinnitus loudness and tinnitus-related distress are only partially separate aspects of the tinnitus with louder tinnitus usually being associated with more distress (see [6] and below).

In summary, whereas both enhanced gamma and delta activity in the (contralateral) auditory cortex (AC) are associated with tinnitus loudness, only gamma activity is seen as a correlate of the tinnitus percept, and it may be related to attention directed towards and emotions generated by this percept.

Tinnitus-related distress

Increases of tinnitus-related distress correlate with increases of power in the delta band. This correlation loses significance, however, when controlled for general psychological distress (GPD). GPD does not exhibit a significant correlation with delta band activity on its own, which might be due to the circumstance that mean SCL-90-R scores were rather low even though depressivity and anxiety scores were significantly elevated in the present patient group. Besides that, content overlap between the TQ and SCL-90-R questionnaires may obscure the association between delta band activity and tinnitus-related distress when controlling for GPD. In addition, the association between tinnitus loudness and delta band power might have obscured the association between tinnitus-related distress and delta power in the global analysis, although according to the electrode specific analysis it has its maximum in the right hemisphere whereas correlation strength between tinnitus-related distress and delta band activity peaks in the left hemisphere.

MEG studies also found enhanced delta band power in tinnitus patients compared to controls [10–12], which along with Llinas et al. [10] was interpreted as the result of sensory deprivation. An alternative interpretation is suggested by the observation of increased delta activity in depressed elderly patients [48], since tinnitus patients are typically of older age and often express enhanced depressivity (e.g. [6]). Moreover, the P300 auditory evoked response correlates positively with delta EEG power and can be enhanced by emotionally relevant salient stimuli. Salience of stimuli in turn appears to be controlled by dopamine release in nucleus accumbens (NAc). Interestingly, in animals delta oscillations correlate with membrane potential changes in NAc [62–64], and D1 agonists of the neurotransmitter dopamine which plays a major role in NAc are known to reduce delta activity [65,66]. In light of the role of NAc in the tinnitus model put forward by Rauschecker et al. [67], it is tentative to speculate that the association between increases of delta activity, tinnitus-related distress, and to a lesser extent tinnitus loudness is related to dopaminergic activity.

Tinnitus patients with high tinnitus-related distress exhibit higher theta oscillatory power than patients with low tinnitus-related distress. Depressiveness itself is associated with enhanced activity in the theta band [47,48]. Moreover, hippocampal theta oscillations were shown to strongly associate with anxiety levels in different animal species during various experimental conditions [68–71], and they are inhibited by several anxiolytics [71–75]. This might explain the higher theta activity in the highly distressed tinnitus patients, while lack of significant correlations between theta power and depressivity as well as anxiety scores of the SCL-90-R may be attributed to their low average level in the present patient population. Whereas gamma oscillations are generated by local circuits, theta oscillations involve larger systems. Slow theta oscillations are generated in a number of brain structures including the hippocampus and parts of the limbic system [76]. They depend on cholinergic input from the medial septum (hippocampal theta) or the basal forebrain (neocortical theta) and are thought to play a role in top-down processing. Theta phase modulation has been implicated in memory retrieval (working memory) and attention [77]. Simultaneous recordings from hippocampus and medial frontal cortex in freely behaving rats indicate that spikes in frontal areas are often phase-locked to the hippocampal theta rhythm, and gamma oscillations generated locally in the neocortex were entrained by this theta rhythm [77]. Furthermore, intracranial recordings in various species and in human epilepsy patients suggest that gamma-theta coupling may contribute to learning and memory formation [77], during which gamma synchrony often couples to the phase of delta or theta oscillations [78]. Therefore, coupling of low frequency and gamma oscillations in tinnitus patients appears likely and it may represent the interaction of the limbic and frontal cortical systems with AC. Enhanced oscillatory brain activity in the gamma range was found to be associated with tinnitus-related distress in some studies [27,79]. An association that could not be substantiated in the present study, however.

Similarly, the reports on a correlation between tinnitus-related distress with alpha and beta band activity [27,28,79] are not supported by the present study. In humans a multitude of factors that are largely independent of tinnitus and are difficult to control for might account for these differences. For example, hunger after overnight fasting is known to influence delta activity [80]. Other reasons could be related to patient selection. This emphasizes the need for a standardization of EEG experiments that investigate tinnitus to allow comparison between studies.

Minimum masking level

Minimum masking level (MML) represents the lowest level at which external sounds completely mask the tinnitus percept. Maskability by environmental sound provides the patient with an important, if not the only tool to influence his tinnitus percept, therefore it is of utmost clinical importance to understand the underlying mechanism [81]. Furthermore MML has been suggested as a measure for treatment outcome [82]. Mechanisms that account for the observed variance in MML between tinnitus patients are largely unknown, but MML are expected to be associated with tinnitus-related distress [8], and also with the perceived tinnitus loudness. In the present study MML was solely but highly significantly related to delta oscillatory power, and the difference between MML and MHL increased with increasing delta power. This points to an association of MML with tinnitus loudness as well as with tinnitus-related distress. We did not find a significant correlation for MML (or the difference of MML and MHL) and tinnitus-related distress, or for MML and the tinnitus loudness TL_{dBSL} and TL_{sones}, however, whereas in an earlier study with a larger number of severely distressed subjects MML was the only audiologically parameter that showed a significant correlation with tinnitus-related distress [8].

In particular because of its clinical importance, mechanisms underlying tinnitus masking and their association with brain oscillatory activity should be addressed in further studies.

Conclusion

This is the first report that finds a significant correlation between psychophysically determined tinnitus loudness and brain activity. In line with previous reports the tinnitus percept loudness correlates with gamma and delta oscillatory activity, but only when tinnitus loudness is estimated with a novel type of sound derived by tinnitus reconstruction. We report an easy to apply synthesization paradigm to generate this sound, which comprehensively reflects the spectral complexity of the tinnitus percept and for which patients report extraordinary similarity to their tinnitus. Because this novel tinnitus reconstruction achieves better results than other

types of sounds, it is suggested to use it for determining tinnitus loudness in future studies.

The results of the present study also support the clinically motivated distinction between tinnitus loudness and tinnitus-related distress which were shown to associate with distinct patterns of gamma and delta oscillatory brain activity. Additionally, tinnitus-related distress correlates with theta oscillatory activity which is known to be associated with depressivity and anxiety. The increase of delta oscillatory power together with increasing minimum masking level should be investigated in more detail in the future because of its high clinical importance as a tool to control the tinnitus percept.

Acknowledgments

The authors would like to thank all volunteers who participated in this study. The excellent technical assistance of Andrea Seegmueller, Joyce Sonny, and the medical student Anne Grieger is gratefully acknowledged.

Author Contributions

Conceived and designed the experiments: TB WD. Performed the experiments: TB WD. Analyzed the data: TB EW WD. Wrote the paper: TB EW WD.

References

1. Sindhusake D, Golding M, Newall P, Rubin G, Jakobsen K, et al. (2003) Risk factors for tinnitus in a population of older adults: the blue mountains hearing study. Ear Hear 24: 501.
2. Weisz N, Dohrmann K, Elbert T (2007) The relevance of spontaneous activity for the coding of the tinnitus sensation. Prog Brain Res 166: 61–70.
3. Roberts LE, Eggermont JJ, Caspary DM, Shore SE, Melcher JR, et al. (2010) Ringing ears: the neuroscience of tinnitus. J Neurosci 30: 14972–14979.
4. Rosenhall U (2003) The influence of ageing on noise-induced hearing loss. Noise Health 5: 47–53.
5. Krog NH, Engdahla B, Tambs K (2010) The association between tinnitus and mental health in a general population sample: results from the hunt study. J Psychosom Res 69: 289–298.
6. Wallhäusser-Franke E, Brade J, Balkenhol T, D'Amelio R, Seegmüller A, et al. (2012) Tinnitus: Distinguishing between subjectively perceived loudness and tinnitus-related distress. PLoS One 7: e34583.
7. Leaver AM, Seydell-Greenwald A, Turesky TK, Morgan S, Kim HJ, et al. (2012) Cortico-limbic morphology separates tinnitus from tinnitus distress. Front Syst Neurosci 6:21.
8. Delb W, D'Amelio R, Schonecke O, Iro H (1999) Are there psychological or audiological parameters determining tinnitus impact? In: Hazell J, editor, Proceedings of the Sixth International Tinnitus Seminar, Cambridge: Oxford University Press. pp. 446–451.
9. Langguth B, Landgrebe M, Kleinjung T, Sand GP, Hajak G (2011) Tinnitus and depression. World J Biol Psychiatry 12: 489–500.
10. Llin'as RR, Ribary U, Jeanmonod D, Kronberg E, Mitra PP (1999) Thalamocortical dysrhythmia: A neurological and neuropsychiatric syndrome characterized by magnetoencephalography. Proc Natl Acad Sci U S A 96: 15222–15227.
11. Weisz N, Moratti S, Meinzer M, Dohrmann K, Elbert T (2005) Tinnitus perception and distress is related to abnormal spontaneous brain activity as measured by magnetoencephalography. PLoS Med 2: e153.
12. Weisz N, Müller S, Schlee W, Dohrmann K, Hartmann T, et al. (2007) The neural code of auditory phantom perception. J Neurosci 27: 1479–1484.
13. Ortmann M, Müller N, Schlee W, Weisz N (2011) Rapid increases of gamma power in the auditory cortex following noise trauma in humans. Eur J Neurosci 33: 568–575.
14. van der Loo E, Gais S, CongedoM, Vanneste S, Plazier M, et al. (2009) Tinnitus intensity dependent gamma oscillations of the contralateral auditory cortex. PLoS One 4: e7396.
15. Vanneste S, Plazier M, van der Loo E, de Heyning PV, Ridder DD (2011) The difference between uni- and bilateral auditory phantom percept. Clin Neurophysiol 122: 578–587.
16. Uhlhaas PJ, Singer W (2006) Neural synchrony in brain disorders: relevance for cognitive dysfunctions and pathophysiology. Neuron 52: 155–168.
17. Buehlmann A, Deco G (2010) Optimal information transfer in the cortex through synchronization. PLoS Comput Biol 6: e1000934.
18. Lorenz I, Müller N, Schlee W, Hartmann T, Weisz N (2009) Loss of alpha power is related to increased gamma synchronization – a marker of reduced inhibition in tinnitus? Neurosci Lett 453: 225–228.
19. Klimesch W, Sauseng P, Hanslmayr S (2007) EEG alpha oscillations: the inhibition-timing hypothesis. Brain Res Rev 53: 63–88.
20. Weisz N, Moratti S, Meinzer M, Dohrmann K, Elbert T (2011) Alpha rhythms in audition: cognitive and clinical perspectives. Front Psychol 2:73.
21. Lehtelä L, Salmelin R, Hari R (1997) Evidence for reactive magnetic 10-Hz rhythm in the human auditory cortex. Neurosci Lett 222: 111–114.
22. Noreña AJ (2011) An integrative model of tinnitus based on a central gain controlling neural sensitivity. Neurosci Biobehav Rev 35: 1089–1109.
23. Dieroff HG (1976) Possibilities of improving the diagnosis of noise-induced hearing damage by means of directional audiometry, the dichotic speech discrimination test, and the EEG. Audiology 15: 152–162.
24. Tyler RS, Stouffer JL (1989) A review of tinnitus loudness. Hear J 42: 52–57.
25. Meikle MB, Henry JA, Griest SE, Stewart BJ, Abrams HB, et al. (2012) The tinnitus functional index: development of a new clinical measure for chronic, intrusive tinnitus. Ear Hear 33: 153–176.
26. Hiller W, Goebel G (2006) Factors influencing tinnitus loudness and annoyance. Arch Otolaryngol Head Neck Surg 132: 1323–1330.
27. Schlee W, Mueller N, Hartmann T, Keil J, Lorenz I, et al. (2009) Mapping cortical hubs in tinnitus. BMC Biol 7:80.
28. Vanneste S, Plazier M, van der Loo E, de Heyning PV, Congedo M, et al. (2010) The neural correlates of tinnitus-related distress. Neuroimage 52: 470–480.
29. Vanneste S, Joos K, Ridder DD (2012) Prefrontal cortex based sex differences in tinnitus perception: same tinnitus intensity, same tinnitus distress, different mood. PLoS One 7: e31182.
30. Hallam RS, Jakes SC, Hinchcliffe R (1988) Cognitive variables in tinnitus annoyance. Br J Clin Psychol 27: 213–222.
31. Goebel G, Hiller W (1998) Tinnitus-Fragebogen [Tinnitus questionnaire]. Göttingen: Hogrefe Verlag.
32. Noreña A, Micheyl C, Chéry-Croze S, Collet L (2002) Psychoacoustic characterization of the tinnitus spectrum: Implications for the underlying mechanisms of tinnitus. Audiol Neurootol 7: 358–369.
33. Tyler RS, Conrad-Armes D (1983) The determination of tinnitus loudness considering the effects of recruitment. J Speech Hear Res 26: 59–72.
34. Derogatis LR (1994) Symptom Checklist-90-Revised (SCL-90-R). Oxford: Pearson Assessment.
35. Franke GH (2002) SCL-90-R – Die Symptom-Checkliste von L.R. Derogatis [SCL-90-R: The symptom checklist of L.R. Derogatis]. Göttingen: Beltz Test GmbH, 2 edition.
36. Kuo SM, Morgan DR (1996) Active Noise Control Systems: Algorithm and DSP Implementations. New York: John Wiley & Sons.
37. Delorme A, Makeig S (2004) EEGLAB: an open source toolbox for analysis of single-trial EEG dynamics including independent component analysis. J Neurosci Methods 134: 9–21.
38. Belouchrani A, Abed-Meraim K, Cardoso JF, Moulines E (1997) A blind source separation technique using second-order statistics. IEEE Trans on Sig Proc 45: 434–444.
39. Mitra PP, Pesaran B (1999) Analysis of dynamic brain imaging data. Biophys J 76: 691–708.
40. Mitra PP, Bokil H (2008) Observed Brain Dynamics. New York: Oxford University Press, 1 edition.
41. Michel CM, Murray MM, Lantz G, Gonzalez S, Spinelli L, et al. (2004) EEG source imaging. Clin Neurophysiol 115: 2195–2222.

42. Gibbons JD, Chakraborti S (2010) Nonparametric Statistical Inference. Boca Raton: Chapman & Hall/CRC Press, 5 edition.

43. Benjamini Y, Hochberg Y (1995) Controlling the false discovery rate: A practical and powerful approach to multiple testing. J Roy Statist Soc Ser B 57: 289–300.

44. Jastreboff PJ (1990) Phantom auditory perception (tinnitus): mechanisms of generation and perception. Neurosci Res 8: 221–254.

45. D'Amelio R, Archonti C, Scholz S, Falkai P, Plinkert PK, et al. (2004) Psychological distress associated with acute tinnitus. HNO 52: 599–603.

46. Langenbach M, Olderog M, Michel O, Albus C, Köhle K (2005) Psychosocial and personality predictors of tinnitus-related distress. Gen Hosp Psychiatry 27: 73–77.

47. Grin-Yatsenko VA, Baas I, Ponomarev VA, Kropotov JD (2010) Independent component approach to the analysis of EEG recordings at early stages of depressive disorders. Clin Neurophysiol 121: 281–289.

48. Köhler S, Ashton CH, Marsh R, Thomas AJ, Barnett NA, et al. (2011) Electrophysiological changes in late life depression and their relation to structural brain changes. Int Psychogeriatr 23: 141–148.

49. Fowler EP (1940) Head noises: Significance, measurement and importance in diagnosis and treatment. Arch Otolaryngol 32: 903–914.

50. Fowler EP (1942) The "illusion of loudness" of tinnitus – its etiology and treatment. Laryngoscope 52: 275–285.

51. Fastl H, Zwicker E (2007) Psychoacoustics – Facts and Models. Berlin Heidelberg: Springer, 3 edition.

52. Llinás R, Urbano FJ, Leznik E, Ramírez RR, van Marle HJ (2005) Rhythmic and dysrhythmic thalamocortical dynamics: Gaba systems and the edge effect. Trends Neurosci 28: 325–333.

53. Vanneste S, de Heyning PV, Ridder DD (2011) Contralateral parahippocampal gamma-band activity determines noise-like tinnitus laterality: a region of interest analysis. Neuroscience 199: 481–490.

54. Adjamian P, Sereda M, Zobay O, Hall DA, Palmer AR (2012) Neuromagnetic indicators of tinnitus and tinnitus masking in patients with and without hearing loss. J Assoc Res Otolaryngol 13: 715–731.

55. Kahlbrock N, Weisz N (2008) Transient reduction of tinnitus intensity is marked by concomitant reductions of delta band power. BMC Biol 6:4.

56. Sukov W, Barth DS (1998) Three-dimensional analysis of spontaneous and thalamically evoked gamma oscillations in auditory cortex. J Neurophysiol 79: 2875–2884.

57. Gourévitch B, Edeline JM (2011) Age-related changes in the guinea pig auditory cortex: relationship with brainstem changes and comparison with tone-induced hearing loss. Eur J Neurosci 34: 1953–1965.

58. Başar E, Başar-Eroğlu C, Karakaş S, Schürmann M (2000) Brain oscillations in perception and memory. Int J Psychophysiol 35: 95–124.

59. Tiitinen H, Sinkkonen J, Reinikainen K, Alho K, Lavikainen J, et al. (1993) Selective attention enhances the auditory 40-Hz transient response in humans. Nature 364: 59–60.

60. Tang Y, Li Y, Wang J, Tong S, Li H, et al. (2011) Induced gamma activity in EEG represents cognitive control during detecting emotional expressions. In: Conf Proc IEEE Eng Med Biol Soc. IEEE, pp. 1717–1720.

61. Domínguez-Borràs J, Garcia-Garcia M, Escera C (2012) Phase re-setting of gamma neural oscillations during novelty processing in an appetitive context. Biol Psychol 89: 545–552.

62. Leung LS, Yim CY (1993) Rhythmic delta-frequency activities in the nucleus accumbens of anesthetized and freely moving rats. Can J Physiol Pharmacol 71: 311–320.

63. O'Donnell P, Grace AA (1995) Synaptic interactions among excitatory afferents to nucleus accumbens neurons: hippocampal gating of prefrontal cortical input. J Neurosci 15: 3622–3639.

64. Grace AA (1995) The tonic/phasic model of dopamine system regulation: its relevance for understanding how stimulant abuse can alter basal ganglia function. Drug Alcohol Depend 37: 111–129.

65. Ferger B, Kropf W, Kuschinsky K (1994) Studies on electroencephalogram (EEG) in rats suggest that moderate doses of cocaine or d-amphetamine activate D1 rather than D2 receptors. Psychopharmacology (Berl) 114: 297–308.

66. Chang AYW, Kuo TBJ, Tsai TH, Chen CF, Chan SH (1995) Power spectral analysis of electroencephalographic desynchronization induced by cocaine in rats: correlation with evaluation of noradrenergic neurotransmission at the medial prefrontal cortex. Synapse 21: 149–157.

67. Rauschecker JP, Leaver AM, Mühlau M (2010) Tuning out the noise: limbic-auditory interactions in tinnitus. Neuron 66: 819–826.

68. Fontani G, Carli G (1997) Hippocampal electrical activity and behavior in the rabbit. Arch Ital Biol 135: 49–71.

69. Gray JA, McNaughton N (2003) The Neuropsychology of Anxiety: An Enquiry into the Functions of the Septo-Hippocampal System. Oxford University Press, 2 edition.

70. Gordon JA, Lacefield CO, Kentros CG, Hen R (2005) State-dependent alterations in hippocampal oscillations in serotonin 1A receptor-deficient mice. J Neurosci 25: 6509–6519.

71. Siok CJ, Taylor CP, Hajós M (2009) Anxiolytic profile of pregabalin on elicited hippocampal theta oscillation. Neuropharmacology 56: 379–385.

72. Caudarella M, Durkin T, Galey D, Jeantet Y, Jaffard R (1987) The effect of diazepam on hippocampal EEG in relation to behavior. Brain Res 435: 202–212.

73. McNaughton N, Gray JA (2000) Anxiolytic action on the behavioural inhibition system implies multiple types of arousal contribute to anxiety. J Affect Disord 61: 161–176.

74. van Lier H, Drinkenburg WHIM, van Eeten YJW, Coenen AML (2004) Effects of diazepam and zolpidem on EEG beta frequencies are behavior-specific in rats. Neuropharmacology 47: 163–174.

75. McNaughton N, Kocsis B, Hajós M (2007) Elicited hippocampal theta rhythm: a screen for anxiolytic and procognitive drugs through changes in hippocampal function? Behav Pharmacol 18: 329–346.

76. Knyazev GG (2007) Motivation, emotion, and their inhibitory control mirrored in brain oscillations. Neurosci Biobehav Rev 31: 377–395.

77. Wang XJ (2010) Neurophysiological and computational principles of cortical rhythms in cognition. Physiol Rev 90: 1195–2268.

78. Schroeder CE, Lakatos P (2009) The gamma oscillation: master or slave? Brain Topogr 22: 24–36.

79. Ridder DD, Vanneste S, Congedo M (2011) The distressed brain: a group blind source separation analysis on tinnitus. PLoS One 6: e24273.

80. Hoffman LD, Polich J (1998) EEG, ERPs and food consumption. Biol Psychol 48: 139–151.

81. Andersson G, Lyttkens L, Larsen HC (1999) Distinguishing levels of tinnitus distress. Clin Otolaryngol Allied Sci 24: 404–410.

82. Jastreboff PJ, Hazell JWP, Graham RL (1994) Neurophysiological model of tinnitus: dependence of the minimal masking level on treatment outcome. Hear Res 80: 216–232.

8

Disentangling Depression and Distress Networks in the Tinnitus Brain

Kathleen Joos, Sven Vanneste*, Dirk De Ridder

Brai²n, Tinnitus Research Initiative Clinic Antwerp, Department of Neurosurgery, University Hospital Antwerp, Belgium

Abstract

Tinnitus is the continuous perception of an internal auditory stimulus. This permanent sound often affects a person's emotional state inducing distress and depressive feelings changes in 6–25% of the affected population. Distress and depression are two distinct emotional states. Whereas distress describes a transient aversive state, interfering with a person's ability to adequately adapt to stressors, depressive feelings should rather be considered as a more constant emotional state. Based on previous observations in chronic pain, posttraumatic stress disorder and depression, we assume that both states are related to separate neural circuits. We used the Dutch version of the Tinnitus Questionnaire to assess the global index of distress together with the Beck Depression Inventory to evaluate the depressive symptoms accompanying tinnitus. Furthermore sLORETA analysis was performed to correlate current density distribution with distress and depression scores, revealing a lateralization effect of depression versus distress. Distress is mainly correlated with alpha 2, beta 1 and beta 2 activity of the right frontopolar cortex and orbitofrontal cortex in combination with beta 2 activation of the anterior cingulate cortex. In contrast, the more permanent depressive alterations induced by tinnitus are associated with activity of alpha 2 activity in the left frontopolar and orbitofrontal cortex. These specific neural circuits are embedded in a greater neural network, with the parahippocampal region functioning as a crucial linkage between both tinnitus related pathways.

Editor: Berthold Langguth, University of Regensburg, Germany

Funding: These authors have no support or funding to report.

Competing Interests: The authors have declared that no competing interests exist.

* E-mail: sven.vanneste@ua.ac.be

Introduction

Tinnitus is the awareness of a tone, a ringing or buzzing sound in the absence of an external auditory stimulus, also defined as a phantom phenomenon [1]. The constant perception of this internal sound frequently causes a considerable amount of distress. It has a prevalence of up to 10%–15% in an adult population, with an increasing prevalence with increasing age [2–4]. About 6% to 25% of tinnitus patients report that their quality of life is reduced [2,5,6], with 2–4% of the total population suffering in the worst degree [3]. Thus, although a considerable amount of people experience tinnitus, 1 out of 5 is emotionally seriously affected by it reporting sleep disturbances, lack of energy and mood disorders [7]. There is no correlation between the amount of distress and the perceived loudness as measured by tinnitus matching [1], suggesting that two separate neural networks might encode tinnitus intensity and tinnitus distress.

Tinnitus can be considered an auditory phantom phenomenon [8] similar to deafferentation pain seen in the somatosensory system [9–11], related to reorganization [12,13] and hyperactivity [14,15] of the auditory central nervous system. New insights into the neurobiology of tinnitus suggest that neuronal changes are not limited to the classical auditory pathways. In particular, the insula [16], anterior cingulate cortex (ACC) [17,18], amygdala, dorsolateral prefrontal cortex [19] and (para)hippocampus (PHC) [20–22] seem to play a specific role in tinnitus as they take part in the neural circuit underlying tinnitus related distress.

Studying the affective dimension of pain and tinnitus, distress has been considered an aversive state in which a person is unable to adapt completely to stressors (i.e. pain or tinnitus) [23,24]. The brain areas involved in tinnitus related distress are also involved in the emotional component of the pain matrix such as the ACC, prefrontal cortex, amygdala, and insula [25–29].

However apart from distress, studies indicate that depressive feelings are an important aspect in pain and tinnitus as well. About 40% of tinnitus patients report to suffer from mood disorders such as depression due to their tinnitus [30]. Mood has been defined as a relatively long lasting emotional state that is less specific, less intense, and less triggered by a particular event [23,24]. As such, mood can be seen as a stable long-term change induced by the persistence of pain and pain distress [29] and depression is a pathological mood state. In pain, the underlying emotional network related to mood or depressive feelings comprises the medial prefrontal cortex, amygdala, PHC, insula and ACC [25,31,32], emphasizing the crucial role of the frontal brain regions, which have been associated with the secondary affect in chronic pain [29].

Chronic pain and tinnitus show many similarities in symptoms [33] and pathophysiology [34,35]. For example, a touch stimulus to the skin can evoke a painful sensation (allodynia) in patients with chronic pain, while tinnitus patients often perceive specific sounds as unpleasant or painful (misophonia) [36]. The generation of these characteristic symptoms is due to a wind-up phenomenon caused by neural plasticity. Furthermore in chronic pain and tinnitus brain areas beyond the somatosensory and auditory brain regions are involved [37]. Furthermoreelectrical stimulation of these sensory cortices has the ability of relieving or masking both pain and tinnitus [38]. Based on the various similarities between pain and tinnitus, we expect that, in analogy to chronic pain [29], distress and depression are generated by distinct neural networks. Hence, the main goal of this study is to disentangle the networks related to distress and depressive feelings caused by tinnitus and to separate these from the observed neural changes associated with the perception of the tinnitus sound using source analysis of the resting-state EEG activity (eyes closed). Depressive feelings are assessed by the Dutch version of the Beck Depression Inventory-II (BDI-II) and the tinnitus related distress by using the Tinnitus Questionnaire (TQ) and correlated to continuous scalp EEG recordings and Low Resolution Electromagnetic Tomography (sLORETA), a tomographic inverse solution imaging technique.

Results

Behavior measures

A significant correlation was obtained between BDI and TQ $r = .29$, $p<.05$. In addition a significant correlation was obtained between TQ and distress as measured with the numeric rating scale (NRS) ($r = .41$, $p<.0$). No significant effect was found between the TQ and respectively age and tinnitus duration, nor was there an association with tinnitus laterality and tinnitus type. A similar analysis with the BDI and distress as measured by the NRS, age, tinnitus duration, tinnitus laterality and tinnitus type yielded no significant effect.

Source localization BDI

Analyzing the results with sLORETA we observed a significant positive correlation ($p<.05$) between BDI scores and alpha 1 ($r = .34$, $p<.05$) and alpha 2 ($r = .37$, $p<.01$) activity in the frontopolar and orbitofrontal cortex (OFC) (Brodmann area (BA) 10 and BA11) and beta 3 ($r = .27$, $p<.05$) activity in the sgACC (BA25) and the PHC (BA35&36) (see figure 1). No significant correlations could be detected between depression severity, assessed by the BDI-II, and other frequency bands.

Source localization. TQA sLORETA analysis demonstrated a significant positive correlation between TQ scores and alpha 2 ($r = .30$, $p<.05$) and beta 2 ($r = .29$, $p<.05$) activity in the frontopolar and OFC (BA10, BA11), subgenual ACC (sgACC)(BA25) and ACC (BA24) (see figure 2). No significant correlations could be detected between the TQ and other frequency bands.

Source localization of distress as measured by the numeric rating scale

sLORETA correlation demonstrated a significant positive effect between the distress using a NRS and respectively alpha 2 activity ($r = .34$, $p<.05$) in the frontopolar and OFC (BA10, BA11) and beta 3 activity ($r = .40$, $p<.05$) subgenual anterior cingulate cortex (BA25), and and parahippocampal area (BA27 & 28) (see figure 3). No significant correlations could be detected between the distress using a NRS and other frequency bands.

Region of interest analysis

The BDI correlates significantly with left and right frontopolar and OFC (BA10 & BA11), the ACC (BA24), and the sgACC (BA25) for the alpha 2 frequency band (see Table 1). By conducting a partial correlation analysis for BDI, controlling for TQ, a significant correlation was only obtained for the left frontopolar and OFC (BA10 & BA11). For beta 3 a significant

positive correlation was found between the left and right PHC (BA35&36). However, when controlling for the TQ this effect did not hold. By conducting a partial correlation analysis for BDI, controlling for distress using a NRS, a significant correlation was only obtained for the left frontopolar and OFC (BA10 & BA11). No correlations could be found for other frequency bands, or with other regions of interest.

For the TQ a significant positive correlation was found between left and right frontopolar and OFC (BA10 & BA11) and the sgACC (BA25) for the alpha 2 frequency band. For the alpha 2 frequency band only a significant positive partial correlation could be found between the right OFC (BA11) and TQ, controlling for BDI, although there is a trend to significance between the TQ and the right frontopolar cortex (BA10). For the beta 1 frequency band a significant positive correlation was found between the right frontopolar and OFC (BA10 & 11) and the TQ. Although only a significant partial correlation could be obtained between the right OFC (BA11) and TQ when controlling for BDI, with a trend to significance for the right frontopolar cortex and the TQ. As for beta 2 significant partial correlations could be obtained between the right frontopolar and OFC (BA10 & 11), the ACC (BA24) and the sgACC (BA25) and TQ.

For distress using a NRS a significant positive correlation was found between left and right frontopolar and OFC (BA10 & BA11) for the alpha 2 frequency band (see Table 2). For the alpha 2 frequency band only a significant positive partial correlation could be found between the right OFC (BA10 & BA11) and distress using a NRS, controlling for BDI. For the beta 3 frequency band a significant positive correlation was obtained for ACC (BA24) and sgACC, this effect remained after controlling for BDI. No correlations could be found for other frequency bands, or with other regions of interest.

Discussion

In this study we focused on the differences between the neural circuits underlying depression and tinnitus-related distress.

A significant correlation was obtained between the BDI and TQ indicated that both questionnaires have some relation. However this correlation was rather weak explaining only .08% of the variance, indicating that both questionnaires e only partly overlie each other, but that they measure other concepts.

Using the TQ to assess the severity of perceived tinnitus related distress, a positive correlation was demonstrated for the frontopolar, OFC and sgACC in the alpha 2 band together with a positive correlation of beta 1 and beta 2 activity in the right frontopolar and OFC cortex. In addition a positive correlation is present with the beta 2 activity in the pgACC and sgACC. These findings indicate that the higher score for tinnitus related distress goes together with increased activity in the frontopolar, OFC, sgACC and pgACC. Partial correlations further demonstrated more precisely that tinnitus related distress correlates exclusively with the right frontopolar and OFC for alpha 2, beta 1 and beta 2, as well as with the ACC and sgACC.

Using the BDI to measure severity of depression, positive correlations could be revealed between BDI-II and respectively alpha 1 and alpha 2 in the frontopolar and OFC, and beta 3 activity in the sgACC, indicating that patients with higher scores on the BDI-II showed an increased synchronized activity in frontopolar and OFC, and sgACC. Partial correlations further demonstrated that depressive feelings exclusively correlates with the left frontopolar and OFC in alpha 2, showing that the higher a patient scores on depressive feelings the more current density is demonstrated in the left OFC for alpha 2. For these latter results

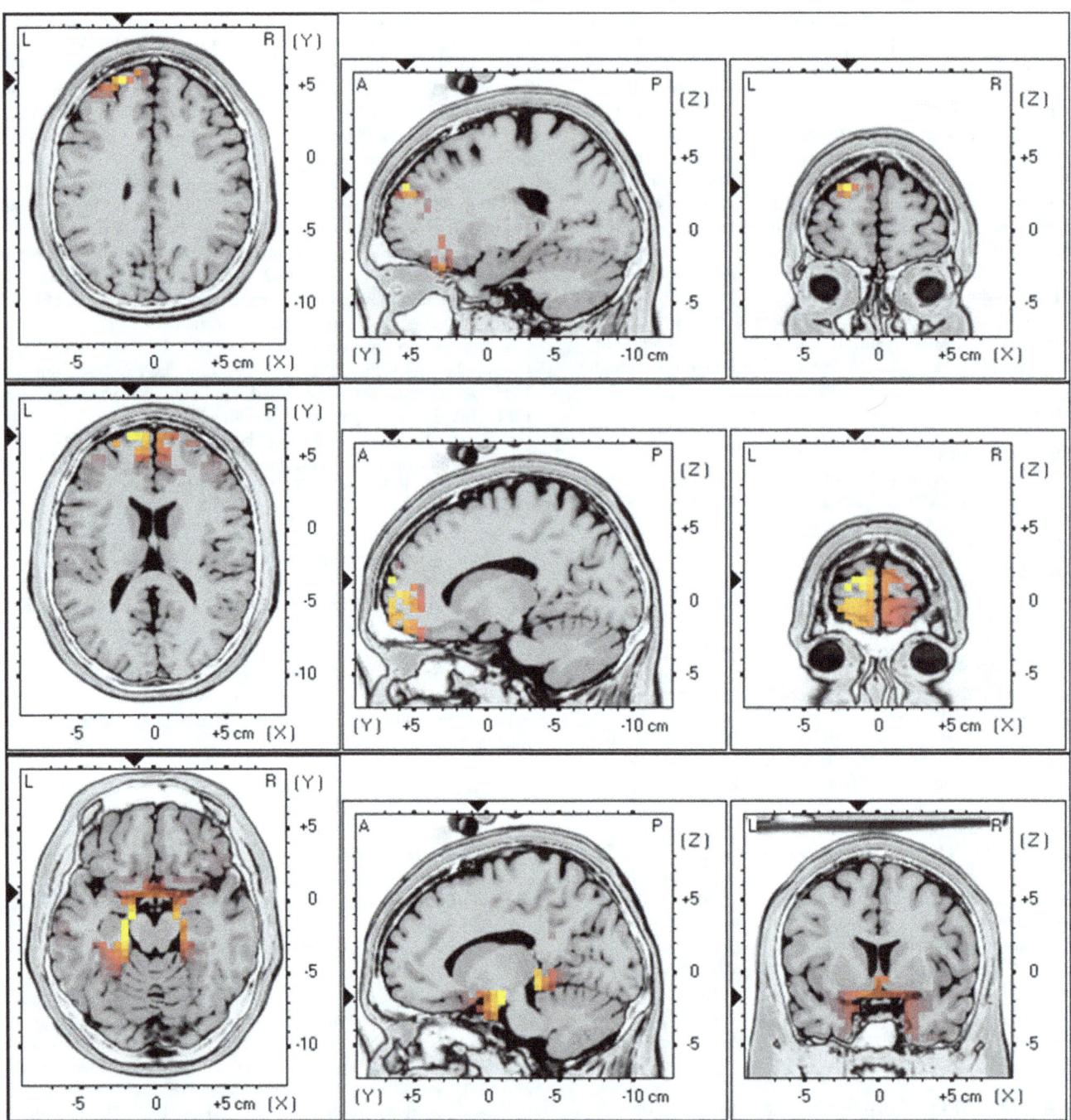

Figure 1. Correlation between the Beck Depression scale and respectively alpha 1 (r=.34) and alpha 2 (r=.37) activity in the frontopolar and orbitofrontal cortex (BA10 & BA11) and beta 3 (r=.27) activity in the subgenual anterior cingulate cortex (BA25) and parahippocampal area (BA35 & 36).

this could be replaced using distress as measured by a NRS. Again is was shown that depressive feelings exclusively correlates with the right frontopolar and OFC in alpha 2 and distress exclusively correlates with the right frontopolar and OFC in alpha 2.

Distress

The neural correlates underlying distress have been explored in different pathologies. One of the most explored fields is distress associated with chronic pain. The ACC has been verified to play a pivotal role in the awareness of pain unpleasantness [29,39]. This

region is associated with a large array of functions such as attention, analysis of sensory information, behavior, emotions and regulation of visceral functions. Moreover altered activity of the ACC can lead to abnormal emotional behavior and might contribute to the depressive symptoms and negative affect [29,39] caused by tinnitus. Previous studies using voxel-based morphometry [40,41], fMRI [42] and positron emission tomography [43] identified the ACC as a critical component of the emotion-processing network underlying the pathophysiology of mood disorders. This is in accordance to findings in this study,

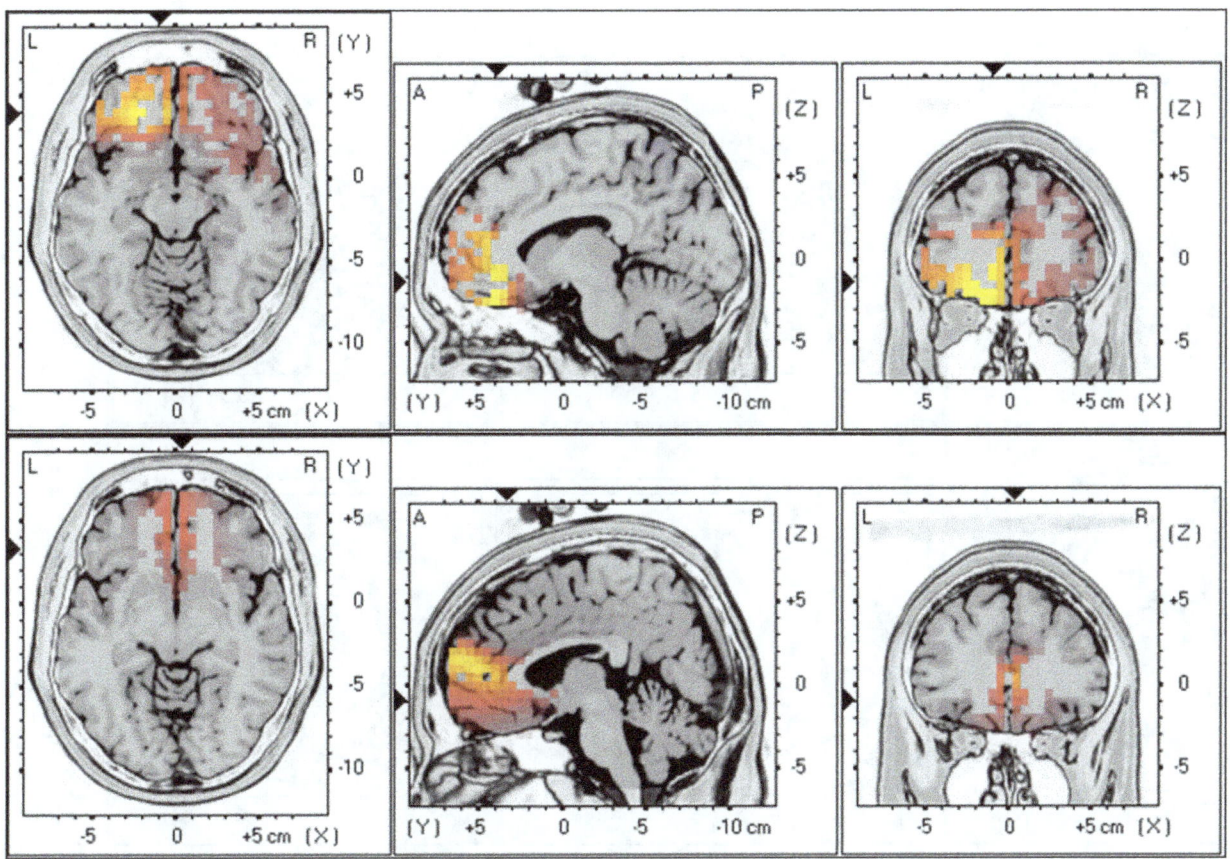

Figure 2. Correlation between the Tinnitus questionnaire and respectively alpha 2 (r = .30) and beta 2 (r = .29) activity in the frontopolar and OFC (BA10, BA11), subgenual anterior cingulate cortex (BA25), pregenual anterior cingulate cortex (BA24).

namely a significant positive correlation with the TQ in the beta 2 frequency band.

Apart from the pregenual ACC, the sgACC showed an increase in alpha 2 and beta 2 frequencies in correlation with TQ scores and increase in alpha 2 and beta 3 in correlation with the NRS measuring distress. Neuroimaging techniques confirmed the critical role of the sgACC in depressive [44,45] and posttraumatic stress disorder [46]. The sgACC has also been associated with storing negatively valenced memories [47], processing of aversive sounds [48] and unpleasant music [49] as well as tinnitus [50] and tinnitus related distress [21]. Severe distress, such as in posttraumatic stress disorder, has already been associated with increased beta activity especially over frontal and central areas [51,52]. In control subjects the dorsal part of the ACC and the prefrontal cortex generate frontal midline theta (alternating with the VMPFC) [53]. In distressed tinnitus patients in contrast to controls alpha and beta activity is increased [21]. In highly distressed versus lowly distressed patients alpha is even more increased, suggesting that the amount of alpha activity correlates with the amount of distress, while it has been hypothesized that beta activity might represent a more general distress activity, compatible with what is known for post-traumatic stress disorders [51,52]. Additionally, based on the findings reported here, it can be assumed that tinnitus related distress mainly correlates with right frontopolar and OFC alpha and beta activity in contrast to more long-standing depressive changes induced by tinnitus.

Depressive feelings

Depressive symptoms are extremely heterogeneous and it is impossible to link these complex neurobehavioral changes to one specific brain structure. Depression can be seen as a dysfunctional limbic-cortical network complementary to failure of intrinsic compensation of the remaining circuit to preserve homeostatic emotional control in stressful situations. An interesting model has been proposed that consists of 7 brain regions, consistently identified by previous studies. Those areas include the anterior thalamus, hippocampus, dorsal prefrontal, medial frontal, OFC, ACC and sgACC [54]. Especially a decreased frontal lobe function, including the frontopolar and OFC (i.e. BA 10 and 11), is consistently identified to play an important contributing factor.

The OFC is not only involved in the pathophysiology of depression [55,56] but also in the storage of implicitly acquired linkages between factual knowledge and bio-regulatory stores, including those that constitute feelings and emotions [57]. Another interesting observation is that this brain area is implicated in the emotional processing of sound [49,58–60]. For example, patients with OFC lesions had reduced self-evaluated perception of the unpleasantness of an acoustic probe stimulus [61].

Lateralization of depression and distress

Distress and depression are two different components of affective disturbances. Whereas depressive feelings are mainly localized to the left frontal side, distress is mostly linked to a change of right frontal brain activity (see Figure 4). This

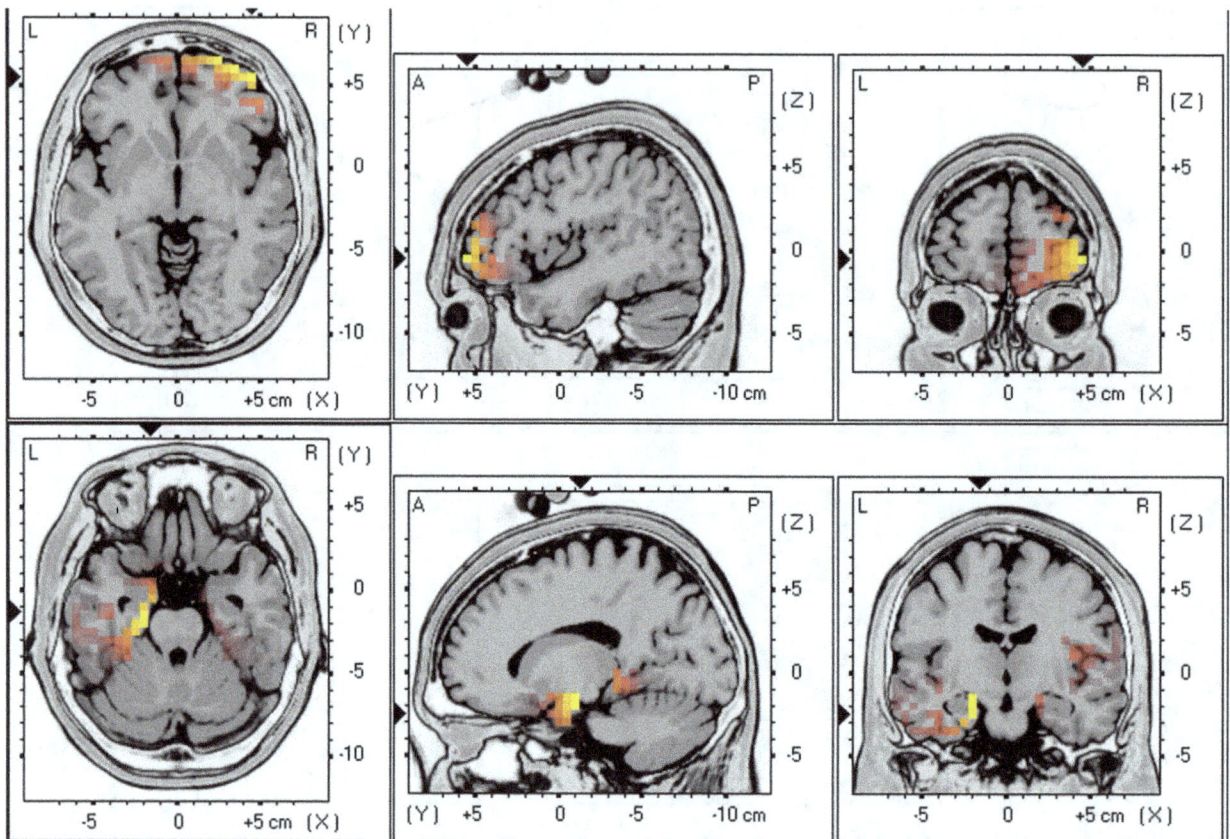

Figure 3. Correlation between the distress using a numeric rating scale and respectively alpha 2 (r = .34) and beta 3 (r = .40) activity in the frontopolar and OFC (BA10, BA11), subgenual anterior cingulate cortex (BA25), and and parahippocampal area (BA27 & 28).

assumption, based on our current results, confirms previous findings in which increased alpha power was related to frontal lateralisation in depression and depressive feelings [62,63]. Moreover, recent studies provide evidence that there is a clear

relationship between EEG activity and depressive feelings with a frontal asymmetry often based on the alpha frequency range [64,65]. More evidence to prove this hypothesis can be found in prior research on transcranial direct current stimulation (tDCS), which is a non-invasive and painless device that modulates cortical excitability in the brain regions of interest through a weak direct electrical current. Depending on the polarity of the stimulation, tDCS can increase or decrease cortical excitability in the brain

Table 1. Significant correlations and partial correlations for the BDI and TQ and regions of interest.

		BDI	TQ	BDI controlled for TQ	TQ controlled for BDI
Alpha2	BA10 Left OFC	.38**	.37**	.28*	.24
	BA10 RightOFC	.32**	.35**	.21	.26†
	BA11 Left OFC	.37**	.37**	.28*	.24
	BA11 RightOFC	.36**	.40**	.23	.30**
	BA24 ACC	.29*	.15	.20	.22
	BA25 sgACC	.28*	.31**	.20	.17
Beta1	BA10 RightOFC	.17	.30**	.06	.26†
	BA11 RightOFC	.19	.33**	.07	.28*
Beta2	BA10 RightOFC	.18	.37**	.04	.33**
	BA11 RightOFC	.20	.43**	.07	.39**
	BA24 ACC	.22	.29*	.13	.27*
	BA25 sgACC	.19	.35**	.05	.31**

†*p*<.10; **p*<.05; ***p*<.01.

Table 2. Significant correlations for distress using a numeric rating scale and BDI for specific regions of interest.

		BDI	Distress	BDI controlled for Distress	Distress controlled for BDI
Alpha2	BA10 Left OFC	.38**	.27*	.36**	.25
	BA10 Right OFC	.32**	.34*	.22	.29*
	BA11 Left OFC	.37**	.25	.35**	.23
	BA11 Right OFC	.36**	.37**	.20	.34**
	BA24 ACC	.29*	.22	.19	.25
	BA25 sgACC	.28*	.27*	.16	.23
Beta 3	BA24 ACC	.22	.32*	.15	.31**
	BA25 sgACC	.19	.36**	.12	.35**

**p*<.05; ***p*<.01.

regions to which it is applied [66]. Using anodal tDCS to the left frontal brain is effective in reducing depressive symptoms [67]. Left anodal stimulation might be successful because it has the ability of restoring hypoactivity of the left prefrontal cortex, further correcting the imbalance between left and right hemisphere, that leads to mood disturbances [68,69].

In contrast to the importance of the left frontopolar and OFC in depressive feelings alterations, distress is mainly generated by the right frontopolar and OFC. For example, bilateral frontal tDCS, placing the anode right and the cathode left, was able to reduce tinnitus intensity and distress although switching the poles couldn't show any significant effect [70].

In addition to the side specificity, depressive feelings were mainly determined by the presence of alpha 2 activity, while distress correlated more with beta 1 and beta 2 frequency in addition to its correlation with the alpha 2 frequency range. Taking these findings together the frontopolar and OFC differentiates the affective component of tinnitus in depressive and distress changes.

Parahippocampal area

Another area, namely the PHC, is most likely implicated in the depressive alterations provoked by the phantom sound. A significant increase in beta 3 activity at the PHC was identified using source localization in patients with higher scores on the BDI-II. In addition, based on a region of interest analysis a significant positive correlation was found between the left and right PHC (BA35) and the BDI. However, when controlling for the TQ this effect did not persist, suggesting that the PHC is important in both tinnitus related distress and depressive feelings.

The PHC together with the auditory and prefrontal cortex, constitutes a network associated with auditory sensory gating [71–74], suppressing irrelevant or abundant noise [75]. It has been hypothesized that the hippocampal region is involved in constantly updating the tinnitus, consequently avoiding habituation of the tinnitus percept [20]. This is based on supraselective amytal testing via the anterior choroidal artery which supplies the amygdalo-hippocampal area, resulting in transient inactivation of the

amygdalohippocampal region. This inactivation has the capability of suppressing tinnitus intensity [20]. Hence, the parahippocampal gyrus may play a crucial role in the presence of tinnitus and has the ability to prevent the tinnitus percept to be constantly updated or to be extracted from the hippocampal memory. Similar to the OFC, activation of the (para)hippocampal region has been observed while listening to unpleasant music during functional magnetic resonance imaging (fMRI) [76]. Considering this, together with the knowledge of parahippocampal connectivity to the sgACC [77] and OFC [78], we assume that the parahippocampal gyrus might be a decisive link between the tinnitus related network and the attention-emotional circuit underlying tinnitus-related emotional disturbances.

Limitations of the study

One major limitation of this and any EEG based approach is that no subcortical activity can be analyzed, limiting network description to cortical sources. The data presented should therefore be viewed acknowledging this limitation.

Depression and distress are related to each other. It is however stated that when there is a low multicollinearity (the correlation among independent variables) it is possible to apply partial correlations [79,80]. As our analysis showed there was only a small correlation between depressive feelings and distress, it is permitted to apply partial correlation analysis. In addition our results were replicated using a NRS measuring distress, and this NRS did not correlate with depression.

Conclusion

In conclusion, tinnitus related distress and more chronic changes in depressive feelings are associated with specific alterations in brain activity of separate neural pathways. We assume that both emotional aspects have their own specific neural circuit embedded within a larger common network. The network responsible for distress is mainly correlated with beta 1 and beta 2 activity of the right frontopolar and OFC, as well as beta 2 frequency in the ACC. The continuous awareness of tinnitus accompanied by distress can induce more long-term changes in depressive feelings. This more constant emotional disturbance, assessed by the BDI-II, can be linked to alpha 2 synchronized activity in the left frontopolar and OFC. Furthermore we assume that the parahippocampal area may be a crucial connection between the tinnitus-related network and the emotion related neural pathways.

Methods

Participants

The patient group included fifty-six patients (N = 56; 27 males and 29 females) with narrow band noise tinnitus, with a mean age of 54.74 (SD = 14.49). As no differences in emotional state nor distress have been demonstrated related to uni- or bilaterality [81] both groups are included in the study. Thirty-six patients have bilateral tinnitus and twenty have unilateral tinnitus. The mean tinnitus duration was 6.92 years (SD = 9.51). Individuals with pulsatile tinnitus, Ménière's disease, otosclerosis, chronic headache, neurological disorders such as brain tumors, and individuals being treated for mental disorders were excluded from the study in order to obtain a more homogeneous sample. To obtain an even more uniform population we only selected patients with narrow band noise. All patients were investigated for the extent of hearing loss using audiograms. Tinnitus patients were tested for the frequency and the minimum masking level of their tinnitus. They were interviewed as to their perceived location of the tinnitus

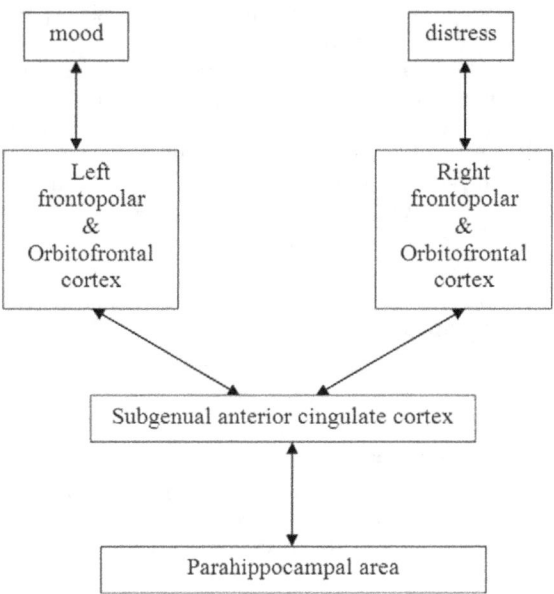

Figure 4. A hypothetical model based on our findings.

(exclusively in the left ear, predominantly in the left ear, in both ears, and centralized in the middle of the head (bilateral), predominantly in the right ear, exclusively in the right ear).

To assess the severity of depression, a chronic pathological negative mood state that frequently accompanies tinnitus, all patients filled out the validated Dutch version of the Beck Depression Inventory-II (BDI-II) [82] originally published in 1961 by Beck et al. This questionnaire was revised in 1996 (BDI-II) following the DSM-IV symptom criteria [83]. The BDI-II is a self-report inventory consisting of 21 items evaluating depressive feelings during the last week. The severity of the depressive feelings is attained by assigning each item with a score ranging between 0–4. Based on the total score of the BDI, patients are categorized in: no or minimal depression (0–9); rand (10–14); mild (15–20); moderate (21–30); severe (31–40); very severe (41–63) depression. The mean BDI score was 10.95 (SD = 9.73).

Patients were also given the validated Dutch version of the Tinnitus Questionnaire [84,85] originally published by Goebel and Hiller [86]. Goebel and Hiller described this TQ as a global index of distress and the Dutch version was further confirmed as a reliable measure for tinnitus-related distress [85]. Based on the total score on the TQ, participants were assigned to a distress category: slight (0–30 points; grade 1), moderate (31–46; grade 2), severe (47–59; grade 3), and very severe (60–84; grade 4) distress. Furthermore, Goebel and Hiller (1994) stated that grade 4 tinnitus patients are psychologically decompensated, indicating that patients categorized into this group cannot cope with their tinnitus. In contrast, patients that have a score lower than 60 on the TQ can cope with their tinnitus. The mean TQ score was 40.93 (SD = 17.03).

Lastly, patients also filled out a NRS measuring distress ("How stressful is your tinnitus? 0 = no distress and 10 = suicidal distress").

The study was approved by the Ethical Committee of the Antwerp University Hospital, Belgium. Patients signed an informed consent.

EEG data collection

EEGs (Mitsar, Nova Tech EEG, Inc, Mesa) were obtained in a fully lighted room with each participants sitting upright in a comfortable chair. The EEG was sampled with 19 electrodes (Fp1, Fp2, F7, F3, Fz, F4, F8, T7, C3, Cz, C4, T8, P7, P3, Pz, P4, P8, O1 O2) in the standard 10–20 international placement referenced to linked lobes and impedances were checked to remain below 5 kΩ. Data were collected for 100 2-s epochs eyes closed, sampling rate = 1024 Hz, and band passed 0.15–200 Hz. Data were resampled to 128 Hz, band-pass filtered (fast Fourier transform filter applying a Hanning window) to 2–44 Hz. These data were transposed into Eureka! Software [87], plotted and carefully inspected for manual for artifact. All episodic artifacts including eye blinks, eye movements, teeth clenching, body movement, or ECG artifacts were removed from the stream of the EEG. In addition, an independent component analysis (ICA) was conducted to further verify if all artifacts were excluded. To investigate the effect possible ICA component rejection we compared the power spectra in two approaches: (1) after visual artifact rejection only (before ICA) and (2) after additional ICA component rejection (after ICA). To test for significant differences between the two approaches we performed a repeated-measure ANOVA, considering mean band power as within-subject variables and groups

(unilateral vs. bilateral tinnitus) as between-subject variable. The mean power in delta (2–3.5 Hz), theta (4–7.5 Hz), alpha1 (8–10 Hz), alpha2 (10–12 Hz), beta1 (13–18 Hz), beta2 (18.5–21 Hz), beta3 (21.5–30 Hz) and gamma (30.5–45 Hz) did not show a statistically significant difference between the two approaches. Therefore, we continued by reporting the results of ICA corrected data.

Source Localization

Standardized low-resolution brain electromagnetic tomography (sLORETA) was used to estimate the intracerebral electrical sources that generated the scalp-recorded activity in each of the eight frequency bands [88]. sLORETA computes electric neuronal activity as current density (A/m^2) without assuming a predefined number of active sources, giving us a global idea of the electrical activity of neuronal cell assemblies with a high temporal resolution. The sLORETA solution space consists of 6239 voxels (voxel size: 5×5×5 mm) and is restricted to cortical gray matter and hippocampi, as defined by digitized MNI brain are derived from the international 10/20 system [89].

Region of interest analysis

The log-transformed electrical current density was averaged across all voxels belonging to the region of interest, Brodmann areas selected on previous research, respectively frontopolar cortex (BA10) [90] left and right separately, OFC (BA11) [90] left and right separately, ACC (BA24; left and right combined) [29], and subgenual ACC (sgACC; BA25; left and right combined) [21] separately for frequency bands delta (2–3,5 Hz), theta (4–7,5 Hz), alpha 1 (8–10 Hz), alpha2 (10,5–12,5 Hz), beta1 (13–18 Hz), beta2 (18.5–21 Hz), beta3 (21.5–30 Hz) and gamma (30.5–45 Hz).

Statistical analyses

For the source localization we used a non-parametric methodology. It is based on estimating, via randomization (i.e. 5000), the empirical probability distribution for the max-statistic, under the null hypothesis. This methodology corrects for multiple testing (i.e., for the collection of tests performed for all voxels, and for all frequency bands). As explained by Nichols and Holmes, the SnPM methodology does not require any assumption of Gaussianity and corrects for all multiple comparisons [91].

In addition, for the region of interest analysis we conducted Pearson correlations and Partial correlations. Partial correlations measure the degree of relationship between two variables, with the effect of a set of controlling variables removed. In our cases we will correlate a region of interest for a certain frequency band with BDI, controlling for TQ and vice versa, thus obtaining source analyzed current density specifically for distress and depressive feelings separately.

Acknowledgments

The authors thank Jan Ost, Bram Van Achteren, Bjorn Devree and Pieter van Looy for their help in preparing this manuscript.

Author Contributions

Conceived and designed the experiments: KJ SV DDR. Performed the experiments: KJ. Analyzed the data: KJ SV. Contributed reagents/materials/analysis tools: KJ SV DDR. Wrote the paper: KJ SV DDR.

References

1. Andersson G (2003) Tinnitus loudness matchings in relation to annoyance and grading of severity. Auris Nasus Larynx 30: 129–133.

2. Heller AJ (2003) Classification and epidemiology of tinnitus. Otolaryngologic Clinics of North America 36: 239–248.

3. Axelsson A, Ringdahl A (1989) Tinnitus-a study of its prevalence and characteristics. BrJAudiol 23: 53–62.

4. Ahmad N, Seidman M (2004) Tinnitus in the older adult – Epidemiology, pathophysiology and treatment options. Drugs & Aging 21: 297–305.

5. Baguley DM (2002) Mechanisms of tinnitus. British Medical Bulletin 63: 195–212.

6. Eggermont JJ, Roberts LE (2004) The neuroscience of tinnitus. Trends in Neurosciences 27: 676–682.

7. Henry JA, Dennis KC, Schechter MA (2005) General review of tinnitus: Prevalence, mechanisms, effects, and management. Journal of Speech Language and Hearing Research 48: 1204–1235.

8. Jastreboff PJ (1990) Phantom Auditory-Perception (Tinnitus) – Mechanisms of Generation and Perception. Neuroscience Research 8: 221–254.

9. De Ridder D, De Mulder G, Menovsky T, Sunaert S, Kovacs S (2007) Electrical stimulation of auditory and somatosensory cortices for treatment of tinnitus and pain. 377–388 p.

10. Moller AR (2010) Similarities between severe tinnitus and chronic pain. Journal of the American Academy of Audiology 11: 115–124.

11. Tonndorf J (1987) The Analogy Between Tinnitus and Pain – A Suggestion for A Physiological-Basis of Chronic Tinnitus. Hearing Research 28: 271–275.

12. Flor H, Elbert T, Knecht S, Wienbruch C, Pantev C, et al. (1995) Phantom-limb pain as a perceptual correlate of cortical reorganization following arm amputation. Nature 375: 482–484.

13. Muhlnickel W, Elbert T, Taub E, Flor H (1998) Reorganization of auditory cortex in tinnitus. Proceedings of the National Academy of Sciences of the United States of America 95: 10340–10343.

14. Kaltenbach JA, Afman CE (2000) Hyperactivity in the dorsal cochlear nucleus after intense sound exposure and its resemblance to tone-evoked activity: a physiological model for tinnitus. Hearing Research 140: 165–172.

15. Salvi RJ, Wang J, Ding D (2000) Auditory plasticity and hyperactivity following cochlear damage. Hearing Research 147: 261–274.

16. Smits M, Kovacs S, de Ridder D, Peeters RR, van Hecke P, et al. (2007) Lateralization of functional magnetic resonance imaging (fMRI) activation in the auditory pathway of patients with lateralized tinnitus. Neuroradiology 49: 669–679.

17. Moazami-Goudarzi M, Michels L, Weisz N, Jeanmonod D (2010) Temporo-insular enhancement of EEG low and high frequencies in patients with chronic tinnitus. QEEG study of chronic tinnitus patients. Bmc Neuroscience 11.

18. Plewnia C, Reimold M, Najib A, Reischl G, Plontke SK, et al. (2007) Moderate therapeutic efficacy of positron emission tomography-navigated repetitive transcranial magnetic stimulation for chronic tinnitus: a randomised, controlled pilot study. Journal of Neurology Neurosurgery and Psychiatry 78: 152–156.

19. Kleinjung T, Eichhammer P, Landgrebe M, Sand P, Hajak G, et al. (2008) Combined temporal and prefrontal transcranial magnetic stimulation for tinnitus treatment: A pilot study. Otolaryngology-Head and Neck Surgery 138: 497–501.

20. De Ridder D, Fransen H, Francois O, Sunaert S, Kovacs S, et al. (2006) Amygdalohippocampal involvement in tinnitus and auditory memory. Acta Oto-Laryngologica 126: 50–53.

21. Vanneste S, Plazier M, van der Loo E, Van de Heyning P, Congedo M, et al. (2010) The neural correlates of tinnitus-related distress. Neuroimage 52: 470–480.

22. Landgrebe M, Langguth B, Rosengarth K, Braun S, Koch A, et al. (2009) Structural brain changes in tinnitus: Grey matter decrease in auditory and non-auditory brain areas. Neuroimage 46: 213–218.

23. Lazarus RS, Folkman S (1984) Stress, appraisal, and coping. New York: Springer.

24. Brown GW, Harris TO (1989) Depression. New York: Guilford.

25. Mobascher A, Brinkmeyer J, Warbrick T, Musso F, Wittsack HJ, et al. (2009) Laser-evoked potential P2 single-trial amplitudes covary with the fMRI BOLD response in the medial pain system and interconnected subcortical structures. Neuroimage.

26. Peyron R, Laurent B, Garcia-Larrea L (2000) Functional imaging of brain responses to pain. A review and meta-analysis (2000). Neurophysiologie Clinique-Clinical Neurophysiology 30: 263–288.

27. Onozawa K, Yagasaki Y, Izawa Y, Abe H, Kawakami Y (2011) Amygdala-prefrontal pathways and the dopamine system affect nociceptive responses in the prefrontal cortex. Bmc Neuroscience 12.

28. Craig ADB (2003) A new view of pain as a homeostatic emotion. Trends in Neurosciences 26: 303–307.

29. Price DD (2000) Neuroscience – Psychological and neural mechanisms of the affective dimension of pain. Science 288: 1769–1772.

30. Zoger S, Svedlund J, Holgers KM (2001) Psychiatric disorders in tinnitus patients without severe hearing impairment: 24 month follow-up of patients at an audiological clinic. Audiology 40: 133–140.

31. Giesecke T, Gracely RH, Williams DA, Geisser ME, Petzke FW, et al. (2005) The relationship between depression, clinical pain, and experimental pain in a chronic pain cohort. Arthritis and Rheumatism 52: 1577–1584.

32. Schweinhardt P, Kalk N, Wartolowska K, Chessell I, Wordsworth P, et al. (2008) Investigation into the neural correlates of emotional augmentation of clinical pain. Neuroimage 40: 759–766.

33. Moller AR (1997) Similarities between chronic pain and tinnitus. Am J Otol 18: 577–585.

34. Tonndorf J (1987) The analogy between tinnitus and pain: a suggestion for a physiological basis of chronic tinnitus. Hear Res 28: 271–275.

35. De Ridder D, Elgoyhen AB, Romo R, Langguth B (2011) Phantom percepts: tinnitus and pain as persisting aversive memory networks. Proc Natl Acad Sci U S A 108: 8075–8080.

36. De Ridder D, Elgoyhen AB, Romo R, Langguth B (2011) Phantom percepts: Tinnitus and pain as persisting aversive memory networks. Proceedings of the National Academy of Sciences of the United States of America 108: 8075–8080.

37. Moller AR (1997) Similarities between chronic pain and tinnitus. American Journal of Otology 18: 577–585.

38. De Ridder D, De Mulder G, Menovsky T, Sunaert S, Kovacs S (2007) Electrical stimulation of auditory and somatosensory cortices for treatment of tinnitus and pain. In: Langguth B, Hajak G, Kleinjung T, Cacace A, Moller AR, editors. Tinnitus: Pathophysiology and Treatment. 377–388.

39. Boggio PS, Zaghi S, Fregni F (2009) Modulation of emotions associated with images of human pain using anodal transcranial direct current stimulation (tDCS). Neuropsychologia 47: 212–217.

40. Li CT, Lin CP, Chou KH, Chen IY, Hsieh JC, et al. (2010) Structural and cognitive deficits in remitting and non-remitting recurrent depression: A voxel-based morphometric study. Neuroimage 50: 347–356.

41. Abe O, Yamasue H, Kasai K, Yamada H, Aoki S, et al. (2010) Voxel-based analyses of gray/white matter volume and diffusion tensor data in major depression. Psychiatry Research-Neuroimaging 181: 64–70.

42. Anand A, Li Y, Wang Y, Wu JW, Gao SJ, et al. (2005) Activity and connectivity of brain mood regulating circuit in depression: A functional magnetic resonance study. Biological Psychiatry 57: 1079–1088.

43. Kennedy SH, Javanmard M, Vaccarino FJ (1997) A review of functional neuroimaging in mood disorders: Positron emission tomography and depression. Canadian Journal of Psychiatry-Revue Canadienne de Psychiatrie 42: 467–475.

44. Drevets WC, Price JL, Furey ML (2008) Brain structural and functional abnormalities in mood disorders: implications for neurocircuitry models of depression. Brain Structure & Function 213: 93–118.

45. Hajek T, Kozeny J, Kopecek M, Alda M, Hoschl C (2008) Reduced subgenual cingulate volumes in mood disorders: a meta-analysis. Journal of Psychiatry & Neuroscience 33: 91–99.

46. Shin LM, Bush G, Whalen PJ, Handwerger K, Cannistraro PA, et al. (2007) Dorsal anterior Cingulate function in posttraurnatic stress disorder. Journal of Traumatic Stress 20: 701–712.

47. Vogt BA (2005) Pain and emotion interactions in subregions of the cingulate gyrus. Nature Reviews Neuroscience 6: 533–544.

48. Zald DH, Mattson DL, Pardo JV (2002) Brain activity in ventromedial prefrontal cortex correlates with individual differences in negative affect. Proceedings of the National Academy of Sciences of the United States of America 99: 2450–2454.

49. Blood AJ, Zatorre RJ, Bermudez P, Evans AC (1999) Emotional responses to pleasant and unpleasant music correlate with activity in paralimbic brain regions. Nature Neuroscience 2: 382–387.

50. Muhlau M, Rauschecker JP, Oestreicher E, Gaser C, Rottinger M, et al. (2006) Structural brain changes in tinnitus. Cerebral Cortex 16: 1283–1288.

51. Jokic-Begic N, Begic D (2003) Quantitative electroencephalogram (qEEG) in combat veterans with post-traumatic stress disorder (PTSD). Nordic Journal of Psychiatry 57: 351–355.

52. Begic D, Hotujac L, Jokic-Begic N (2001) Electroencephalographic comparison of veterans with combat-related post-traumatic stress disorder and healthy subjects. International Journal of Psychophysiology 40: 167–172.

53. Asada H, Fukuda Y, Tsunoda S, Yamaguchi M, Tonoike M (1999) Frontal midline theta rhythms reflect alternative activation of prefrontal cortex and anterior cingulate cortex in humans. Neuroscience Letters 274: 29–32.

54. Mayberg HS (2003) Modulating dysfunctional limbic-cortical circuits in depression: towards development of brain-based algorithms for diagnosis and optimised treatment. British Medical Bulletin 65: 193–207.

55. Rolls ET, Grabenhorst F (2008) The orbitofrontal cortex and beyond: From affect to decision-making. Progress in Neurobiology 86: 216–244.

56. Drevets WC (2007) Orbitofrontal cortex function and structure in depression. 499–527 p.

57. Volz KG, von Cramon DY (2009) How the orbitofrontal cortex contributes tot decision making – a view from neuroscience. Progress in Brain Researsch 174: 61–71.

58. Dias R, Robbins TW, Roberts AC (1996) Dissociation in prefrontal cortex of affective and attentional shifts. Nature 380: 69–72.

59. Wheeler RE, Davidson RJ, Tomarken AJ (1993) Frontal Brain Asymmetry and Emotional Reactivity – A Biological Substrate of Affective Style. Psychophysiology 30: 82–89.

60. Damasio AR (1996) The somatic marker hypothesis and the possible functions of the prefrontal cortex. Philosophical Transactions of the Royal Society B-Biological Sciences 351: 1413–1420.

61. Angrilli A, Bianchin M, Radaelli S, Bertagnoni G, Pertile M (2008) Reduced startle reflex and aversive noise perception in patients with orbitofrontal cortex lesions. Neuropsychologia 46: 1179–1184.

62. Vogt T, Schneider S, Brümmer V, Strüder HK (2010) Frontal EEG asymmetry: The effects of sustained walking in the elderly. Neuroscience Letters.

63. Kemp Ah, Griffiths K, Felmingham KL, Shankman SA, Drinkenburg W, et al. (2010) Disorder specificity despite comorbidity: Resting EEG alpha asymmetry

in major depressive disorder and post-traumatic stress disorder. Biological Psychiatry 85: 350–354.

64. Davidson RJ (1998) Anterior electrophysiological asymmetries, emotion, and depression: Conceptual and methodological conundrums. Psychophysiology 35: 607–614.

65. Allen JJB, Kline JP (2004) Frontal EEG asymmetry, emotion, and psychopathology: the first, and the next 25 years. Biological Psychology 67: 1–5.

66. Miranda PC, Lomarev M, Hallett M (2006) Modeling the current distribution during transcranial direct current stimulation. Clinical Neurophysiology 117: 1623–1629.

67. Vanneste S, Plazier M, Ost J, van der Loo E, Van de Heyning P, et al. (2010) Bilateral dorsolateral prefrontal cortex modulation for tinnitus by transcranial direct current stimulation: a preliminary clinical study. Exp Brain Res 202: 779–785.

68. Grimm S, Beck J, Schuepbach D, Hell D, Boesiger P, et al. (2008) Imbalance between left and right dorsolateral prefrontal cortex in major depression is linked to negative emotional judgment: An fMRI study in severe major depressive disorder. Biological Psychiatry 63: 369–376.

69. Fales CL, Barch DM, Rundle MA, Mintun MA, Mathews J, et al. (2009) Antidepressant treatment normalizes hypoactivity in dorsolateral prefrontal cortex during emotional interference processing in major depression. Journal of Affective Disorders 112: 206–211.

70. Vanneste S, Plazier M, Ost J, van der Loo E, Van de Heyning P, et al. (2010) Bilateral dorsolateral prefrontal cortex modulation for tinnitus by transcranial direct current stimulation: a preliminary clinical study. Experimental Brain Research 202: 779–785.

71. Boutros NN, Mears R, Pflieger ME, Moxon KA, Ludowig E, et al. (2008) Sensory gating in the human hippocampal and rhinal regions: regional differences. Hippocampus 18: 310–316.

72. Boutros N, Rukov OAK, Rosburg T, Trautner P, Kurthen M (2005) Sensory gating in the human hippocampal and rhinal regions. Biological Psychiatry 57: 597.

73. Grunwald T, Boutros NN, Pezer N, von Oertzen J, Fernandez G, et al. (2003) Neuronal substrates of sensory gating within the human brain. Biological Psychiatry 53: 511–519.

74. Korzyukov O, Pflieger ME, Wagner M, Bowyer SM, Rosburg T, et al. (2007) Generators of the intracranial P50 response in auditory sensory gating. Neuroimage 35: 814–826.

75. Tulving E, Markowitsch HJ (1997) Memory beyond the hippocampus. Current Opinion in Neurobiology 7: 209–216.

76. Koelsch S, Fritz T, Von Cramon DY, Muller K, Friederici AD (2006) Investigating emotion with music: An fMRI study. Human Brain Mapping 27: 239–250.

77. Kahn I, Andrews-Hanna JR, Vincent JL, Snyder AZ, Buckner RL (2008) Distinct cortical anatomy linked to subregions of the medial temporal lobe revealed by intrinsic functional connectivity. J Neurophysiol 100: 129–139.

78. Powell HWR, Guye M, Parker GJM, Symms MR, Boulby P, et al. (2004) Noninvasive in vivo demonstration of the connections of the human parahippocampal gyrus. Neuroimage 22: 740–747.

79. Waliczek TM (1996) A primer on partial correlation coefficients. New Orleans, :LA: Southwest Educational Research Association.

80. Cramer D (2003) A cautionary tale of two statistics: partial correlation and standardized partial regression. J Psychol 137: 507–511.

81. Lim JJ, Lu PK, Koh DS, Eng SP (2010) Impact of tinnitus as measured by the Tinnitus Handicap Inventory among tinnitus sufferers in Singapore. Singapore Med J 51: 551–557.

82. Bouman TK, Luteijn F, Albersnagel FA, van der Ploeg FAE (1985) Enige ervaringen met de Beck Depression Inventory. Gedrag: tijdschrift voor psychologie 13: 13–24.

83. Beck AT, Steer RA, Brown GK (1996) Manual for the Beck Depression Inventory-II. San Antonio, TX: Psychological Corporation.

84. Meeus O, Blaivie C, Van de Heyning P (2007) Validation of the Dutch and the French version of the Tinnitus questionnaire. B-Ent: 11–17.

85. Vanneste S, Plazier M, van der Loo E, Ost J, Meeus O, et al. (2010) Validation of the Mini-TQ in a Dutch-speaking population. A rapid assessment for tinnitus-related distress. B-Ent.

86. Goebel G, Hiller W (1994) The Tinnitus Questionnaire (Tq) – A Standardized Instrument for Grading the Severity of Tinnitus – Results of A Multicenter Study Using the Tq. Hno 42: 166–172.

87. Novatech EEG Inc. website. EureKa! (Version 3.0) Computer Software. Available: http://www.novatecheeg.com/downloads.html. Accessed 2012 June 21.

88. Pascal-Marqui RD (2002) Standarized low-resolution brain electromagnetic tomography (sLORETA): technical details. Methods and Findings in Experimental and Clinical Pharmacology 24 Suppl D: 5–12.

89. Jurcak V, Tsuzuki D, Dan I (2007) 10/20, 10/10, and 10/5 systems revisited: their validity as relative head-surface-based positioning systems. Neuroimage 34: 1600–1611.

90. Vanneste S, Joos K, De Ridder D (2012) Prefrontal Cortex Based Sex Differences in Tinnitus Perception: Same Tinnitus Intensity, Same Tinnitus Distress, Different Mood. Plos One 7.

91. Nichols TE, Holmes AP (2002) Nonparametric permutation tests for functional neuroimaging: a primer with examples. Hum Brain Mapp 15: 1–25.

rTMS Induced Tinnitus Relief is Related to an Increase in Auditory Cortical Alpha Activity

Nadia Müller[1]*, **Isabel Lorenz**[2], **Berthold Langguth**[3], **Nathan Weisz**[1,4]

1 Università degli Studi di Trento, Center for Mind/Brain Sciences, Mattarello, Italy, 2 University of Konstanz, Department of Psychology, Konstanz, Germany, 3 University Hospital Regensburg, Department of Psychiatry and Psychotherapy, Regensburg, Germany, 4 Zukunftskolleg, University of Konstanz, Konstanz, Germany

Abstract

Chronic tinnitus, the continuous perception of a phantom sound, is a highly prevalent audiological symptom. A promising approach for the treatment of tinnitus is repetitive transcranial magnetic stimulation (rTMS) as this directly affects tinnitus-related brain activity. Several studies indeed show tinnitus relief after rTMS, however effects are moderate and vary strongly across patients. This may be due to a lack of knowledge regarding how rTMS affects oscillatory activity in tinnitus sufferers and which modulations are associated with tinnitus relief. In the present study we examined the effects of five different stimulation protocols (including sham) by measuring tinnitus loudness and tinnitus-related brain activity with Magnetoencephalography before and after rTMS. Changes in oscillatory activity were analysed for the stimulated auditory cortex as well as for the entire brain regarding certain frequency bands of interest (delta, theta, alpha, gamma). In line with the literature the effects of rTMS on tinnitus loudness varied strongly across patients. This variability was also reflected in the rTMS effects on oscillatory activity. Importantly, strong reductions in tinnitus loudness were associated with increases in alpha power in the stimulated auditory cortex, while an unspecific decrease in gamma and alpha power, particularly in left frontal regions, was linked to an increase in tinnitus loudness. The identification of alpha power increase as main correlate for tinnitus reduction sheds further light on the pathophysiology of tinnitus. This will hopefully stimulate the development of more effective therapy approaches.

Editor: André Mouraux, Université catholique de Louvain, Belgium

Funding: This work was supported by a grant from the Deutsche Forschungsgemeinschaft (grant number: 4156/2-1) and the Tinnitus Research Initiative. The funders had no role in study design, data collection and analysis, decision to publish, or preparation of the manuscript.

Competing Interests: The authors have read the journal's policy and have no conflicts of interest.

* E-mail: nadia.muller@unitn.it

Introduction

Tinnitus is defined as the subjective perception of a sound in the absence of any physical sound source. If persisting longer than a certain amount of time, conventionally between six and twelve months, it is usually regarded as 'chronic', reflecting clinical experience that the phantom sound will persist. Chronic tinnitus is a common phenomenon with a prevalence of 5–15% of the population in western societies [1,2]. In 1–3% of the population, tinnitus is associated with severe distress including psychiatric problems (e.g., depression), sleep disturbances, concentration problems or work impairment [1]. To date, there is no effective treatment that reliably eliminates tinnitus [1], partly because the processes that generate and maintain tinnitus and its associated problems are not completely understood. A broad consensus, however, is that tinnitus is generated in central brain structures rather than in the peripheral auditory system. Evidence comes from clinical studies showing that the tinnitus percept persists even after transection of the auditory nerve fibres [3,4].

In most cases, tinnitus is associated with a damage of hair cells in the inner ear [5,6], resulting in pathological neuronal activity in central structures [7–10]. Various neurophysiological processes at different levels of the auditory system that are elicited by hearing loss have been suggested as being involved in the generation of tinnitus [9]. Hearing loss, for instance, results in a loss of inhibition and a reorganisation of the tonotopic map [11,1]. Studies in

animals and humans demonstrate that the tinnitus sensation is associated with hyperactivity in subcortical and cortical auditory brain structures. This hyperactivity is reflected in an enhanced spontaneous firing rate [12–14], elevated bursting activity [13,15] and increases in neural synchrony that have been shown to correspond closely to hearing loss [16]. Roberts et al. (2010) postulate that, among these processes, the increase in neural synchrony seems to be most relevant for the actual generation of tinnitus as it has the potential to impact postsynaptic targets and recruit cortical and downstream neurons into a tinnitus percept. The role of altered synchrony in tinnitus is strongly supported by studies that report changes in oscillatory brain activity associated with tinnitus [7,17–19] on a subcortical and cortical level. On a subcortical level, for instance, abnormal low-frequency activity in the thalamus can lead to disturbances in the thalamo–cortico–thalamic network (thalamocortical dysrhythmia, TCD) and thereby influence perception [20]. On the cortical level it has been shown that oscillatory activity in the so-called alpha band (8–12 Hz), which has been related to inhibitory processes [21], is reduced in the auditory cortex of tinnitus patients [10]. Power increases were found for low frequencies in the delta [10] to theta range [20,22,23,24] and in gamma power compared to normal hearing controls [7,18,25].

A promising treatment approach for chronic tinnitus is transcranial magnetic stimulation (TMS) [26,27] as this affects brain activity directly, thereby holding the potential to influence abnormal ongoing brain activity related to tinnitus. Particularly in its repetitive form (rTMS; [28,29]), it has been shown (mostly in the motor system) that stimulation-induced changes of excitability and plasticity outlast the period of stimulation. A growing number of studies indeed point to tinnitus relief after a series of ten rTMS sessions (for an overview see [30]), with effects lasting for up to four years [31]. However, the effects show great interindividual variability [27,32] and only moderate effect sizes [33]. Only few studies have investigated the effects of rTMS on auditory cortical activity in tinnitus sufferers and which aspects of these modulations are relevant for tinnitus relief. In a previous study, we were able to demonstrate that various forms of single session rTMS (particularly cTBS, iTBS and 1 Hz rTMS) could reduce the auditory Steady State Response (aSSR), which is in turn correlated with subjectively perceived tinnitus loudness [34]. In the context of the same study we also collected resting MEG activity. To date, no published reports have investigated the impact of rTMS on spontaneous oscillatory brain activity in tinnitus patients - a potentially fundamental element in the generation of tinnitus [9,10]. In order to better understand the pathophysiology of tinnitus and also to systematically advance tinnitus therapies, it is essential to know if and how oscillatory brain activity in tinnitus patients is modulated by rTMS and what changes in oscillatory activity are crucial for tinnitus suppression. This view is also strongly supported by Fuggetta and colleagues who emphasized that we will gain further insight into therapy approaches and the pathophysiology of a variety of neurological disorders by investigating rTMS effects on TCD-like EEG patterns [23]. With the current data we are able to show - on the level of group as well as single subject statistics - that tinnitus relief after rTMS is associated with an increase in alpha activity in the auditory cortex, thus supporting the relevance of alpha activity for tinnitus [10].

Methods

1. Participants

Ten patients with chronic tinnitus participated in the current study (7 males, 3 females). The mean age of the participants was 49.8 years (range: 21–70). Patients were recruited via advertisements in the local newspaper and flyers posted at the University of Konstanz. Tinnitus severity was assessed with Hallam's [35] Tinnitus Questionnaire (*Tinnitus-Fragebogen*; [36]), revealing a mean score of 29.9 (range: 8–59). Half of the patients reported unilateral tinnitus (4 with left-sided tinnitus, 1 with right-sided tinnitus), while the other half indicated having perceived the tinnitus bilaterally. We only included patients with a maximum tinnitus duration of four years, as the impact of rTMS on chronic tinnitus declines with longer tinnitus duration [26]. All patients were informed about the content of the study as well as the potential risk factors and underwent a thorough anamnesis concerning potential contraindications for TMS (previous personal or family history of epileptic seizures, cardiac pacemaker, pregnancy, neurodegenerative diseases, brain injuries). Furthermore, patients with psychiatric or neurological disorders according to the M.I.N.I. (Mini International Neuropsychiatric Interview, German Version 5.0.0) and with anticonvulsant or tranquilizer medication were excluded from the study. The Ethics Committee of the University of Konstanz approved the experimental procedure and the participants gave their written informed consent prior to taking part in the study.

2. Experimental Design

Patients underwent five sessions of rTMS, including the measurement of tinnitus loudness and brain activity with MEG before and after rTMS, resulting in a dataset of 100 MEG and 100 tinnitus loudness measurements ($10 \times 5 \times 2$). In the five sessions, five different rTMS protocols were applied, with a minimum interval of one week between sessions and using a randomized, single-blind, placebo-controlled design. For an overview of the study design, see Figure 1.

3. Measurement of Tinnitus Loudness

Before the first and after the second MEG recording, patients were asked to match the loudness of their tinnitus to a reference tone of 1 kHz (tinnitus intensity matching; TIM). This procedure considers the absolute hearing threshold of the 1-kHz tone so that the matched tinnitus intensity is expressed in 'sensation level'. Additional to this psychoacoustic assessment, the patients estimated their perceived tinnitus loudness on a visual analogue scale (VAS) ranging from 0 ('not loud at all') to 10 ('extremely loud').

4. Data Acquisition with MEG

The MEG recordings were carried out using a 148-channel whole-head magnetometer system (MAGNESTM 2500 WH, 4D Neuroimaging, San Diego, USA) installed in a magnetically shielded chamber (Vakuumschmelze Hanau). Prior to the recording, individual head shapes were collected using a digitiser. Participants lay in a supine position and were asked to keep their eyes open and to focus on a fixed point on the ceiling during the recording. The recording time was five minutes. MEG signals were recorded with a sampling rate of 2034.51 Hz and a hard-wired high-pass filter of 0.1 Hz. MEG measurements were conducted before and after TMS. The time interval between the end of the TMS session and the start of the second MEG recording did not exceed five minutes.

5. Brain Stimulation with TMS

TMS stimulation (biphasic magnetic pulses) was administered with a figure-of-eight coil (coil winding diameter 2×75 mm; Magnetic Coil Transducer C-B60, Medtronic) connected to a MagPro X 100 TMS stimulator (Medtronic A/S, Skovlunde, Denmark).

Five different stimulation protocols were applied in randomized order over five sessions separated by at least one week: 1-Hz rTMS (1 train with 1000 pulses, frequency 1 Hz), individual alpha frequency rTMS (IAF; 20 trains with 50 pulses and 25 seconds inter-train interval, peak frequency ranging between 8 and 12 Hz), continuous theta burst stimulation (cTBS; 200 bursts at a frequency of 5 Hz with bursts consisting of 3 pulses at 50 Hz), intermittent theta burst stimulation (iTBS; 10 trains of 10 bursts at a frequency of 5 Hz with bursts consisting of 3 pulses at 50 Hz and an 8 seconds inter-train interval), and a placebo sham stimulation (45° coil angulation, applying the IAF protocol). Individual alpha frequency was defined as the peak of the power spectrum (between 8 and 12 Hz) at temporal sensors in the first MEG recording. For an illustration of the different protocols see right upper panel of Figure 1. The patients were blind to the TMS condition. The intensity of the stimulation was adjusted according to the resting motor threshold (RMT) –a common procedure in TMS studies [37]. RMT was measured by delivering single pulses at the optimal site over the motor cortex and defined as the lowest stimulation intensity required for producing visible hand muscle contractions in at least five out of ten trials as it has been done in previous studies [37]. For

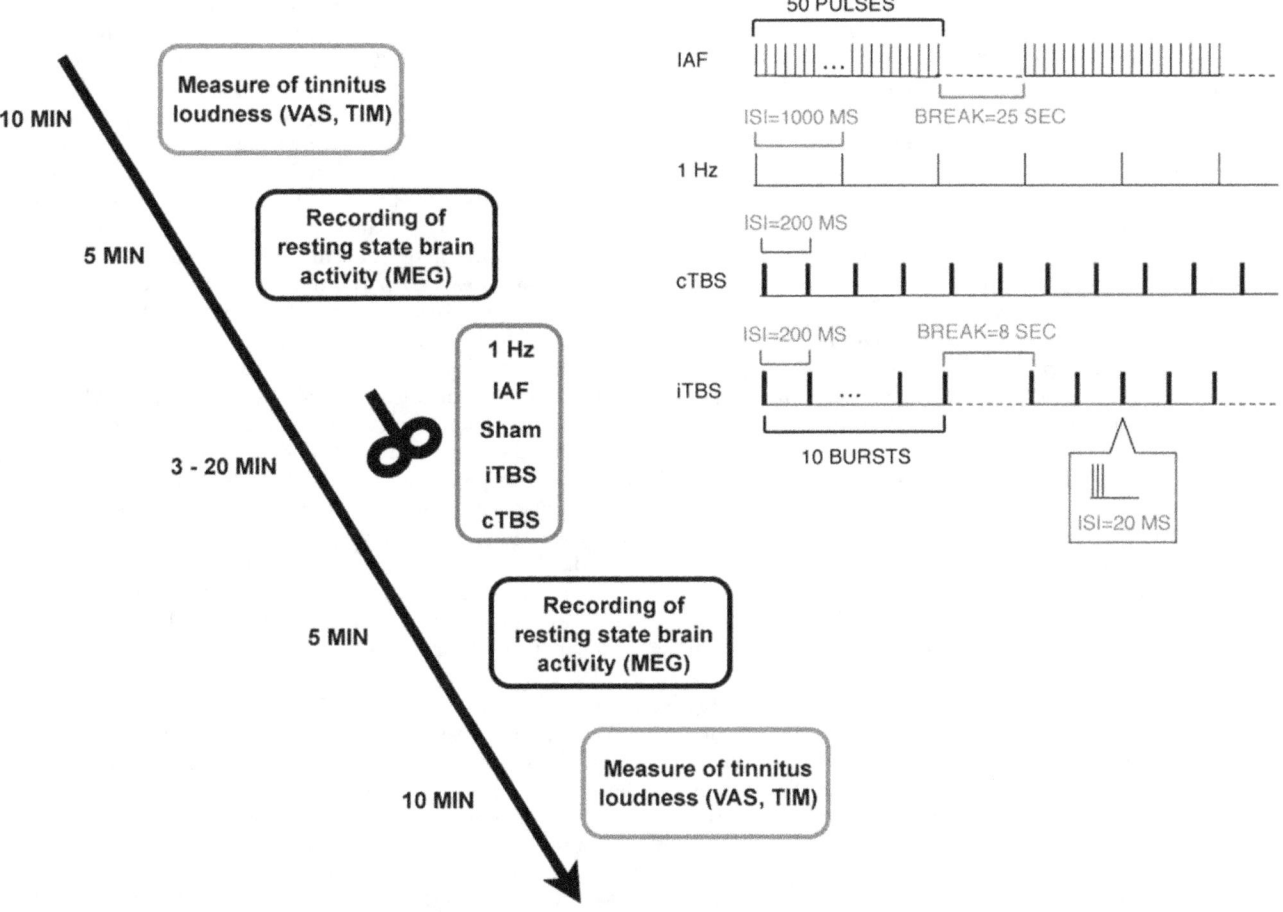

Figure 1. Experimental design. Patients underwent five sessions with five different rTMS protocols (including Sham). In each session, tinnitus loudness and oscillatory brain activity were measured before and after rTMS. The right upper panel illustrates the different stimulation protocols.

1-Hz rTMS, IAF, and sham stimulation, intensity was set to 110% of the RMT and for iTBS and cTBS to 80% of the RMT. Thus, the intensities we applied were slightly higher than those used by Huang et al. [87] for motor cortex stimulation. To prevent hearing damage caused by the loud clicking sound of the TMS device, patients were required to use earplugs. Patients were seated in a comfortable chair while the TMS coil was fixated with a mechanical arm. The handle of the coil always pointed upwards. In case of right-ear or bilateral tinnitus, the coil was placed over left Heschl's gyrus by moving 2.5 cm upwards from T3 on the line between T3 and Cz and then 1.5 cm perpendicularly in a posterior direction, analogously over right Heschl's Gyrus in case of left-ear tinnitus. This procedure has been proven to reliably position the TMS coil over the auditory cortex [38].

6. Data Analysis

6.1. Preprocessing. We analysed the data sets using Matlab (The MathWorks, Natick, MA, Version 7.5.0 R 2007b) and the Fieldtrip toolbox [39]. We separately extracted two-second epochs from the continuously recorded MEG signal for the measurements, resulting in 150 trials for the pre (baseline) and post-TMS condition, respectively. We then performed artefact rejection in two steps. First, we visually inspected trials for eye movements, muscle artefacts or channel jumps and rejected the affected trials. Furthermore, we eliminated dead and very noisy channels. Two

out of 100 data sets (one from the cTBS and one from the IAF protocol) had to be excluded because of very poor data quality. In a second step, the data sets were processed using an Independent Component Analysis (ICA; http://sccn.ucsd.edu/eeglab/) to correct for heartbeat-related artefacts. We entered 80 randomly sampled trials into the ICA in order to get independent components with a distinct time course and spatial topography. We identified those components (two in the majority of cases) that captured cardiac activity through visual inspection. Afterwards, the respective weights of the ICA were applied to the whole data set, artefact components were removed and the original data were reconstructed without the impact of the artefact. To ensure similar signal-to-noise-ratio for direct comparisons between the placebo (sham) and active TMS conditions, the trial number was adjusted to the minimum remaining trial number for the two time points (pre and post) and the compared conditions (sham and the respective active TMS protocols). To keep trial numbers in a comparable range, maximum trial number was set to 90.

6.2. Spectral power analyses derived from auditory cortex. As patients had to leave the MEG between pre and post-TMS sessions, all analyses were performed at source level in order to obtain robust effects, in contrast to a potential analysis at sensor level, which would have been more susceptible to altered head positions in the sensor helmet (from pre to post as well as over different days).

For each patient, we created a head model fitted to the head shape of the first MEG measurement using a multisphere approach [40]. This yielded a grid covering the entire brain with a resolution of 1 cm and assured that the same grid would be used in a single participant across all sessions. The leadfield for each grid point, however, was separately calculated for each session to account for potentially altered positioning of the sources with respect to the sensors.

Data were then analysed for the region of interest, defined as the auditory cortex (Brodman Area 41 & 42; Talairach atlas) ipsilateral to the TMS stimulation side. We also investigated oscillatory brain activity contralateral to the stimulation side. This analysis did not reveal any consistent effects; we thus do not describe them in further detail. In order to estimate power spectra for the region of interest, we employed a multitaper spectral estimation method [41] to the ICA-corrected raw data and kept the complex Fourier coefficients. We used a different smoothing for low (2–12 Hz) and high frequencies (30–90 Hz) so that the data were multiplied with a set of orthogonal Slepian tapers, yielding a frequency smoothing of $+/-1$ Hz for low and $+/-5$ Hz for high frequencies. We then constructed spatial filters (with fixed orientation) using the lcmv-algorithm (lcmv beamformer; [42]) for each grid point within the region of interest. This was again accomplished for low and high frequencies respectively by filtering the non-ICA corrected data in the corresponding frequency bands (2–12 Hz, 30–90 Hz). Afterwards, we projected the complex values into source space by multiplying them with the accordant spatial filters and by calculating the complex modulus of the values. We thereby obtained absolute power values for each voxel within the region of interest. By averaging the values in the region of interest we obtained one single value for each frequency. This procedure was repeated for each patient, for both time points (pre and post) and for the five different conditions (4 active TMS protocols & sham). Finally, spectral source estimates were normalized for each patient and condition by calculating a (post-pre)/pre ratio, reflecting the modulation of oscillatory power from pre to post TMS intervention. It should be noted that we focused on frequencies of interest that were derived from previous studies on altered auditory oscillatory power in tinnitus patients: delta (1–3 Hz; [10]), theta (4–6 Hz; [20,22]; alpha (8–12 Hz; [10]), gamma ([7,18,25]) subdivided in low gamma (30–70 Hz) and high gamma (70–90 Hz). In the next step, these values were statistically tested.

6.3. Statistical analyses of the pre-post modulations. Statistical analyses were performed using R version 2.11.1 for Mac OS X (www.r.project.org). As the complex study design entailed a small sample size and we identified various 'outliers' that, after precise investigation, we did not wish to treat as real outliers, we used a bootstrap approach for the statistical analysis. The 'outliers' or extreme values were not due to poor data quality, but rather reflect strong interindividual differences in the different stimulation protocols with somehow systematic patterns (only for specific TMS protocols and in patients with very short tinnitus duration; see Figure S1 in the supplemental material for comparison). Therefore, we decided not to exclude these cases and instead use robust statistics. We always compared the pre-post ratios of the active TMS conditions against sham using a bootstrap approach ('boot' package included in R). Thus, the sham values were subtracted from the activation values for each patient. After that we created 1000 new samples from the original sample (by drawing with replacement). For each of these new samples (having the same size as the original sample) the median was calculated. We thereby obtained a distribution of

1000 bootstrapped medians. The median was used in order to not overemphasize extreme values. We subsequently extracted the 95% confidence intervals (CI) for the median for each stimulation form respectively. If the confidence interval did not include 0, the effect could be considered as significant (power modulation significantly different in the active TMS vs sham TMS condition).

We performed this procedure for both, the modulation of tinnitus loudness and the modulation of auditory oscillatory activity in the frequency bands of interest.

6.4. Signatures of auditory brain activity reducing tinnitus loudness. Apart from analyses that focused on consistent modulations of tinnitus loudness and oscillatory activity after the different TMS protocols, we wanted to identify the signatures of oscillatory brain activity that are decisive for a strong reduction or an enhancement of tinnitus loudness. Hence, we defined the most effective stimulation protocol (among active TMS conditions) in *reducing* tinnitus loudness according to the TIM scores for each patient and analysed the according modulations in oscillatory activity. We repeated this procedure for the stimulation protocols that *increased* tinnitus loudness. For the selection of the according TMS protocol we used the TIM scores as they clearly separated the different protocols, whereas the VAS scores were more ambiguous (i.e., different protocols lead to identical modulations of tinnitus loudness). Note that we obtained similar results when excluding the ambiguous cases in the VAS assignment compared to the TIM assignment.

We conducted a further bootstrap statistic (the same method as described above) for the five frequency bands of interest (delta, theta, alpha, low gamma, high gamma) and for both increasing and decreasing tinnitus loudness protocols. We thereby defined the signatures of neuronal activity resulting in tinnitus loudness decreases/increases within the same participants.

6.5. Auditory alpha power modulation for the individual patients. The group results showed a high inter-individual variance for all investigated stimulation protocols, but also hinted at the potential of rTMS for treating tinnitus when it is applied in an individually optimized way (i.e. selecting protocol that increases auditory alpha power, see results section; see also Discussion indicating that this issue needs more definite confirmation). In order to address the clinically highly relevant question of the neuronal changes on an individual level we decided to add a single subject analysis. This was done to elucidate the pattern of how auditory alpha activity is modulated in the individual patients by the different stimulation protocols, in order to obtain information how the high variability within the protocols is made up. We therefore repeated the same analysis as described in the section on 'Spectral power analyses derived from auditory cortex', focussing on alpha power (as this was the most illuminating frequency band based on the group level results; see results section) however this time projecting the complex fourier spectra of the *single trials* onto our sources of interest. We then performed a single patient statistic by comparing the pre-post ratios of the single trials for each patient and TMS condition separately. Therefore, 5000 bootstrap replicates of the median were generated. We subsequently extracted the upper and lower quantiles corresponding to a probability of 5% and obtained the confidence intervals (CI) for each patient and stimulation form, respectively. This bootstrap procedure was in line with the one described above. Note that we here did not control for multiple comparisons so that the results should be interpreted on an explorative level only.

In a second step, we defined the most effective stimulation protocol in *reducing* tinnitus loudness according to the TIM (as already described for the group level in the section on 'Signatures of auditory brain activity reducing tinnitus loudness') for each patient separately and performed a single patient statistic quantifying the auditory alpha power modulation for the selected stimulation protocols. We further related the extent of the auditory alpha power modulation to the extent of the tinnitus loudness reduction (ranked from 1 to 10 with 1 reflecting the strongest loudness reduction). This procedure was repeated for the stimulation protocols that increased tinnitus loudness.

6.6. Signatures of whole brain activity reducing tinnitus loudness. Although it was not the focus of the present study, we examined the signatures of oscillatory brain activity in non-auditory regions that are decisive for a strong decrease or increase in tinnitus loudness. We thus performed a whole brain analysis for the stimulation protocol (individually selected) that most effectively reduced or enhanced tinnitus loudness according to the TIM and analysed power modulations from pre to post-TMS in the frequency bands of interest (delta, theta, alpha, low gamma, high gamma). For this purpose, we performed Dynamic Imaging of Coherent Sources (DICS), introduced by Gross and colleagues [43]. This beamformer technique optimally estimates the power for a certain location while suppressing activity at all other locations. The headmodel and leadfield were taken from the prior ROI analysis. For each grid point, we constructed a spatial filter from the cross-spectral density matrix of the MEG signal (not ICA-cleaned) at the frequency of interest (delta, theta, alpha, low and high gamma) and the respective leadfield. Thereafter we applied the spatial filters to the Fourier-transformed ICA-cleaned data (multitaper analysis) for the frequency of interest and divided the values by an estimate of the spatially inhomogenous noise (obtained for each gridpoint on the basis of the smallest value of the covariance matrix) in order to normalise this across participants. Afterwards we interpolated the resulting activation volumes to the individual MRI of the patients and normalised them to a template MNI brain provided by the SPM2 toolbox (http://www.fil.ion.ucl.ac.uk/spm/software/spm2). For statistical analysis, we calculated (post-pre)/pre ratios for each voxel of the source solutions respectively and tested these relative values against zero by applying a voxel-wise t-statistic. To correct for multiple comparisons, we defined a minimum cluster size (minimum number of neighbouring voxels above a given threshold that are required for a significant cluster) with AlphaSim provided by the Afni Package (http://afni.nimh.nih.gov/afni/doc/manual/AlphaSim.pdf). We thereby preserved the main non-auditory regions (>770 voxels) that were modulated by an effective tinnitus loudness-reducing or enhancing TMS stimulation in the frequency bands of interest.

Results

1. Individual Tolerance of the TMS Stimulation

None of the patients showed serious side effects of rTMS apart from transient mild to moderate discomfort due to muscle contractions, involuntary movements of the jaw and cutaneous sensations during TMS stimulation. One patient experienced a mild headache after stimulation, which disappeared without medication after several hours. Another patient reported periods of complete absence of the tinnitus lasting for several minutes after 1 Hz rTMS. Three patients reported a worsening of their tinnitus after IAF stimulation lasting for several hours up to a few days.

2. Tinnitus Loudness Modulations for the Different Stimulation Protocols Compared to Sham

Matched tinnitus loudness (TIM) was significantly reduced for 1-Hz rTMS (median: $-.15$, 95% CI: $-.04$ to $-.27$) and not modulated for the other stimulation protocols (Figure 2; upper panel). The reduction of subjective tinnitus loudness (VAS) was marginally significant for the 1-Hz (95% CI: -0.4 to 0) and cTBS protocols (95% CI: $-.25$ to 0), whereas it turned out to be marginally enhanced for the IAF stimulation (95% CI: 0 to.26). ITBS did not consistently change the tinnitus loudness (see Figure 2 (lower panel) for comparison). TIM (median:.08) and VAS (median:.06) values were not significantly modulated by sham stimulation.

3. Modulations of Auditory Oscillatory Brain Activity for the Different Stimulation Protocols Compared to Sham

Auditory oscillatory activity was not consistently modulated for the delta (1–3 Hz), theta (4–6 Hz) and low gamma (30–70 Hz) frequency bands (data shown in Figure S2 in the supplemental material)–that is, the confidence interval of all bootstrap statistics crossed the zero line. In contrast to this, power modulations in the alpha band were significantly reduced for the IAF stimulation (median: $-.07$, 95% CI: $-.54$ to $-.02$) and iTBS (median: $-.10$, 95% CI: $-.20$ to $-.004$), while no consistent differences were apparent in the cTBS and 1-Hz protocols (see Figure 3 upper panel). Furthermore, oscillatory power in the high gamma band (70–90 Hz) was significantly reduced for 1-Hz rTMS (median: $-.11$, 95% CI: $-.24$ to $-.004$) and iTBS (median: $-.10$, 95% CI: $-.21$ to $-.02$), while no consistent differences were apparent in cTBS and IAF stimulation (Figure 3, lower panel). Note, that we did not control for multiple comparisons, so that the results should be interpreted at an explorative level only.

Power modulations after sham stimulation were not significant (median of alpha power: .08; median of high gamma power.06).

4. Signatures in Auditory Oscillatory Power that Result in Strong Modulations of Tinnitus Loudness

Selecting the stimulation protocol (only active TMS protocols were considered, not sham) that was best in reducing tinnitus loudness for each patient individually resulted in a strong tinnitus reduction from pre to post rTMS for both the subjective (VAS; median: $-.27$, 99% CI: $-.9$ to $-.14$, only unambiguous cases included) and objective (TIM; median: $-.13$, 99% CI: $-.30$ to $-.03$) loudness measure. We would like to stress that this result was expected as we by definition selected the most effective stimulation protocols. However, by including this analysis we could in a next step derive the signatures in oscillatory activity, which were related to tinnitus relief. Importantly, for every patient, we could identify a 'real' TMS protocol that was better at reducing tinnitus compared to the placebo sham stimulation (according to TIM scores). Loudness reductions and a distribution of the contributing stimulation protocols are shown in Figure 4.

Analogously, we selected the stimulation protocols that consistently increased objective tinnitus loudness (TIM; median: .10, 99% CI: .01 to.24). It should be noted that as we could not select the stimulation protocols that enhanced tinnitus loudness unambiguously with the VAS scores for the majority of patients (only possible in 4 of 10 patients), we disregarded these values in further analyses. The loudness increase and a distribution of the contributing stimulation protocols are illustrated in Figure 5.

We could not identify any signatures of oscillatory activity in the stimulated auditory cortex related to a strong *increase* in tinnitus loudness (see Figure 6). However, when looking at the modulations of oscillatory power that were associated with a strong tinnitus loudness *reduction*, it turned out that a significant power enhancement in the *alpha* band was related to the tinnitus reduction (TIM

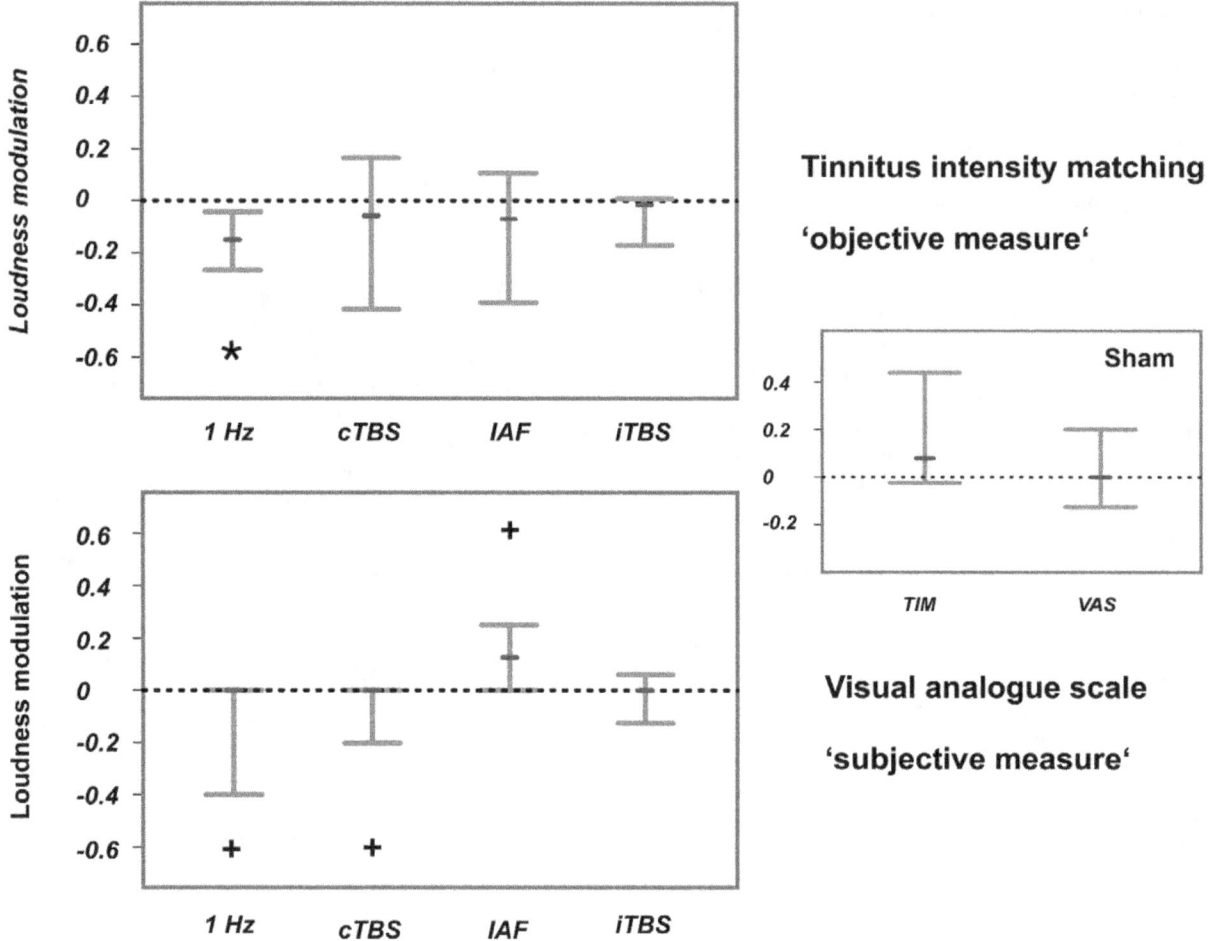

Figure 2. Consistent changes in tinnitus loudness after the four active TMS protocols compared to sham. The upper panel displays tinnitus loudness modulations that were measured with a matched-intensity approach (TIM), while the lower panel illustrates tinnitus loudness modulations that were quantified with a visual analogue scale (VAS). Sham effects are visualised in the right panel. Shown are the 95% confidence intervals. The small bars display the median. The asterisk indicates significant modulations, while the cross points to marginally significant modulations. According to the TIM, tinnitus loudness was reduced after 1-Hz rTMS. A trend pointing to a tinnitus reduction was revealed after 1-Hz rTMS and cTBS, while tinnitus loudness was marginally enhanced after IAF rTMS.

alpha: median: .03, 95% CI: .01 to.04, VAS alpha: median:.15, 95% CI: .03 to.21). Delta, theta and gamma (low and high) power were not consistently modulated and varied strongly (confidence intervals included zero). This was true for both, subjective tinnitus loudness (VAS) in the six patients that could be unambiguously assigned to one stimulation protocol as well as objective tinnitus loudness (TIM) (see Figure 6 for comparison).

5. Auditory Alpha Power Modulation for the Individual Patients

Following the group results that showed a big variance within the stimulation protocols concerning tinnitus loudness modulations and also oscillatory activity modulations together with a potential key role of enhancing auditory alpha power in reducing tinnitus loudness (see section above) it is now depicted how the *individual* patients reacted to the different stimulation protocols. We thereby focussed on auditory alpha power. This statistic should be interpreted at an explorative level only as we did not control for multiple comparisons. The single subject statistics point to a high interindividual variability within the stimulation protocols. Overall, each stimulation protocol had a significant effect on auditory

alpha power for a *subgroup* of the patients (95% confidence interval not including zero). In detail, alpha power was significantly modulated after application of 1 Hz rTMS in 4 of 10 patients (against sham 2 of 10), after IAF rTMS for 4 of 10 patients (against sham: 4 of 10), after cTBS in 10 of 10 patients (against sham: 5 of 10) and after iTBS in 3 of 10 patients (against sham: 3 of 10). However, the direction of the effects was not consistent resulting in the high variance and the lack of an effect on group level. This leads to the important conclusion that the variance is not due to individual participants with extreme values (this risk was already reduced by choosing the median), but that the effects of specific stimulation protocols on different patients are indeed highly variable. An overview of the auditory alpha power modulations for the single patients is given in Figure 7.

To investigate if the association between auditory alpha power modulations and tinnitus loudness modulations is also visible on a single subject level we investigated the auditory alpha power modulations for the individually most effective stimulation protocol in reducing tinnitus loudness for the individual patients separately (as done before on a group level). We thereby disclosed an interesting pattern of auditory alpha power modulations for the 'tinnitus reducers': In particular the patients with a very strong

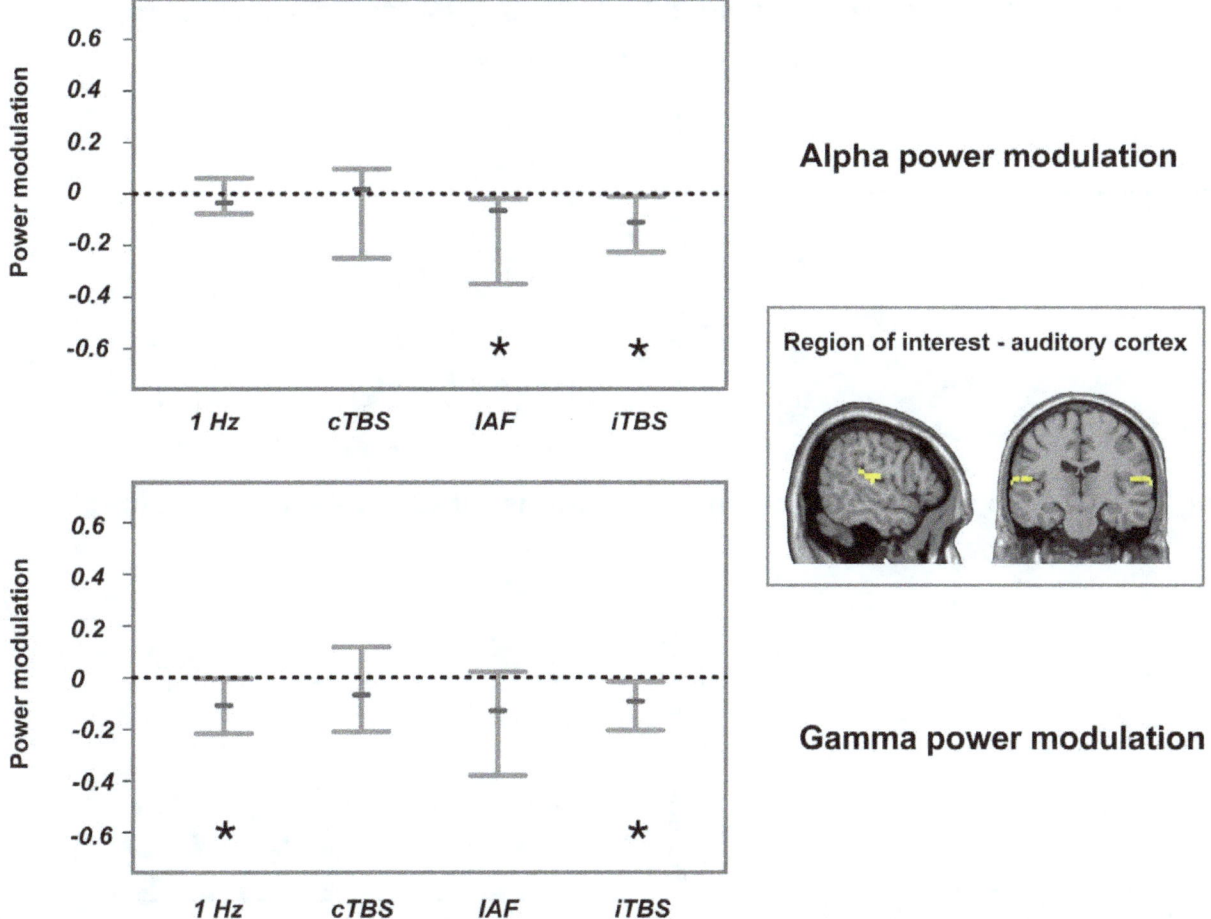

Figure 3. Consistent changes in oscillatory activity after the four active TMS protocols compared to sham. The upper panel displays alpha power modulations, while the lower panel illustrates modulations of high gamma power at the stimulated auditory cortex. The stimulated region and region of interest are displayed on the right side. Shown are the 95% confidence intervals. The small bars display the median while the asterisks indicate that the modulations were significant. Alpha power was significantly reduced after IAF rTMS and iTBS, while gamma power was significantly decreased by 1-Hz rTMS and iTBS (uncorrected).

tinnitus loudness reduction showed a strong auditory alpha power increase. The correlation between the individual auditory alpha power increase and the concomitant tinnitus loudness decrease was significant (Spearman's rank correlation rho $= -.61$, p$<$.05). In contrast, the stimulation protocols that were most effective in enhancing tinnitus loudness revealed a rather inconsistent pattern (Spearman's rank correlation rho $= -.37$, p not significant) what is in line with the inconsistent auditory cortex group results for the 'tinnitus enhancers'. The individual alpha power modulations related to a strong reduction (and enhancement) of tinnitus loudness are displayed in Figure 8.

6. Signatures of Non-auditory Oscillatory Power that Result in a Strong Tinnitus Loudness Modulation

We did not reveal any consistent non-auditory modulations of oscillatory activity associated with a strong tinnitus loudness decrease. However, we could identify left-hemispheric dominant reductions in oscillatory activity related to an increase in tinnitus loudness. Gamma power was significantly (p$<$.01, corrected) reduced in a left prefrontal (ventromedial frontal), a left precentral and a left parieto-temporo-occipital region. Furthermore, alpha power was reduced (p$<$.01, corrected) in a left superior frontal

area. The power modulations in non-auditory regions related to a tinnitus worsening are displayed in Figure 9.

Discussion

In the current study, we show how oscillatory brain activity is modulated in tinnitus patients by the application of four different TMS protocols (compared to sham) that are currently explored for treatment. We first focused on short-term modulations of oscillatory activity and tinnitus loudness that were consistent across patients for the specific TMS protocols, though overall effects were relatively small and varied strongly across patients. In a second step we identified the most effective stimulation protocols in decreasing (and increasing) tinnitus loudness and looked at associated modulations of oscillatory activity in auditory and non-auditory brain regions. As the increase of auditory alpha power turned out to be the main factor being related to a reduction of tinnitus loudness and as the most efficient stimulation protocol differed across patients we added a single-patient auditory alpha power analysis to further corroborate at an explorative level how the individual patients reacted to the different rTMS protocols. As expected from the group results, there was a high interindividual variability of the different rTMS protocols on alpha power and,

Reducing tinnitus with most effective stimulation forms - TIM (objective measure)

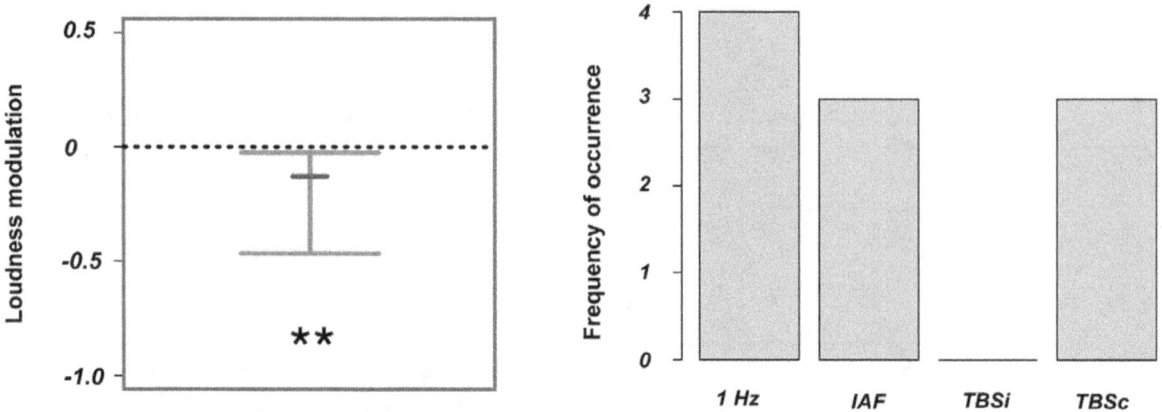

Reducing tinnitus with most effective stimulation forms - VAS (subjective measure)

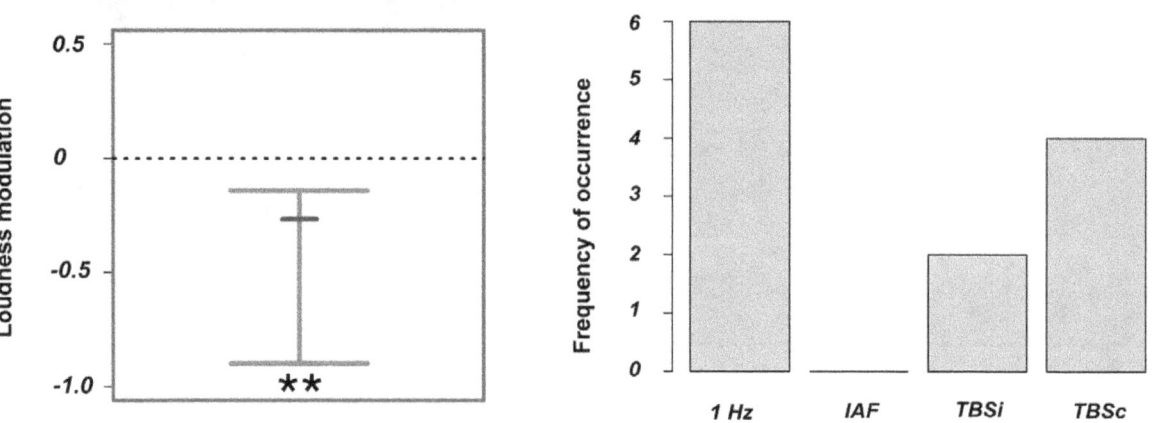

Figure 4. Changes in tinnitus loudness after application of the individually most effective stimulation protocol. The upper panel displays tinnitus loudness modulations that were measured with the tinnitus intensity matching procedure (TIM), while the lower panel illustrates tinnitus loudness modulations that were quantified with a visual analogue scale (VAS). The 99% confidence intervals are shown on the left side. The small bars display the median. The asterisks indicate significant modulations. As expected tinnitus loudness was significantly reduced after application of the individually selected protocol that was best in reducing tinnitus. The distribution of these protocols is displayed on the right side. Note that, as the ambiguous cases (when selecting the most effective protocol with VAS) were included for this illustration, the summed frequency of occurrence can be higher than the total number of patients.

importantly, the extent of the auditory alpha power increase was crucial for the extent of the tinnitus loudness reduction. This finding is of direct clinical relevance, since it suggests the potential of auditory cortex alpha power as a predictor for treatment outcome on an individual level.

1. Consistent Modulations of Tinnitus Loudness

We demonstrate that 1-Hz rTMS most consistently reduced tinnitus loudness (measured with a subjective and objective measure) compared to sham. However, the effects were relatively small and varied across subjects. This is in line with current literature on rTMS in tinnitus treatment that reports an impact of repeated 1-Hz rTMS sessions at the auditory cortex, albeit with moderate effect sizes and great interindividual variability [26,30,44]. Regarding the subjective estimates of tinnitus loudness, we additionally observed a trend for an overall reduction in tinnitus loudness after cTBS and, furthermore, an increase in tinnitus loudness after IAF rTMS. Again results were only moderate and varied strongly across patients (significant only on

a trend level). The trend of a tinnitus relief after cTBS is consistent with the few reports on this relatively new stimulation paradigm tested for the treatment of tinnitus [45,46]. At first glance, the trend pointing to an average increase in tinnitus loudness after IAF stimulation was rather unexpected, as most studies using high-frequency rTMS demonstrated a transient reduction of the tinnitus percept in the majority of the patients [47–50]. However, these discrepancies were likely due to differences in the experimental designs. In most studies, alterations in tinnitus loudness were assessed immediately after rTMS, whereas we assessed changes about 10–15 minutes after rTMS. Moreover, the duration of stimulation may play a role [51] as we measured tinnitus loudness after the application of 1000 pulses, in contrast to a maximum of 200 pulses in all previous studies on tinnitus. Consistent with the present data, that in average point to a disinhibition of the auditory cortex and increased tinnitus loudness after prolonged high-frequency rTMS, studies in the motor system show increased excitability and facilitated motor responses after such an extensive stimulation [52–54].

Increasing tinnitus with disadvantageous stimulation forms - TIM (objective measure)

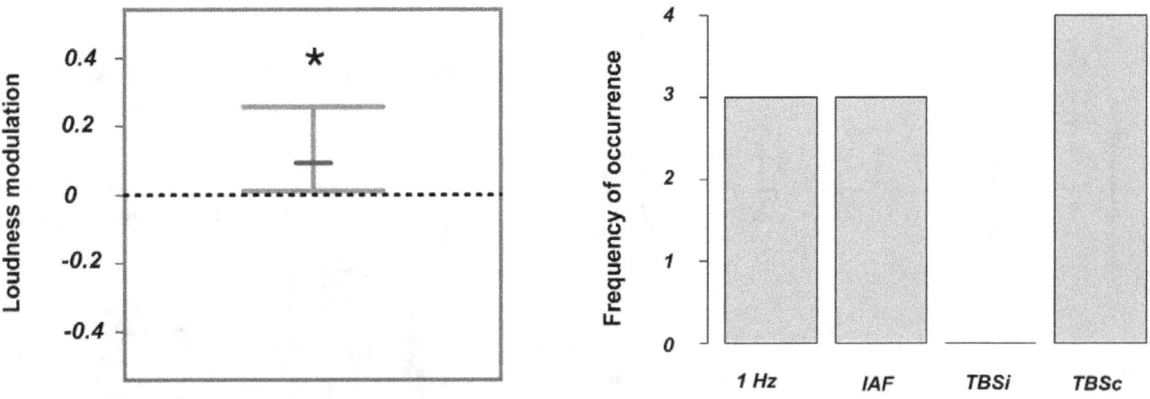

Increasing tinnitus with disadvantageous stimulation forms - VAS (subjective measure)

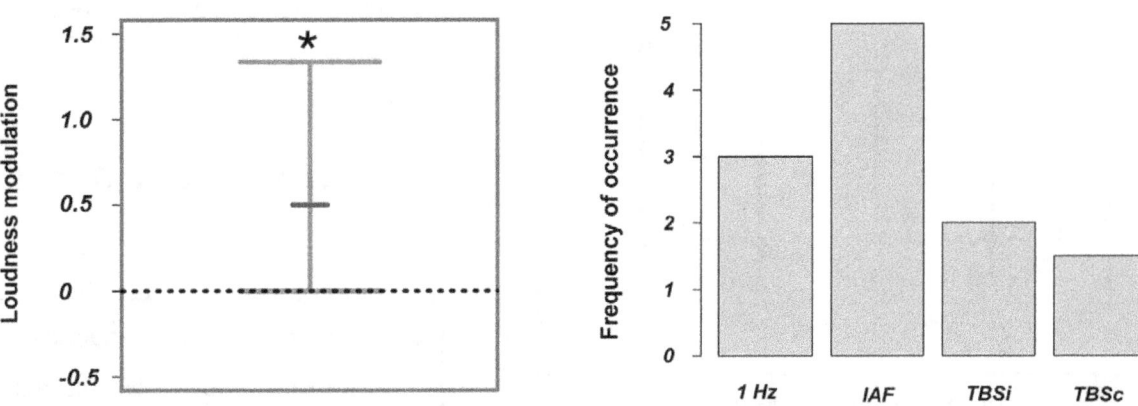

Figure 5. Changes in tinnitus loudness after application of the stimulation protocol that enhanced tinnitus loudness. The upper panel displays tinnitus loudness modulations that were measured with the tinnitus intensity matching procedure (TIM), while the lower panel illustrates tinnitus loudness modulations that were quantified using a visual analogue scale (VAS). The 95% confidence intervals are shown on the left side. The small bars display the median. The asterisks indicate significant modulations. As expected tinnitus loudness was significantly reduced after application of the individually selected protocol that worsened tinnitus. The distribution of these protocols is displayed on the right side. Note that, as the ambiguous cases (when selecting the most effective protocol with VAS) were included for this illustration, the summed frequency of occurrence can be higher than the total number of patients.

2. Consistent Modulations of Oscillatory Activity

We would like to emphasize that the group effects on auditory oscillatory activity were in general very small and should be rather interpreted at an explorative level. Alpha power (8–12 Hz) was significantly reduced (uncorrected) after treatment with IAF rTMS and iTBS in the auditory cortex ipsilateral to rTMS. It has been demonstrated that a decrease in alpha power is linked to disinhibition, whereas an increase in alpha power reflects active inhibition of the underlying neuronal tissue [19,21,55–60]. Regarding oscillatory activity in tinnitus patients, it has been shown that tinnitus patients exhibit a reduced alpha peak compared to normal controls, which is putatively linked to reduced inhibition in the auditory cortex [10,19]. Thus, we suggest that the decrease in alpha power after rTMS is related to a disinhibition and hence an increase in excitability of the stimulated auditory cortex.

To our knowledge, the impact of high-frequency rTMS or iTBS on *auditory* cortex excitability has not yet been investigated, despite the presence of the above-mentioned studies on tinnitus. Research in the motor system usually reports an enhancement

in excitability after high-frequency (in the alpha range) rTMS and iTBS [29,54,61–63]. Therefore, the decrease in alpha power after rapid-rate rTMS and iTBS fits well into the literature and furthermore extends the role of high-frequency rTMS and iTBS in increasing excitability from the motor to the auditory system.

It has to be mentioned here that the described effects of reduced auditory alpha power after high-frequency rTMS and iTBS were only moderate. However, this weak (IAF rTMS, iTBS) or also absent (1 Hz rTMS, cTBS) group effects were not due to absent effects in the individual patients but rather to a great interindividual variability as reflected by the single-patient analysis. The most powerful stimulation protocol, in the sense of affecting brain activity in most patients, for instance was cTBS: 10 of 10 patients (5 of 10 when testing against sham) showed a significant modulation (uncorrected) of auditory alpha power after the application of cTBS, 3 of them reducing and 7 of them enhancing significantly auditory alpha power. For every stimulation protocol we could find such a subgroup of patients that showed a strong modulation of auditory alpha power, albeit the direction of the

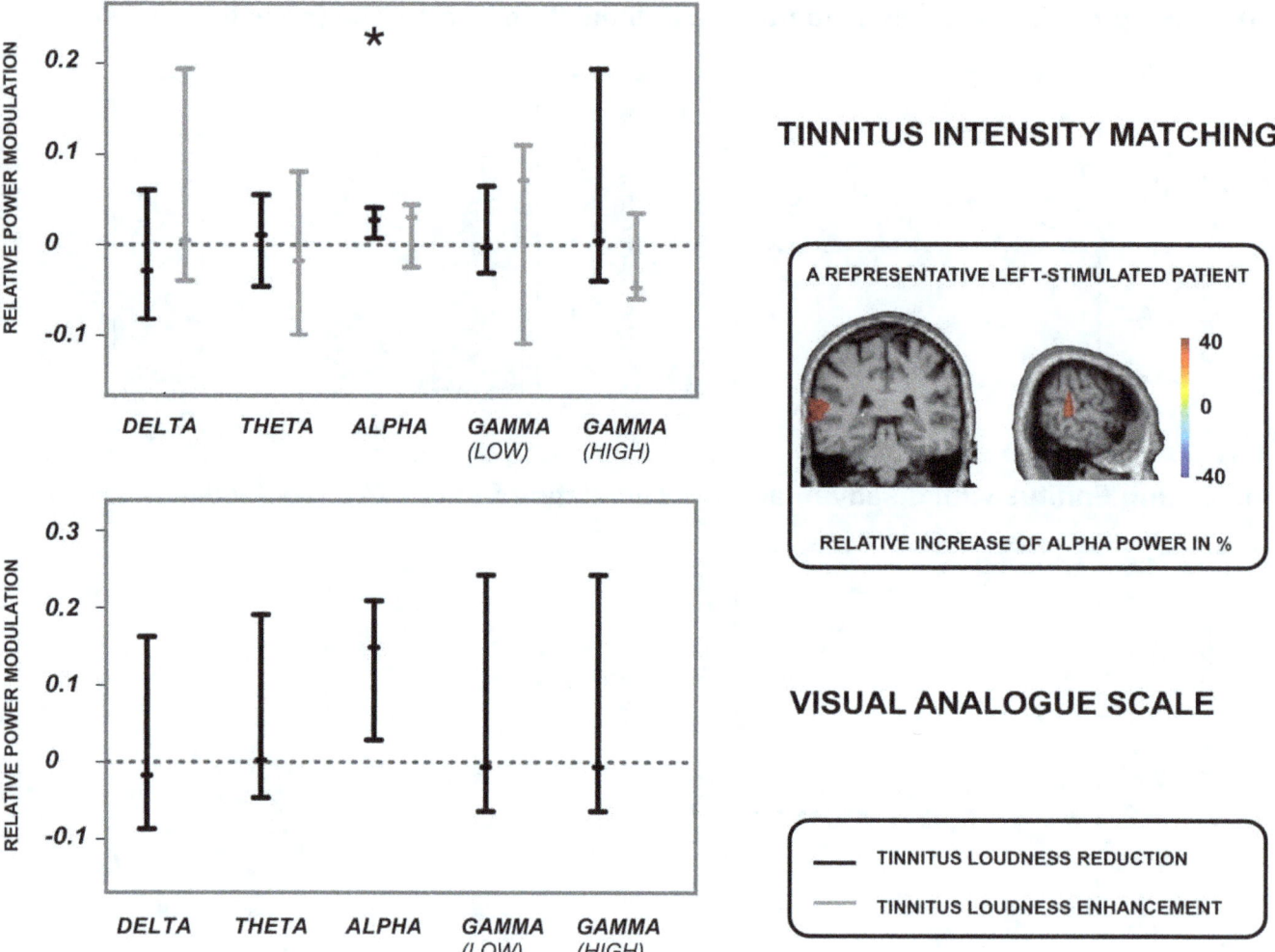

Figure 6. Modulation of oscillatory activity for the most effective TMS protocols. Shown are changes in oscillatory activity at the stimulated auditory cortex after application of the rTMS protocols that were best in reducing (black bars) and enhancing (grey bars) tinnitus loudness. The upper panel displays power modulations that were associated with the tinnitus intensity matching procedure (TIM), while the lower panel illustrates power modulations that were related to the visual analogue scale (VAS). Displayed are the 95% confidence intervals for power modulations in the stimulated auditory cortex and the different frequency bands (delta, theta, alpha, low gamma, high gamma). The small bars show the median, while the asterisk indicates the power modulations as significant. Note that we observed too many ambiguous cases for the VAS with respect to an increase in tinnitus loudness; we could thus not specify the according signature in oscillatory activity. Alpha power was significantly enhanced when tinnitus loudness was most effectively reduced by rTMS.

effect (decrease or increase) was rather inconsistent. This finding can explain the high interindividual variability in treatment effects observed in many clinical trials [27,30] on a neuronal basis and puts into question the possibility to develop a 'standard therapy' for the treatment of tinnitus. As the different stimulation protocols had specific effects on brain activity dependent on the individual patient, different patients may profit from different stimulation protocols. However, this assumption has still to be tested more conclusively by assessing the re-test reliability of the results.

High gamma power (70–90 Hz) was consistently modulated after two of the 4 active rTMS protocols: we detected a significant reduction (uncorrected) after 1-Hz rTMS as well as after iTBS in the stimulated auditory cortex. In contrast to the alpha rhythm, gamma oscillations are associated with higher-order functions and active sensory processing [64,65]. It has been demonstrated that tinnitus patients exhibit enhanced auditory gamma power compared to controls [7,20,25] and that auditory gamma activity is also increased during transient tinnitus after noise trauma [17].

Furthermore, gamma power in the auditory cortex contralateral to the tinnitus percept has been suggested to reflect the loudness of the tinnitus percept [18].

Several studies have investigated the impact of low-frequency rTMS (≤ 1 Hz) on neuronal and behavioural outcomes. It has been demonstrated that low-frequency rTMS decreases cortical excitability [28,61] (for an overview see [66]), reduces gamma activity in schizophrenic patients [67], improves inhibitory function in tinnitus patients [26,27], reduces auditory metabolic activity in tinnitus patients [68] and reduces tinnitus loudness when applied during repeated sessions [26]. This is consistent with results from the present study that demonstrate a decrease in gamma power in the stimulated area and thus a reduction in auditory cortical activity after 1-Hz rTMS.

The effects of iTBS are rather variable and inconsistent regarding different stimulation areas: iTBS has been related to an enhanced motor cortex excitability [62] and an increased gamma power in the sensory-motor cortex of rats [69] which is in

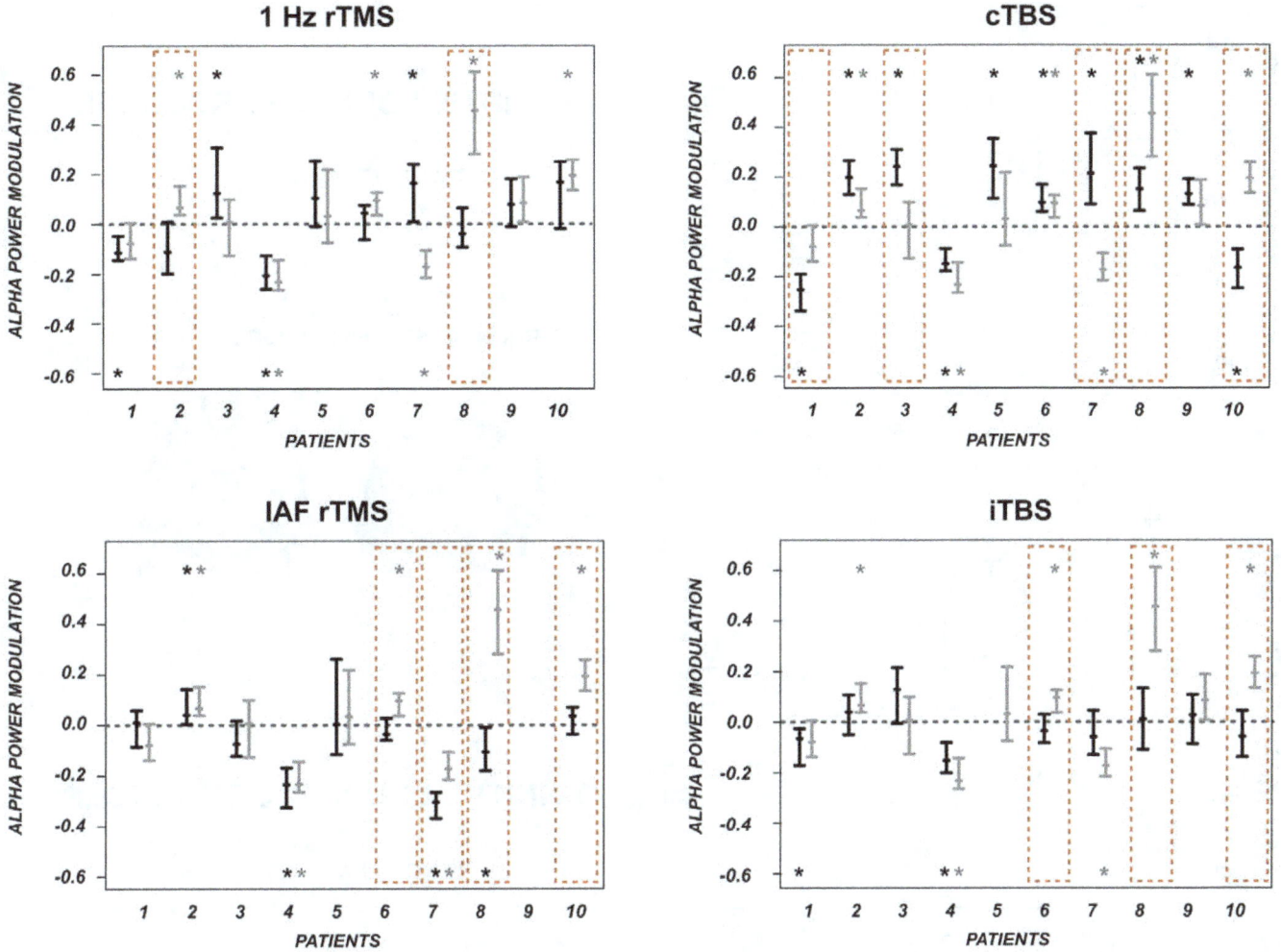

Figure 7. Modulation of auditory alpha power in the individual patients. Depicted are modulations of auditory alpha power in the individual patients and for the four active TMS protocols (black bars) and sham (grey bars). Shown are the 95% confidence intervals (uncorrected). The small bars display the median. The asterisks indicate significant modulations from pre to post TMS. The orange boxes point to significant modulations against sham stimulation. TMS modulates alpha activity significantly already in individual patients: 1 Hz rTMS (4 of 10, against Sham: 2 of 10), cTBS (10 of 10, against sham 5 of 10), IAF rTMS (4 of 10, against sham 4 of 10), iTBS (2 of 10, against Sham 3 of 10), however, not consistently into the same direction (increase vs decrease of alpha power).

opposition to our finding of reduced gamma power after iTBS. However, studies also report an increased cortical inhibition [69,70] as well as a reduction in the auditory steady-state response after iTBS [34]. In general, reports on the effects of iTBS on excitability of cortical regions apart from the human motor cortex are rare and suggest that the effects are not simply transferable to non-motor brain regions [71,72]. The only study investigating the effect of iTBS on tinnitus loudness did not reveal any consistent effects [45]. Furthermore, a reduction in auditory gamma activity after iTBS does not necessarily point to a generally reduced excitability since we also detected a decrease in alpha power (rather pointing to increased excitability) following iTBS as described above.

All these inconsistencies in sum, we emphasize that the relationship of alpha power, gamma power and the perception of tinnitus loudness is not sufficiently understood to date and would require further research. In the following section we, however, attempt to further enlighten the role of auditory alpha power as a prerequisite for a change of tinnitus perception.

3. Signatures of Oscillatory Activity Associated with a Reduction in Tinnitus Loudness after rTMS in Auditory Brain Regions

As expected tinnitus loudness was most effectively reduced by individually selected stimulation protocols implying that different patients profited from different protocols. Importantly, for every patient, sham stimulation was worse at reducing tinnitus loudness than the best 'real' rTMS protocol. For about half of the patients 1 Hz rTMS was most successful while the other half profited from other protocols such as IAF rTMS and cTBS. However, we would like to stress here that the identification of individually most effective specific stimulation protocols might have been confounded by spontaneous fluctuations in tinnitus loudness. Despite being possible, this is unlikely as sham stimulation in no case was identified as the most successful protocol. For definitively ruling out this alternative explanation assessment of test re-test reliability by further studies will be needed.

Having selected the most effective stimulation protocol for each patient, we were then able to elucidate if the different rTMS protocols having in common to effectively reduce tinnitus loudness

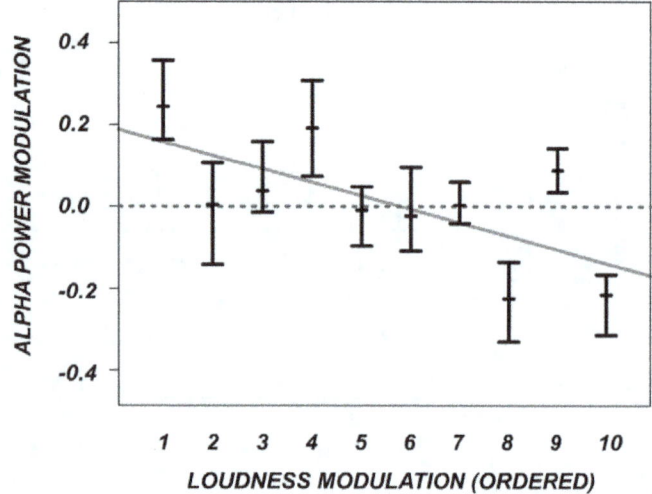

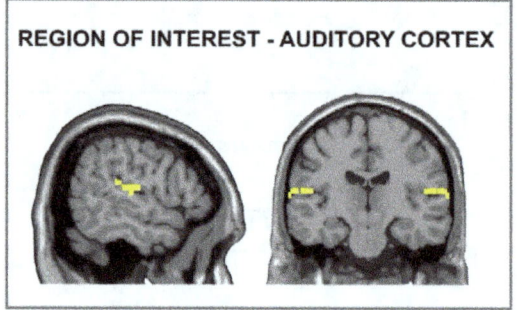

'TINNITUS LOUDNESS REDUCER'

RANGE (TIM): -0.63 – 0

REGION OF INTEREST - AUDITORY CORTEX

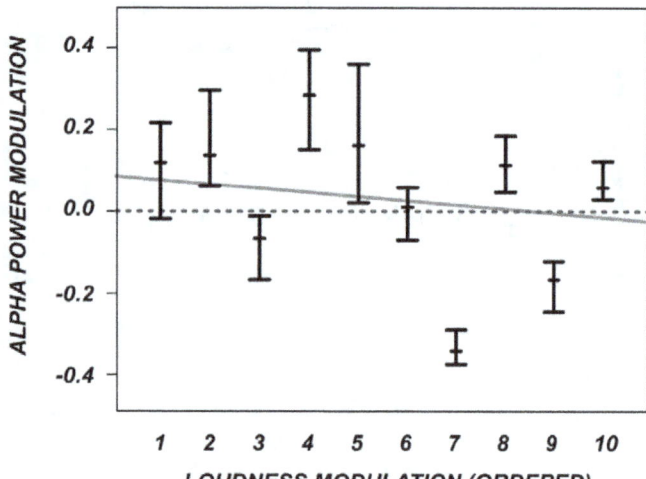

'TINNITUS LOUDNESS ENHANCER'

RANGE (TIM): -0.06 – 0.56

Figure 8. Modulation of oscillatory activity for the most effective TMS protocols and the individual patients. Shown are the changes in oscillatory activity at the stimulated auditory cortex for the individual patients after application of the rTMS protocols that were best in reducing (upper panel) and enhancing (lower panel) tinnitus loudness. Shown are the 95% confidence intervals for the individual patients. The small bars display the median. Patients are ordered according to the strength of the tinnitus loudness decrease (upper panel) or increase (lower panel). The grey line illustrates the correlation between the extent of the alpha power modulation and the extent of the tinnitus loudness modulation (ordered from 1 to 10). When tinnitus loudness is maximally reduced (range of TIM values: −0.63–0) the extent of the alpha power modulation is negatively correlated with the extent of the loudness reduction (RHO: −.61, p<. 05), thus the patients with the strongest alpha power increase were the patients with the strongest tinnitus loudness decrease. In contrast, When tinnitus loudness was maximally increased no such correlation was evident (RHO: −.37, p not significant).

also affect ongoing auditory cortical activity in a specific way. Our findings demonstrate that a strong reduction in tinnitus loudness was associated with an enhancement of alpha power in the stimulated auditory cortex (ipsilateral to rTMS), while delta, theta and gamma power were not consistently modulated and varied strongly. Therefore, we suppose that an increase in alpha power in the auditory cortex is crucial for the reduction of tinnitus loudness, whereas auditory delta, theta and gamma power seem to be related to more unspecific effects. This is in line with studies that have demonstrated a normalisation in alpha power after successful tinnitus treatment using a neurofeedback approach [73,74]. Importantly, the specific role of auditory *alpha* power does not contradict the results on the *average* modulations of tinnitus loudness and oscillatory activity described in the first part of the discussion where on average effective stimulation protocols (such as 1 Hz rTMS) were not associated with increases in auditory

alpha power. Due to the fact that within categories patients that profit and do not profit from a specific protocol are automatically intermingled such an analysis is less sensitive in detecting tinnitus relief specific modulations than an individualised analysis. It rather focuses on modulations that are specific for the selected stimulation protocol regardless of its potential to strongly reduce tinnitus. We therefore think that the individualised analysis is more powerful to derive the features associated with tinnitus relief. It suggests the importance of alpha power increases in the auditory cortex as such a relevant feature to effectively reduce tinnitus.

Notably, due to the correlational approach of the current study we are not able to draw any conclusions about the directionality of the effects. Thus further studies are needed to clarify whether an increase in auditory alpha power indeed causes tinnitus relief, whether it rather reflects reduced auditory processing when

Modulation of alpha power

left superior frontal gyrus

Modulation of gamma power

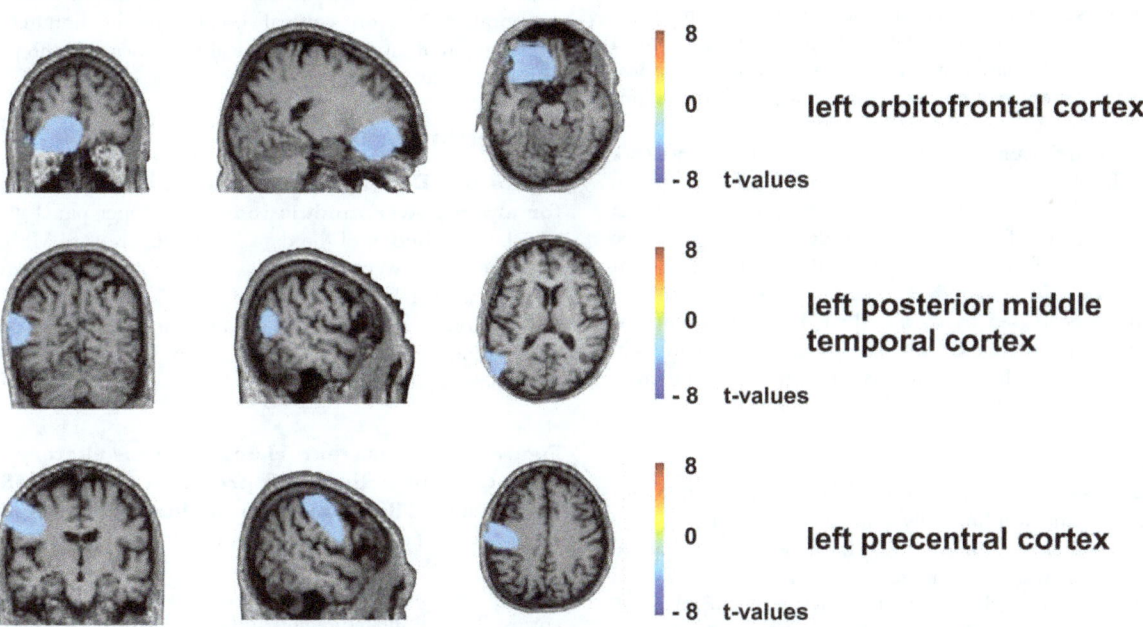

left orbitofrontal cortex

left posterior middle temporal cortex

left precentral cortex

Figure 9. Changes in oscillatory activity in non-auditory brain areas for the most effective stimulation protocols. Shown are the changes in oscillatory activity in non-auditory brain areas after application of the rTMS protocols that were most effective in enhancing tinnitus loudness. The upper panel displays brain regions with power modulations in the alpha band, while the lower panel illustrates the areas exhibiting modulations in gamma power. Displayed are comparisons from pre to post rTMS and are quantified in t-values. Gamma power was significantly (p<.01; corrected) reduced in a left prefrontal, a left precentral and a left parieto-temporo-occipital region. Alpha power was reduced (p<.01; corrected) in a left superior frontal area.

tinnitus is reduced spontaneously or whether both effects are caused by a third mechanism.

We would like to point out that most studies on signatures in oscillatory activity related to tinnitus include comparisons between tinnitus patients and normal hearing controls [7,10,22,23,25]. The observed differences in neuronal activity are therefore not unequivocal and could be due to many unspecific mechanisms appearing in the tinnitus patients related to emotional or cognitive processes such as attention and evaluation. It is thus of great interest to identify the specific neuronal signatures in tinnitus patients (in this case oscillatory activity) that are related to a strong decrease (or increase) in tinnitus loudness compared to the 'normal' tinnitus perception and to find out which of these signatures must be modulated in order to successfully reduce tinnitus [88]. With respect to our data, we again emphasise the importance of an alpha power increase in the auditory cortex for an alleviation of the tinnitus percept. This is further substantiated by the single-patient auditory alpha power analysis showing that the patients with the strongest tinnitus loudness decrease were also the patients with the strongest alpha power increase. The association between high auditory alpha power and tinnitus relief

further corroborates the role of alpha power in the active inhibition of cortical brain regions [19,21,56,58,60] and extends its role in the pathophysiology of brain diseases with an excitatory-inhibitory imbalance such as tinnitus [1,10]. As tinnitus is predominantly characterised by a hyperexcitation in auditory brain regions [30], we suggest that enhancing auditory alpha activity is most relevant for the relief of tinnitus, putatively by increasing ongoing inhibitory mechanisms.

4. Signatures in Oscillatory Activity Associated with an Increase in Tinnitus Loudness after rTMS in Non-auditory Brain Regions

In this study we were not able to identify any extra-auditory signatures in oscillatory activity related to tinnitus loudness reduction. However, we found that an increase in tinnitus loudness was associated with a decrease in gamma and alpha power predominantly in left frontal regions. Specifically, tinnitus loudness increases were related to reduced alpha power in the left superior middle frontal region, which is in line with findings of increased activity in middle frontal and superior frontal regions in tinnitus patients [75]. The increase in tinnitus was further associated with gamma power reductions in the left prefrontal, left precentral and left posterior temporal cortex pointing to a deactivation of these regions when tinnitus loudness increased. Various studies underpin the relevance of a frontoparietal network in tinnitus perception [76–79]. It has been postulated that the prefrontal cortex integrates sensory and emotional aspects of tinnitus [8] and is part of a network associated with conscious tinnitus perception [10,79]. Transcranial direct current stimulation [80] and transcranial magnetic stimulation [81] of the prefrontal cortex led to a decrease in tinnitus intensity and distress. A deactivation of the left prefrontal cortex associated with reduced positive affect [82,83] and an increase in pain perception [84] is in line with the worsening of the tinnitus found in the present study. The precentral region has been related to the attentional control for the selection of auditory stimuli [85] and parieto-temporo-occipital regions were active during verbal auditory hallucinations [86].

However, the relevance of the observed top-down network including left frontal and centro-parietal regions for the generation of tinnitus and the significance of reduced alpha and gamma power in the sense of activation and deactivation must be investigated through further studies. It should also be noted that the lack of effects in non-auditory regions related to tinnitus reduction might be biased by the fact that the intervention was targeted at the auditory cortex. One may speculate that changes in tinnitus loudness through interventions focussing on other brain areas may reveal different patterns of network alterations.

5. Conclusion

The present results have shed further light on the pathophysiology of tinnitus and will hopefully stimulate the development of more effective therapy approaches. It appears essential to determine the signatures in auditory and non-auditory brain regions that are associated with the tinnitus percept in order to better understand this complex disease and to be able to develop more effective treatments. In this study we focused on the relationship of tinnitus loudness changes and changes in oscillatory activity in the stimulated auditory cortex and in other cortical regions. Our study confirmed that a reduction in tinnitus loudness is possible using conventional rTMS approaches; however, in line with most other studies, the general relief of the tinnitus percept was small and varied strongly across patients [27]. This pattern was also reflected in the neurophysiological data.

Beyond that we identified the signatures in oscillatory brain activity that relate to tinnitus relief. *Reductions* in the tinnitus sensation were associated with increases in alpha power in the stimulated auditory cortex, meaning that the intervention had specific effects. The identification of alpha power increases in the stimulated area as the relevant mechanisms of action for tinnitus

relief is of high relevance as it provides an initial orientation for an individualized treatment approach. Future clinical studies may aim at identifying the optimal rTMS protocol having the potential to reliably increase alpha activity in the temporal cortex in the individual patient in order to enhance clinical efficacy. On the other hand, *increases* in the tinnitus sensation were related to alterations in a left-lateralised fronto-centro-parietal network, confirming the relevance of this network for tinnitus perception. Increase in tinnitus loudness may thus either result from propagated rTMS effects on non-auditory (mostly left frontal) brain regions or may be unspecific. More comprehensive clinical trials are needed in order to further explore the observed effects of temporal rTMS on cortical oscillations in tinnitus patients, regarding in addition to this clinical relevance and the persistence of these effects.

Supporting Information

Figure S1   Distribution of extreme values, exemplary for alpha power modulations. The upper panel illustrates a boxplot distribution of the data for the different rTMS protocols. Extreme values were detected after cTBS, IAF rTMS and iTBS, and not after 1-Hz rTMS and sham. The lower panel illustrates the relation between tinnitus duration and auditory alpha power modulation. Extreme values are exclusively associated with very short tinnitus duration.

Figure S2   Consistent changes in oscillatory activity after the four active TMS protocols (1 Hz rTMS, cTBS, IAF rTMS, iTBS) compared to sham. The upper left panel displays delta power modulations, the upper right panel illustrates theta power modulations and the lower left panel shows modulations of low gamma power at the stimulated auditory cortex. The stimulated region and region of interest is displayed on the lower right side. Shown are the 95% confidence intervals. The small bars display the median. No significant power modulations were found either in the delta, theta or in the low gamma band.

Acknowledgments

We thank Thomas Elbert for helpful discussions during the design of the study and Ursula Lommen for help in acquiring the data.

Author Contributions

Conceived and designed the experiments: NM IL BL NW. Performed the experiments: NM IL. Analyzed the data: NM. Contributed reagents/materials/analysis tools: NM BL NW. Wrote the paper: NM.

References

1. Eggermont JJ, Roberts LE (2004) The neuroscience of tinnitus. Trends in neurosciences 27: 676–682.
2. Shargorodsky J, Curhan GC, Farwell WR (2010) Prevalence and characteristics of tinnitus among US adults. The American journal of medicine 123: 711–718.
3. Baguley DM, Axon P, Winter IM, Moffat DA (2002) The effect of vestibular nerve section upon tinnitus. Clinical otolaryngology and allied sciences 27: 219–226.
4. Zacharek MA, Kaltenbach JA, Mathog TA, Zhang J (2002) Effects of cochlear ablation on noise induced hyperactivity in the hamster dorsal cochlear nucleus: implications for the origin of noise induced tinnitus. Hearing research 172: 137–143.
5. Rajan R, Irvine DR (1998) Neuronal responses across cortical field A1 in plasticity induced by peripheral auditory organ damage. Audiology & neuro-otology 3: 123–144.
6. Salvi RJ, Wang J, Ding D (2000) Auditory plasticity and hyperactivity following cochlear damage. Hearing research 147: 261–274.
7. Ashton H, Reid K, Marsh R, Johnson I, Alter K, et al. (2007) High frequency localised "hot spots" in temporal lobes of patients with intractable tinnitus: a quantitative electroencephalographic (QEEG) study. Neuroscience letters 426: 23–28.
8. Jastreboff PJ (1990) Phantom auditory perception (tinnitus): mechanisms of generation and perception. Neuroscience research 8: 221–254.
9. Roberts LE, Eggermont JJ, Caspary DM, Shore SE, Melcher JR, et al. (2010) Ringing ears: the neuroscience of tinnitus. The Journal of neuroscience: the official journal of the Society for Neuroscience 30: 14972–14979.
10. Weisz N, Moratti S, Meinzer M, Dohrmann K, Elbert T (2005) Tinnitus perception and distress is related to abnormal spontaneous brain activity as measured by magnetoencephalography. PLoS medicine 2: e153.
11. Dietrich V, Nieschalk M, Stoll W, Rajan R, Pantev C (2001) Cortical reorganization in patients with high frequency cochlear hearing loss. Hearing research 158: 95–101.

12. Kaltenbach JA (2006) Summary of evidence pointing to a role of the dorsal cochlear nucleus in the etiology of tinnitus. Acta oto-laryngologica Supplementum 20–26.

13. Noreña AJ, Eggermont JJ (2003) Changes in spontaneous neural activity immediately after an acoustic trauma: implications for neural correlates of tinnitus. Hearing research 183: 137–153.

14. Mulders WH, Robertson D (2009) Hyperactivity in the auditory midbrain after acoustic trauma: dependence on cochlear activity. Neuroscience 164: 733–746.

15. Finlayson PG, Kaltenbach JA (2009) Alterations in the spontaneous discharge patterns of single units in the dorsal cochlear nucleus following intense sound exposure. Hearing research 256: 104–117.

16. Seki S, Eggermont JJ (2003) Changes in spontaneous firing rate and neural synchrony in cat primary auditory cortex after localized tone-induced hearing loss. Hearing research 180: 28–38.

17. Ortmann M, Müller N, Schlee W, Weisz N (2011) Rapid increases of gamma power in the auditory cortex following noise trauma in humans. The European journal of neuroscience 33: 568–575.

18. van der Loo E, Gais S, Congedo M, Vanneste S, Plazier M, et al. (2009) Tinnitus intensity dependent gamma oscillations of the contralateral auditory cortex. PLoS ONE 4: e7396.

19. Weisz N, Dohrmann K, Elbert T (2007) The relevance of spontaneous activity for the coding of the tinnitus sensation. Progress in brain research 166: 61–70.

20. Llinás RR, Ribary U, Jeanmonod D, Kronberg E, Mitra PP (1999) Thalamocortical dysrhythmia: A neurological and neuropsychiatric syndrome characterized by magnetoencephalography. Proceedings of the National Academy of Sciences of the United States of America 96: 15222–15227.

21. Klimesch W, Sauseng P, Hanslmayr S (2007) EEG alpha oscillations: the inhibition-timing hypothesis. Brain research reviews 53: 63–88.

22. Moazami-Goudarzi M, Michels L, Weisz N, Jeanmonod D (2010) Temporo-insular enhancement of EEG low and high frequencies in patients with chronic tinnitus. QEEG study of chronic tinnitus patients. BMC neuroscience 11: 40.

23. Fuggetta G, Noh NA (2012) A neurophysiological insight into the potential link between transcranial magnetic stimulation, thalamocortical dysrhythmia and neuropsychiatric disorders. Experimental Neurology. ScienceDirect website. Available: http://dx.doi.org/10.1016/j.expneurol.2012.10.010. Accessed 2012 Dec.

24. Ramirez RR, Kopell BH, Butson CR, Gaggl W, Friedland DR, et al. (2009) Neuromagnetic source imaging of abnormal spontaneous activity in tinnitus patient modulated by electrical cortical stimulation. Conference proceedings: Annual International Conference of the IEEE Engineering in Medicine and Biology Society IEEE Engineering in Medicine and Biology Society Conference 2009: 1940–1944.

25. Weisz N, Müller S, Schlee W, Dohrmann K, Hartmann T, et al. (2007) The neural code of auditory phantom perception. The Journal of neuroscience: the official journal of the Society for Neuroscience 27: 1479–1484.

26. Kleinjung T, Steffens T, Londero A, Langguth B (2007) Transcranial magnetic stimulation (TMS) for treatment of chronic tinnitus: clinical effects. Progress in brain research 166: 359–367.

27. Langguth B, Ridder D, Dornhoffer JL, Eichhammer P, Folmer RL, et al. (2008) Controversy: Does repetitive transcranial magnetic stimulation/transcranial direct current stimulation show efficacy in treating tinnitus patients? Brain Stimulation 1: 192–205.

28. Chen R, Classen J, Gerloff C, Celnik P, Wassermann EM, et al. (1997) Depression of motor cortex excitability by low-frequency transcranial magnetic stimulation. Neurology 48: 1398–1403.

29. Pascual-Leone A, Valls-Solé J, Wassermann EM, Hallett M (1994) Responses to rapid-rate transcranial magnetic stimulation of the human motor cortex. Brain: a journal of neurology 117: 847–858.

30. Plewnia C (2010) Brain Stimulation: New Vistas for the Exploration and Treatment of Tinnitus. CNS neuroscience & therapeutics 00: 1–13.

31. Khedr EM, Rothwell JC, El-Atar A (2009) One-year follow up of patients with chronic tinnitus treated with left temporoparietal rTMS. European journal of neurology: the official journal of the European Federation of Neurological Societies 10.1111/j.1468-1331.2008.02522.x.

32. Londero A, Langguth B, De Ridder D, Bonfils P, Lefaucheur JP (2006) Repetitive transcranial magnetic stimulation (rTMS): a new therapeutic approach in subjective tinnitus? Neurophysiologie clinique = Clinical neurophysiology 36: 145–155.

33. Kleinjung T, Langguth B (2009) Strategies for enhancement of transcranial magnetic stimulation effects in tinnitus patients. The international tinnitus journal 15: 154–160.

34. Lorenz I, Müller N, Schlee W, Langguth B, Weisz N (2010) Short-term effects of single repetitive TMS sessions on auditory evoked activity in patients with chronic tinnitus. Journal of neurophysiology 104: 1497–1505.

35. Hallam RS, Jakes SC, Hinchcliffe R (1988) Cognitive variables in tinnitus annoyance. The British journal of clinical psychology/the British Psychological Society 27: 213–222.

36. Goebel G, Hiller W (1994) The tinnitus questionnaire. A standard instrument for grading the degree of tinnitus. Results of a multicenter study with the tinnitus questionnaire. HNO 42: 166–172.

37. Pridmore S, Fernandes Filho JA, Nahas Z, Liberatos C, George MS (1998) Motor threshold in transcranial magnetic stimulation: a comparison of a neurophysiological method and a visualization of movement method. The journal of ECT 14: 25–27.

38. Langguth B, Zowe M, Landgrebe M, Sand P, Kleinjung T, et al. (2006) Transcranial magnetic stimulation for the treatment of tinnitus: a new coil positioning method and first results. Brain topography 18: 241–247.

39. Oostenveld R, Fries P, Maris E, Schoffelen JM (2011) FieldTrip: Open source software for advanced analysis of MEG, EEG, and invasive electrophysiological data. Computational intelligence and neuroscience 2011: 156869.

40. Huang MX, Mosher JC, Leahy RM (1999) A sensor-weighted overlapping-sphere head model and exhaustive head model comparison for MEG. Physics in medicine and biology 44: 423–440.

41. Percival DB, Walden AT (1993) Spectral Analysis for Physical Applications: Multitaper and Conventional Univariate Techniques. Cambridge: Cambridge University Press.

42. Van Veen BD, van Drongelen W, Yuchtman M, Suzuki A (1997) Localization of brain electrical activity via linearly constrained minimum variance spatial filtering. IEEE transactions on bio-medical engineering 44: 867–880.

43. Gross J, Kujala J, Hämäläinen M, Timmermann L, Schnitzler A, et al. (2001) Dynamic imaging of coherent sources: Studying neural interactions in the human brain. Proceedings of the National Academy of Sciences of the United States of America 98: 694–699.

44. Kleinjung T, Vielsmeier V, Landgrebe M, Hajak G, Langguth B (2008) Transcranial magnetic stimulation: a new diagnostic and therapeutic tool for tinnitus patients. The international tinnitus journal 14: 112–118.

45. Poreisz C, Paulus W, Moser T, Lang N (2009) Does a single session of theta-burst transcranial magnetic stimulation of inferior temporal cortex affect tinnitus perception? BMC neuroscience 10: 54.

46. Soekadar SR, Arfeller C, Rilk A, Plontke SK, Plewnia C (2009) Theta burst stimulation in the treatment of incapacitating tinnitus accompanied by severe depression. CNS spectrums 14: 208–211.

47. Plewnia C, Bartels M, Gerloff C (2003) Transient suppression of tinnitus by transcranial magnetic stimulation. Annals of neurology 53: 263–266.

48. Fregni F, Marcondes R, Boggio PS, Marcolin MA, Rigonatti SP, et al. (2006) Transient tinnitus suppression induced by repetitive transcranial magnetic stimulation and transcranial direct current stimulation. European journal of neurology: the official journal of the European Federation of Neurological Societies 13: 996–1001.

49. De Ridder D, Verstraeten E, Van der Kelen K, De Mulder G, Sunaert S, et al. (2005) Transcranial magnetic stimulation for tinnitus: influence of tinnitus duration on stimulation parameter choice and maximal tinnitus suppression. Otology & neurotology: official publication of the American Otological Society, American Neurotology Society and European Academy of Otology and Neurotology 26: 616–619.

50. Folmer RL, Carroll JR, Rahim A, Shi Y, Hal Martin W (2006) Effects of repetitive transcranial magnetic stimulation (rTMS) on chronic tinnitus. Acta oto-laryngologica Supplementum 96–101.

51. Gamboa OL, Antal A, Moliadze V, Paulus W (2010) Simply longer is not better: reversal of theta burst after-effect with prolonged stimulation. Experimental brain research Experimentelle Hirnforschung Expérimentation cérébrale 204: 181–187.

52. Quartarone A, Bagnato S, Rizzo V, Morgante F, Sant'angelo A, et al. (2005) Distinct changes in cortical and spinal excitability following high-frequency repetitive TMS to the human motor cortex. Experimental brain research Experimentelle Hirnforschung Expérimentation cérébrale 161: 114–124.

53. Peinemann A, Reimer B, Löer C, Quartarone A, Münchau A, et al. (2004) Long-lasting increase in corticospinal excitability after 1800 pulses of subthreshold 5 Hz repetitive TMS to the primary motor cortex. Clinical neurophysiology: official journal of the International Federation of Clinical Neurophysiology 115: 1519–1526.

54. Fitzgerald PB, Fountain S, Daskalakis ZJ (2006) A comprehensive review of the effects of rTMS on motor cortical excitability and inhibition. Clinical neurophysiology: official journal of the International Federation of Clinical Neurophysiology 117: 2584–2596.

55. Foxe JJ, Simpson GV, Ahlfors SP (1998) Parieto-occipital approximately 10 Hz activity reflects anticipatory state of visual attention mechanisms. Neuroreport 9: 3929–3933.

56. Jensen O, Mazaheri A (2010) Shaping functional architecture by oscillatory activity: gating by inhibition. Frontiers in Human Neuroscience 4: 186.

57. Rihs TA, Michel CM, Thut G (2007) Mechanisms of selective inhibition in visual spatial attention are indexed by alpha-band EEG synchronization. The European journal of neuroscience 25: 603–610.

58. Romei V, Rihs T, Brodbeck V, Thut G (2008) Resting electroencephalogram alpha-power over posterior sites indexes baseline visual cortex excitability. Neuroreport 19: 203–208.

59. Worden MS, Foxe JJ, Wang N, Simpson GV (2000) Anticipatory biasing of visuospatial attention indexed by retinotopically specific alpha-band electroencephalography increases over occipital cortex. The Journal of neuroscience: the official journal of the Society for Neuroscience 20: RC63.

60. Foxe JJ, Snyder AC (2011) The role of alpha-band brain oscillations as a sensory suppression mechanism during selective attention. Frontiers in Psychology 2: 1–13.

61. Di Lazzaro V, Dileone M, Pilato F, Capone F, Musumeci G, et al. (2011) Modulation of Motor Cortex Neuronal Networks by rTMS: Comparison of Local and Remote Effects of Six Different Protocols of Stimulation. Journal of neurophysiology 10.1152/jn.00781.2010.

62. Huang YZ, Edwards MJ, Rounis E, Bhatia KP, Rothwell JC (2005) Theta burst stimulation of the human motor cortex. Neuron 45: 201–206.

63. Takano B, Drzezga A, Peller M, Sax I, Schwaiger M, et al. (2004) Short-term modulation of regional excitability and blood flow in human motor cortex following rapid-rate transcranial magnetic stimulation. NeuroImage 23: 849–859.

64. Gray CM, König P, Engel AK, Singer W (1989) Oscillatory responses in cat visual cortex exhibit inter-columnar synchronization which reflects global stimulus properties. Nature 338: 334–337.

65. Singer W (1999) Neuronal synchrony: a versatile code for the definition of relations? Neuron 24: 49–65, 111–25.

66. Thut G, Miniussi C (2009) New insights into rhythmic brain activity from TMS-EEG studies. Trends in cognitive sciences 13: 182–189.

67. Ferrarelli F, Massimini M, Peterson MJ, Riedner BA, Lazar M, et al. (2008) Reduced evoked gamma oscillations in the frontal cortex in schizophrenia patients: a TMS/EEG study. The American journal of psychiatry 165: 996–1005.

68. Marcondes RA, Sanchez TG, Kii MA, Ono CR, Buchpiguel CA, et al. (2009) Repetitive transcranial magnetic stimulation improve tinnitus in normal hearing patients: a double-blind controlled, clinical and neuroimaging outcome study. European journal of neurology: the official journal of the European Federation of Neurological Societies 10.1111/j.1468-1331.2009.02730.x.

69. Benali A, Trippe J, Weiler E, Mix A, Petrasch-Parwez E, et al. (2011) Theta-burst transcranial magnetic stimulation alters cortical inhibition. The Journal of neuroscience: the official journal of the Society for Neuroscience 31: 1193–1203.

70. Trippe J, Mix A, Aydin-Abidin S, Funke K, Benali A (2009) Theta burst and conventional low-frequency rTMS differentially affect GABAergic neurotransmission in the rat cortex. Experimental brain research Experimentelle Hirnforschung Expérimentation cérébrale 31(4): 1193–203.

71. Franca M, Koch G, Mochizuki H, Huang YZ, Rothwell JC (2006) Effects of theta burst stimulation protocols on phosphene threshold. Clinical neurophysiology: official journal of the International Federation of Clinical Neurophysiology 117: 1808–1813.

72. Poreisz C, Antal A, Boros K, Brepohl N, Csifcsák G, et al. (2008) Attenuation of N2 amplitude of laser-evoked potentials by theta burst stimulation of primary somatosensory cortex. Experimental brain research Experimentelle Hirnforschung Expérimentation cérébrale 185: 611–621.

73. Dohrmann K, Weisz N, Schlee W, Hartmann T, Elbert T (2007) Neurofeedback for treating tinnitus. Progress in brain research 166: 473–485.

74. Weiler EW, Brill K, Tachiki KH, Schneider D (2002) Neurofeedback and quantitative electroencephalography. The international tinnitus journal 8: 87–93.

75. Wunderlich AP, Schönfeldt-Lecuona C, Wolf RC, Dorn K, Bachor E, et al. (2010) Cortical activation during a pitch discrimination task in tinnitus patients and controls–an fMRI study. Audiology & neuro-otology 15: 137–148.

76. Lanting CP, de Kleine E, van Dijk P (2009) Neural activity underlying tinnitus generation: results from PET and fMRI. Hearing research 255: 1–13.

77. Mirz F, Gjedde A, Ishizu K, Pedersen CB (2000) Cortical networks subserving the perception of tinnitus–a PET study. Acta oto-laryngologica Supplementum 543: 241–243.

78. Plewnia C, Reimold M, Najib A, Reischl G, Plontke SK, et al. (2007) Moderate therapeutic efficacy of positron emission tomography-navigated repetitive transcranial magnetic stimulation for chronic tinnitus: a randomised, controlled pilot study. Journal of neurology, neurosurgery, and psychiatry 78: 152–156.

79. Schlee W, Mueller N, Hartmann T, Keil J, Lorenz I, et al. (2009) Mapping cortical hubs in tinnitus. BMC biology 7: 80.

80. Vanneste S, Plazier M, Ost J, van der Loo E, van de Heyning P, et al. (2010) Bilateral dorsolateral prefrontal cortex modulation for tinnitus by transcranial direct current stimulation: a preliminary clinical study. Experimental brain research Experimentelle Hirnforschung Expérimentation cérébrale 202: 779–785.

81. Kleinjung T, Eichhammer P, Landgrebe M, Sand P, Hajak G, et al. (2008) Combined temporal and prefrontal transcranial magnetic stimulation for tinnitus treatment: a pilot study. Otolaryngology–head and neck surgery: official journal of American Academy of Otolaryngology-Head and Neck Surgery 138: 497–501.

82. Davidson RJ, Pizzagalli D, Nitschke JB, Putnam K (2002) Depression: perspectives from affective neuroscience. Annual review of psychology 53: 545–574.

83. Kringelbach ML (2005) The human orbitofrontal cortex: linking reward to hedonic experience. Nature reviews Neuroscience 6: 691–702.

84. Moont R, Crispel Y, Lev R, Pud D, Yarnitsky D (2011) Temporal changes in cortical activation during conditioned pain modulation (CPM), a LORETA study. Pain 60: 709–719.

85. Westerhausen R, Moosmann M, Alho K, Belsby SO, Hämäläinen H, et al. (2010) Identification of attention and cognitive control networks in a parametric auditory fMRI study. Neuropsychologia 48: 2075–2081.

86. Jardri R, Pouchet A, Pins D, Thomas P (2011) Cortical activations during auditory verbal hallucinations in schizophrenia: a coordinate-based meta-analysis. The American journal of psychiatry 168: 73–81.

87. Huang YZ, Edwards MJ, Rounis E, Bhatia KP, Rothwell JC (2005) Theta burst stimulation of the human motor cortex. Neuron 45(2): 201–6.

88. Sedley W, Teki S, Kumar S, Barnes GR, Bamiou DE, et al. (2012) Single-subject oscillatory gamma response in tinnitus. Brain 135: 3089–100.

10

Auditory Resting-State Network Connectivity in Tinnitus: A Functional MRI Study

Audrey Maudoux[1,2]*, Philippe Lefebvre[2], Jean-Evrard Cabay[3], Athena Demertzi[1], Audrey Vanhaudenhuyse[1], Steven Laureys[1,4], Andrea Soddu[1]*

1 Coma Science Group, Cyclotron Research Centre, University of Liège, Liège, Belgium, 2 OtoRhinoLaryngology Head and Neck Surgery Department, University of Liège, Liège, Belgium, 3 Radiology Department, CHU Sart Tilman Hospital, University of Liège, Liège, Belgium, 4 Neurology Department, CHU Sart Tilman Hospital, University of Liège, Liège, Belgium

Abstract

The underlying functional neuroanatomy of tinnitus remains poorly understood. Few studies have focused on functional cerebral connectivity changes in tinnitus patients. The aim of this study was to test if functional MRI "resting-state" connectivity patterns in auditory network differ between tinnitus patients and normal controls. Thirteen chronic tinnitus subjects and fifteen age-matched healthy controls were studied on a 3 tesla MRI. Connectivity was investigated using independent component analysis and an automated component selection approach taking into account the spatial and temporal properties of each component. Connectivity in extra-auditory regions such as brainstem, basal ganglia/NAc, cerebellum, parahippocampal, right prefrontal, parietal, and sensorimotor areas was found to be increased in tinnitus subjects. The right primary auditory cortex, left prefrontal, left fusiform gyrus, and bilateral occipital regions showed a decreased connectivity in tinnitus. These results show that there is a modification of cortical and subcortical functional connectivity in tinnitus encompassing attentional, mnemonic, and emotional networks. Our data corroborate the hypothesized implication of non-auditory regions in tinnitus physiopathology and suggest that various regions of the brain seem involved in the persistent awareness of the phenomenon as well as in the development of the associated distress leading to disabling chronic tinnitus.

Editor: Bogdan Draganski, Centre Hospitalier Universitaire Vaudois Lausanne - CHUV, UNIL, Switzerland

Funding: This research was funded by the Belgian National Funds for Scientific Research (FNRS),the Tinnitus Prize 2011 (FNRS 9.4501.12), the European Commission, the James McDonnell Foundation, the Mind Science Foundation, the French Speaking Community Concerted Research Action (ARC-06/11-340), the Public Utility Foundation "Université Européenne du Travail," "Fondazione Europea di Ricerca Biomedica," and the University and University Hospital of Liège. AM is a Research Fellow; AV and AS are Post-Doctoral Fellows, and SL is a Senior Research Associate at the FNRS. The funders had no role in study design, data collection and analysis, decision to publish, or preparation of the manuscript.

Competing Interests: The authors have declared that no competing interests exist.

* E-mail: amaudoux@doct.ulg.ac.be (AM); Andrea.Soddu@ulg.ac.be (AS)

Introduction

Tinnitus is defined as a perception of sound in the absence of any external auditory stimuli [1]. It is sometimes referred to as 'phantom' auditory experience. About 15% of the population is affected by chronic tinnitus and tinnitus severely affects quality of life of 1 to 3% of the population [2]. Despite its high prevalence, there is little consensus regarding the neuropathological origin of tinnitus. The prevailing opinion is that tinnitus is a perceptual consequence of altered patterns of intrinsic neural activity generated along the central auditory pathway following damage to peripheral auditory structures [2]. While the loss of afferent input to the central auditory system can initiate tinnitus, thereafter, central mechanisms are thought to play an important role in its maintenance [3]. That surgical section of the eight cranial nerve in tinnitus patients is not successful in suppressing tinnitus in 38 to 85% of the cases further supports this hypothesis [4,5]. A better characterization of central neural processing abnormalities in tinnitus can offer a better understanding of the physiopathology and may contribute to the development of therapeutic intervention procedures.

Few studies on tinnitus have assessed cerebral functional connectivity changes. Previous electrophysiological studies suggested evidence of modified connectivity in tinnitus subjects [6,7,8,9]. However, the use of magnetoencephalography (MEG) or electroencephalography (EEG), while providing high temporal resolution, is known to have a poor anatomical resolution making difficult precise interpretation on the exact location of the source of the signal. One way to overcome this limitation is to use a functional brain imaging technique which, even if more limited concerning temporal resolution, has better structural resolution (e.g. functional MRI).

Since it has been shown that correlation of low frequency fluctuations (0.01–0.05 Hz) of resting BOLD activity reflect functional connectivity [10], an increased focus has been directed to functional MRI studies of the brain's baseline activity (i.e., "resting state" acquisitions) [11]. Indeed, these fluctuations are shown to be coherent across widely separated (although functionally related) brain regions, constituting "resting state networks" [12,13]. Past studies in healthy volunteers showed that it is possible to identify consistent resting-state networks that have a functional relevance. "Default" network or networks involved in visual, motor, language, and auditory processing can be consistently found in healthy subjects [14,15] and can be separated from each other from a single resting-fMRI dataset using their distinct temporal characteristics. Maps of spontaneous network correlations have been proposed to provide tools for the understanding of clinical conditions. fMRI resting-state paradigms have, for example, been applied to the study of hypnosis [16], anesthesia [17] and various neurological disorders including dementia [18,19], depression [20] disorder of consciousness [21,22] and auditory hallucinations [23]. The aim of this study was to investigate auditory resting state network connectivity in chronic tinnitus patients.

Materials and Methods

Subjects and MRI acquisition

Two independent groups were included. The data of the first healthy control group (group 1) were analyzed in order to select auditory regions of interest (ROIs) subsequently used for auditory independent component selection in group 2. Data from the second group (group 2) were analyzed to compare the auditory resting-state fMRI activity of healthy subjects and tinnitus patients. Healthy volunteers and patients were free of major neurological, neurosurgical or psychiatric history. Head movements were minimized using customized cushions.

Group 1 included 12 control subjects (4 women; mean age 21 yrs, SD = 3). Resting state BOLD data were acquired on a 3T magnetic resonance scanner (Siemens, Allegra, Germany) with a gradient echo-planar sequence using axial slice orientation (32 slices; voxel size = $3.4 \times 3.4 \times 3$ mm^3; matrix size = $64 \times 64 \times 32$; repetition time = 2460 ms, echo time = 40 ms, flip angle = 90°; field of view = 220 mm). A protocol of 350 scans was performed. A T1-weighted MPRAGE sequence was also acquired for registration with functional data on each subject.

Group 2 included 13 patients (6 women; mean age 52 yrs, SD = 11), with chronic tinnitus present either constantly or intermittently for at least 1 year, and 15 age-matched healthy volunteers (6 women; mean age 51 yrs, SD = 13). Patients with hyperacusis or phonophobia were excluded. Hearing levels were assessed using audiological testing. Pure tones ranging from 250 Hz to 8 kHz were presented to each ear until the threshold of detection was reached. Tinnitus patients were tested to identify the best match to the perceived frequency of their tinnitus. Patients identified the pure tone or white noise from the audiological examination that best matched the center frequency of their tinnitus sensation. Self-reported severity of tinnitus impact was measured using the Tinnitus Handicap Inventory (THI) [24] and the Tinnitus Questionnaire (TQ) [25]. We asked the tinnitus patients to score the tinnitus loudness they experienced during the scanning session directly after the session on a numeric rating scale, ranging from of 0 (none) to 10 (loudest imaginable tinnitus). In group 2, resting state BOLD data were acquired on a 3T magnetic resonance scanner (Siemens, Trio Tim, Germany) with a gradient echo-planar sequence using axial slice orientation (32 slices; voxel size = $3.0 \times 3.0 \times 3.75$ mm^3; matrix size = $64 \times 64 \times 32$; repetition time = 2000 ms, echo time = 30 ms, flip angle = 78°; field of view = 192 mm). A protocol of 300 scans lasting 600 seconds was performed. A T1-weighted MPRAGE sequence was also acquired for registration with functional data on each subject.

Written informed consent was obtained from all patients and healthy volunteers. The study was approved by the Ethics Committee of the Faculty of Medicine of the University of Liège.

Data preprocessing and analysis

fMRI data were preprocessed and analyzed using the "BrainVoyager" software package (Brain Innovation, Maastricht, The Netherlands) and a previously published method [26]. Preprocessing of functional scans included 3D motion correction, linear trend removal, slice scan time correction and filtering out low frequencies of up to 0.005 Hz. The data were spatially smoothed with a Gaussian filter of full width at half maximum value of 8 mm. The functional images from each subject were aligned to the participant's own anatomical scan and warped into the standard anatomical space of Talairach and Tournoux (1988). The spatial transformation was performed in two steps. The first step consisted in rotating the 3-D data set of each subject to be aligned with stereotaxic axes (for this step the location of the anterior commissure, the posterior commissure and two rotation parameters for midsagittal alignment were specified manually). In the second step, the extreme points of the cerebrum were specified. These points together with the anterior commissure and posterior commissure coordinates were then used to scale the 3-D data sets into the dimensions of the standard brain of the Talairach and Tournoux (1988) atlas using a piecewise affine and continuous transformation.

Auditory component selection

Before investigating spontaneous brain activity, it is necessary to correct the fMRI data for physiological and non-physiological artifacts. To be sure that the further analyzed signal is neurobiologically meaningful and corresponds to the spontaneous brain activity of interest (i.e. the auditory spontaneous activity), we applied independent component analysis. The selection of the components of interest was based on a previously validated selection method which takes advantage of the capability of independent component analysis to decompose the signal in neuronal and artifactual sources while preserving the concept of connectivity in a defined network of ROIs [26]. In order to select the independent component which represent the auditory spontaneous activity, our selection method employed ROIs that were representative regions of previously described auditory resting state network [11,12,13,14]. The ROIs were defined on an average auditory map calculated on a group of twelve independent healthy subjects (group 1). We performed self organizing ICA as implemented in Brain Voyager [27] grouping the 30 independent components of the 12 healthy subjects of group 1 in 30 clusters of spatially similar components. Subsequently, we averaged the maps belonging to the cluster which was selected as auditory by visual inspection. Fourteen ROIs were selected as representative clusters of the Heschl gyrus (Brodman area 41/42), secondary/associative auditory cortices (Brodman area 22) and the insula of our average auditory map *(table S1)*. The ROIs were set initially to a cubic shape $10 \times 10 \times 10$ mm^3, and the center was chosen accordingly to the mean auditory map extracted from group 1 but once the ROI was saved in Brain Voyager only the ROI's voxels belonging to the auditory map end up making the saved ROI. Similarly to the targets ROIs of the auditory component, we then selected six other ROIs representing the most representative regions appearing as anti-correlated regions in the auditory average map calculated on the group 1 of healthy subjects *(table S1)*. These ROIs were used in order to rule out the global signal from the selection. Finally, we picked as auditory component the component that was selected using a compromise between spatial and temporal properties *(figure 1)*.

The methodology used, as described by Soddu et al [26], allows building for each independent component a connectivity graph which summarizes the level of connectivity for a defined network

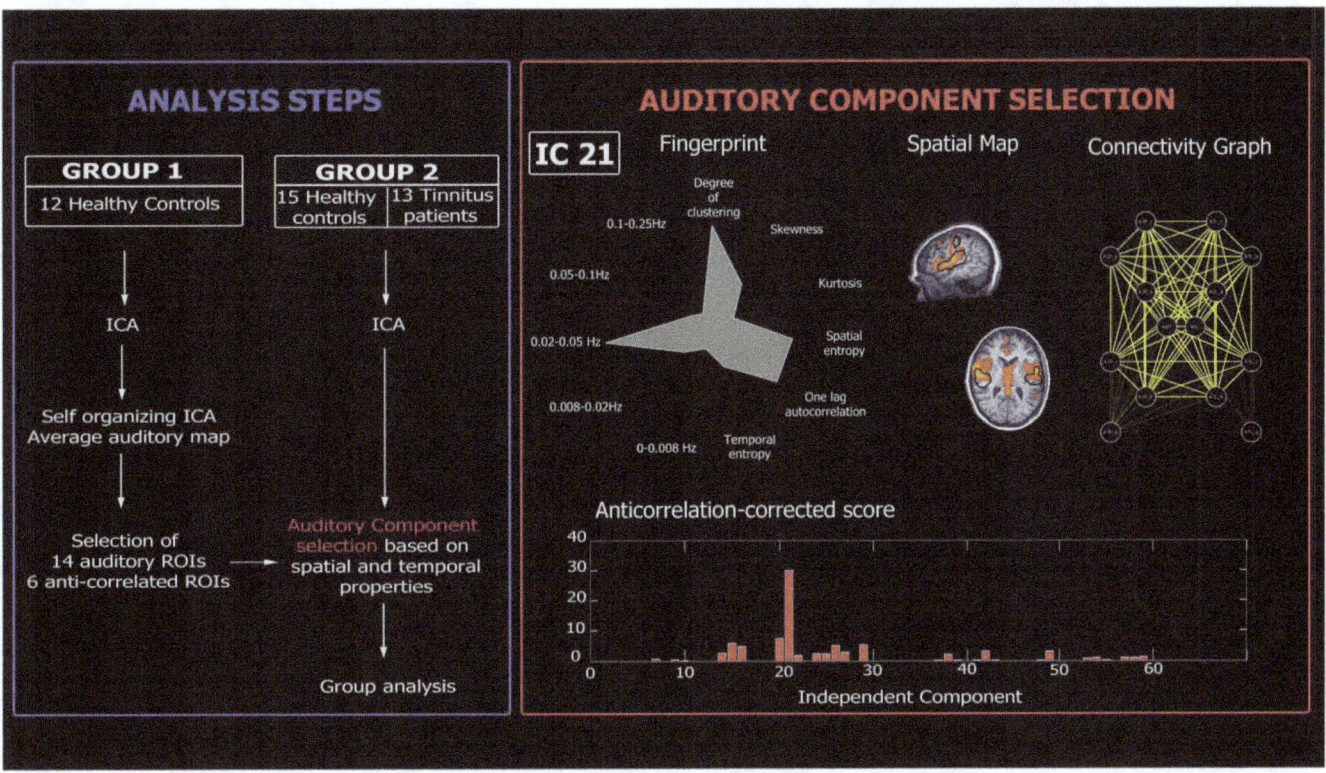

Figure 1. Analysis steps (Blue Box). For the analysis, two independent groups were included. The data of the first group (group 1, healthy controls) were analyzed in order to define auditory regions of interest (ROIs) subsequently used to select the auditory independent component in the second group (group 2, healthy controls and tinnitus patients). Data from group 2 were used to compare the auditory resting-state fMRI activity of healthy subjects and tinnitus patients. **Auditory component selection (Red Box).** The independent component (IC) reflecting the auditory network was selected based on both spatial and temporal properties. *Upper panel (from left to right):* Fingerprint of the selected IC; Spatial map of the selected IC (black contours indicate average auditory map calculated on group 1); Connectivity graph representing significant connectivity edges between the selected ROIs of the auditory network. *Lower panel:* Anticorrelation-corrected score of each graph vs. the corresponding IC number. The component with the highest score will be selected as the auditory network (IC 21 in the present example).

of ROIs according to the time behavior described by the correspondent independent component time course. After running ICA with thirty components, we used the corresponding time courses to regress in the BOLD signal in each of the fourteen ROIs. The time courses from each ROI were extracted as the arithmetic mean of the time courses of the voxels belonging to the same ROI. For each component we then obtained fourteen parameter estimates (beta values) indicating the weight of each regressor and the corresponding T-values. In order to build a connectivity graph we drew an edge between each pair of target points with $T>T_{th}$ with T_{th} corresponding to 1-p/91 for p = 0.05 with 267 degrees of freedom (Bonferroni correction for multiple comparisons was performed dividing p by the number of possible edges between the thirteen nodes; $14*(14-1)/2 = 91$). To account for the fact that ICA does not predict the sign of the independent components, the condition $T<-T_{th}$ was also used. This allowed us to end up with two connectivity graphs for each of the thirty components (1–30 for the condition $T>T_{th}$ and 31–60 for $T<-T_{th}$). We hypothesized that the number of edges E for each of the 60 connectivity graphs should be the highest for the auditory component. But given that no regressing out of the global signal was applied, we did not pick the component corresponding to the graph with the largest number of total edges (i.e., the global component could appear as the main source of connectivity). Therefore, we implemented the "anticorrelation-corrected number of edges". The anticorrelation-corrected number of edges was

obtained by multiplying the total number of edges of each graph by a weight "w" which measures the anti-correlation of the auditory activity with the set of selected anti-correlated ROIs (w will be around zero for the global component for which all the ROIs are positively correlated). However, to be sure to select a component of neuronal origin one also needs to take into account the temporal properties of the component. To do so, we selected the component with the highest "anticorrelation-corrected score", built by multiplying the number of anticorrelation-corrected edges by a new weight "w_F" which measures the distance of its fingerprint [28] from the average fingerprint of the auditory component in healthy controls (group 1). The weight w_F is close to 0 for components which have "artefactual" source and close to 1 for components with "neuronal" origin - the latter assumes that in healthy controls ICA was able to fully separate artefactual from neuronal sources *(figure 1)*.

Group analysis

Spatial maps were obtained by running a two step analysis. First, the time courses of all components but that of interest (i.e. the independent component selected as auditory) were used to regress out the BOLD signal; the saved residuals represented the BOLD activity which can possibly be explained by the auditory component. Then, by using the time course of the component of interest as a predictor of this residual BOLD activity, beta-values were obtained.

Table 1. Tinnitus Population.

Participant	Sex	Age (years)	Tinnitus Ear	Tinnitus duration (years)	Tinnitus frequency (Hz)	THI/TQ Score	Initial onset related to	Tinnitus loudness during scan (0–10)
Patient #1	F	44	Right	9	8000	58/35	Unknown	7
Patient #2	M	47	Right	33	3000	38/22	Unknown	10
Patient #3	M	36	Left	1.75	2500	84/58	Sudden deafness	6.5
Patient #4	M	66	Left	2	4000	80/56	Earwax extraction	8
Patient #5	M	67	Left	3.75	1500	30/26	Noise trauma	5
Patient #6	M	57	Bilateral	2	8000	50/52	Unknown	6.5
Patient #7	M	50	Right	10	6000	38/29	Stress	3
Patient #8	F	60	Bilateral	>20	4000	20/20	Fatigue	3
Patient #9	F	42	Right	2.4	3000	40/34	Noise trauma	2.5
Patient #10	M	33	Left	3.5	8000	32/22	Unknown	4
Patient #11	F	60	Bilateral	5	3000	36/21	Unknown	4.5
Patient #12	F	66	Left	2	6000	16/18	Hypoacousis	4
Patient #13	F	52	Left	5	6000	44/22	Arnold's neuralgia	5

At a second-level analysis, the estimated beta-values entered a multi-subject random effect analysis providing group-level statistical T-maps. Maps were thresholded at a false discovery rate corrected p<0.05. A contrast T-test map was also estimated comparing controls and tinnitus patients. Statistical parametric maps resulting from the voxel wise analysis were considered significant for statistical values that survived a cluster-based correction for multiple comparisons as implemented in Brain Voyager [29] using the "cluster-level statistical threshold estimator" plug-in, which is based on a 3D extension of the randomization procedure described by Forman and colleagues [30]. First, voxel-level threshold was set at t = 2.772 (p = 0.01, uncorrected). After 1000 iterations, the minimum cluster size threshold that yielded a cluster-level false positive rate of 5% was applied to the statistical maps.

Results

Patients had chronic tinnitus for a mean period of 8 years (SD 9). Tinnitus matched frequencies ranged from 150 Hz to 8 kHz (mean = 4846 Hz, SD = 2276 Hz). Tinnitus Handicap Inventory score [24] varied across patients, from slight to catastrophic (Range: 16–84) as did the Tinnitus Questionnaire (Range: 18–58) [25] *(Table 1)*. According to the World Health Organization grades of hearing impairment [31], only one tinnitus patient had a grade 1 impairment (slight impairment) all the other had a grade 0 impairment (no impairment). No patients showed profound hearing loss at any frequency (>90 dB above threshold). Four patients didn't exhibit any degree of hearing loss at any of the tested frequencies. The remaining patients exhibited a mild or moderate hearing loss at one or more frequencies (20–40 dB or 40–60 dB above threshold, respectively), and two of these patients demonstrated severe hearing loss in at least one tested frequency (60–90 dB above threshold, on the 4 and 8 kHz).

In controls, the identified auditory resting state network encompassed bilateral primary and associative auditory cortices, insula, prefrontal, sensorimotor, anterior cingulate and left occipital cortices *(Table 2, figure 2)*. In tinnitus patients, the identified auditory network encompassed all previously mentioned areas (excluding the anterior cingulate cortex) and included also the brainstem, thalamus, nucleus accumbens (NAc), isthmus of cingulate gyrus, right occipital, parietal and prefrontal cortices *(Table 3, figure 2)*.

Chronic tinnitus patients, as compared to controls, showed increased connectivity in the brainstem, cerebellum, right basal ganglia/NAc, parahippocampal areas, right frontal and parietal areas, left sensorimotor areas and left superior temporal region. Tinnitus patients showed decreased connectivity in right primary auditory cortex, left fusiform gyrus, left frontal and bilateral occipital regions *(Table 4, figure 3, figure S1)*.

Discussion

When analyzing spontaneous BOLD fluctuations using fMRI, special care should be taken to disentangle signal changes related to spontaneous neural activity from those related to scanner instability or physiological artifacts due to respiratory, cardiac or motor activity. We here employed the independent component analysis algorithm, decomposing the acquired BOLD signal into different neuronal and non-neuronal components. The selection of the auditory network component was based on a previously published method that allows us to take into account both the spatial and temporal properties of the fMRI signal in order to automatically select the neuronal component of interest in a user-independent manner [26]. The prospectively studied convenience

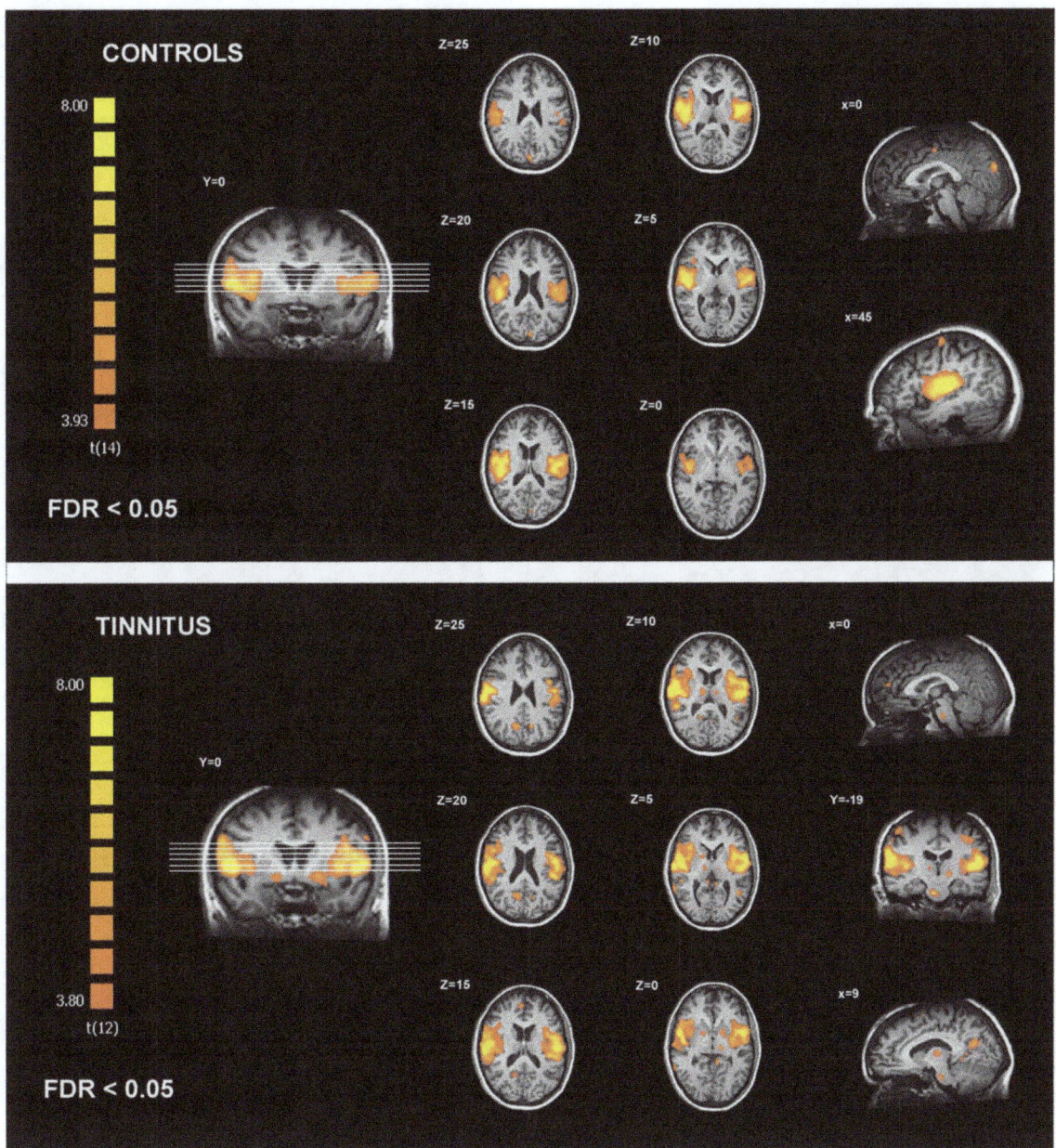

Figure 2. Regions of the auditory resting state network identified in controls and chronic tinnitus patients.

sample of chronic tinnitus patients included subjects with different characteristics regarding tinnitus laterality, frequency and type (pure tone or white noise). Moreover, when looking at the Tinnitus Handicap Inventory and the Tinnitus Questionnaire scores, one could argue that our population was not homogenous regarding the impact of tinnitus on patients' life. This patient inhomogeneity could affect our results mainly by increasing variance and hence decreasing sensitivity. Future studies in larger patient cohorts should aim to correlate specific tinnitus characteristics (such as intensity, localization, type of sound, duration, coping, treatment response) with fMRI BOLD activity.

With the present study we provide evidence for a distributed cerebral network associated with tinnitus. Our data corroborate the hypothesized implication of non-auditory regions in tinnitus physiopathology as proposed by Jastreboff et al [32,33] (including participation of auditory, limbic, prefrontal areas and autonomic nervous system); Rauschecker et al [34] (suggesting the implication of the NAc and associated paralimbic structures) and De Ridder et al [35] (considering phantom perception -including tinnitus- as a consequence of dysfunction in multiple parallel overlapping dynamic networks -i.e., perception, salience, distress and memory networks-).

The auditory network identified in healthy controls is in line with previous studies using "resting state" fMRI [11,12,13,36]. The observed connectivity impairment in auditory cortex corroborates previous human studies. MEG [37] and EEG studies [38] have demonstrated gamma band activity changes in auditory areas of tinnitus patients and several PET studies have identified primary auditory cortex dysfunction in tinnitus [39,40,41,42].

Table 2. Peak voxels and local maxima of the auditory resting state network identified in controls.

Brain region (area)	x	y	z	t	p
R Superior & transverse temporal gyrus (41/42/22)	49	−18	11	10.81	<0.0001
Insula	46	−12	11	10.76	
Precentral gyrus (6)	58	−6	11	9.59	
Inferior frontal gyrus (45)	40	21	11	5.17	
L Superior & transverse temporal gyrus (41/42/22)	−44	−6	11	10.56	<0.0001
Transverse temporal gyrus (42)	−59	−21	17	4.93	
Insula	−41	−18	11	10.12	
Supramarginal gyrus (40)	−47	−15	14	8.43	
Precentral gyrus (6)	−53	−6	8	8.50	
L Cuneus (18)	−6	−88	37	7.35	<0.0001
R Precentral gyrus (4)	45	−13	58	6.11	<0.0001
R Anterior Cingulate Cortex (24)	6	−7	43	5.37	<0.0001

Stereotaxic coordinates are in normalized Talairach space, p values are corrected for multiple comparisons at the whole brain level (FDR<0.05).

Our finding of increased connectivity in tinnitus encompassing parahippocampal areas is in accordance with a previous PET study showing increased blood flow in hippocampal areas during tinnitus modified by oral facial movement [40]. Similarly, using EEG, Vanneste et al [8] reported an increase in gamma band frequency in parahippocampal regions and an increase in connectivity between the latter and auditory cortices in tinnitus patients as compared to controls. In fact, primate anatomical studies demonstrated reciprocal connections between parahippocampal regions and associative auditory cortices [43]. Interestingly, De Ridder et al [44], showed that selective amobarbital

Table 3. Peak voxels and local maxima of the auditory resting state network identified in the tinnitus patients.

Brain region (area)	x	y	z	t	p
R Superior & transverse temporal gyrus (41/42/22)	62	−18	23	13.97	<0.0001
Middle Temporal Gyrus (37)	64	−48	5	6.26	
Insula	40	−18	11	7.16	
Precentral Gyrus (4)	55	−9	26	10.48	
Inferior Frontal Gyrus (44)	49	9	23	6.98	
L Superior & transverse temporal gyrus (41/42/22)	−50	−15	11	11.09	<0.0001
Insula	−50	−33	20	9.04	
Precentral Gyrus (4)	−56	6	5	10.59	
Postcentral Gyrus (3,1,2)	−52	−9	20	9.96	
Inferior Frontal Gyrus (44)	−50	0	17	7.80	
Basal ganglia/NAc	−29	−9	8	7.12	
R Cuneus/Precuneus (19/31)	9	−64	25	5.88	<0.0001
L Cuneus/Precuneus (19/31)	−15	−64	25	6.20	0.0002
L Middle occipital gyrus (19)	−45	−52	7	6.13	<0.0001
L Precentral gyrus (4)	−33	−19	46	5.27	<0.0001
R Superior frontal gyrus (6)	6	5	46	4.31	<0.0001
R Prefrontal cortex (10)	3	47	16	5.24	0.001
R Superior parietal cortex (7)	54	−22	52	5.61	0.0001
R Basal ganglia/NAc	15	−1	−5	5.61	0.0001
L Isthmus of Cingulate Gyrus	−9	−40	1	5.72	0.0003
R Thalamus	9	−13	10	5.11	<0.0001
L Thalamus	−15	−19	−2	6.44	<0.0001
R Brainstem	6	−19	−23	7.77	<0.0001

Stereotaxic coordinates are in normalized Talairach space, p values are corrected for multiple comparisons at the whole brain level (FDR<0.05).

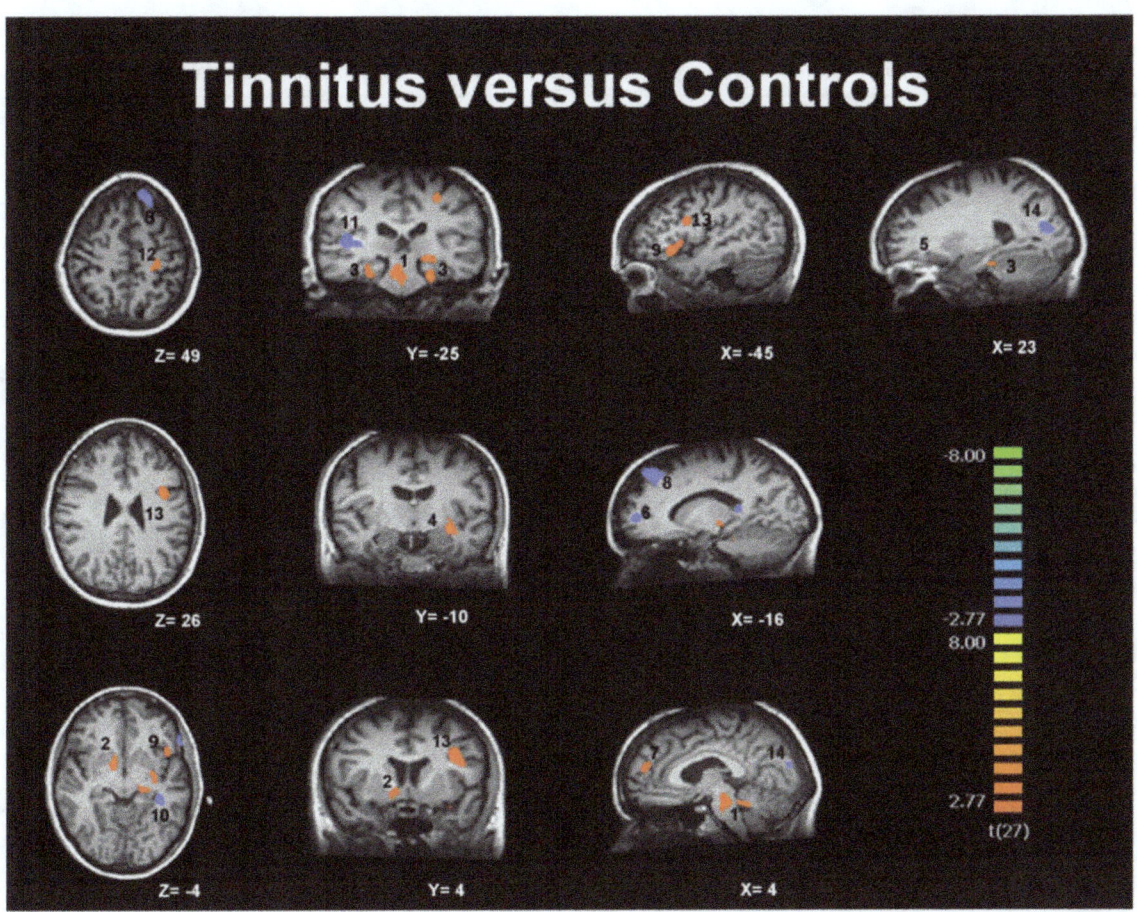

Figure 3. Increased (in red) and decreased (in blue) functional connectivity in the auditory resting-state network in tinnitus. Results are thresholded at cluster level corrected p<0.05. 1- Brainstem/Cerebellum, 2-Basal ganglia/NAc, 3-Parahippocampal gyri, 4-Superior temporal gyrus, 5-Orbitofrontal cortex, 6-Prefrontal cortex, 7-Prefrontal cortex, 8-Superior frontal gyrus, 9-Inferior frontal gyrus, 10-Fusiform gyrus, 11-Superior temporal gyrus, 12-Postcentral gyrus, 13-Precentral gyrus, 14-Cuneus/Precuneus.

injections in the anterior choroidal artery (which supplies the amygdalohippocampal region) can suppress tinnitus.

We also found evidence of increased connectivity in the basal ganglia in a region close to the NAc, in line with a fMRI study using auditory stimulations reporting increased activation of the NAc in chronic tinnitus [45]. Rauschecker proposed a tinnitus model in which the NAc and its associated paralimbic networks in the medial prefrontal cortex play an important role. This theory suggests that, under normal circumstances, the tinnitus signal is cancelled out at the level of the thalamus by an inhibitory feedback loop originating in paralimbic structures. If the paralimbic regions are compromised, inhibition of the tinnitus signal at the thalamus gate is lost allowing the signal to reach the auditory cortex where it leads to permanent reorganization and chronic tinnitus [34]. Recently, Larson and colleagues [46] showed that electrical stimulation of the caudate nucleus triggered phantom sounds and modulated tinnitus loudness. These results indicate that the basal ganglia and the NAc might play a key role in tinnitus physiopathology, allowing or not the phantom auditory percept to reach conscious awareness.

The observed tinnitus-related connectivity changes involving the higher-order prefrontal and parietal associative cortices are in line with previous PET [39] and MEG studies [6,7,47]. Kleinjung and colleagues showed that tinnitus treatment with repetitive

transcranial magnetic stimulation applied on the temporal cortex is enhanced by additional stimulation of the prefrontal cortex [48]. The activation of these regions in tinnitus is consistent with the hypothesis that tinnitus might be associated with an inappropriate allocation of attentional resources, which maintain a sustained state of alertness. Indeed, a multimodal network consisting of temporo-parietal, frontal, and cingulate components is thought to play a key role in identifying and evaluating salient events in the sensory environment, independently of the stimulus modality [49]. Moreover, frontal lobe functioning has also been associated with emotions. An early study, by Beard et al [50], described the effect of frontal leucotomy as a treatment for tinnitus. The effect of frontal lobotomy on tinnitus distress is similar to the effect of lobotomy on pain perception [51]; it was believed to produce asymbolia for pain [52]. Similarly, frontal lobotomy might not alter the tinnitus percept but makes it bearable, dealing with the emotional-behavioral aspect of tinnitus.

Even if considered as the center of motor control, the cerebellum is known to play a role in purely sensory auditory processing [53]. The identified increased functional connectivity in the cerebellum confirms previous PET studies showing increased regional cerebral blood flow in cerebellum when the tinnitus is perceived [39,54,55]. At present, few neuroimaging studies in tinnitus reported our observed brainstem involvement. In humans,

Table 4. Peak voxels of areas showing increased and decreased connectivity in tinnitus as compared to controls.

Brain region (area)		x	y	z	t	p
INCREASED CONNECTIVITY						
L	Parahippocampal gyrus	−21	−28	−17	4.53	0.0001
R/L	Brainstem/Cerebellum	2	−21	−19	4.09	0.0004
L	Precentral gyrus (6)	−42	2	25	4.58	<0.0001
L	Superior temporal gyrus	−30	−10	−8	4.51	0.0001
L	Inferior frontal gyrus (47)	−45	14	−5	3.74	0.0009
R	Basal ganglia/Nucleus accumbens	9	−1	−5	4.37	0.0002
R	Prefrontal cortex (10)	3	50	19	3.81	0.0007
L	Postcentral gyrus (3,1,2)	−33	−16	43	3.69	0.001
R	Parahippocampal gyrus	27	−25	−14	3.47	0.002
R	Orbitofrontal cortex (11)	30	20	−11	3.83	0.0007
R	Inferior parietal lobe (39)	42	−52	40	3.29	0.003
DECREASED CONNECTIVITY						
L	Superior frontal gyrus (8)	−21	38	46	−4.20	0.0003
L	Fusiform gyrus	−39	−31	−8	−4.67	<0.0001
R	Superior temporal gyrus (41)	39	−28	10	−4.06	0.0004
R	Occipital cortex (18)	21	−76	16	−4.74	<0.0001
L	Occipital cortex (18)	−12	−85	13	−3.57	0.001
L	Prefrontal cortex (10)	−15	53	4	−4.17	0.0003

Stereotaxic coordinates are in normalized Talairach space (p values are cluster level corrected).

Lockwood et al [55] used PET to show increased blood flow in the brainstem (supposedly encompassing the cochlear nuclei) correlating with increased tinnitus induced by eye-movements. Finally, the shown connectivity changes within sensorimotor and visual areas could be seen in light of clinical studies showing that tinnitus can be evoked directly or modulated by inputs from somatosensory, somatomotor, and visual-motor systems in a proportion of individuals [56]. These observations give support to the concept that tinnitus could result from, or could be modified by crossmodal neural interactions.

In conclusion, we here provide fMRI evidence for a distributed network of auditory and non-auditory cortical and sub-cortical regions associated with chronic tinnitus. Our results suggest that the tinnitus percept is not only linked to activity in sensory auditory areas but is also associated to connectivity changes in limbic/parahippocampal areas, basal ganglia/NAc, higher-order prefrontal/parietal associative networks, infratentorial brainstem/cerebellar and sensory-motor/visual-motor systems. These results show that there is a modification of cortical and subcortical functional connectivity in tinnitus encompassing attentional, mnemonic and emotional networks. Various tinnitus models suggested the implication of non-auditory regions in tinnitus physiopathology. Our data corroborate these hypotheses and suggest that, even if tinnitus can initially be a perceptual consequence of altered patterns of intrinsic neural activity generated along the central auditory pathway, various regions of the brain seem involved in the persistent awareness of the phenomenon as well as in the development of associated distress leading to disabling chronic tinnitus.

Supporting Information

Figure S1 Individual and mean beta-values for each of the cluster found to show significant increased and decreased connectivity in tinnitus as compared to controls. L Para- Left Parahippocampal gyrus; B/C- Brainstem/Cerebellum; L Pre-Left Precentral gyrus; L STG-Left Superior temporal gyrus; L IFG-Left Inferior frontal gyrus; R BG/NAc-Right Basal ganglia/Nucleus accumbens; R Prefr-Right Prefrontal cortex; L Post-Left Postcentral gyrus; R Para-Right Parahippocampal gyrus; R Orbito-Right Orbitofrontal cortex; R IP-Rigth Inferior parietal lobe; L SFG-Left Superior frontal gyrus; L Fusi-Left Fusiform gyrus; R STG-Rigth Superior temporal gyrus; R Occ-Right Occipital cortex; L Occ- Left Occipital cortex; L Prefr-Left Prefrontal cortex.

Table S1 Regions of interest used for the auditory component selection.

Acknowledgments

The authors thank the technicians of the Department of Radiology for their active participation in the MRI studies in tinnitus patients.

Author Contributions

Conceived and designed the experiments: AM PL AV SL AS. Performed the experiments: AM JC. Analyzed the data: AM AS AD SL. Contributed reagents/materials/analysis tools: AV JC PL AS. Wrote the paper: AM AS SL.

References

1. Moller (2011) Textbook of Tinnitus. New York: Springer.
2. Eggermont JJ, Roberts LE (2004) The neuroscience of tinnitus. Trends Neurosci 27: 676–682.
3. Adjamian P, Sereda M, Hall DA (2009) The mechanisms of tinnitus: perspectives from human functional neuroimaging. Hear Res 253: 15–31.
4. Barrs D, Brackmann D (1984) Translabyrinthine nerve section: effect on tinnitus. The Journal of Laryngology & Otology (Supplement). pp 287–293.
5. House JW, Brackmann DE (1981) Tinnitus: surgical treatment. Ciba Found Symp 85: 204–216.
6. Schlee W, Mueller N, Hartmann T, Keil J, Lorenz I, et al. (2009) Mapping cortical hubs in tinnitus. BMC Biol 7: 80.
7. Schlee W, Weisz N, Bertrand O, Hartmann T, Elbert T (2008) Using auditory steady state responses to outline the functional connectivity in the tinnitus brain. PLoS One 3: e3720.
8. Vanneste S, van de Heyning P, De Ridder D (2011) The neural network of phantom sound changes over time: a comparison between recent-onset and chronic tinnitus patients. Eur J Neurosci 34: 718–731.
9. Vanneste S, Focquaert F, Van de Heyning P, De Ridder D (2011) Different resting state brain activity and functional connectivity in patients who respond and not respond to bifrontal tDCS for tinnitus suppression. Exp Brain Res 210: 217–227.
10. Biswal B, Yetkin FZ, Haughton VM, Hyde JS (1995) Functional connectivity in the motor cortex of resting human brain using echo-planar MRI. Magn Reson Med 34: 537–541.
11. Damoiseaux JS, Rombouts SA, Barkhof F, Scheltens P, Stam CJ, et al. (2006) Consistent resting-state networks across healthy subjects. Proc Natl Acad Sci U S A 103: 13848–13853.
12. De Luca M, Beckmann CF, De Stefano N, Matthews PM, Smith SM (2006) fMRI resting state networks define distinct modes of long-distance interactions in the human brain. Neuroimage 29: 1359–1367.
13. Beckmann CF, DeLuca M, Devlin JT, Smith SM (2005) Investigations into resting-state connectivity using independent component analysis. Philos Trans R Soc Lond B Biol Sci 360: 1001–1013.
14. van den Heuvel M, Mandl R, Hulshoff Pol H (2008) Normalized cut group clustering of resting-state FMRI data. PLoS One 3: e2001.
15. Laird AR, Fox PM, Eickhoff SB, Turner JA, Ray KL, et al. (2011) Behavioral interpretations of intrinsic connectivity networks. J Cogn Neurosci 23: 4022–4037.
16. Demertzi A, Soddu A, Faymonville ME, Bahri MA, Gosseries O, et al. (2011) Hypnotic modulation of resting state fMRI default mode and extrinsic network connectivity. Prog Brain Res 193: 309–322.
17. Boveroux P, Vanhaudenhuyse A, Bruno MA, Noirhomme Q, Lauwick S, et al. (2010) Breakdown of within- and between-network resting state functional magnetic resonance imaging connectivity during propofol-induced loss of consciousness. Anesthesiology 113: 1038–1053.
18. Zhou J, Greicius MD, Gennatas ED, Growdon ME, Jang JY, et al. (2010) Divergent network connectivity changes in behavioural variant frontotemporal dementia and Alzheimer's disease. Brain 133: 1352–1367.
19. Greicius MD, Srivastava G, Reiss AL, Menon V (2004) Default-mode network activity distinguishes Alzheimer's disease from healthy aging: evidence from functional MRI. Proc Natl Acad Sci U S A 101: 4637–4642.
20. Greicius MD, Flores BH, Menon V, Glover GH, Solvason HB, et al. (2007) Resting-state functional connectivity in major depression: abnormally increased contributions from subgenual cingulate cortex and thalamus. Biol Psychiatry 62: 429–437.
21. Vanhaudenhuyse A, Noirhomme Q, Tshibanda LJ, Bruno MA, Boveroux P, et al. (2010) Default network connectivity reflects the level of consciousness in non-communicative brain-damaged patients. Brain 133: 161–171.
22. Boly M, Tshibanda L, Vanhaudenhuyse A, Noirhomme Q, Schnakers C, et al. (2009) Functional connectivity in the default network during resting state is preserved in a vegetative but not in a brain dead patient. Hum Brain Mapp 30: 2393–2400.
23. Hunter MD, Eickhoff SB, Miller TW, Farrow TF, Wilkinson ID, et al. (2006) Neural activity in speech-sensitive auditory cortex during silence. Proc Natl Acad Sci U S A 103: 189–194.
24. Newman CW, Jacobson GP, Spitzer JB (1996) Development of the Tinnitus Handicap Inventory. Arch Otolaryngol Head Neck Surg 122: 143–148.
25. Hallam RS (1996) Manual of the Tinnitus Questionnaire (TQ). London: Psychological Corporation.
26. Soddu A, Vanhaudenhuyse A, Bahri MA, Bruno MA, Boly M, et al. (2011) Identifying the default-mode component in spatial IC analyses of patients with disorders of consciousness. Hum Brain Mapp 33(4): 778–796.
27. Esposito F, Scarabino T, Hyvarinen A, Himberg J, Formisano E, et al. (2005) Independent component analysis of fMRI group studies by self-organizing clustering. Neuroimage 25: 193–205.
28. De Martino F, Gentile F, Esposito F, Balsi M, Di Salle F, et al. (2007) Classification of fMRI independent components using IC-fingerprints and support vector machine classifiers. Neuroimage 34: 177–194.
29. Goebel R, Esposito F, Formisano E (2006) Analysis of functional image analysis contest (FIAC) data with brainvoyager QX: From single-subject to cortically aligned group general linear model analysis and self-organizing group independent component analysis. Hum Brain Mapp 27: 392–401.
30. Forman SD, Cohen JD, Fitzgerald M, Eddy WF, Mintun MA, et al. (1995) Improved assessment of significant activation in functional magnetic resonance imaging (fMRI): use of a cluster-size threshold. Magn Reson Med 33: 636–647.
31. WHO (1991) Grades of hearing impairment. Hearing Network News 1.
32. Jastreboff PJ (1990) Phantom auditory perception (tinnitus): mechanisms of generation and perception. Neurosci Res 8: 221–254.
33. Jastreboff PJ, Hazell JW (1993) A neurophysiological approach to tinnitus: clinical implications. Br J Audiol 27: 7–17.
34. Rauschecker JP, Leaver AM, Muhlau M (2010) Tuning out the noise: limbic-auditory interactions in tinnitus. Neuron 66: 819–826.
35. De Ridder D, Elgoyhen AB, Romo R, Langguth B (2011) Phantom percepts: tinnitus and pain as persisting aversive memory networks. Proc Natl Acad Sci U S A 108: 8075–8080.
36. Smith SM, Fox PT, Miller KL, Glahn DC, Fox PM, et al. (2009) Correspondence of the brain's functional architecture during activation and rest. Proc Natl Acad Sci U S A 106: 13040–13045.
37. Weisz N, Muller S, Schlee W, Dohrmann K, Hartmann T, et al. (2007) The neural code of auditory phantom perception. J Neurosci 27: 1479–1484.
38. van der Loo E, Gais S, Congedo M, Vanneste S, Plazier M, et al. (2009) Tinnitus intensity dependent gamma oscillations of the contralateral auditory cortex. PLoS One 4: e7396.
39. Mirz F, Pedersen B, Ishizu K, Johannsen P, Ovesen T, et al. (1999) Positron emission tomography of cortical centers of tinnitus. Hear Res 134: 133–144.
40. Lockwood AH, Salvi RJ, Coad ML, Towsley ML, Wack DS, et al. (1998) The functional neuroanatomy of tinnitus: evidence for limbic system links and neural plasticity. Neurology 50: 114–120.
41. Smits M, Kovacs S, de Ridder D, Peeters RR, van Hecke P, et al. (2007) Lateralization of functional magnetic resonance imaging (fMRI) activation in the auditory pathway of patients with lateralized tinnitus. Neuroradiology 49: 669–679.
42. Reyes SA, Salvi RJ, Burkard RF, Coad ML, Wack DS, et al. (2002) Brain imaging of the effects of lidocaine on tinnitus. Hear Res 171: 43–50.
43. Engelien A, Stern E, Isenberg N, Engelien W, Frith C, et al. (2000) The parahippocampal region and auditory-mnemonic processing. Ann N Y Acad Sci 911: 477–485.
44. De Ridder D, Fransen H, Francois O, Sunaert S, Kovacs S, et al. (2006) Amygdalohippocampal involvement in tinnitus and auditory memory. Acta Otolaryngol Suppl. pp 50–53.
45. Leaver AM, Renier L, Chevillet MA, Morgan S, Kim HJ, et al. (2011) Dysregulation of limbic and auditory networks in tinnitus. Neuron 69: 33–43.
46. Larson PS, Cheung SW (2011) Deep brain stimulation in area LC controllably triggers auditory phantom percepts. Neurosurgery 70(2): 398–405.
47. Weisz N, Moratti S, Meinzer M, Dohrmann K, Elbert T (2005) Tinnitus perception and distress is related to abnormal spontaneous brain activity as measured by magnetoencephalography. PLoS Med 2: e153.
48. Kleinjung T, Eichhammer P, Landgrebe M, Sand P, Hajak G, et al. (2008) Combined temporal and prefrontal transcranial magnetic stimulation for tinnitus treatment: a pilot study. Otolaryngol Head Neck Surg 138: 497–501.
49. Knight RT, Grabowecky MF, Scabini D (1995) Role of human prefrontal cortex in attention control. Adv Neurol 66: 21–34; discussion 34-26.
50. Beard AW (1965) Results of leucotomy operations for tinnitus. J Psychosom Res 9: 29–32.
51. Murphy JP (1951) Frontal lobe surgery in treatment of intractable pain; a critique. Yale J Biol Med 23: 493–500.
52. Watts JW, Freeman W (1946) Psychosurgery for the relief of unbearable pain. J Int Coll Surg 9: 679–683.
53. Petacchi A, Laird AR, Fox PT, Bower JM (2005) Cerebellum and auditory function: an ALE meta-analysis of functional neuroimaging studies. Hum Brain Mapp 25: 118–128.
54. Osaki Y, Nishimura H, Takasawa M, Imaizumi M, Kawashima T, et al. (2005) Neural mechanism of residual inhibition of tinnitus in cochlear implant users. Neuroreport 16: 1625–1628.
55. Lockwood AH, Wack DS, Burkard RF, Coad ML, Reyes SA, et al. (2001) The functional anatomy of gaze-evoked tinnitus and sustained lateral gaze. Neurology 56: 472–480.
56. Cacace AT (2003) Expanding the biological basis of tinnitus: crossmodal origins and the role of neuroplasticity. Hear Res 175: 112–132.

11

The Distressed Brain: A Group Blind Source Separation Analysis on Tinnitus

Dirk De Ridder[1]*, Sven Vanneste[1], Marco Congedo[2]

1 Brai²n, TRI & Department of Neurosurgery, Antwerp University Hospital, Antwerp, Belgium, **2** Team ViBS (Vision and Brain Signal Processing), GIPSA-lab, National Center for Scientific Research, Grenoble University, Grenoble, France

Abstract

Background: Tinnitus, the perception of a sound without an external sound source, can lead to variable amounts of distress.

Methodology: In a group of tinnitus patients with variable amounts of tinnitus related distress, as measured by the Tinnitus Questionnaire (TQ), an electroencephalography (EEG) is performed, evaluating the patients' resting state electrical brain activity. This resting state electrical activity is compared with a control group and between patients with low (N = 30) and high distress (N = 25). The groups are homogeneous for tinnitus type, tinnitus duration or tinnitus laterality. A group blind source separation (BSS) analysis is performed using a large normative sample (N = 84), generating seven normative components to which high and low tinnitus patients are compared. A correlation analysis of the obtained normative components' relative power and distress is performed. Furthermore, the functional connectivity as reflected by lagged phase synchronization is analyzed between the brain areas defined by the components. Finally, a group BSS analysis on the Tinnitus group as a whole is performed.

Conclusions: Tinnitus can be characterized by at least four BSS components, two of which are posterior cingulate based, one based on the subgenual anterior cingulate and one based on the parahippocampus. Only the subgenual component correlates with distress. When performed on a normative sample, group BSS reveals that distress is characterized by two anterior cingulate based components. Spectral analysis of these components demonstrates that distress in tinnitus is related to alpha and beta changes in a network consisting of the subgenual anterior cingulate cortex extending to the pregenual and dorsal anterior cingulate cortex as well as the ventromedial prefrontal cortex/orbitofrontal cortex, insula, and parahippocampus. This network overlaps partially with brain areas implicated in distress in patients suffering from pain, functional somatic syndromes and posttraumatic stress disorder, and might therefore represent a specific distress network.

Editor: Thomas Koenig, University of Bern, Switzerland

Funding: The authors have no support or funding to report.

Competing Interests: The authors have declared that no competing interests exist.

* E-mail: dirk.de.ridder@uza.be

Introduction

At some point in life most people experience a sound in their ears or head although no external sound is present [1]. This has been related to listening to loud music[2], sudden sensorineural hearing loss[3], use of medication[4], trauma[5] or other causes. Typically, this sensation is reversible and subsides approximately between a few seconds to a few days. The early explorers of Africa titrated the dose of quinine to the reversible presence of a phantom sound, as was done for aspirin in the treatment for rheumathoid arthritis and gout[6]. This phantom sound is also called tinnitus. To date, no FDA approved pharmacological treatment exists for this auditory phantom phenomenon [7].

In an adult population 10 to 15% of the population perceives tinnitus chronically and about 6 to 25% of the affected people report interference with their daily living, as tinnitus can cause a considerable amount of distress, involving sleep deprivation[8,9], depression[10], annoyance, cognitive problems[11], and work impairment [1,9,12,13,14].

Therefore, tinnitus is usually evaluated for both its intensity or loudness by tinnitus matching or VAS scores and for its annoyance or distress, using validated tinnitus questionnaires. One of the surprising findings in tinnitus research is that the perceived tinnitus intensity as determined by tinnitus matching correlates poorly with the associated distress [15–16], suggesting that separable networks might be involved in both aspects of tinnitus. This is clinically well known from the 1930's and 1940's when frontal lobotomies were performed for the treatment of tinnitus, resulting in unchanged tinnitus intensity but markedly decreased tinnitus annoyance [17,18].

Magnetoencephalography (MEG) studies have demonstrated that tinnitus is correlated to decreased alpha [19] and associated increased gamma band activity in the contralateral auditory cortex [20,21]. Furthermore, the amount of contralateral gamma band activity as estimated by EEG current density correlates with the perceived intensity of the phantom sound.

On the other hand, a recent study, using LORETA source localization in EEG, revealed that distress in tinnitus patients is related to increased beta activity in the dorsal part of the anterior cingulate cortex (ACC) and the amount of distress correlates with an alpha activity in several brain areas such as the amygdala, ACC, insula and parahippocampus [22]. A MEG study further showed that long-range coupling between frontal, parietal and cingulate brain areas in 'alpha and gamma networks' is related to tinnitus distress [23]. Due to the low spatial resolution of this MEG study (based on a coarse inverse solution) it cannot be deduced whether the frontal area also incorporates the anterior insula found in the source localization EEG study. The distress in tinnitus patients also correlates with an increase in incoming and outgoing connections in the gamma band in the prefrontal cortex, the orbitofrontal cortex and the parieto-occipital region [24]. The available spectral EEG and network MEG literature suggests that the increased spontaneous resting state activity and connectivity present in tinnitus distress is the result of a 'distress network' separable from a tinnitus intensity network. Thus the question arises whether the increased alpha activity in the amygdala, anterior cingulate cortex, parahippocampus and insula and the beta activity in the dorsal anterior cingulate form one 'distress network' of functionally interconnected areas, as one separable component of multiple overlapping tinnitus networks each defining a specific tinnitus characteristic such as laterality [25], tinnitus type (pure tone vs noise-like tinnitus) [26] etc. Two main data analysis approaches have been used to study functional connectivity, i.e., the correlations between spatially remote neurophysiological events in resting state networks by fMRI [27]; a seed-based connectivity analysis and independent component analysis (ICA). The latter is currently enjoying increasing popularity thanks to its complete data-driven nature [28,29,30]. Another source separation method similar to ICA has recently been extended to group analysis of resting state EEG, test-retesting two independent EEG databases in normal population. This resulted in the discovery of seven replicable groups blind source separation (BSS) components explaining about 92% of the variance [31](Table 1). As any other source separation method of this family, the BSS approach we use decomposes the whole EEG in a number of elementary statistically independent components, each one characterised by its time course and spatial pattern, therein used as input to source localization by the sLORETA inverse solution [32].

This study analyzes the group BSS networks in tinnitus and tinnitus distress, by comparing the resting state electrical activity of a very homogeneous group of tinnitus patients with controls and by comparing low and high distress, with the clinical groups not different for tinnitus type, tinnitus duration or tinnitus laterality (Table 1). This 'functional network' is further verified by performing a multivariate lagged coherence analysis between the brain areas defined by the group BSS results.

Results

Normative Group Blind Source Separation

Comparisons for the components generated on the normative database and compared with the two tinnitus groups (low and high distress) revealed significant differences for the relative power ($p<.01$) for two of the seven components: IC5 and IC6. An overview is given in Figure 1. Table 1 specifies the Brodmann areas involved in each component. For both components more activity was revealed in all frequencies bands (delta, theta, alpha, beta and gamma) for both the low and high tinnitus distress in comparison to normative database. Since we analyzed relative power measures (with respect to the total power of the seven components) this shows that these two components are overall predominant in the EEG of the patients as compared to the normative group, irrespective to frequency.

A comparison between low and high distress for the different components revealed only a significant effect for component 6 for the frequency band 14–18 Hz ($t=2.57$, $p<.05$) and 22–26 Hz ($t=2.82$, $p<.05$). No other component did obtain significance.

Additional analysis

An additional analysis was conducted comparing the normative group with age-matched tinnitus patients (Table S1) for respectively low and high distress. Similar results were obtained as for the whole group and for the older tinnitus patients (Figures S1, S2).

For IC5, Visual inspection indicate that for the young tinnitusgroup had less delta, theta, alpha activity compared to the older tinnitus group for patients with low distress. However, there were no significant effect differences for the young and old group For patients with high distress, visual inspection indicicates that young tinnitus group had less delta and theta compared to the older tinnitus group. Again, no significant effect was obtained when comparing the young and old tinnitus group with high distress. Yet, both the low and high distress patients showed, independently of belonging to theyoung or old tinnitus group, significantly increased activity compared the normative database.

For IC6 visual inspection indicates a difference between theyoung tinnitus group in comparison to the older tinnitus group with high distress in delta and theta. However, a statistical comparison between both groups showed no significant differences. Both groups showed significantly increased activity in comparison to the normative database.

Table 1. Anatomical Structures and Brodmann Areas of the sevec normative independent components (IC) [67].

IC1	Anterior Cingulate (BA 23/24/32/33/25), Insula (BA 13), Middle/Superior Frontal Gyrus and Paracentral Lobule (BA 4/5/6), Parahippocampal/Subcallosal Gyrus (BA 28/34/35/36)
IC2	Cuneus/Precuneus/ (BA 7/31/18/19/), Post-central gyrus (BA 3/4/5), Superior Parietal and Paracentral Lobule (BA 5/7), Posterior Cingulate Gyrus (BA 23/31)
IC3	Cuneus/Precuneus/ (BA 30/31/7), Right superior parietal lobule (BA 7), Posterior Cingulate (BA 30), Lyngual/Parahippocampal Gyrus (BA 18/19/30), Right Fusiform Gyrus (BA 19)
IC4	Cuneus/Precuneus/Posterior Cingulate (BA 23/30/31), Lyngual Gyrus/Fusiform Gyrus/Middle and Inferior Occipital Gyrus (Occipital Pole) (BA 17/18/19)
IC5	Anterior Cingulate (BA 24/25/32), Medial Frontal Gyrus (BA 32/9/10/11), Rectal/Orbital Gyrus (BA 11/47), Inferior Frontal Gyrus (BA 47), Parahippocampal Gyrus (BA 28/34)
IC6	Medial Frontal/Rectal Gyrus/Anterior Cingulate (BA 11, 25), Middle Frontal Gyrus (BA 11), Inferior Frontal Gyrus (BA 47), Parahippocampal Gyrus (BA 28/34), Insula (BA 13)
IC7	Post-central Gyrus (BA 1/2/3), Supramarginal Gyrus/Inferior Parietal Lobule (BA 40), Precentral Gyrus (BA 6), Cuneus/Precuneus (BA 17/18/19/31), Middle Occipital Gyrus (BA 18), Superior and Middle temporal Gyrus (BA 21/22/39/41), Insula (BA 13), Angular Gyrus (BA 39)

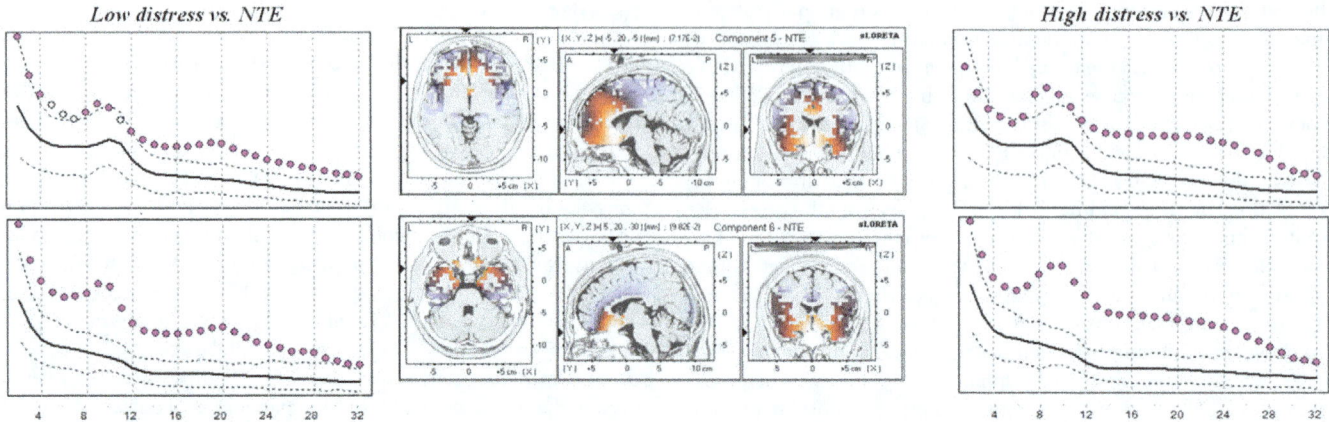

Figure 1. Comparison for the normative independent components IC5 and IC6. Left and right panels: Relative Power (arbitrary units) of components along frequencies in the range 2–32 Hz for low distress (left) and high distress (right) in tinnitus patients. Black solid and dotted lines represents the mean and 95% confidence intervals, respectively, for the normative group. Disks represent the mean of the clinical group. Pink disks flag a statistically higher power (p<0.01) in the relative mean power of the patients as compared to the normative database. Middle power: the sLORETA source localization of IC5 and IC6 (Congedo et al., 2010).

Correlation analysis

Correlation analysis revealed a significant (p<0.05) positive correlation between the log-power of two components and the TQ-scores: a significant positive correlation was found in the alpha (8–12 Hz) and beta (12–16 Hz and 16–20 Hz) range for component 5 and in the alpha (8–12 Hz) and beta (12–16 Hz and 16–20 Hz as well as 22–26 Hz) range for component 6 (Table 2 and Figures S3, S4). Also after exclusion of potential outliers, correlations remained significant. No other component reached significance.

Group Blind Source Separation on the Tinnitus Sample

For the group BSS on the tinnitus group the Akaike information criterion (AIC) suggested to retain the four most energetic components, explaining 52% of the total variance (Figure 2). Component 1 and 2 showed increased activity in the posterior cingulate cortex (BA23, BA33), precuneus (BA7), retrosplenial

Table 2. Correlation analysis between TQ and BSS components.

	Frequencies	r
IC5	8–12 Hz	.28*
	12–16 Hz	.32**
	16–20 Hz	.24*
IC6	8–12 Hz	.25*
	12–16 Hz	.36**
	16–20 Hz	.26*
	22–26 Hz	.34**
Tinnitus IC4	8–12 HZ	.28*
	12–16 Hz	.28*
	16–20 Hz	.27*
	20–24 Hz	.30*

See additional figure in supplementary material (Figures S3S, S4, S5).
*p<.05;
**p<.01.

posterior cingulate cortex (BA29, BA30), and subgenual anterior cingulate cortex (BA25). Component 3 revealed activity in parahippocampal area (BA19, BA30), while component 4 demonstrated activity in subgenual anterior cingulate cortex (BA25) extending into right inferior frontal gyrus (BA47). Significant positive correlations (p<0.05) were found between components obtained for the tinnitus group and the TQ-scores for alpha (8–12 Hz), beta (12–16 Hz, 16–20 Hz, 20–24 Hz) for component 4 (Table 2 and Figure S5). No other component did obtain significance.

Multivariate Functional Connectivity Analysis

We verified the group BSS defined functional networks with a functional connectivity analysis evaluating lagged coherence between the areas defined by the BSS analysis. These additional analyses revealed an increased functional connectivity between the (para)hippocampus, subgenual anterior cingulate cortex, orbito-frontal cortex and the inferior frontal gyrus for alpha (8–12 Hz) (Figure 3) and for beta (12–16 Hz and 16–20 Hz) (Figure 4).

Hearing loss

No significant correlation was found for hearing loss as measured by the loss in decibels (dB SPL) at the tinnitus frequency and the independent components.

Discussion

Based on the Aikake information criterium tinnitus is characterized by at least four independent components, two of which are posterior cingulate based, one based on the subgenual anterior cingulate and one based on the parahippocampal area. The anterior cingulate has been implicated in emotional [33], attentional [34], reward [35] and executive [36] processing, whereas the posterior cingulate seems to be related more to cognitive and memory aspects of information processing [36].

The posterior based components found in this analysis might thus be related to cognitive and memory related aspects of the tinnitus percept, as the retrosplenial PCC (BA 29& 30) is implicated in auditory memory [37,38] and the PCC is involved in cognitive aspects of auditory processing [39]. Activity in the precuneus and adjacent retrosplenial and posterior cingulate

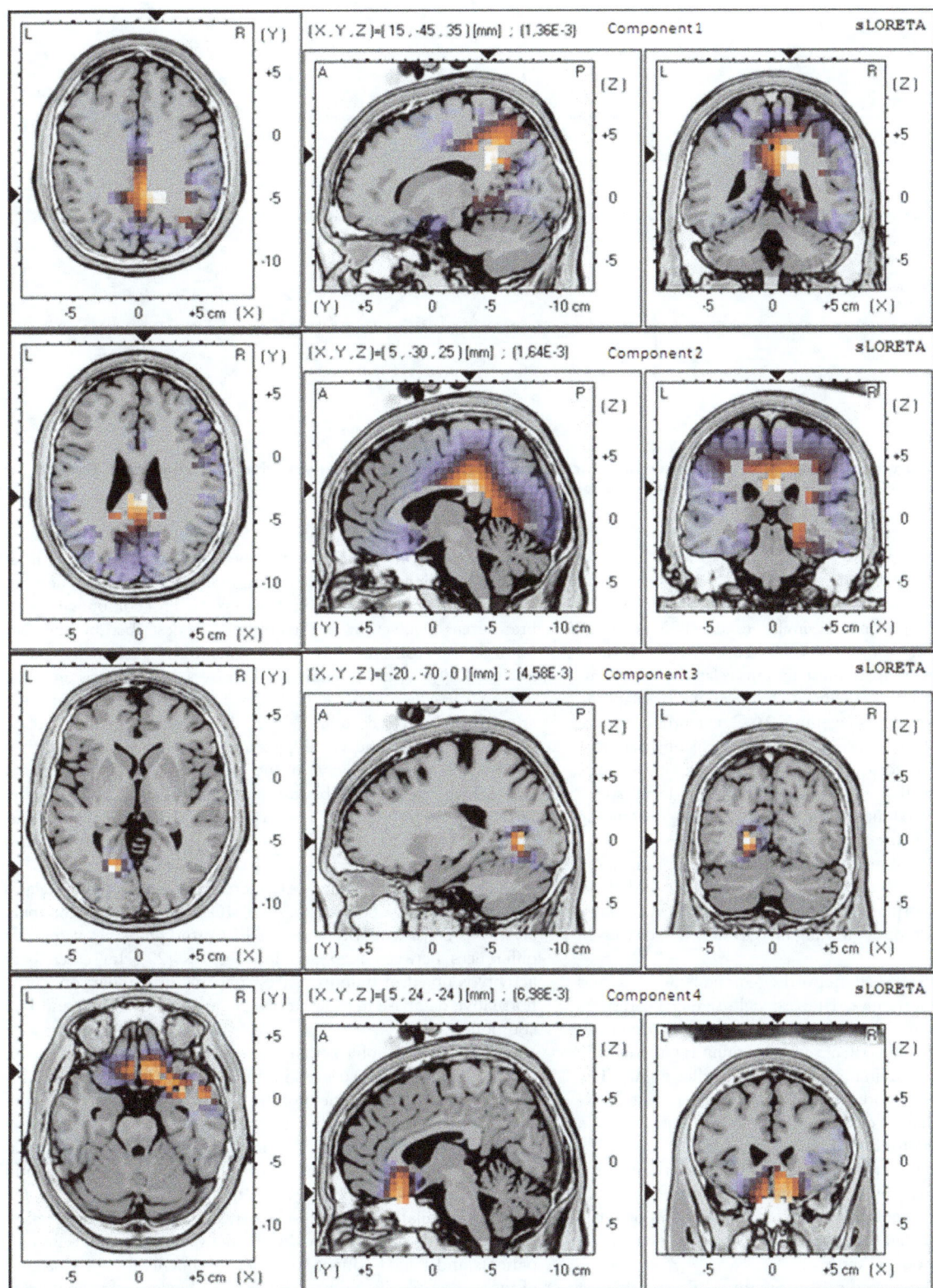

Figure 2. The four most energetic components obtained by applying group Blind Source Separation on the tinnitus group.

cortex has indeed been linked to successful retrieval from auditory (and visual) memory [40,41]. The PCC/precuneus component has been proposed to exert a salience based cognitive auditory comparator function [39]. When the PCC component is deficient or less active, such as in tinnitus distress [22], this could reflect an incapacity of the PCC/precuneus to exert its salience based comparator function, pulling irrelevant auditory (tinnitus)sound from hippocampal memory [42], via dysfunctional parahippo-

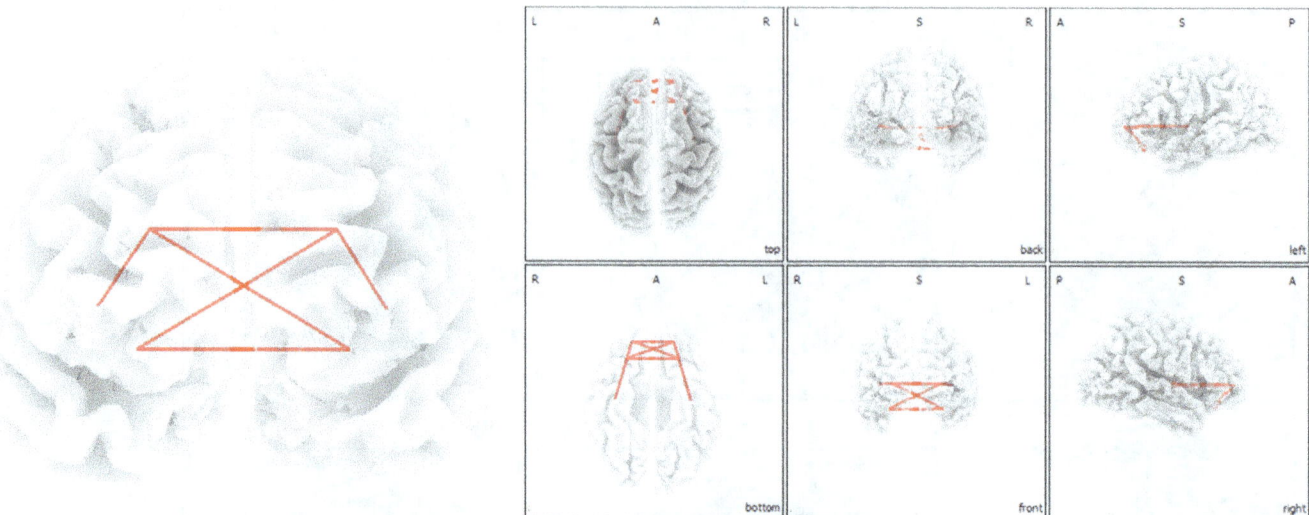

Figure 3. Phase synchronization analysis demonstrating increased functional connectivity within the region of interest of component 5 and 6 for 8–12 Hz for tinnitus patients in comparison to normative database.

campal auditory sensory gating [43], analogous to what has been proposed for auditory hallucinations [44].

The subgenual anterior cingulate (BA25) based independent component in tinnitus patients is similar to the IC5 and IC6 (Table 1) described in a normative database [31], and it is therefore interesting to compare these tinnitus related components to a normative database. IC5 and IC6 make up overlapping networks consisting of the subgenual ACC extending to the pregenual and dorsal ACC as well as the ventromedial and ventrolateral prefrontal cortex/orbitofrontal cortex, insula, and parahippocampal area. IC5 is more centered on the dorsal ACC, whereas IC6 is centered on the subgenual cingulate, extending into the orbitofrontal cortex and insula.

The comparison of mild and very severe distress in tinnitus and their comparison to a normative ICA EEG database yields both spatial and spectral information distinguishing distress in tinnitus patients from norms and distinguishing mild from severe distress in this patient group.

Two anatomically specified networks (components IC5 and IC6, Table 1) of the normative database yield significant distress related differences in tinnitus patients in comparison to controls and one of these components (IC6) separates tinnitus patients who suffer a lot from those who do not suffer or only suffer mildly. The fact that distress is a network property fits with a recent MEG study using network analysis demonstrating multiple hubs [24] in a large scale network involved in tinnitus distress [45].

The subgenual component found in the tinnitus group is the only component correlating to the tinnitus distress (Table 2), adding further data and confirming the concept that components 5 and 6 in the normative database constitute networks which can be involved in the generation of distress.

It has been recently proposed that tinnitus is the result of a deficient noise cancellation mechanism originating in the nucleus accumbens-subgenual cingulate area [46]. This area would modulate thalamocortical dysrhythmic activity via the reticular nucleus of the thalamus [46]. Thus stress could modulate this putative noise-cancelling mechanism, explaining potentially both the fact that many people attribute their tinnitus and pain to stress, and that distress often accompanies phantom perceptions [47].

The IC6, which differentiates between distressed and non-distressed patients, represents an emotion and autonomic nervous system binding network (Table 1, Figure 1). This component binds brain areas involved in tinnitus distress, as described in a smaller set of patients using a different technique [22]. In this study, source analyzed FFT spectral analysis of distress in comparison to no distress correlated with beta activity in the dorsal ACC, and the amount of distress correlated with alpha activity in the sgACC, insula, amygdala, and parahippocampal area, associated with a decrease in alpha activity in the PCC. FFT based functional connectivity, as analyzed by instantaneous coherence between the areas defined by the ICA analysis (IC5 and IC6) further reveals that the brain areas involved in distress [22], really form a functional network.

In these IC5 and IC6 networks increasing distress also correlates with increasing beta activity. The IC5 and IC6 related beta activity is consistent with a recent EEG study looking at spectral differences between high and low distress [22]. Increased beta activity is noted in tinnitus distress patients in comparison to the normative database in the anterior cingulated based IC5 and IC6 components [22].

The increased alpha activity in the subgenual ACC noted in that study[22] is also retrieved in this analysis, but only in the FFT on the subgenual component of the tinnitus, which correlates with the perceived amount of distress.

Severe distress such as in posttraumatic stress disorder is associated with increased beta activity especially over frontal and central areas (C3,C4,F3,F4) [48,49]. The beta activity in the anterior cingulate-anterior insula network might therefore reflect the expression of an aspecific distress network, common to tinnitus patients and PTSD patients. Further arguments for the existence of such a non-specific distress network can be derived from the fact that pain distress [50,51], distress in asthmatic dyspnea [52] and distress in functional somatic syndromes such as electro-sensitivity for mobile phones [53] as well as social rejection distress [54] also correlate with activity in some of these areas (insula, anterior cingulate). Furthermore, in pain, beta activity is increased in the insula and anterior cingulate [55], in accordance with this hypothesis.

(A)

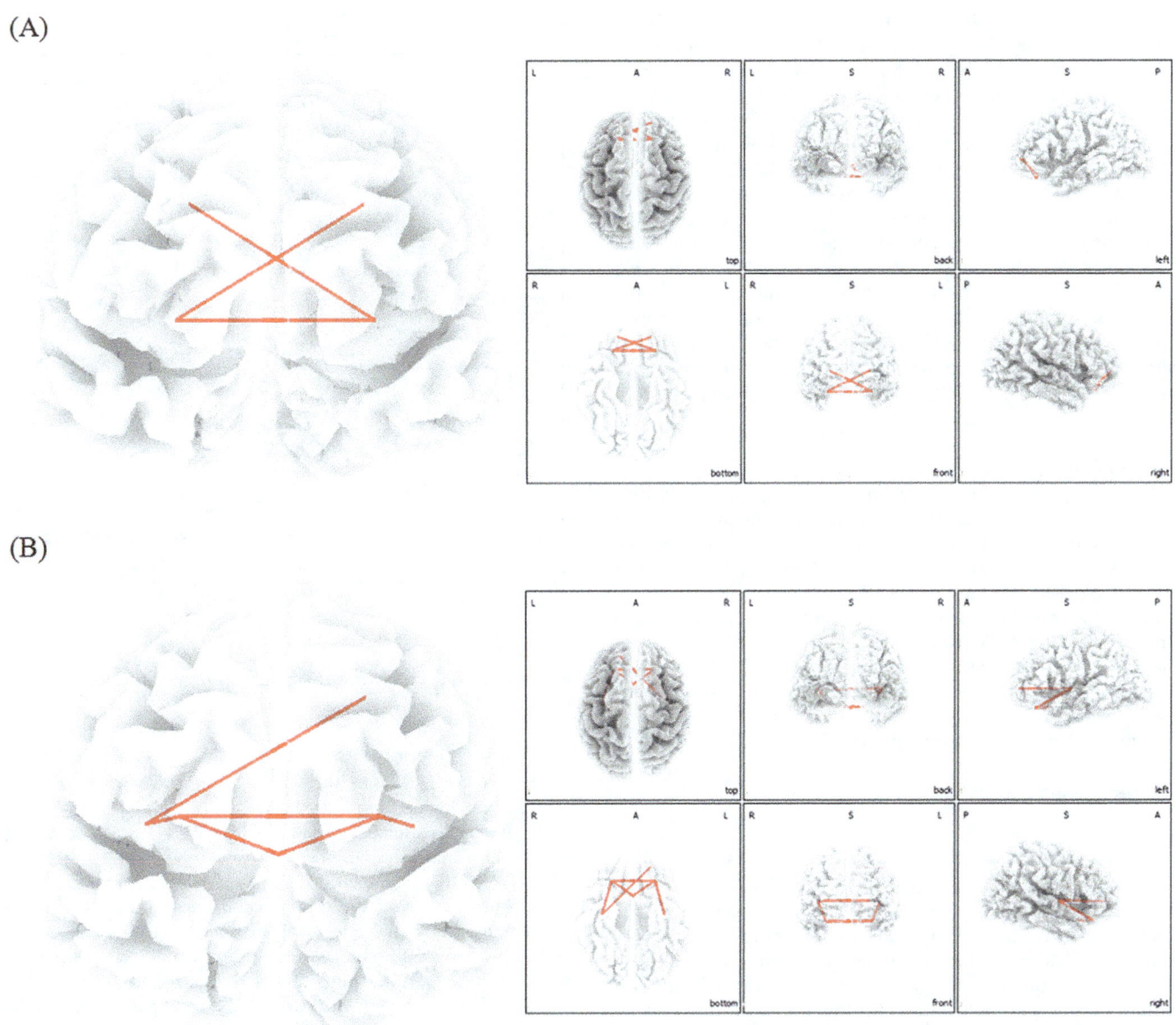

(B)

Figure 4. Phase synchronization analysis demonstrating increased functional connectivity within the region of interest of component 5 and 6 for 12–16 Hz (A) and 16–20 Hz (B) for tinnitus patients in comparison to normative database.

On the other hand, in posterior cingulate based components no increased power is found. This might reflect the predominant autonomic-emotional-attentional aspects of distress (ACC based) and the limited influence of PCC based cognition [36,56] Thus whereas the PCC is involved in tinnitus, as reflected by the ICA analysis, it seems it is not involved in tinnitus distress, but possibly forms part of a separable cognitive-memory related tinnitus network.

Contrary to expectation, no increased power is found in component 1 (Table 1), a dorsal ACC related network, extending to the insula, parahippocampus and DLPFC. As IC1 reflects an attentional network focusing on salient information it could be hypothesized that this network predominantly is involved in the intensity coding of the tinnitus. It has been shown that the intensity of perceived pain [57] and auditory [41] stimuli depends on fluctuations of activity in the dACC and anterior insula. The parahippocampal area, which acts as a sensory auditory gate [43],

is involved in the percept of tinnitus [25,58], as is the DLPFC [59,60,61]. As there is no significant difference in the perceived intensity in the different distress groups, this component will not differ between the different distress groups.

Limitations of the study

One major limitation of this and any EEG based approach is that no subcortical activity can be analyzed, limiting network description to cortical sources. The data presented should therefore be viewed acknowledging this limitation. Another limitation of the present study relates to age differences between the tinnitus group and the control group. However, an analysis comparing age-matched tinnitus patients with low and high distress with respectively older patients with low and high distress showed no statistical differences. Furthermore, no prior research has shown that independent components change with age in resting state EEG, although power changes over age are expected.

Secondly, as the control group was collected at a different lab it is possible that cultural background could also have an influence on our results. However, cross-cultural differences on independent components have not yet been shown across different continents [62]. Finally, the normative and clinical data have been acquired using different EEG machine, which may engender systematic distortions in the comparisons due to the different amplifiers response. However, we have analyzed relative measures, excluding confounding factors due to overall gain differences. On the other hand, frequency-specific distortions, if any, should appear in all components, which is not what we have observed. Hence, we think that differences demonstrated between both tinnitus group and the control group in our study might be reliable and valid, however further research is needed. This study demonstrates the need for a large normative database containing a large sample of all ages, and applicable to multiple EEG machines by calibration correction factors.

Conclusion

Comparing patients with mild and very severe tinnitus distress to a normative BSS EEG database and comparing low with high distress permits to evaluate brain activity differences in functional networks associated with tinnitus distress. Based on this analysis it can be proposed that tinnitus distress results from alpha and beta abnormal activity in subgenual ACC extending to the pregenual and dorsal ACC and VM&VLPFC/OFC, insula, and parahippo-campal area. This network overlaps partially with brain areas implicated in distress in patients suffering from pain, dyspnea, functional somatic syndromes and posttraumatic stress disorder, and might therefore represent an aspecific distress network.

Materials and Methods

Patients

Fifty-five tinnitus patients were selected from the multidisciplin-ary Tinnitus Research Initiative (TRI) Clinic of the University Hospital of Antwerp, Belgium (Table 3). The average age was 51 years ($SD = 13$). Individuals with pulsatile tinnitus, Ménière disease, otosclerosis, chronic headache, neurological disorders such as brain tumors, and individuals being treated for mental disorders were not included in the study in order to promote sample homogeneity. The patients selected for this study were not included in a previous study on tinnitus related distress conducted by the same research group [22].

All patients were investigated for the extent of hearing loss using audiograms. Tinnitus matching was performed looking for tinnitus pitch (frequency) and tinnitus intensity. Participants were request-ed to refrain from alcohol consumption 24 hours prior to recording, and from caffeinated beverages consumption on the day of recording.

Patients were also given the validated Dutch version of the Tinnitus Questionnaire [63,64] originally published by Goebel and Hiller [65]. Goebel and Hiller described this TQ as a global index of distress and the Dutch version was further confirmed as a reliable measure for tinnitus-related distress [64]. Based on the total score on the TQ, participants were assigned to a low distress (0–46) points and high distress (47–84) category. Patient distribution in all groups for tinnitus laterality, tinnitus type, tinnitus duration and tinnitus intensity is represented in Table 2. No significant results were obtained between the two groups.

This study was approved by the local ethical committee (Antwerp University Hospital) and was in accordance with the declaration of Helsinki. We did not obtain an informed consent as this EEG recording was obtained for further diagnosis of the

Table 3. Tinnitus Characteristics.

		Grade		statistic
		Low distress	High distress	
Tinnitus laterality	Left	8	8	$\chi^2 = .24$, n.s.
	Right	7	6	
	Bilateral	15	11	
Tinnitus type	Pure Tone	7	8	$\chi^2 = .52$, n.s.
	Narrow Band Noise	23	17	
Tinnitus duration		M = 5.01	M = 5.10	t = −.10, n.s.
		Sd = 3.49	Sd = 3.32	
Tinnitus Intensity		M = 6.05	M = 6.27	t = −.66, n.s.
		Sd = 2.02	Sd = 1.90	
TQ		M = 32.90	M = 56.39	t = −.7.47, n.s.
		Sd = 12.57	Sd = 9.50	

n.s.: not significant.

tinnitus patients and was a standard procedure for ongoing investigation.

EEG data collection

EEG recordings (Mitsar-201, NovaTech http://www.novatecheeg.com/) were obtained in a fully lighted room with each participant sitting upright on a small but comfortable chair. The actual recording lasted approximately 5 min. The EEG was sampled with 19 electrodes (Fp1, Fp2, F7, F3, Fz, F4, F8, T7, C3, Cz, C4, T8, P7, P3, Pz, P4, P8, O1 O2) in the standard 10–20 International placement referenced to digitally linked ears, analogous to what is done in the normative group, and impedances were checked to remain below 5 kΩ. Data were collected eyes-closed (sampling rate = 1024 Hz, band passed 0.15–200 Hz). Data were resampled to 128 Hz, band-pass filtered in the range 2–32 Hz and subsequently transposed into Eureka! software [66], plotted and carefully inspected for manual artifact-rejection. All episodic artifacts including eye blinks, eye movements, teeth clenching, body movement, or ECG artifact were removed from the stream of the EEG. We only removed episodic artifacts. Maximum 1 minute of artifact was removed. It is however difficult to say the number of artifacts that are removed for each patient as there is a relative large variability between patients.

Normative database

Also the normative database of the Nova Tech EEG (NTE), Inc, Mesa, AZ (N = 84) was used (http://www.novatecheeg.com/). None of these subjects was known to suffer from tinnitus. Exclusion criteria for the NTE database were known psychiatric or neurological illness, psychiatric history of drug/alcohol abuse in a participant or any relative, current psychotropic/CNS active medications, history of head injury (with loss of consciousness) or seizures, headache, physical disability. To build the database about 3–5 min of EEG was continuously recorded while participant sat with the eyes closed on a comfortable chair in a quiet and dimly lit room. EEG data were acquired at the 19 standard leads prescribed by the 10–20 international system (FP1, FP2, F7, F3, FZ, F4, F8, T3, C3, CZ, C4, T4, T5, P3, PZ, P4, T6,

O1, O2) using both earlobes as reference and enabling a 60 Hz notch filter to suppress power line contamination. The resistance of all electrodes was kept below 5 kΩ. Data of the NTE database were acquired using the 12-bit A/D NeuroSearch-24 acquisition system (Lexicor Medical Technology, Inc. Boulder, CO) and sampled at 128. The data were subsequently band-pass filtered in the region 2–32 Hz and artifact rejection was carried out using the same software and procedures as per the clinical data.

sLORETA imaging

Standardized low-resolution brain electromagnetic tomography (sLORETA; Pascual-Marqui, 2002) was used to estimate the intracerebral electrical sources that generated the seven NICA components. As a standard procedure a common average reference transformation (see Pascual-Marqui [32]) is performed before applying the sLORETA algorithm. That is, the coordinates of the 19 electrode positions were applied to a digitized MRI version of the Talairach Atlas (McConnell Brain Imaging Centre, Montréal Neurological Institute, McGill University). These Talairach coordinates were then used to compute the sLORETA transformation matrix. More technical details can be found in [32].

sLORETA computes electric neuronal activity as current density (A/m2) without assuming a predefined number of active sources. The solution space used in this study and associated leadfield matrix are those implemented in the LORETA-Key software (freely available at URL http://www.uzh.ch/keyinst/loreta.htm).This software implements revisited realistic electrode coordinates (Jurcak et al. 2007) and the lead field produced by Fuchs et al. (2002) applying the boundary element method on the MNI-152 (Montreal neurological institute, Canada) template of Mazziotta et al. (2001). The sLORETA-key anatomical template divides and label the neocortical (including hippocampus and anterior cingulated cortex) MNI-152 volume in 6,239 voxels of dimension 5 mm³, based on probabilities returned by the Demon Atlas (Lancaster et al. 2000). The coregistration makes use of the correct translation from the MNI-152 space into the Talaiach and Tournoux (1988) space (Brett et al. 2002).

Group Blind Source Separation

We employed the group blind source separation approach consisting in the approximate joint diagonalization of grand-average Fourier co-spectral matrices [31,67]. Such method can separate uncorrelated sources with non-proportional power spectra [68] and is analogous to the averaging group ICA approach described for fMRI by Schmithorst and Holland [69]. Only co-spectra in the range of 2–32 Hz were diagonalized because in this band-pass region continuous EEG features the highest signal-to-noise ratio. Following previous work (Congedo et al., 2010) we extracted the seven most energetic components. The demixing matrix was used to extract the power of the seven normative components in both the normative sample and in the low and high distress group, as described in details in Congedo et al. [67,70]. In addition, a group BSS analysis was conducted on the tinnitus group. We used the Aikake Information Criterium (AIC) to determine the number of components [71].

Comparison between BSS components of normative database, low and high distressed tinnitus group

For each of the seven components (Table 1) relative power was computed with 1 Hz resolution with respect to the total energy across all components. Then the relative power for each frequency and each component was compared between the normative

sample and the two Tinnitus groups (low and high distress). Multiple comparison Student-t tests were performed separately for each component. The significance threshold was based on a permutation test with 5000 permutations. The methodology used is non-parametric. It is based on estimating, via randomization, the empirical probability distribution for the max-statistic, under the null hypothesis [72]. This methodology corrects for multiple testing across frequencies and guarantees that the probability of falsely rejecting even only one hypothesis is less than the chosen alpha level.

Correlation analysis

A correlation analysis was conducted between the relative power of the seven components and the TQ-scores. TQ-scores are used and not the TQ grade to have a continuous variable that can be correlated to the specific independent component. This analysis has as advantage that the tinnitus group is not divided in to two separate groups (low vs high distress). Analysis was performed in all 4 Hz spaced discrete Fourier frequencies in the range 2–32 Hz (2–4 Hz, 4–8 Hz, 8–12 Hz, 12–16 Hz, 16–20 Hz, 20–24 Hz, 24–28 Hz, 28–32 Hz). Corrections were performed for multiple comparisons across eight frequencies bands using a Bonferroni method and testing separately for each component.

Functional Connectivity

Functional connectivity between time series corresponding to different spatial locations is calculated using lagged coherence [73]. Based on the method introduced by Pascual-Marqui, this measure of dependence can be applied to any number of brain areas jointly, that is, they reflect a global functional connectivity between all series included in the analysis. Time-series were extracted for different ROIs using sLORETA. The measures are non-negative and take the value zero only when there is independence. They were defined in the frequency domain in the range 2–32 Hz (2–4 Hz, 4–8 Hz, 8–12 Hz, 12–16 Hz, 16–20 Hz, 20–24 Hz, 24–28 Hz, 28–32 Hz). Regions of interest were defined based upon the areas involved in IC5 and IC6 (Table 2).

Supporting Information

Figure S1   Comparison for the independent components C5 generated from the normative database (middle) and compared with an aged-matched and older tinnitus group. Left and right panels: Relative Power (arbitrary units) of component along frequencies in the range 2–32 Hz for low distress (left) and high distress (right) in tinnitus patients. Black solid line represents the mean, dotted black lines 95% confidence intervals. Pink dots represent statistically significant (p<0.05) increased power, plotted for each frequency (on X-axis) and the relative power on the Y-Axis.

Figure S2   Comparison for the independent components C6 generated from the normative database (middle) and compared with an aged-matched and older tinnitus group. Left and right panels: Relative Power (arbitrary units) of component along frequencies in the range 2–32 Hz for low distress (left) and high distress (right) in tinnitus patients. Black solid line represents the mean, dotted black lines 95% confidence intervals. Pink dots represent statistically significant (p<0.05) increased power, plotted for each frequency (on X-axis) and the relative power on the Y-Axis.

Figure S3 Scatterplots for respectively the alpha frequency band (8–12 Hz) and the beta frequency band (12–20 Hz) between TQ and the relative power for IC5.

Figure S4 Scatterplot for respectively the alpha frequency band (8–12 Hz) and the beta frequency band (12–26 Hz) between TQ and the relative power for IC6.

Figure S5 Scatterplots for respectively the alpha frequency band (8–12 Hz) and the beta frequency band (12–

24 Hz) between TQ and the relative power for Tinnitus IC4.

Table S1 Young and Old Tinnitus patients.

Author Contributions

Conceived and designed the experiments: DDR SV MC. Performed the experiments: DDR SV MC. Analyzed the data: DDR SV MC. Contributed reagents/materials/analysis tools: DDR SV MC. Wrote the paper: DDR SV MC.

References

1. Eggermont JJ, Roberts LE (2004) The neuroscience of tinnitus. Trends Neurosci 27: 676–682.
2. Axelsson A, Prasher D (2000) Tinnitus induced by occupational and leisure noise. Noise Health 2: 47–54.
3. Schreiber BE, Agrup C, Haskard DO, Luxon LM (2010) Sudden sensorineural hearing loss. Lancet 375: 1203–1211.
4. Dille MF, Konrad-Martin D, Gallun F, Helt WJ, Gordon JS, et al. (2010) Tinnitus onset rates from chemotherapeutic agents and ototoxic antibiotics: results of a large prospective study. J Am Acad Audiol 21: 409–417.
5. Folmer RL, Griest SE (2003) Chronic tinnitus resulting from head or neck injuries. Laryngoscope 113: 821–827.
6. Clark WW (1991) Noise exposure from leisure activities: a review. J Acoust Soc Am 90: 175–181.
7. Dobie RA (1999) A review of randomized clinical trials in tinnitus. Laryngoscope 109: 1202–1211.
8. Alster J, Shemesh Z, Ornan M, Attias J (1993) Sleep disturbance associated with chronic tinnitus. Biol Psychiatry 34: 84–90.
9. Cronlein T, Langguth B, Geisler P, Hajak G (2007) Tinnitus and insomnia. Prog Brain Res 166: 227–233.
10. Dobie RA (2003) Depression and tinnitus. Otolaryngol Clin North Am 36: 383–388.
11. Hallam RS, McKenna L, Shurlock L (2004) Tinnitus impairs cognitive efficiency. Int J Audiol 43: 218–226.
12. Baguley DM (2002) Mechanisms of tinnitus. Br Med Bull 63: 195–212.
13. Heller AJ (2003) Classification and epidemiology of tinnitus. Otolaryngol Clin North Am 36: 239–248.
14. Langguth B, Kleinjung T, Fischer B, Hajak G, Eichhammer P, et al. (2007) Tinnitus severity, depression, and the big five personality traits. Prog Brain Res 166: 221–225.
15. Moller A (1994) Tinnitus. In: Jackler R, Brackmann D, eds. Neurotology. St Louis: Mosby. pp 153–166.
16. van der Loo E, Gais S, Congedo M, Vanneste S, Plazier M, et al. (2009) Tinnitus intensity dependent gamma oscillations of the contralateral auditory cortex. PLoS One 4: e7396.
17. Beard AW (1965) Results of leucotomy operations for tinnitus. J Psychosom Res 9: 29–32.
18. Elithorn A (1953) Prefrontal leucotomy in the treatment of tinnitus. Proc R Soc Med 46: 832–833.
19. Lorenz I, Muller N, Schlee W, Hartmann T, Weisz N (2009) Loss of alpha power is related to increased gamma synchronization-A marker of reduced inhibition in tinnitus? Neurosci Lett 453: 225–228.
20. Llinas RR, Ribary U, Jeanmonod D, Kronberg E, Mitra PP (1999) Thalamocortical dysrhythmia: A neurological and neuropsychiatric syndrome characterized by magnetoencephalography. Proc Natl Acad Sci U S A 96: 15222–15227.
21. Weisz N, Muller S, Schlee W, Dohrmann K, Hartmann T, et al. (2007) The neural code of auditory phantom perception. J Neurosci 27: 1479–1484.
22. Vanneste S, Plazier M, der Loo E, de Heyning PV, Congedo M, et al. (2010) The neural correlates of tinnitus-related distress. Neuroimage 52: 470–480.
23. Schlee W, Weisz N, Bertrand O, Hartmann T, Elbert T (2008) Using auditory steady state responses to outline the functional connectivity in the tinnitus brain. PLoS ONE 3: e3720.
24. Schlee W, Mueller N, Hartmann T, Keil J, Lorenz I, et al. (2009) Mapping cortical hubs in tinnitus. BMC Biol 7: 80.
25. Vanneste S, Plazier M, van der Loo E, Van de Heyning P, De Ridder D (2011) The difference between uni- and bilateral auditory phantom percept. Clin Neurophysiol.
26. Vanneste S, Plazier M, van der Loo E, Van de Heyning P, De Ridder D (2010) The differences in brain activity between narrow band noise and pure tone tinnitus. PLoS One 5: e13618.
27. Buckner RL, Andrews-Hanna JR, Schacter DL (2008) The brain's default network: anatomy, function, and relevance to disease. Ann N Y Acad Sci 1124: 1–38.
28. Bluhm RL, Osuch EA, Lanius RA, Boksman K, Neufeld RW, et al. (2008) Default mode network connectivity: effects of age, sex, and analytic approach. Neuroreport 19: 887–891.
29. Greicius MD, Srivastava G, Reiss AL, Menon V (2004) Default-mode network activity distinguishes Alzheimer's disease from healthy aging: evidence from functional MRI. Proc Natl Acad Sci U S A 101: 4637–4642.
30. Scheeringa R, Bastiaansen MC, Petersson KM, Oostenveld R, Norris DG, et al. (2008) Frontal theta EEG activity correlates negatively with the default mode network in resting state. Int J Psychophysiol 67: 242–251.
31. Congedo M, John RE, De Ridder D, Prichep L (2010) Group independent component analysis of resting state EEG in large normative samples. Int J Psychophysiol.
32. Pascual-Marqui RD (2002) Standardized low-resolution brain electromagnetic tomography (sLORETA): technical details. Methods Find Exp Clin Pharmacol 24(Suppl D): 5–12.
33. Sinha R, Lacadie C, Skudlarski P, Wexler BE (2004) Neural circuits underlying emotional distress in humans. Ann N Y Acad Sci 1032: 254–257.
34. Cohen RA, Kaplan RF, Moser DJ, Jenkins MA, Wilkinson H (1999) Impairments of attention after cingulotomy. Neurology 53: 819–824.
35. Bush G, Vogt BA, Holmes J, Dale AM, Greve D, et al. (2002) Dorsal anterior cingulate cortex: a role in reward-based decision making. Proc Natl Acad Sci U S A 99: 523–528.
36. Vogt BA, Finch DM, Olson CR (1992) Functional heterogeneity in cingulate cortex: the anterior executive and posterior evaluative regions. Cereb Cortex 2: 435–443.
37. Grasby PM, Frith CD, Friston KJ, Bench C, Frackowiak RS, et al. (1993) Functional mapping of brain areas implicated in auditory—verbal memory function. Brain 116(Pt 1): 1–20.
38. Fletcher PC, Frith CD, Grasby PM, Shallice T, Frackowiak RS, et al. (1995) Brain systems for encoding and retrieval of auditory-verbal memory. An in vivo study in humans. Brain 118(Pt 2): 401–416.
39. Laufer I, Negishi M, Constable RT (2009) Comparator and non-comparator mechanisms of change detection in the context of speech—an ERP study. Neuroimage 44: 546–562.
40. Shannon BJ, Buckner RL (2004) Functional-anatomic correlates of memory retrieval that suggest nontraditional processing roles for multiple distinct regions within posterior parietal cortex. J Neurosci 24: 10084–10092.
41. Sadaghiani S, Hesselmann G, Kleinschmidt A (2009) Distributed and antagonistic contributions of ongoing activity fluctuations to auditory stimulus detection. J Neurosci 29: 13410–13417.
42. De Ridder D, Fransen H, Francois O, Sunaert S, Kovacs S, et al. (2006) Amygdalohippocampal involvement in tinnitus and auditory memory. Acta Otolaryngol Suppl. pp 50–53.
43. Boutros NN, Mears R, Pflieger ME, Moxon KA, Ludowig E, et al. (2008) Sensory gating in the human hippocampal and rhinal regions: regional differences. Hippocampus 18: 310–316.
44. Diederen KM, Neggers SF, Daalman K, Blom JD, Goekoop R, et al. (2010) Deactivation of the Parahippocampal Gyrus Preceding Auditory Hallucinations in Schizophrenia. Am J Psychiatry 167: 427–435.
45. Schlee W, Hartmann T, Langguth B, Weisz N (2009) Abnormal resting-state cortical coupling in chronic tinnitus. BMC Neurosci 10: 11.
46. Rauschecker JP, leaver AM, Muhlau M (2010) Tuning Out the Noise: Limbic-Auditory Interactions in Tinnitus. Neuron 66: 819–826.
47. De Ridder D, Elgoyhen AB, Romo R, Langguth B (2011) Phantom percepts: Tinnitus and pain as persisting aversive memory networks. Proc Natl Acad Sci U S A 108: 8075–8080.
48. Begic D, Hotujac L, Jokic-Begic N (2001) Electroencephalographic comparison of veterans with combat-related post-traumatic stress disorder and healthy subjects. Int J Psychophysiol 40: 167–172.
49. Jokic-Begic N, Begic D (2003) Quantitative electroencephalogram (qEEG) in combat veterans with post-traumatic stress disorder (PTSD). Nord J Psychiatry 57: 351–355.
50. Price DD (2000) Psychological and neural mechanisms of the affective dimension of pain. Science 288: 1769–1772.
51. Moisset X, Bouhassira D (2007) Brain imaging of neuropathic pain. Neuroimage 37(Suppl 1): S80–88.
52. von Leupoldt A, Sommer T, Kegat S, Baumann HJ, Klose H, et al. (2009) Dyspnea and pain share emotion-related brain network. Neuroimage 48: 200–206.

53. Landgrebe M, Barta W, Rosengarth K, Frick U, Hauser S, et al. (2008) Neuronal correlates of symptom formation in functional somatic syndromes: A fMRI study. Neuroimage 41: 1336–1344.

54. Kross E, Egner T, Ochsner K, Hirsch J, Downey G (2007) Neural dynamics of rejection sensitivity. J Cogn Neurosci 19: 945–956.

55. Stern J, Jeanmonod D, Sarnthein J (2006) Persistent EEG overactivation in the cortical pain matrix of neurogenic pain patients. Neuroimage 31: 721–731.

56. Vogt BA (2005) Pain and emotion interactions in subregions of the cingulate gyrus. Nat Rev Neurosci 6: 533–544.

57. Boly M, Balteau E, Schnakers C, Degueldre C, Moonen G, et al. (2007) Baseline brain activity fluctuations predict somatosensory perception in humans. Proc Natl Acad Sci U S A 104: 12187–12192.

58. Moazami-Goudarzi M, Michels L, Weisz N, Jeanmonod D (2010) Temporo-insular enhancement of EEG low and high frequencies in patients with chronic tinnitus. QEEG study of chronic tinnitus patients. BMC Neurosci 11: 40.

59. Kleinjung T, Eichhammer P, Landgrebe M, Sand P, Hajak G, et al. (2008) Combined temporal and prefrontal transcranial magnetic stimulation for tinnitus treatment: a pilot study. Otolaryngol Head Neck Surg 138: 497–501.

60. Mirz F, Gjedde A, Sodkilde-Jrgensen H, Pedersen CB (2000) Functional brain imaging of tinnitus-like perception induced by aversive auditory stimuli. Neuroreport 11: 633–637.

61. Vanneste S, Plazier M, Ost J, van der Loo E, Van de Heyning P, et al. (2010) Bilateral dorsolateral prefrontal cortex modulation for tinnitus by transcranial direct current stimulation: a preliminary clinical study. Exp Brain Res 202: 779–785.

62. Paul RH, Gunstad J, Cooper N, Williams LM, Clark CR, et al. (2007) Cross-cultural assessment of neuropsychological performance and electrical brain function measures: additional validation of an international brain database. Int J Neurosci 117: 549–568.

63. Meeus O, Blaivie C, Van de Heyning P (2007) Validation of the Dutch and the French version of the Tinnitus Questionnaire. B-ENT 3(Suppl 7): 11–17.

64. Vanneste S, Plazier M, van der Loo E, Ost J, Meeus O, et al. (2010) Validation of the Mini-TQ in a Dutch-speaking population. A rapid assessment for tinnitus-related distress. B-ENT.

65. Goebel G, Hiller W (1994) [The tinnitus questionnaire. A standard instrument for grading the degree of tinnitus. Results of a multicenter study with the tinnitus questionnaire]. HNO 42: 166–172.

66. Congedo M (2002) EureKa! (Version 3.0) [Computer Software]. Knoxville, TN: NovaTech EEG Inc. Available: www.NovaTechEEG. Accessed: 2011 Aug 28.

67. Congedo M, John RE, De Ridder D, Prichep L, Isenhart R (2010) On the "dependence" of "independent" group EEG sources; an EEG study on two large databases. Brain Topogr 23: 134–138.

68. Congedo M, Gouy-Pailler C, Jutten C (2008) On the blind source separation of human electroencephalogram by approximate joint diagonalization of second order statistics. Clin Neurophysiol 119: 2677–2686.

69. Schmithorst VJ, Holland SK (2004) Comparison of three methods for generating group statistical inferences from independent component analysis of functional magnetic resonance imaging data. J Magn Reson Imaging 19: 365–368.

70. Congedo M, John RE, De Ridder D, Prichep L (2010) Group independent component analysis of resting state EEG in large normative samples. Int J Psychophysiol.

71. Waldorp LJ, Huizenga HM, Nehorai A, Grasman RP, Molenaar PC (2005) Model selection in spatio-temporal electromagnetic source analysis. IEEE Trans Biomed Eng 52: 414–420.

72. Nichols TE, Holmes AP (2002) Nonparametric permutation tests for functional neuroimaging: a primer with examples. Hum Brain Mapp 15: 1–25.

73. Pascual-Marqui R (2007) Instantaneous and lagged measurements of linear and nonlinear dependence between groups of multivariate time series: frequency decomposition. ;Available: http://arxiv.org/abs/0711.1455. Accessed 2011 Aug 28.

12

The Reduced Cochlear Output and the Failure to Adapt the Central Auditory Response Causes Tinnitus in Noise Exposed Rats

Lukas Rüttiger[9], **Wibke Singer**[9], **Rama Panford-Walsh**[9], **Masahiro Matsumoto**, **Sze Chim Lee**, **Annalisa Zuccotti**, **Ulrike Zimmermann**, **Mirko Jaumann**, **Karin Rohbock**, **Hao Xiong**, **Marlies Knipper***

Department of Otolaryngology, Hearing Research Centre Tübingen (THRC), Molecular Physiology of Hearing, University of Tübingen, Tübingen, Germany

Abstract

Tinnitus is proposed to be caused by decreased central input from the cochlea, followed by increased spontaneous and evoked subcortical activity that is interpreted as compensation for increased responsiveness of central auditory circuits. We compared equally noise exposed rats separated into groups with and without tinnitus for differences in brain responsiveness relative to the degree of deafferentation in the periphery. We analyzed (1) the number of CtBP2/RIBEYE-positive particles in ribbon synapses of the inner hair cell (IHC) as a measure for deafferentation; (2) the fine structure of the amplitudes of auditory brainstem responses (ABR) reflecting differences in sound responses following decreased auditory nerve activity and (3) the expression of the activity-regulated gene Arc in the auditory cortex (AC) to identify long-lasting central activity following sensory deprivation. Following moderate trauma, 30% of animals exhibited tinnitus, similar to the tinnitus prevalence among hearing impaired humans. Although both tinnitus and no-tinnitus animals exhibited a reduced ABR wave I amplitude (generated by primary auditory nerve fibers), IHCs ribbon loss and high-frequency hearing impairment was more severe in tinnitus animals, associated with significantly reduced amplitudes of the more centrally generated wave IV and V and less intense staining of Arc mRNA and protein in the AC. The observed severe IHCs ribbon loss, the minimal restoration of ABR wave size, and reduced cortical Arc expression suggest that tinnitus is linked to a failure to adapt central circuits to reduced cochlear input.

Editor: Berthold Langguth, University of Regensburg, Germany

Funding: This work was supported by the Marie Curie Research Training Network CavNET MRTN-CT-2006–035367, the Deutsche Forschungsgemeinschaft DFG-Kni-316-4-1 and Hahn Stiftung (Index AG). The authors acknowledge support by Deutsche Forschungsgemeinschaft and the Open Access Publishing Fund of Tuebingen University. The funders had no role in study design, data collection and analysis, decision to publish, or preparation of the manuscript.

Competing Interests: The authors have declared that no competing interests exist.

* E-mail: marlies.knipper@uni-tuebingen.de

9 These authors contributed equally to this work.

Introduction

Tinnitus is a brain disorder causally linked to noise-induced hearing loss, cochlear damage [1], and stress [2,3,4,5,6,7]. Due to demographic changes and to increasing use of personal headsets, especially by young people [8], tinnitus is a cumulative challenge. In both tinnitus patients and tinnitus animal models, cochlear damage has been suggested to be associated with subcortical and cortical hyperactivity [1,9,10,11,12,13,14]. Subcortical hyperactivity was observed as increases in spontaneous and evoked spike activity at the level of the dorsal cochlear nucleus (DCN), ventral cochlear nucleus (VCN) and the inferior colliculus (IC) following cochlear damage [12,15,16,17,18,19,20].

To study central responsiveness to auditory trauma related to tinnitus, we used a tinnitus animal model that was designed to minimize stress based on access to sugar water as a positive reward [21,22]. Unlike most previous studies on tinnitus, we analyzed equally hearing-impaired animals which, based on their behavior, were separated into groups with and without tinnitus [23]. These groups were compared for (i) the number of CtBP2/RIBEYE-positive particles in ribbon synapses of the inner hair cell (IHC) as

a measure for deafferentation [24], (ii) the fine structure of the amplitudes of auditory brainstem response (ABR) waves that may reflect crucial differences in sound responses following decreased auditory nerve (AN) activity [25], and (iii) the expression pattern of the rapid immediate early gene Arc/Arg3.1 (activity-regulated cytoskeleton-associated protein/activity-regulated gene 3.1, for simplicity henceforth referred to as Arc) in the auditory cortex (AC).

Arc expression is involved in acute and long-lasting alterations of network activity as a consequence of altered sensory input [26,27]. Most importantly Arc mobilization is essential for homeostatic adaptation of responsiveness following visual deprivation during development [28,29]. In order to identify a tinnitus-specific trait rats were exposed to noise and were behaviorally separated into tinnitus and no-tinnitus animals. Animals were analyzed 1–4 weeks after exposure for hearing loss, damage of the IHC synapse, changes in ABR wave amplitude and cortical Arc expression. IHCs ribbon loss (deafferentation) did not lead to tinnitus when brainstem responses were restored and Arc was mobilized in the AC. When brainstem responses remain reduced and Arc was not mobilized, IHC ribbon loss resulted in tinnitus.

Both response patterns were found independent of low frequency threshold loss. The results are discussed in the context of a facilitating adaptive (no tinnitus) or non-adaptive (tinnitus) brain response following injury.

Materials and Methods

In order to identify a tinnitus-specific difference between equally acoustically exposed animals with and without tinnitus (tinnitus-trait), we exposed rats binaurally to noise and behaviorally identified animals with tinnitus. In this model, rats are trained to associate white noise with a sugar water reward and silence with no reward [22]. When rats perceive tinnitus after noise trauma, they incorrectly access the liquid reward because they hear their tinnitus. This access behavior is expressed as silence activity.

To increase the likelihood of detecting a tinnitus-trait, we used various noise conditions. To assure specificity, tinnitus was evaluated in both groups by the same criteria (silence activity >0.1), independently of the hearing loss of individuals. One group of animals was exposed to noise at a sound pressure level of 120 decibels (dB sound pressure level, SPL) at 10 kilo Hertz (kHz) for 1 hour (h) and analyzed 6 days (d) post exposure, when no further recovery of hearing was expected to occur. Another group of animals was exposed to 120 dB SPL for 1.5 h. Since the exposure for 1.5 h resulted in a stronger trauma, we analyzed these animals 30 d post exposure to make certain that the hearing and the tinnitus had recovered at its best and no further recovery of threshold was expected.

Hearing function was studied by ABRs evoked with short acoustic stimuli before and after noise exposure, at the same day as behavioral testing. ABRs represent the summed activity of neurons in the ascending auditory pathway and are measured by averaging the evoked electrical response recorded via subcutaneous electrodes.

1.1 Ethics Statement, Animals, and Noise Exposure

Animal care, procedures, and treatments were performed in accordance with institutional and national guidelines following approval by the University of Tübingen, Veterinary Care Unit, and the Animal Care and Ethics Committee of the regional board of the Federal State Government of Baden-Württemberg, Germany (approval number HN5/05).

Adult female Wistar rats weighing 200–300 g were exposed in anesthesia to sound (120 dB SPL), or sham exposed with loud speaker switched off, for either 1 h or 1.5 h, at 10 kHz and sacrificed 6 d, or 30 d after [23].

Animals were anesthetized with a mixture of ketamine–hydrochloride (75 mg/kg body weight, Ketavet 100, Pharmacia, Erlangen, Germany) and xylazine hydrochloride (5 mg/kg body weight, Rompun 290, Bayer, Leverkusen, Germany), injected i.p. Anesthetized rats were binaurally exposed to free field inside a reverberating chamber (a chamber of ca. 50×50×50 cm with tilted, non-parallel walls to avoid standing waves and to achieve a mostly homogeneous sound field). To eliminate furthermore the effects of any possible inhomogeneity in the acoustic field and to avoid that ear were positioned at sites of pressure wave extinction animals were slowly constantly moved through the sound field by means of a rotating turntable and were repositioned on this table in intervals of 30 minutes to ensure a homogeneous exposure of all animals on both ears. The reverberating chamber was equipped with top and side wall mounted speakers (DR48, Visaton, Haan, Germany, and Piezo Horn 335835, Conrad Electronic, Hirschau, Germany). The loudness and spectrum of the traumatizing sound was constantly monitored my means of a microphone placed in the centre of the chamber and customized computer software analyzing the frequency spectrum by fast fourier transformation (FFT). The traumatizing sound had a narrow peak at 10 kHz and sidebands at 20 kHz (−40 dB) and 30 kHz (−60 dB). Additional side bands were below 50 dB SPL and therefore did not exceed the normal laboratory background noise.

Additional doses of anaesthetics were administered if needed and body temperature maintained by heating pads and lamps.

1.2 Hearing Measurements

ABRs were measured in a soundproof chamber (IAC 400-A, Industrial Acoustics Company GmbH, Niederkrüchten, Germany) as described [30,31,32]. In short, ABRs were recorded in anesthetized adult animals. Electrical brainstem responses to free field click (100 µs, 0–90 dB SPL), and pure tone (1–45 kHz in half-octave steps, 20–100 dB SPL in steps of 5 dB, 3 ms, 1 ms cosine squared rise-fall envelope) acoustic stimuli of alternating polarity (compression and rarefaction) were recorded with subdermal silver wire electrodes at the ear (positive, active), the vertex (negative, reference) and the back of the animals (ground). Recordings were made for 10 ms with stimulus presentations of alternating polarity to eliminate electrical artefacts. In each case, stimulus presentation was at time 0 ms. The click stimulus was a broadband stimulus with a center frequency at 4.9 kHz (50th percentile) and the 25th and 75th percentiles at 2.2 kHz and 13.8 kHz, respectively. Signals were amplified (50,100-fold, 94 dB), bandpass filtered (0.2–5 kHz 6-pole Butterworth filter, Wulf Elektronik, Frankfurt, Germany), averaged across 64–256 repetitions (dependent on the signal to noise ratio, but always the same repetition time at close threshold stimulation) at each sound pressure presented (usually 0–100 dB SPL in steps of 5 dB), and recorded at 10 kHz sample frequency. Stimuli were delivered to the ear in a calibrated open system by a loudspeaker (DT-911, Beyerdynamic, Heilbronn, Germany) placed 3 cm lateral to the animal's pinna. Sound pressure was calibrated online prior to each measurement with a microphone (B&K 4191, Bruel & Kjaer, Naerum, Denmark) placed near the animal's ear.

For stimulus generation and recording of ABRs, a multifunction IO-Card (PCI-6052E or PCI-MIO-16E1, National Instruments, Austin, Texas, USA) was used, housed in an IBM compatible computer. Sound pressure level was controlled with an attenuator and amplifier (Wulf Elektronik). Filter settings, ABR spectral components (by FFT), potential stimulus artefacts were examined beforehand to ensure that ABR signal waveform, amplitude and latencies of distinct peaks in the ABR were not affected by the chosen hardware and software parameters. In particular, to reduce physical stress of the animals by long lasting anaesthesia to a minimum, ABR measurement times were reduced to a minimum by increasing stimulus repetition rates to 80/s, minimizing repetition numbers for clearly suprathreshold signals (when ABR wave amplitudes were exceeding ±4 µV), and reducing sample rates to 10 kHz to reduced delay times by computer online analyses. In control studies it was validated that the protocols that were finally used (64–256 repetitions, 0.2–5 kHz bandpass filtering, 10 kHz sampling rate), gave homogeneous results as compared to higher repetition numbers (512) and higher (100 kHz) sample rates.

Hearing threshold was determined by the lowest sound pressure that produced visually distinct evoked potentials from above threshold to near threshold.

1.3 ABR Analysis

For each individual ear, the auditory brainstem response (ABR) waveform to click stimuli (*waveform analysis*), and the peak input-output function (*peak I/O*) was analyzed.

Waveform analysis. The ABR wave functions of individuals were averaged. Average curves were built for four different groups: (1) no-tinnitus rats before exposure, (2) no-tinnitus rats after exposure, (3) tinnitus rats before exposure, and (4) tinnitus rats after exposure. For all four groups, the ABR functions were analyzed at a stimulus level of 90 dB SPL (a high stimulus level) and at 40 dB above hearing threshold (40 dB hearing level). The average waveforms gave a qualitative and temporal assessment of changes in amplitude ranges in the ABR function.

Peak I/O analysis. The ABR wave data for the click stimuli were analyzed for peak and through amplitudes and the latencies by customized computer programs.

From individual ABR waves to click stimuli, peak amplitudes and peak latencies were collected, grouped in clusters of similar peak amplitude and latencies, and averaged for ABR wave input-output (I/O) analysis. Wave amplitudes were defined as peak to peak amplitude of a negative peak (n) followed by a positive (p) peak. Clusters of peaks were found at average latencies n0.9-p1.2, n1.3-p1.6, n1.9-p2.4 or p2.7, n3.6-p4.9, and n7.1-p9.4. The ABR recordings are presented for the first 10 ms recording time. To affirm that the peak at p9.4 was not missed out due to a peak latency longer than 10 ms, the whole recording cycle consisting of a compression and a rarefaction stimulus (lasting 20 ms, see above: hearing measurements) was analyzed and the peak position approved within the first 10 ms. For selected peaks and troughs the I/O functions were derived from the peak-to-peak amplitudes at all recorded stimulus sound pressure levels. Three peak classes were selected: (1) early peaks (at 0.9–1.2 ms, with the "wave I" interpreted as the sum of the first stimulus-related action potential within the auditory nerve); (2) delayed peaks (at 3.6–4.9 ms), found in the range of the greatest loss of the ABR waveform (as determined by analyzing the square difference between ABR curves before and after noise exposure, not shown); and (3) late peaks (at 7.1–9.4 ms), as these peaks fall into the time range of thalamic activation.

Waveform correlation analysis. The similarity in the waveform of the ABR before and after an acoustic noise exposure is founded on changes of all peak amplitudes and all peak latencies. In human tinnitus studies, often the relation of wave-I to wave-V is reported [33]. Since these parameters are circumstantial to describe in the rat ABR data, we applied a general measure for the "similarity" of ABR waves: As an estimation for the recovery of click-ABR waves after acoustic noise exposure, correlation of ABR waves before and after recovery (6–30 d) were analyzed by the correlation factor (CorF):

$$CorF = \frac{Cov(A_{Pre}, A_{Post})}{Var_{Pre}}$$

where

Cov: covariance of the click-ABR waves before exposure and after recovery

A_{Pre}: the amplitudes at point 1 to 100 (0–10 ms) before exposure

A_{Post}: the amplitudes at point 1 to 100 (0–10 ms) after exposure

Var_{Pre} variance of the click-ABR wave before exposure

CorF: correlation factor (covariance/variance) $\in R$

The CorF therefore provides a normalization of the covariance with respect to the variance of the measurement before exposure.

In contrast to the correlation by the Pearson Momentum Coefficient that is not sensitive to overall amplitude changes, the CorF reflects changes in waveform and amplitude. Typical values are 1.0 for optimal correlation between waveforms of similar amplitude values. Loss of similarity and loss of amplitude typically result in CorF values approaching null.

1.4 Behavioral Animal Model

Within 3–4 months before the noise exposure, rats were trained using operant conditioning to perform a specific motor task (foraging behavior for sugar water, on average 1–3 timely randomized rewards per minute) when perceiving an external sound cue (presented for 1–3 minutes) and to cease this motor activity during periods of silence (lasting 40–120 seconds, accesses during silence were randomly paired with electrical foot shocks of 0.1–0.4 mA, 100 µs). A conditioning session lasted 20–60 minutes containing 10–30 silence and sound periods, sound stimuli were varied between 70 and 10 dB SPL (in steps of 10 dB), and 32–38 sessions were required to train the rats to meet the training criterion. Correct indication of tinnitus of either rats was tested by transient tinnitus induction after salicylate injection (350 mg/kg bodyweight) [22] In test situation, rewards and foot shocks were omitted and sound (broad band noise sound of 60 dB SPL) and silence periods (60 s each) were presented interleaved for 23 minutes, as described [22]. Animals with tinnitus actively execute the motor task even when the external sound cue has not been presented, for details see [22]. A detailed protocol for noise-induced tinnitus is described in [23]. The motor task was quantified by the ratio of activity during external sound and the activity during periods of silence (silence activity). Typical values for silence activity are below 0.1 for no-tinnitus and above 0.1 for tinnitus animals, dependent on the conditioning level. White noise sound stimuli were presented for operant conditioning and testing in the experimental phase. These stimuli could easily be generalized by rats with their induced tinnitus percept, even if (for our particular method of induction) this tinnitus percept was of unknown frequency and loudness.

1.5 Tissue Preparation

Cochlear and brain tissues were dissected as previously described [23]. For detection of mRNA and protein, brains were fixed for 48 h in 4% paraformaldehyde, embedded in 4% agarose and stored at 4°C. The tissue was sectioned at 60 µm with the Leica VT 1000S vibratome (Wetzlar, Germany).

1.6 Immunohistochemistry and Ribbon Counts

Rat cochleae were isolated, fixed, cryosectioned, and stained as described in [23]. Mouse monoclonal anti-CtPB2/RIBEYE antibody (BD Transduction Laboratories, San Jose, CA, USA) and rabbit polyclonal anti-GluR4 antibody (Millipore, Schwalbach, Germany) were used as primary antibodies. Image acquisition and CtBP2/RIBEYE-immunopositive spot counting were carried out as previously described [34]. In brief, cryosectioned cochleae were imaged over a distance of 8 µm covering the entire IHC nucleus and areas beyond it in an image stack along the z-axis (z-stack). One z-stack consisted of 30 layers with a z-increment of 0.28 µm; for each layer, one image per fluorochrome was acquired. To display spatial protein distribution, z-stacks were three-dimensionally deconvoluted using Cell F's RIDE module with the Nearest Neighbor Algorithm, Voxel Viewer, and Slice Viewer (Cell F, OSIS 231 GmbH, Münster, Germany).

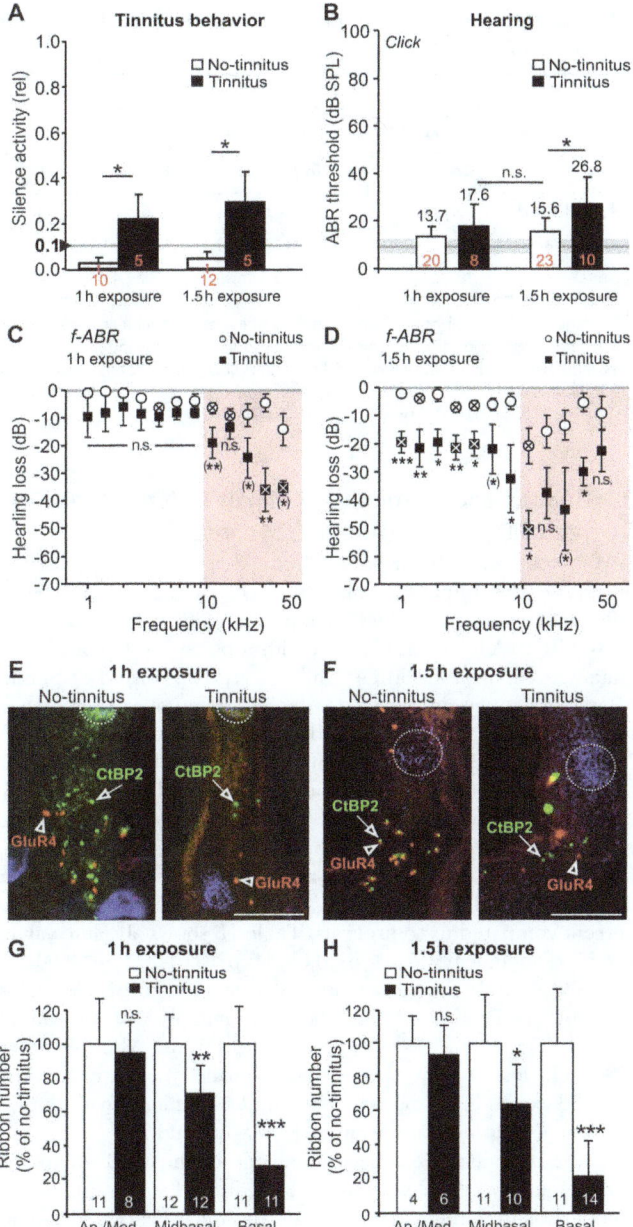

Figure 1. Development of tinnitus in equally sound-exposed animals correlates with altered structure of the IHC synapse. (**A**) Following exposure to 120 dB SPL at 10 kHz for 1 h (assessed at 6 d after exposure) or for 1.5 h (assessed at 30 d after exposure), tinnitus occurred in ~30% of the animals. Mean silence activity (± S.D.) as a measure for tinnitus for no-tinnitus (white) and tinnitus animals (black). The criterion for tinnitus was a silence activity above 0.1 (horizontal grey line, black triangle on ordinate). Number of animals is given in or below the bars. (**B**) A significant difference in the hearing threshold to click stimuli was only observed between animals with or without tinnitus after 1.5 h exposure. Mean (± S.D.) ABR thresholds for click stimuli of no-tinnitus (white) and tinnitus animals (black), tinnitus judged from their silence activity. Hearing threshold is depicted above each bar. Number of animals is given within each bar. The grey horizontal line and area illustrates the mean ABR threshold (± S.D.) before exposure. (**C, D**) High-frequency hearing is impaired following noise exposure, more pronounced in tinnitus animals than in no-tinnitus animals. Following 1.5 h exposure (**D**), also low-frequency hearing is impaired in tinnitus animals. Mean ABR threshold loss (dB, ± S.E.M.) to frequency-specific tone bursts for no-tinnitus (circles) and tinnitus animals (squares). The grey line at the top of each panel shows the normal

hearing threshold before exposure. Frequencies with a significant hearing loss (>99% confidence interval of hearing threshold before exposure) are marked by crossed symbols. Frequencies with a significantly different loss between no-tinnitus and tinnitus animals are indicated by asterisks (Student's t-Test with Bonferroni-Holms adjustments for alpha-shifts). Asterisks in brackets indicate descriptive statistics for p-values from t-tests that fail to meet the Bonferroni-Holms criterion. n.s. not significant. (**E, F**) Antibody staining for GluR4 (red, open arrowhead) and ribbon synapses (CtBP2, green, open arrow) are shown for the IHCs of the midbasal turn for the animals used in (A, B). Cell nuclei are stained with DAPI (blue). Scale bars, 10 μm. (**G**) IHC ribbon numbers of control and no-tinnitus animals were not significantly different. IHC ribbon numbers of hearing-impaired tinnitus animals were significantly reduced in the midbasal and basal turns in comparison to no-tinnitus animals. Ribbon counts were compared for statistical significance using the 1-way ANOVA, p-values were corrected for alpha-shift by multiple testing using the Bonferroni-Holms procedure, df = 8.
doi:10.1371/journal.pone.0057247.g001

1.7 Co-localization of mRNA and Protein in Brain Sections

Riboprobes were designed as described in [23]. mRNA and protein were co-localized on free-floating sections. Following pre-hybridization for 1 h at 37°C, sections were incubated overnight with Arc riboprobes at 56°C, incubated with anti-digoxigenin antibody conjugated to alkaline phosphatase (anti-Dig-AP, Roche, Mannheim, Germany) and developed as previously described [35]. For protein detection, streptavidin-biotin was blocked according to the manufacturer's instructions (Streptavidin-Biotin Blocking Kit, Vector Laboratories, Burlingame, CA, USA) after blocking endogenous peroxidase. Sections were incubated overnight at 4°C with the primary antibodies against Arc (Synaptic Systems, Göttingen, Germany), followed by incubation with the secondary antibody (biotinylated goat anti-rabbit, Vector Laboratories) and chromogenic detection (AEC, 3-amino-9-ethylcarbazole, Vector Laboratories). Sections were counterstained with the nuclear marker methyl-green (Vector Laboratories), embedded with gelatin, and analyzed using an Olympus AX70 microscope.

1.8 Data Analysis

Statistical analysis. Correlation factors and hearing loss were compared using Student's t-Test. The statistical significance at the alpha level of 0.05 is indicated in the figure legends.

Tinnitus behavior was compared using the Mann-Whitney-U Test. For the ribbon counts of apical, medial and basal cochlear turns, P-values were corrected for alpha-shift by multiple testing using the Bonferroni-Holms procedure.

Ribbon numbers from 3–5 animals from 3 independent experiments per group were counted and compared by 1-way ANOVA. For the ribbon counts of apical, medial and basal cochlear turns, P-values were corrected for alpha-shift by multiple testing using the Bonferroni-Holms procedure.

Quantification of Arc/Arg3.1 positive cells in the AC. Arc mRNA expressing cells were counted in the AC as previously described [35]. In brief, Arc immunoreactive cells were counted in the AC of coronal brain sections using an integrated microscopic counting chamber to fix the area of interest delineated by a square of 2,450 μm2. The number of Arc positive cells from eight 2,450 μm2 squares on four rat brain sections for each treatment group (between 4.2 and 5.2 mm posterior to Bregma) [36] including the 10 kHz region of the auditory cortex were counted throughout the thickness of the slice, and the average was taken. These squares were placed with respect to the cellular anatomy of the AC: they covered cortical layers II to VI and spanned the bulk of the area designated as the primary AC according to Doron et al. [36]. Data are expressed as mean cell count ± S.E.M. Statistical analysis was performed using the two-tailed Student's *t* test, with alpha = 0.05. Cells were counted in 3 animals per group in three independent experiments.

Results

Behavioral testing [22,23] showed that ca. 30% of the animals in both groups (5 of 15 rats and 5 of 17 rats for the 1 h and 1.5 h exposure, respectively) had developed a significantly elevated silence activity, indicating occurrence of tinnitus (Fig. 1A, difference for both groups: p<0.02 for the Mann-Whitney-U Test).

ABR thresholds for click-stimuli (Fig. 1B, Table 1A) and frequency-specific stimuli (Fig. 1C and D, Table 1A) revealed a permanent, though mild, threshold loss in all animals that increased with exposure duration (Table 1A). ABR threshold loss for click stimuli was mild but significant for all groups (p = 0.0115, 0.0403, 0.0074 and 0.0004 for 1 h no-tinnitus, 1 h tinnitus, 1.5 h no-tinnitus, and 1.5 h tinnitus, respectively for the Student's t-Test). This indicates that a hearing loss to broadband click stimuli was not necessarily leading to tinnitus (studied by behavioral testing). Since the click stimulus contained frequencies predominantly in the lower frequency range of the hearing range of a rat (1–10 kHz), a loss of these frequencies may not be of relevance for inducing tinnitus. However, the group of tinnitus rats exposed to 1.5 h had a significantly larger hearing loss than no-tinnitus rats (Table 1A, 18.20±4.23; n = 5 for tinnitus rats), and also individual animals in both no-tinnitus groups showed significant hearing loss at isolated low frequencies (Fig. 1 C, D, crossed circles), what raises the question how hearing loss for low and high frequencies might contribute to the generation of tinnitus. To specify the hearing function in the high frequency hearing range of the rats we performed frequency specific ABR measurements. When frequency-specific ABR thresholds between tinnitus and no-tinnitus groups were compared, we consistently observed that in both tinnitus groups, hearing loss for frequencies above 11.3 kHz was significantly increased compared to no-tinnitus groups (Fig. 1C and D; Table 1A). After the more intense noise exposure (1.5 h), threshold loss in tinnitus animals was also significantly greater for low stimulus frequencies (Fig. 1D, *: p<0.05, **: p<0.01, ***: p<0.001, Student's t-Test with alpha correction for multiple comparison).

Although the various intensities of sound exposure led to a variable amount of hearing loss, the 1 h exposed tinnitus rats and the 1.5 h exposed tinnitus-free rats had a similar low frequency hearing function (Fig. 1B), though both groups had significant frequency specific hearing loss after noise exposure. This suggests that threshold loss at low frequencies per se is not leading to tinnitus. Animals with tinnitus had a characteristic threshold loss in the high-frequency regions.

Table 2. Number of inner hair cell ribbons in no-tinnitus and tinnitus animals.

	unexposed	1–1.5 h, 120 dB SPL		
	Control	No-tinnitus	Tinnitus	P
Apical/Med.	16.4±3.5	15.4±2.4 (n.s.)	14.6±1.2 (n.s.)	n.s.
Midbasal	20.7±4.0	18.6±2.8 (n.s.)	12.6±2.7 (***)	*
Basal	18.8±3.5	15.5±3.1 (n.s.)	4.3±2.4 (***)	***

Average number of ribbons counted in IHCs of indicated cochlear turns from 3–5 animals (corresponding to animals measured in A) from 3 independent experiments. Statistics in brackets indicate differences in comparison to control, P indicates differences between no-tinnitus and tinnitus animals (n.s.: not significant, *: p<0.05, **: p<0.01, ***: p<0.001).

2.1 Tinnitus and No-tinnitus Animals Differ in their Degree of Damage at the IHC Synapse

We counted IHC ribbons from 3–5 animals per group (unexposed, no-tinnitus, tinnitus) as a correlate of the number of afferent auditory fibers [24,37] using antibodies directed against CtBP2/RIBEYE in combination with a postsynaptic marker, the glutamate receptor isoform 4 (GluR4) [24] (Fig. 1E and F). Similar to previous studies in mice [24], the highest number of ribbons in rats was detected in the midbasal cochlear turn (Table 1B). Number of IHC ribbons for unexposed control and no-tinnitus animals were not significantly different (Fig. 1 G, Table 1 B). Animals with tinnitus showed a significantly stronger loss of ribbons (up to 82%), most pronounced in the basal turn, covering frequencies above 17 kHz, and midbasal turn, covering frequencies above ~11 kHz [38] (Fig. 1G show ribbon numbers in percent compared to control rats, Table 1B shows absolute values, n = 35, done in triplicate, *: p<0.05, **: p<0.01, ***: p<0.001, 1-way ANOVA). In the apical and medial cochlear turns, ribbon loss was not significantly different between animals with or without tinnitus (Fig. 1G, Table 1B, n.s., not significant, Mann-Whitney Test). The loss of afferent fibers was confirmed qualitatively by the reduced expression of postsynaptic GluR4 in animals with tinnitus as compared to no-tinnitus animals (Fig. 1E and F).

These data indicate a severe damage of the IHC synapse in high-frequency cochlear turns of animals with tinnitus in comparison to tinnitus-free animals with similar hearing thresholds for click auditory stimuli (Fig. 1B).

Table 1. Hearing loss in no-tinnitus and tinnitus animals.

	Click-ABR		F-ABR >11.3 kHz	
	1 h, 120 dB SPL	1.5 h, 120 dB SPL	1 h, 120 dB SPL	1.5 h, 120 dB SPL
No-tinnitus	3.4±3.2; n = 10	6.1±4.2; n = 12	7.9±5.6; n = 10	11.5±10.6; n = 12
Tinnitus	7.4±5.5; n = 5	18.2±8.1; n = 5	22.8±8.5; n = 5	38.7±15.1; n = 5
Significance	n.s.	***	**	**

Hearing loss (in dB) in no-tinnitus and tinnitus animals following 1 h or 1.5 h exposure using click- and frequency-specific stimuli. Animals were either exposed to 120 dB SPL, 10 kHz for 1 h and analyzed after 6 d or exposed for 1.5 h and analyzed after 30 d. The groups are subdivided in tinnitus animals and no-tinnitus animals. A significant difference in hearing threshold was observed between no-tinnitus and tinnitus animals following exposure at stimulus frequencies of 11.3 kHz and above (*: p<0.05, **: p<0.01, ***: p<0.001).

2.2 Tinnitus and No-tinnitus Animals Differ in their ABR Wave Size (Synaptic Responses) Following Auditory Deprivation

IHC ribbons determine the generation of spikes in afferent auditory fibers [39]. The summed activity of the auditory nerve is determined by the synchronicity and the reliability of spikes within active fibers [40]. This activity propagates in the ascending auditory pathway and generates the ABR waves in the ventral cochlear nucleus (VCN, wave II, Fig. 2, <p1.2), superior olivary complex (SOC, wave III, Fig. 2<p3.6), responses in the lateral lemniscus and the IC (wave IV, Fig. 2>p4.9) as well as the IC output activity (wave V, Fig. 2>p7.1) [41].

Click-evoked ABR waveform amplitudes before and after noise exposure were compared for differences in signal amplitudes for 1 h (no-tinnitus: n = 10 animals; tinnitus: n = 5 animals) and 1.5 h exposure duration (no-tinnitus: n = 12 animals; tinnitus: n = 5 animals) at 40 dB above threshold and 90 dB SPL (Fig. 2A and B). These conditions allow to distinguish between response amplitudes derived from low-threshold fibers (~60%) with a high spontaneous rate (high-SR) that have a fast saturation at about 40 dB SPL, and amplitudes from high-threshold fibers (~40%) with a low spontaneous rate (low-SR) that respond to higher SPLs [42], in this case to a 90 dB SPL stimulus.

As expected from the permanent, although mild, hearing loss to click stimuli within both groups (Fig. 1B, Table 1A), a reduction in the overall amplitude of the sound-evoked signals compared to the waveform prior to exposure was observed in animals with and without tinnitus (Fig. 2A and B) for 90 dB SPL (upper row) and 40 dB (lower row). For both stimuli conditions the correlation analysis of the ABR waves (CorF) revealed a reduced recovery for tinnitus animals in comparison to tinnitus-free animals (Fig. 2C and D) across the whole input/output (I/O) range of stimulus levels (Fig. 2E).

This suggests that both, high-SR, low level and low-SR, high level auditory fibers might be affected. This was studied by the I/O growth of the dominant peaks (indicated in Fig. 2A, arrowheads) before and after exposure (Fig. 3). Importantly, the amplitude waves of the early peaks (Fig. 3, Early), corresponding to the AN or cochlear nucleus (CN), were reduced in animals with and without tinnitus following both exposure protocols (1 h or 1.5 h, 120 dB SPL, 10 kHz). ABR amplitude wave size remained reduced particularly at lower threshold levels up to 60 dB SPL (Fig. 3, Early), indicating that responsiveness of afferent fibers with both high-SR (low-threshold) and low-SR (high-threshold) are affected.

We need to point out that click stimuli are used that are dominated by frequencies lower than 10 kHz (see methods 2.2). As shown by [43] for cats following middle to high frequency noise trauma, units with low characteristic frequencies (CFs) still respond at threshold, though amplitudes of compound action potential (CAP) responses are reduced. In accordance, we found a moderate ABR threshold loss using the click stimuli which are predominately stimulating cochlear regions below 10 kHz. We therefore would not expect to find differences of early peak amplitudes (ABR wave I) between tinnitus and no-tinnitus rats.

However, for tinnitus-free animals, amplitude functions improved at delayed peaks and showed nearly complete recovery at late peaks compared to animals with tinnitus (compare Fig. 3, *Delayed* and *Late*). This suggested that in tinnitus-free animals, responsiveness to sound at the level of the lateral lemniscus and inferior colliculus (IC) (*Delayed*) or at the level of the IC output and medial geniculate body (MGB) (*Late*) is enhanced, in comparison to animals with tinnitus. As cochlear CF regions of best hearing of the animals are the main source

of ABR waves generated in higher brain regions (wave V, [44], the difference in high-frequency CF regions above 11.3 kHz between tinnitus-free and tinnitus animals is likely the drive for less or more elevated late peaks in higher brain regions of these animals. Pure tone stimuli with frequencies above 10 kHz would be expected to result in differential growth function also in early peaks between tinnitus and no-tinnitus animals. In future studies this aspect will be analyzed in detail. However, due to the hearing loss at higher frequencies, ABR wave I response for high-frequency and moderate sound pressure stimulation is expected to be small in case of trauma.

2.3 Tinnitus and No-tinnitus Animals Differ in Arc Levels in Sensory-deprived Cortical Regions

To further analyze to what extent the differences in ABR wave sizes may be linked to gain in central auditory circuits, we studied the expression of Arc mRNA and protein to trace neurons that are long-lastingly activated [26,27,45]. We used a method that permits the simultaneous monitoring of expression changes in Arc mRNA and protein.

A significant decline of Arc expression in neurons was found in all layers of the AC of animals with tinnitus monitored following both exposure protocols (1 h, 120 dB SPL, 10 kHz, Fig. 4A and C and 1.5 h, 120 dB SPL, 10 kHz, Fig. 4B and C) in comparison to no-tinnitus animals (n = 3 animals, p<0.001 for unpaired Student's t-test, α = 0.05).

The observation that Arc expression levels are reduced in the AC only in those animals that also exhibit reduced IHC ribbon numbers, reduced ABR wave size and tinnitus, strengthens the argument that animals with tinnitus have developed a rather reduced (instead of enhanced) responsiveness of central circuits.

Discussion

The present study compared markers for deafferentation, brainstem responsiveness and homeostatic plasticity in equally acoustically exposed animals that were behaviorally separated into groups of animals with and without tinnitus. A characteristic pattern of severe IHCs ribbon loss, insufficiently restored late ABR wave and a failure to mobilize Arc in the cortex could be linked to high-frequency hearing impairment and tinnitus. This finding is discussed in the context of a failure to recruit central gain following cochlear deprivation as a correlate of tinnitus.

3.1 Behaviorally-tested Tinnitus is Associated with IHC Ribbon Loss

To assure the specificity of a tinnitus-specific trait, this trait should be a discrete property, independent of hearing loss. The rats with tinnitus after a mild trauma (1 h) and the rats in the no-tinnitus group after mild (1 h) and a more extensive trauma (1.5 h) had a similar low frequency hearing. This indicates that the amount of threshold loss required for tinnitus induction is not necessarily of a uniform dimension, as already suggested by other authors [46,47,48,49]. Indeed various investigations show tinnitus to occur even when hearing impairment cannot be detected by hearing threshold tests [47,50,51].

Irrespective of the amount of hearing impairment, we observed that tinnitus was coupled to severe IHC ribbon loss after both exposure durations in 30% of animals, an incidence also observed among hearing-impaired humans [1] but different from the 50–70% of tinnitus animals depicted using gap-detection methods [16,52].

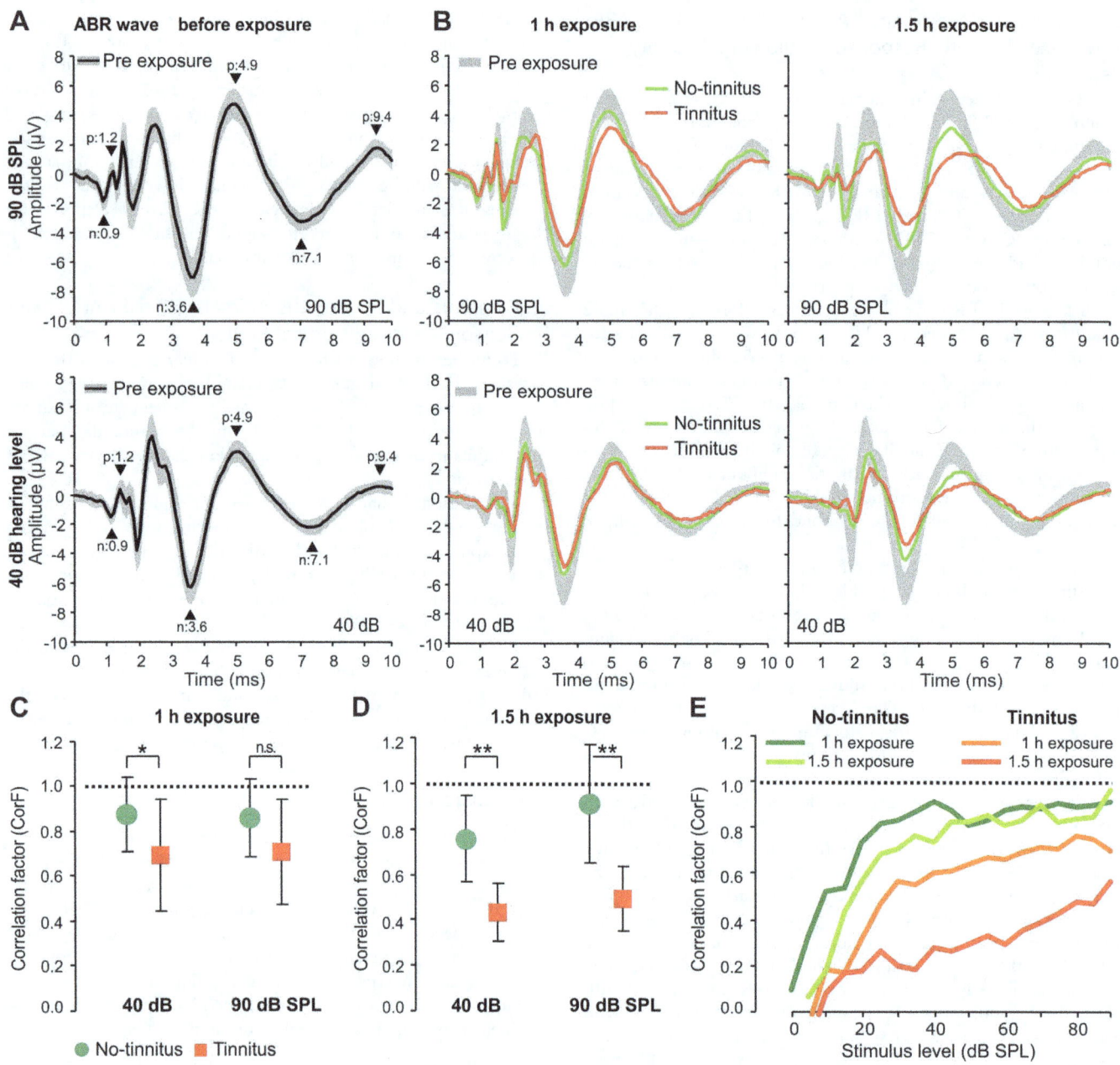

Figure 2. Changes in ABR waveforms following noise exposure is more pronounced in animals with tinnitus. (A) Average ABR waveform before exposure at stimulation level 90 dB SPL (upper panel) and 40 dB above hearing threshold (lower panel). Mean (black line) ± S.D (grey area) of n = 32 animals. **(B)** ABR waves illustrating the difference in ABR waveform after 1 h (left panels) or 1.5 h (right panels) noise exposure for animals with (red) or without tinnitus (green) in comparison with the waveforms before noise exposure (mean ± S.D., black line and grey area) depicted for 90 dB SPL (upper panels) and 40 dB above the hearing threshold (lower panels). **(C)** Correlation of ABRs to click stimuli before and after 1 h noise exposure of individual animals (expressed as the correlation factor (CorF) for close to threshold (40 dB hearing level) and at high stimulation levels (90 dB SPL). Mean (± S.D.) derived from n = 10 (No-tinnitus, green circles) and n = 5 (Tinnitus, red squares) rats. The correlation factor of 1 (dashed horizontal line) indicates a perfect similarity of ABR waveforms before and after noise exposure. Correlation was significantly lower in tinnitus animals at 40 dB. At 90 dB SPL, the difference was not quite significant (p = 0.055). **(D)** Correlation of ABRs to click stimuli before and after 1.5 h noise exposure. At both 40 dB and 90 dB SPL, the correlation factor of ABRs from animals with tinnitus was significantly reduced. n = 12 and 5 for no-tinnitus and tinnitus animals, respectively. * p 0.05, ** p<0.01, 1-sided t-Test. **(E)** Correlation of averaged ABRs to click stimuli as a function of stimulus levels (dB SPL). In all four groups, the correlation factor steeply increased at supra-threshold levels. For tinnitus animals, the ABR waveform correlation did not reach the value of no-tinnitus animals, indicating reduced amplitude and waveform recovery after noise exposure.

3.2 Differential IHC Ribbon Loss is Linked to Different ABR Wave Size in Higher Brain Regions

Approximately 20 ribbons tether synaptic vesicles in the active zones of an IHC [53], each driving a postsynaptic AN fiber [54]

and determining through the maintenance of a large releasable pool of synaptic vesicles the reliability and precision of spikes [39]. Typically, the spike response of AN runs through a maximal rate before approaching adapted rates [55]. As peak rates influence

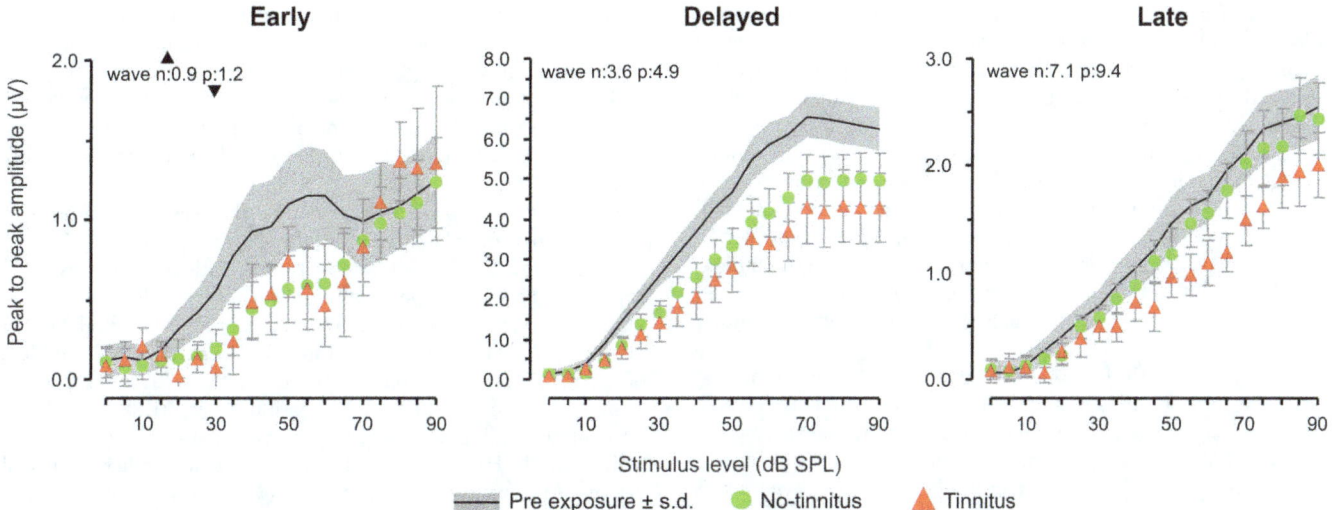

Figure 3. Peak-to-peak amplitudes of late peaks of ABR waves remain reduced following noise exposure in animals with tinnitus. Mean peak growth input/output (I/O) function (± S.D.) for early, delayed and late peaks before exposure (black line and grey shaded area) after 1 h or 1.5 h exposure. Three selected peak-to-peak amplitude growth functions (µV) with increasing stimulus levels (dB SPL) are shown for rats with tinnitus (green) or without tinnitus (red). In the rats with tinnitus, the peak-to-peak amplitudes remain reduced up to late peaks (right panel). The peak latencies are given in each panel for negative (n) and positive (p) peaks.

ABR thresholds, severe ribbon loss would lead to worsened thresholds despite intact outer hair cell (OHC) function [39]. This would explain why tinnitus animals with severe ribbon loss exhibit higher ABR thresholds in affected regions (Fig. 1C and D). ABR threshold loss in high-frequency regions was also detected in subjectively normal-hearing tinnitus patients [56].

Using click stimuli spectrally dominated by frequencies below 10 kHz, we found mild and similar but significant hearing loss (3–18 dB, Fig. 1B, Table 1A) and ABR wave I reduction in tinnitus and no-tinnitus animals (Fig. 3), indicating that units with low characteristic frequencies (CFs) were only slightly affected following moderate noise trauma, independent of a strong damage of units with high CFs, as also shown for cats [43]. High CF regions

of the cochlea participate in the generation of ABR waves in higher brain regions [44] and may thus be directly linked to differences in ABR wave size at delayed (lateral lemniscus, IC) and late peaks (IC output, MGB) in animals with tinnitus (Fig. 3). The 82% ribbon loss in animals with tinnitus must include low-threshold afferent fibers with high-SR since this fiber class comprises 60% of afferent fibers [42]. A loss of high-SR fibers has been already previously observed in tinnitus studies [46]. Based on computational models of tinnitus development [15,57,58], it was hypothesized that deafferentation of a substantial fraction of the AN fibers, as observed in mice following "temporary" hearing loss [24], could trigger the development of elevation of central spontaneous firing rates [57,58,59]. This

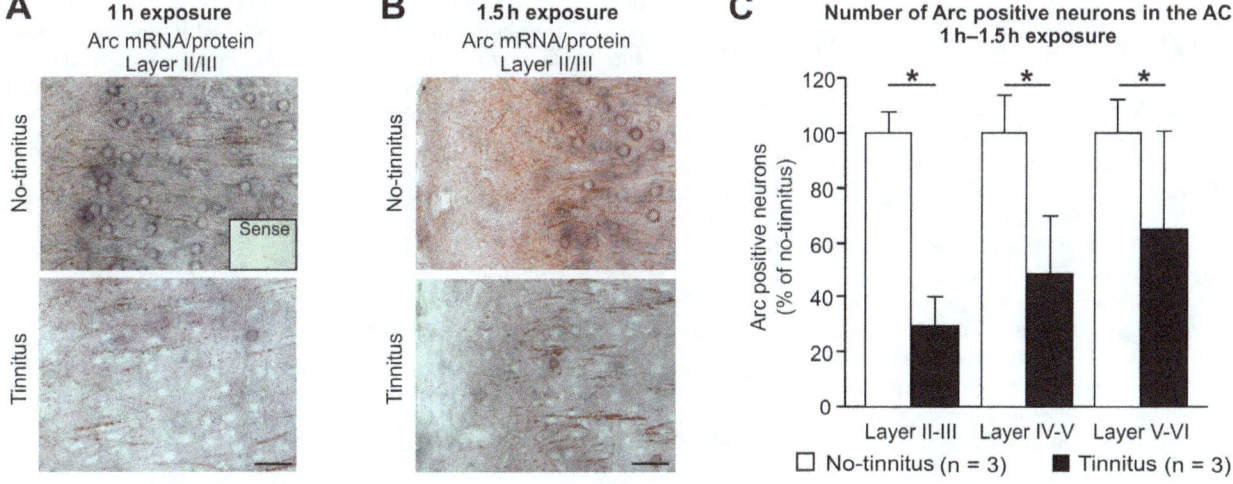

Figure 4. Silencing of Arc expression in auditory cortex (AC) in animals with tinnitus. (A, B) Double detection of Arc mRNA (blue) and Arc protein (red) in the AC of equally noise-exposed rats shows a significantly reduced expression in animals with tinnitus in all cortical layers, quantified in **(C**, unpaired Students t-test, p<0.001, alpha = 0.05, df = 6). Scale bars, 50 µm. n = 3 animals per group in three independent experiments. Images correspond to coronal sections 2.5 and 3.6 mm posterior to Bregma. Hybridization with sense riboprobes plus omission of the primary antibody produced no signals (insert in A, Sense).

elevation of central spontaneous firing rates following deafferentation would be accompanied by enhancement of neural synchrony [57] in the ascending auditory pathway leading to increased central gain, as suggested in a gain adaptation model for tinnitus [15]. This model suggests that increased central gain in the frequency range that is affected by hearing loss [60] is generated through deficit in AN function manifested as a reduction in nerve output at high sound levels, indicating deafferentation of high-threshold low-SR AN fibers [17]. Whether increased central gain fails to be generated when a critical number of low-threshold high-SR AN fibers is lost, as suggested in the present study to occur in tinnitus animals, needs to be analyzed in more detail in future studies.

The restored ABR waves observed here in hearing impaired animals without tinnitus mainly reflect spreading activity through the VCN but not DCN [41]. Higher discharge rates generated in the VCN following acoustic trauma have been shown to lead to steeply increasing loudness recruitment during hyperacusis [61,62,63]. We therefore hypothesize that the differences in Delayed and Late ABR waves observed here between tinnitus and tinnitus–free animals reflect differences in compensating increases in VCN activity between tinnitus and hyperacusis animals both occurring as a consequence of reduced cochlear input [61].

As our results show that ABR waves are restored in the tinnitus-free situation, the findings do not support the idea that increased responsiveness in CN target neurons is a correlate for tinnitus. [17,60]. In this context it must be considered that previous studies never compared the central responsiveness in equally traumatized animals, and so far no patients with hearing loss (reduced wave I) but without tinnitus have been studied [17].

The more restored ABR waves in tinnitus-free animals may reflect a form of loudness recruitment or hyperacusis and the less restored ABR waves in tinnitus animals a reduced capacity to compensate missing gain in the ascending pathway. Data would thereby experimentally support a recent computational model that suggests steeper rate level function in brainstem neurons as the source of non-linear gain that produces loudness recruitment and hyperacusis [64]. Accordingly, in patients with both tinnitus and hyperacusis, steeper than normal loudness growth functions were found, while tinnitus patients without threshold loss had normal loudness growth at the tinnitus frequency [65].

3.3 Reduced ABR Wave Size is Correlated with Reduced Arc Levels in the AC

In the cortex, Arc mRNA is expressed in non-GABAergic glutamatergic neurons [26,27,66,67,68,69].

Arc mRNA is directly transported within minutes to distal dendrites following LTP like activity [70], where through sustained translation for 2–4 h, Arc protein scales surface AMPA receptors in dendritic spines up and down, a process essential for LTP consolidation, for review see [27,45,70,71,72,73,74]. Moreover, Arc mediated synaptic scaling is an essential need for a system to respond to continuous changes in activity, maintain averaged firing rate [75,76,77] and regulate cell-wide responses to long-term changes in activity including responses to reduced input [78] or e.g. visual deprivation [29]. (see for a review [45]. Arc mobilization has also been described in pyramidal neurons of layer II-III

following e.g. environmental enrichment [79] Furthermore, Arc mobilization is linked to higher density of dendritic spines [79] or increased sensitivity to glutamate and synaptic strength [28].

Since Arc protein is rapidly degraded [27] the long-lasting changes in Arc mRNA and protein observed in previous studies [80,81,82] and in the present study likely reflect permanently altered network activity.

While Arc mobilization in the cortex may elevate the sensitivity of cortical pyramidal neurons [28] the sensitivity after the failure to mobilize Arc, as observed here in tinnitus animals, remains to be explored. Plasticity, specifically homeostatic scaling, is highly sensitive to Arc levels. The scaling responses to manipulation of neuronal activity in vitro are lost in Arc KO neurons [73] and loss of Arc is disrupting the ability of spine formation [83]. Arc deletion has been shown to lead to an increase in basic mEPSCs [29] and development of highly synchronized epileptic-like cortical network activity [84]. High synchronization and epileptic-like neuronal activity in sensory-deprived frequency regions of the primary auditory cortex are also assumed to be associated with cortical activity changes during tinnitus [51,85,86,87]. Arc decline has been observed in cortical regions with reduced thalamo-cortical input in regions >8 kHz (determined by cortical field potentials) [23] tonotopically related to the regions where a decline of IHC ribbon numbers in the cochlea occurred (Fig. 1 G and F, see also [88] and where the most pronounced hearing deficit was observed (Fig. 1 C and D). The failure to mobilize Arc could explain the perception of the tinnitus pitch within the frequency deprived region [51,89]. Since we found a reduction of IHC ribbons and ABR waves that correlate with reduced Arc levels in the AC as a feature of tinnitus, we may conclude that potentiating activity essential to drive Arc mobilization [70,73,74] is obviously missing in the frequency deprived region during tinnitus.

The rapid deafferentation [24,90,91], and the rapid changes of Arc mobilization [27,45] would moreover be in line with the immediate and transient appearance of tinnitus and hyperacusis [92,93,94,95,96,97].

3.4 Conclusion

In conclusion, the current findings provide a rationale for the altered responsiveness of central circuitries after different degrees of IHC synapse and auditory fiber damage. The observed severe decline of ribbon numbers, the changes in ABR wave amplitudes and the failure to mobilize Arc in the AC strongly support the idea that increased neuronal activity in the auditory periphery is a compensation of peripheral input – avoiding tinnitus – rather than a correlate or even the origin of tinnitus.

Acknowledgments

We gratefully thank Prof. Jos Eggermont for critically reading an earlier version of this manuscript.

Author Contributions

Conceived and designed the experiments: LR WS RPW MK. Performed the experiments: LR WS RPW MM AZ HX. Analyzed the data: LR WS RPW MM SCL AZ MJ HX MK. Contributed reagents/materials/analysis tools: AZ UZ KR. Wrote the paper: LR WS RPW MK.

References

1. Lockwood AH, Salvi RJ, Burkard RF (2002) Tinnitus. N Engl J Med 347: 904–910.
2. Møller AR (2003) Pathophysiology of tinnitus. Otolaryngol Clin North Am 36: 249–266, v-vi.
3. Jastreboff PJ (2007) Tinnitus retraining therapy. Prog Brain Res 166: 415–423.
4. Zenner HP, Pfister M, Birbaumer N (2006) Tinnitus sensitization: Sensory and psychophysiological aspects of a new pathway of acquired centralization of chronic tinnitus. Otol Neurotol 27: 1054–1063.
5. Puel JL, Guitton MJ (2007) Salicylate-induced tinnitus: molecular mechanisms and modulation by anxiety. Prog Brain Res 166: 141–146.

6. Leaver AM, Renier L, Chevillet MA, Morgan S, Kim HJ, et al. (2011) Dysregulation of limbic and auditory networks in tinnitus. Neuron 69: 33–43.

7. Meltser I, Tahera Y, Canlon B (2009) Glucocorticoid receptor and mitogen-activated protein kinases activity after restraint stress and acoustic trauma. J Neurotrauma 26: 1835–1845.

8. Langguth B, Salvi R, Elgoyhen AB (2009) Emerging pharmacotherapy of tinnitus. Expert Opin Emerg Drugs 14: 687–702.

9. Roberts LE, Eggermont JJ, Caspary DM, Shore SE, Melcher JR, et al. (2010) Ringing ears: the neuroscience of tinnitus. J Neurosci 30: 14972–14979.

10. Knipper M, Zimmermann U, Müller M (2010) Molecular aspects of tinnitus. Hear Res 266: 60–69.

11. Rauschecker JP, Leaver AM, Mühlau M (2010) Tuning out the noise: limbic-auditory interactions in tinnitus. Neuron 66: 819–826.

12. Salvi RJ, Wang J, Ding D (2000) Auditory plasticity and hyperactivity following cochlear damage. Hear Res 147: 261–274.

13. Brozoski TJ, Bauer CA, Caspary DM (2002) Elevated fusiform cell activity in the dorsal cochlear nucleus of chinchillas with psychophysical evidence of tinnitus. J Neurosci 22: 2383–2390.

14. Kaltenbach JA (2007) The dorsal cochlear nucleus as a contributor to tinnitus: mechanisms underlying the induction of hyperactivity. Prog Brain Res 166: 89–106.

15. Schaette R, Kempter R (2009) Predicting tinnitus pitch from patients' audiograms with a computational model for the development of neuronal hyperactivity. J Neurophysiol 101: 3042–3052.

16. Middleton JW, Kiritani T, Pedersen C, Turner JG, Shepherd GM, et al. (2011) Mice with behavioral evidence of tinnitus exhibit dorsal cochlear nucleus hyperactivity because of decreased GABAergic inhibition. Proc Natl Acad Sci USA 108: 7601–7606.

17. Schaette R, McAlpine D (2011) Tinnitus with a normal audiogram: physiological evidence for hidden hearing loss and computational model. J Neurosci 31: 13452–13457.

18. Yang S, Weiner BD, Zhang LS, Cho SJ, Bao S (2011) Homeostatic plasticity drives tinnitus perception in an animal model. Proc Natl Acad Sci USA 108: 14974–14979.

19. Dehmel S, Pradhan S, Koehler S, Bledsoe S, Shore S (2012) Noise overexposure alters long-term somatosensory - auditory processing in the dorsal cochlear nucleus–possible basis for tinnitus-related hyperactivity? J Neurosci 32: 1660–1671.

20. Dong S, Mulders WH, Rodger J, Robertson D (2009) Changes in neuronal activity and gene expression in guinea-pig auditory brainstem after unilateral partial hearing loss. Neuroscience 159: 1164–1174.

21. Turner JG (2007) Behavioral measures of tinnitus in laboratory animals. Prog Brain Res 166: 147–156.

22. Rüttiger L, Ciuffani J, Zenner HP, Knipper M (2003) A behavioral paradigm to judge acute sodium salicylate-induced sound experience in rats: a new approach for an animal model on tinnitus. Hear Res 180: 39–50.

23. Tan J, Rüttiger L, Panford-Walsh R, Singer W, Schulze H, et al. (2007) Tinnitus behavior and hearing function correlate with the reciprocal expression patterns of BDNF and Arg3.1/arc in auditory neurons following acoustic trauma. Neuroscience 145: 715–726.

24. Kujawa SG, Liberman MC (2009) Adding insult to injury: cochlear nerve degeneration after "temporary" noise-induced hearing loss. J Neurosci 29: 14077–14085.

25. Zuccotti A, Kuhn S, Johnson SL, Franz C, Singer W, et al. (2012) Lack of brain-derived neurotrophic factor hampers inner hair cell synapse physiology, but protects against noise induced hearing loss. J Neurosci 32, 8545–8553.

26. Ramirez-Amaya V, Vazdarjanova A, Mikhael D, Rosi S, Worley PF, et al. (2005) Spatial exploration-induced Arc mRNA and protein expression: evidence for selective, network-specific reactivation. J Neurosci 25: 1761–1768.

27. Bramham CR, Alme MN, Bittins M, Kuipers SD, Nair RR, et al. (2010) The Arc of synaptic memory. Exp Brain Res 200: 125–140.

28. Goel A, Lee HK (2007) Persistence of experience-induced homeostatic synaptic plasticity through adulthood in superficial layers of mouse visual cortex. J Neurosci 27: 6692–6700.

29. Gao M, Sossa K, Song L, Errington L, Cummings L, et al. (2010) A specific requirement of Arc/Arg3.1 for visual experience-induced homeostatic synaptic plasticity in mouse primary visual cortex. J Neurosci 30: 7168–7178.

30. Knipper M, Zinn C, Maier H, Praetorius M, Rohbock K, et al. (2000) Thyroid hormone deficiency before the onset of hearing causes irreversible damage to peripheral and central auditory systems. J Neurophysiol 83: 3101–3112.

31. Schimmang T, Tan J, Müller M, Zimmermann U, Rohbock K, et al. (2003) Lack of Bdnf and TrkB signalling in the postnatal cochlea leads to a spatial reshaping of innervation along the tonotopic axis and hearing loss. Development 130: 4741–4750.

32. Engel J, Braig C, Rüttiger L, Kuhn S, Zimmermann U, et al. (2006) Two classes of outer hair cells along the tonotopic axis of the cochlea. Neuroscience 143: 837–849.

33. Kehrle HM, Granjeiro RC, Sampaio AL, Bezerra R, Almeida VF, et al. (2008) Comparison of auditory brainstem response results in normal-hearing patients with and without tinnitus. Arch Otolaryngol Head Neck Surg 134: 647–651.

34. Heidrych P, Zimmermann U, Kuhn S, Franz C, Engel J, et al. (2009) Otoferlin interacts with myosin VI: implications for maintenance of the basolateral synaptic structure of the inner hair cell. Hum Mol Genet 18: 2779–2790.

35. Panford-Walsh R, Singer W, Rüttiger L, Hadjab S, Tan J, et al. (2008) Midazolam reverses salicylate-induced changes in brain-derived neurotrophic factor and arg3.1 expression: implications for tinnitus perception and auditory plasticity. Mol Pharmacol 74: 595–604.

36. Doron NN, Ledoux JE, Semple MN (2002) Redefining the tonotopic core of rat auditory cortex: physiological evidence for a posterior field. J Comp Neurol 453: 345–360.

37. Sheets L, Trapani JG, Mo W, Obholzer N, Nicolson T (2011) Ribeye is required for presynaptic Ca(V)1.3a channel localization and afferent innervation of sensory hair cells. Development 138: 1309–1319.

38. Müller M (1991) Frequency representation in the rat cochlea. Hearing Research 51: 247–254.

39. Buran BN, Strenzke N, Neef A, Gundelfinger ED, Moser T, et al. (2010) Onset coding is degraded in auditory nerve fibers from mutant mice lacking synaptic ribbons. J Neurosci 30: 7587–7597.

40. Johnson DH, Kiang NY (1976) Analysis of discharges recorded simultaneously from pairs of auditory nerve fibers. Biophys J 16: 719–734.

41. Melcher JR, Kiang NY (1996) Generators of the brainstem auditory evoked potential in cat. III: Identified cell populations. Hear Res 93: 52–71.

42. Yates GK, Winter IM, Robertson D (1990) Basilar membrane nonlinearity determines auditory nerve rate-intensity functions and cochlear dynamic range. Hear Res 45: 203–219.

43. Pettigrew AM, Liberman MC, Kiang NY (1984) Click-evoked gross potentials and single-unit thresholds in acoustically traumatized cats. Ann Otol Rhinol Laryngol Suppl 112: 83–96.

44. Don M, Eggermont JJ (1978) Analysis of the click-evoked brainstem potentials in man unsing high-pass noise masking. Journal of the Acoustical Society of America 63: 1084–1092.

45. Korb E, Finkbeiner S (2012) Arc in synaptic plasticity: from gene to behavior. Trends Neurosci 34: 591–598.

46. Bauer CA, Brozoski TJ, Myers K (2007) Primary afferent dendrite degeneration as a cause of tinnitus. J Neurosci Res 85: 1489–1498.

47. Weisz N, Hartmann T, Dohrmann K, Schlee W, Noreña A (2006) High-frequency tinnitus without hearing loss does not mean absence of deafferentation. Hear Res 222: 108–114.

48. Geven LI, de Kleine E, Free RH, van Dijk P (2011) Contralateral suppression of otoacoustic emissions in tinnitus patients. Otol Neurotol 32: 315–321.

49. Knipper M, Müller M, Zimmermann U (2012) Molecular Mechanism of Tinnitus. In: Fay RR, Popper AN, Eggermont JJ, editors. Springer Handbook of Auditory Research: Neural Correlates of Tinnitus. New York. Springer: 49–82.

50. Roberts LE, Moffat G, Baumann M, Ward LM, Bosnyak DJ (2008) Residual inhibition functions overlap tinnitus spectra and the region of auditory threshold shift. J Assoc Res Otolaryngol 9: 417–435.

51. Noreña AJ, Eggermont JJ (2003) Changes in spontaneous neural activity immediately after an acoustic trauma: implications for neural correlates of tinnitus. Hear Res 183: 137–153.

52. Engineer ND, Riley JR, Seale JD, Vrana WA, Shetake JA, et al. (2011) Reversing pathological neural activity using targeted plasticity. Nature 470: 101–104.

53. Glowatzki E, Fuchs PA (2002) Transmitter release at the hair cell ribbon synapse. Nat Neurosci 5: 147–154.

54. Matthews G, Fuchs P (2010) The diverse roles of ribbon synapses in sensory neurotransmission. Nat Rev Neurosci 11: 812–822.

55. Westerman LA, Smith RL (1984) Rapid and short-term adaptation in auditory nerve responses. Hear Res 15: 249–260.

56. Kim DK, Park SN, Kim HM, Son HR, Kim NG, et al. (2011) Prevalence and significance of high-frequency hearing loss in subjectively normal-hearing patients with tinnitus. Ann Otol Rhinol Laryngol 120: 523–528.

57. Dominguez M, Becker S, Bruce I, Read H (2006) A spiking neuron model of cortical correlates of sensorineural hearing loss: Spontaneous firing, synchrony, and tinnitus. Neural Comput 18: 2942–2958.

58. König O, Schaette R, Kempter R, Gross M (2006) Course of hearing loss and occurrence of tinnitus. Hear Res 221: 59–64.

59. Parra LC, Pearlmutter BA (2007) Illusory percepts from auditory adaptation. J Acoust Soc Am 121: 1632–1641.

60. Schaette R, Kempter R (2012) Computational models of neurophysiological correlates of tinnitus. Front Syst Neurosci 6: 34.

61. Cai S, Ma WL, Young ED (2009) Encoding intensity in ventral cochlear nucleus following acoustic trauma: implications for loudness recruitment. J Assoc Res Otolaryngol 10: 5–22.

62. Qiu C, Salvi R, Ding D, Burkard R (2000) Inner hair cell loss leads to enhanced response amplitudes in auditory cortex of unanesthetized chinchillas: evidence for increased system gain. Hear Res 139: 153–171.

63. Szczepaniak WS, Møller AR (1996) Evidence of neuronal plasticity within the inferior colliculus after noise exposure: a study of evoked potentials in the rat. Electroencephalography and Clinical Neurophysiology 100: 158–164.

64. Zeng FG (2012) An active loudness model suggesting tinnitus as increased central noise and hyperacusis as increased nonlinear gain. Hear Res.

65. Penner MJ (1986) Tinnitus as a source of internal noise. J Speech Hear Res 29: 400–406.

66. Vazdarjanova A, Ramirez-Amaya V, Insel N, Plummer TK, Rosi S, et al. (2006) Spatial exploration induces ARC, a plasticity-related immediate-early gene, only in calcium/calmodulin-dependent protein kinase II-positive principal excitatory and inhibitory neurons of the rat forebrain. J Comp Neurol 498: 317–329.

67. Kelly MP, Deadwyler SA (2002) Acquisition of a novel behavior induces higher levels of Arc mRNA than does overtrained performance. Neuroscience 110: 617–626.

68. Daberkow DP, Riedy MD, Kesner RP, Keefe KA (2007) Arc mRNA induction in striatal efferent neurons associated with response learning. Eur J Neurosci 26: 228–241.

69. Lonergan ME, Gafford GM, Jarome TJ, Helmstetter FJ (2010) Time-dependent expression of Arc and zif268 after acquisition of fear conditioning. Neural Plast 2010: 139891.

70. Link W, Konietzko U, Kauselmann G, Krug M, Schwanke B, et al. (1995) Somatodendritic expression of an immediate early gene is regulated by synaptic activity. Proc Natl Acad Sci USA 92: 5734–5738.

71. Bramham CR, Worley PF, Moore MJ, Guzowski JF (2008) The immediate early gene arc/arg3.1: regulation, mechanisms, and function. J Neurosci 28: 11760–11767.

72. Tzingounis AV, Nicoll RA (2006) Arc/Arg3.1: linking gene expression to synaptic plasticity and memory. Neuron 52: 403–407.

73. Shepherd JD, Rumbaugh G, Wu J, Chowdhury S, Plath N, et al. (2006) Arc/Arg3.1 mediates homeostatic synaptic scaling of AMPA receptors. Neuron 52: 475–484.

74. Guzowski JF, McNaughton BL, Barnes CA, Worley PF (1999) Environment-specific expression of the immediate-early gene Arc in hippocampal neuronal ensembles. Nat Neurosci 2: 1120–1124.

75. Moga DE, Shapiro ML, Morrison JH (2006) Bidirectional redistribution of AMPA but not NMDA receptors after perforant path simulation in the adult rat hippocampus in vivo. Hippocampus 16: 990–1003.

76. Steward O, Wallace CS, Lyford GL, Worley PF (1998) Synaptic activation causes the mRNA for the IEG Arc to localize selectively near activated postsynaptic sites on dendrites. Neuron 21: 741–751.

77. Okuno H, Akashi K, Ishii Y, Yagishita-Kyo N, Suzuki K, et al. (2012) Inverse synaptic tagging of inactive synapses via dynamic interaction of Arc/Arg3.1 with CaMKIIbeta. Cell 149: 886–898.

78. Beique JC, Na Y, Kuhl D, Worley PF, Huganir RL (2010) Arc-dependent synapse-specific homeostatic plasticity. Proc Natl Acad Sci U S A 108: 816–821.

79. Pinaud R, Penner MR, Robertson HA, Currie RW (2001) Upregulation of the immediate early gene arc in the brains of rats exposed to environmental enrichment: implications for molecular plasticity. Brain Res Mol Brain Res 91: 50–56.

80. Kozlovsky N, Matar MA, Kaplan Z, Kotler M, Zohar J, et al. (2008) The immediate early gene Arc is associated with behavioral resilience to stress exposure in an animal model of posttraumatic stress disorder. Eur Neuropsychopharmacol 18: 107–116.

81. Ons S, Rotllant D, Marin-Blasco IJ, Armario A (2010) Immediate-early gene response to repeated immobilization: Fos protein and arc mRNA levels appear to be less sensitive than c-fos mRNA to adaptation. Eur J Neurosci 31: 2043–2052.

82. Yilmaz-Rastoder E, Miyamae T, Braun AE, Thiels E (2011) LTP- and LTD-inducing stimulations cause opposite changes in arc/arg3.1 mRNA level in hippocampal area CA1 in vivo. Hippocampus 21: 1290–1301.

83. Peebles CL, Yoo J, Thwin MT, Palop JJ, Noebels JL, et al. (2010) Arc regulates spine morphology and maintains network stability in vivo. Proc Natl Acad Sci U S A 107: 18173–18178.

84. Porcher C, Hatchett C, Longbottom RE, McAinch K, Sihra TS, et al. (2011) Positive feedback regulation between gamma-aminobutyric acid type A (GABA(A)) receptor signaling and brain-derived neurotrophic factor (BDNF) release in developing neurons. J Biol Chem 286: 21667–21677.

85. Ochi K, Eggermont JJ (1997) Effects of quinine on neural activity in cat primary auditory cortex. Hear Res 105: 105–118.

86. Eggermont JJ, Roberts LE (2004) The neuroscience of tinnitus. Trends Neurosci 27: 676–682.

87. Borsello T, Clarke PG, Hirt L, Vercelli A, Repici M, et al. (2003) A peptide inhibitor of c-Jun N-terminal kinase protects against excitotoxicity and cerebral ischemia. Nat Med 9: 1180–1186.

88. Singer W, Zuccotti A, Jaumann M, Lee SC, Panford-Walsh R, et al. (2012) Noise-Induced Inner Hair Cell Ribbon Loss Disturbs Central Arc Mobilization: A Novel Molecular Paradigm for Understanding Tinnitus. Mol Neurobiol.

89. Schecklmann M, Vielsmeier V, Steffens T, Landgrebe M, Langguth B, et al. (2012) Relationship between Audiometric slope and tinnitus pitch in tinnitus patients: insights into the mechanisms of tinnitus generation. PLoS One 7: e34878.

90. Lin HW, Furman AC, Kujawa SG, Liberman MC (2011) Primary neural degeneration in the Guinea pig cochlea after reversible noise-induced threshold shift. J Assoc Res Otolaryngol 12: 605–616.

91. Wang Y, Liberman MC (2002) Restraint stress and protection from acoustic injury in mice. Hear Res 165: 96–102.

92. Loeb M, Smith RP (1967) Relation of induced tinnitus to physical characteristics of the inducing stimuli. J Acoust Soc Am 42: 453–455.

93. Atherley GR, Hempstock TI, Noble WG (1968) Study of tinnitus induced temporarily by noise. J Acoust Soc Am 44: 1503–1506.

94. McFeely WJ, Jr., Bojrab DI, Davis KG, Hegyi DF (1999) Otologic injuries caused by airbag deployment. Otolaryngol Head Neck Surg 121: 367–373.

95. Mrena R, Paakkonen R, Back L, Pirvola U, Ylikoski J (2004) Otologic consequences of blast exposure: a Finnish case study of a shopping mall bomb explosion. Acta Otolaryngol Suppl 124: 946–952.

96. Nottet JB, Moulin A, Brossard N, Suc B, Job A (2006) Otoacoustic emissions and persistent tinnitus after acute acoustic trauma. Laryngoscope 116: 970–975.

97. Schreiber BE, Agrup C, Haskard DO, Luxon LM (2010) Sudden sensorineural hearing loss. Lancet 375: 1203–1211.

13

Tinnitus Severity is Reduced with Reduction of Depressive Mood

Sylvie Hébert[1]*, Barbara Canlon[4], Dan Hasson[2,4], Linda L. Magnusson Hanson[2], Hugo Westerlund[2], Töres Theorell[2,3]

1 École d'orthophonie et d'audiologie, Faculté de médecine, Université de Montréal, BRAMS, International Laboratory for Brain, Music, and Sound Research, and Centre de recherche de l'Institut universitaire de gériatrie de Montréal, Montréal, Québec, Canada, 2 Stress Research Institute, Stockholm University, Stockholm, Sweden, 3 Department of Public Health, Karolinska Institute, Stockholm, Sweden, 4 Department of Physiology and Pharmacology, Karolinska Institute, Stockholm, Sweden

Abstract

Tinnitus, the perception of sound without external source, is a highly prevalent public health problem with about 8% of the population having frequently occurring tinnitus, and about 1–2% experiencing significant distress from it. Population studies, as well as studies on self-selected samples, have reported poor psychological well-being in individuals with tinnitus. However, no study has examined the long-term co-variation between mood and tinnitus prevalence or tinnitus severity. In this study, the relationship between depression and tinnitus prevalence and severity over a 2-year period was examined in a representative sample of the general Swedish working population. Results show that a decrease in depression is associated with a decrease in tinnitus prevalence, and even more markedly with tinnitus severity. Hearing loss was a more potent predictor than depression for tinnitus prevalence, but was a weaker predictor than depression for tinnitus severity. In addition, there were sex differences for tinnitus prevalence, but not for tinnitus severity. This study shows a direct and long-term association between tinnitus severity and depression.

Editor: Berthold Langguth, University of Regensburg, Germany

Funding: Swedish Council for Working Life and Social Research (FAS). DH is supported by a grant from FAS Centre for Research on Hearing Problems in Working Life and Tysta Skolan. BC is supported from the Swedish Medical Research Council, FAS Centre for Research on Hearing Problems in Working Life, the Karolinska Institute, and Tysta Skolan. SH is supported by Fondation Caroline-Durand. The funders had no role in study design, data collection and analysis, decision to publish, or preparation of the manuscript.

Competing Interests: The authors have declared that no competing interests exist.

* E-mail: sylvie.hebert@umontreal.ca

Introduction

Tinnitus is an increasing public health problem in modern societies. Its prevalence is estimated to be about 25% in the general population [1] and about 8% for frequently occurring tinnitus [2]. Tinnitus prevalence is increasing in young adults [3] and it is presumed to be related with exposure to high volume music in portable devices as well as to noisy environments [4]. Another important etiological factor among older men is a history of exposure to noise in heavy industry and military operations [2,5,6]. Indeed, the most important predictor of tinnitus is hearing loss, especially at high frequencies, and recent estimates of the prevalence of hearing loss range from 2% to 93% depending on gender and age, with an overall rate of 31% for the whole US population [5]. Hearing loss has been found to predict tinnitus and to a lesser extent tinnitus severity [7,8]. Tinnitus severity indicates the extent to which the individual is bothered, upset or worried by the tinnitus. Hearing pathology has been linked to tinnitus even when there is no measurable hearing loss in the audiogram [9,10].

During recent years [11,12], the relationship between psychological well-being and tinnitus has been emphasized. There are many symptoms of long-lasting stress that are associated with tinnitus. A recent population study reported that emotional exhaustion is a strong predictor of tinnitus severity [7]. However

cross-sectional studies do not allow ascertaining the causality of such relationships, or how well-being co-varies over time with tinnitus severity. Tinnitus may cause distress, giving rise to a deterioration of psychological well-being. The reverse relationship could also prevail [13]. Feelings of distress, associated with tinnitus, may increase during periods of poor psychological well-being. Population studies have found associations between tinnitus and generalized anxiety disorders [2] and depressive symptoms [14]. However, individuals with tinnitus may have depressive symptoms but not meet the clinical diagnosis of major depressive disorder [2]. Indirect evidence suggests that reducing tinnitus-related distress also reduces psychopathological symptoms. A recently published Cochrane review [15] came to the conclusion that cognitive behavioral therapy (CBT) is not likely to reduce the subjective loudness of tinnitus using a visual analogue scale (VAS). The value of using these scale types for tinnitus severity assessment has been questioned [16]. However, in six randomized trials, CBT has been shown to improve tinnitus-related distress scores and in five other similar studies to improve the quality of life in tinnitus patients. Another recent systematic review, involving nine additional trials and 806 patients, demonstrated that CBT had a further positive effect on mood scores and stress reduction [17]. Tinnitus-related distress was still reduced at 18 months follow-up, although effect sizes decreased over time. Mood was not assessed beyond 12 months, and effect sizes varied substantially. In addition, it was not possible to know whether the positive effects of the therapy were due to a reduction in anxiety and/or depression symptoms since depression and anxiety measures were combined into a single mood construct. Nevertheless, there is some evidence that tinnitus severity and mood co-vary, at least over the short-term, although direct relationships or long-term assessments have not yet been reported.

The focus of the present study is to investigate the relationship between depression and tinnitus prevalence and severity. More specifically, the study is longitudinal and conducted on a representative sample of the general Swedish working population. It is therefore possible to examine the relationship between a two-year change in depression score and a change in tinnitus or tinnitus severity during the same period. Our hypothesis was that an improvement in depression symptoms would be associated with an improvement in tinnitus prevalence and severity, and vice versa.

Methods

Population

Respondents from the 2003 and 2005 Swedish Work Environment Survey (SWES) conducted biennially by Statistics Sweden (SCB) were invited to enroll in the Swedish Longitudinal Occupational Survey of Health (SLOSH) [18], which was initiated by the Stress Research Institute in 2006. These are subsamples of gainfully employed people and stratified by county, sex, citizenship, and inferred employment status. Data collection was conducted in April 2008. A total of 18,734 individuals were mailed self-completion questionnaires in 2008, out of which 11,441 (61%) responded. However, the present study use only 9,756 (52% of the sample) who were working at the time of the survey (the rest being retired, unemployed or otherwise working less than 30% of full-time). In 2010 the total response rate was 57%. Table 1 shows the numbers of subjects responding to different parts of the present study in 2006 and 2008. For the final prospective analyses, 6,215 individuals who had complete data from both 2008 and 2010 for all the variables in this study were included in the analyses:

Socioeconomic (SES) status in 2008 (SEK/year). The variable corresponding to SES was annual income (taken from the tax registry). This variable was markedly skewed and was subjected to n-logarithmic transformation that provided a perfect normal distribution (range after transformation 0–8.23). Adjustments were also made for age and sex.

Tinnitus in 2008 and 2010 (range 1–4). The single question for determining tinnitus was: Have you during the most recent time experienced sound in any of the ears, without there being an external source (so-called tinnitus) lasting more than five minutes? (No, Yes sometimes, Yes often, Yes all the time). This variable was slightly skewed (skewness 1.94 in 2008 and 1.90 in 2010). The questions about tinnitus were adapted from Davis [19] and Palmer et al. [20].

Tinnitus severity in 2008 and 2010 (range 1–4). The single item for determining tinnitus severity was: How much do you feel that the tinnitus sounds worry, bother or upset you? (Not at all, A little, Moderately, Severely). The questions about tinnitus were adapted from Davis [19]and Palmer et al. [20]. The tinnitus severity item was answered only by those who reported that they experienced tinnitus (skewness 0.36 in 2008 and 0.45 in 2010).

Depressive symptoms in 2008 and 2010 (range 6–30). Depressive symptoms were measured with a brief subscale from the Hopkins Symptom Checklist [21]. This particular version was based upon clinical validity, and focused on the six items corresponding to the Hamilton Depression sub-scale HAM-D_6 [22]. Feeling blue? Feeling no interest in things? Feeling lethargy or low in energy? Worrying too much about things? Blaming yourself for things? Feeling everything is an effort? (last week; $0 =$ not at all to $4 =$ extremely). A sum score was used and it was nearly normally distributed (skewness 1.14 in 2008 and 1.19 in 2010).

Subjective hearing loss in 2008 and 2010 (range 0–3). Subjective hearing loss was assessed with the question: How difficult is it for you to (without hearing aid) hear what is said in a conversation between several persons? ($0 =$ not difficult at all to $3 =$ very difficult). In this study, *subjective* hearing loss reflects difficulties in communicating. The question about hearing loss was derived from Statistics Sweden and has been used in several population studies (see for instance [1] 2010).

Statistical Analyses

Paired t-tests were conducted in order to assess possible changes in outcome variables between 2008 and 2010. Since all variables, explanatory as well as outcome, were close to normally distributed, multiple linear regressions were computed with all explanatory variables entered in one single step. Changes in depression and hearing loss were obtained by subtracting the 2008 scores from the respective depression and hearing loss 2010 scores. All the study variables have skewness estimates between -1.0 and 1.2 which is regarded as acceptably close to normal distributions with one important exception, the tinnitus variable which has skewness 1.9 for both years, which could possibly give rise to error. However,

Table 1. Characteristics of male and female participants.

	Men				Women			
	2008		2010		2008		2010	
	M (± SD)	n	M (± SD)	n	M (± SD)	n	M (± SD)	n
Age (20–70)	49.8 (11.5)	5,086	53.3 (11.1)	3,778	48.7 (11.7)	6,355	51.8 (11.3)	4,993
Income (elog)	5.74 (0.50)	5,061	5.84 (0.49)	3,762	5.47 (0.49)	6,331	5.55 (0.52)	4,971
Tinnitus	1.58 (0.98)	4,969	1.63 (1.01)	3,735	1.35 (0.75)	6,234	1.36 (0.77)	4,919
Tinnitus severity	2.14 (0.82)	1,397	2.07 (0.85)	1,348	2.15 (0.78)	1,179	2.02 (0.81)	1,223
Depression symptoms	11.08 (4.96)	4,365	10.51 (4.66)	2,908	12.03 (5.45)	5,171	11.88 (5.37)	3,821
Hearing loss	0.65 (0.73)	4,354	0.72 (0.78)	3,699	0.56 (0.70)	5,164	0.58 (0.73)	4,886

we also tested an ordinal multiple logistic regression using an ordinal version of tinnitus in 2008 as explanatory and similarly an ordinal version of tinnitus 2010 as dependent variables. This analysis showed that the same variables came out as significant independent predictors for tinnitus in 2010 as in the multiple linear regression. For the tinnitus severity variable there was no such problem (skewness 0.36 in 2008 and 0.45 in 2010), and for simplicity we therefore use the same statistical model for both outcomes. We chose linear regression since this seems to provide an adequate albeit not perfect solution.

We first regressed tinnitus score in 2010 on sex, age, income (n log transformed), depression score in 2008, change in depression score from 2008 to 2010, hearing loss in 2008, change in hearing loss from 2008 to 2010, and tinnitus score in 2008. Restricting the analysis to only those who reported tinnitus in 2008, we then regressed tinnitus severity in 2010 on the same explanatory variables, except that tinnitus score in 2008 was replaced by tinnitus severity in 2008. The variable income was markedly skewed to the right (which is typical of this variable in population studies), with a small number of participants with a very high income. Since these participants could give rise to distortion in analyses including income this variable was transformed logarithmically.

The software JMP®, Version 9 (SAS Institute Inc., Cary, NC) was used for all statistical analyses. Significance level was set at $p < 0.05$.

The Regional Research Ethics Committee in Stockholm (Ref no 2006/158-31) has approved the study. There was written consent from every participant and the committee perused the conditions of the study after which they gave their consent. No children or relatives participated.

Results

The characteristics of the participants are presented in Table 1, which is based upon participants in each wave separately. All numbers (n) of respondents for each variable (divided into men and women) are given in the table. The depression score decreased significantly in the population as a whole between 2008 and 2010 (paired samples t-test, $t = 3.91$, $p = 0.0001$, N = 6,340). The tinnitus score, on the other hand, did not change significantly. During the two years there was a significant increase in the mean value for the self-rated hearing loss ($t = 2.13$, $p = 0.034$, N = 7,173).

Predictors of Tinnitus

Table 2 shows the results of a multiple linear regression analysis with tinnitus in 2010 as the dependent variable. The independent variables were: age, gender (m = 1, f = 2), income, tinnitus in 2008, depressive symptoms in 2008 and change in depressive symptoms from 2008 to 2010 as well as hearing loss in 2008 and change in hearing loss 2008–2010. The results demonstrated that sex (men have a higher prevalence of tinnitus) as well as baseline (2008) levels of tinnitus, depressive symptoms and hearing loss as well as change in depressive symptoms and hearing loss (2008–2010) were all statistically significant predictors of tinnitus in 2010. Age and income had no significant explanatory value. Analyses were then performed with men and women separately, yielding similar results to the combined model. The exception was that the predictive power of depressive symptom level in 2008 was statistically significant only in men ($p = 0.039$) but not in women ($p = 0.137$). Since all other factors that were highly predictive in the combined model were sex-independent (all $p < 0.002$), we therefore present the results from the combined model. This model described 63% of the explained variance.

Table 3 is limited to participants with tinnitus and depicts the results of multiple regression analysis with tinnitus severity in 2010 as the dependent variable. The independent variables were: age, sex, income, tinnitus severity, depressive symptoms and hearing loss in 2008 and change in depressive symptoms and hearing loss (2008–2010). The results showed that tinnitus severity, depressive symptoms and hearing loss in 2008 as well as changes in depressive symptoms and hearing loss (2008–2010) were statistically significant predictors of tinnitus severity in 2010. Sex, age and income had no statistically significant explanatory value. Analyses were also performed with men and women separately. The results were very similar to the combined model, with the only observation that the predictive power of depressive symptom level in 2008 reached statistical significance only in women ($p = 0.002$) but not in men ($p = 0.144$). All factors that were highly significant predictors in the combined model were also predictive for women and men separately (all $ps < 0.001$). Therefore we present the whole model, which describes 63% of the explained variance.

Discussion

The main finding of the present study is that, within a random sample of Swedish workers, depression co-varies with tinnitus prevalence and tinnitus severity over time. That is, a decrease in

Table 2. Tinnitus score in 2010 as dependent variable in relation to predictors.

	Standardized β	B	SEM(B)	t	p	Chi square (p)
Intercept		0.801	0.113	7.06	<0.0001	
Sex (m = 1, f = 2)	−0.0315	−0.056	0.015	3.84	0.0001	12.80 (0.0003)
Age (10 y)	−0.0107	−0.008	0.007	1.10	0.27	2.65 (0.104)
Income 2008 (elog)	0.0025	0.004	0.016	0.26	0.79	0.07 (0.791)
Depressive symptoms 2008	0.0214	0.004	0.002	2.27	0.023	13.41 (0.0002)
Change in depressive symptoms (2010–2008)	0.0421	0.008	0.002	4.67	<0.0001	29.23 (0.0001)
Tinnitus score 2008	0.7451	0.752	0.008	90.67	<0.0001	2982.96 (0.0001)
Hearing loss 2008	0.1088	0.109	0.011	9.66	<0.0001	79.87 (0.0001)
Change in hearing loss (2010–2008)	0.0577	0.088	0.013	6.88	<0.0001	36.48 (0.0001)

Multiple linear regression (n = 6,095).
Adjusted r^2 was 62.8%. Chi square and p values in the last column are obtained from ordinal logistic regression analysis.
(df = 3 for tinnitus score in 2008 and df = 1 for all other explanatory variables).

Table 3. Tinnitus severity score in 2010 as dependent variable in relation to predictors.

	Standardized β	B	SEM(B)	t	p	Chi square (p)
Intercept		1.623	0.319	5.09	<0.0001	
Sex (m = 1, f = 2)	−0.0118	−0.020	0.039	0.51	0.61	0.218 (0.641)
Age (10 y)	−0.0285	0.020	0.021	0.93	0.63	2.197 (0.138)
Income 2008 (elog)	−0.0288	−0.047	0.047	0.99	0.98	1.021 (0.312)
Depressive symptoms 2008	0.0848	0.013	0.004	3.22	0.005	8.876 (0.003)
Change in depressive symptoms (2010–2008)	0.1324	0.023	0.004	5.24	<0.0001	27.138 (0.0001)
Tinnitus severity score 2008	0.5027	0.523	0.025	20.74	<0.0001	385.95 (0.0001)
Hearing loss 2008	0.0406	0.196	0.026	7.59	<0.0001	144.874 (0.0001)
Change in hearing loss (2010–2008)	0.1030	0.148	0.032	4.66	<0.0001	17.698 (0.0001)

Multiple linear regression (n = 1,233). Adjusted r^2 was 62.5%. Chi square and p values in the last column are obtained from ordinal logistic regression analysis (df = 3 for tinnitus score in 2008 and df = 1 for all other explanatory variables).

depression is associated with a decrease in tinnitus prevalence, and even more markedly with severity, over a two-year period. Hearing loss and change in hearing loss are stronger predictors than depressive symptoms and change in depressive symptoms for *tinnitus prevalence*. However, hearing loss is a much less important predictor than depressive symptoms for *tinnitus severity*. To our knowledge, this is the first study to show a direct and long-term association between tinnitus severity and depression.

Langguth and colleagues [23] have recently argued that there are common pathways in the pathophysiology of tinnitus (especially tinnitus-related distress) and depression. Therefore, it is unlikely that these disorders are co-morbid only by chance and that depression is a direct reaction to tinnitus. However, depressive symptoms will make the tinnitus-related handicap more pronounced. In addition, in both depression and tinnitus, personality factors such as neuroticism and traits such as anxiety can also be predisposing factors [24,25].

Tinnitus patients may not present signs of clinical depression, but rather a number of distress-related symptoms. Indeed, Ooms et al [26] found that the somatic depressive subscale of the Beck Depression Inventory II (BDI-II) [27] (not including the affective or cognitive subscales) predicted tinnitus severity. These authors challenged the idea that tinnitus is related to depression and instead proposed that the relationship between tinnitus handicap and depressive symptoms is a result of content overlap between the questionnaires BDI-II and the Tinnitus handicap inventory (THI). In our study, however, tinnitus severity and depression scores did not overlap. Tinnitus-related distress was assessed by a question related to somatic problems (i.e., How much do you feel that the tinnitus sounds worry, bother or upset you?), whereas depressive symptoms were assessed by questions mixing affective (e.g., Feeling blue? Feeling no interest in things? Blaming yourself for things) and somatic (e.g., Feeling lethargy or low in energy? Feeling everything is an effort?) items. Our study therefore does not support the idea that the association between depression and tinnitus severity is an artifact, but rather associated disorders that share core symptomatology or stem from a common etiology.

A recent study on 755 normal hearing individuals showed that tinnitus debut in older ages was more distressful than when the incidence occurred in younger ages [28]. Our population study

could not corroborate this finding because data of the debut of tinnitus onset were not available. Furthermore, an effect of age on tinnitus prevalence or severity was not found. One explanation for this might be that our population was on the average below 50 years of age in 2008, and that the older age groups (>50 years), where prevalence rates of tinnitus typically increase with presbyacusis, were less represented here than in other studies.

Finally, another interesting finding of the present study was that sex predicted tinnitus prevalence, conditional on a number of other factors, but sex did not predict tinnitus severity. This finding is compatible with a recent population study showing a higher prevalence of frequent tinnitus in men than in women [2], and the reasons for this may be due to the higher prevalence of hearing loss in men compared to women. In contrast, hearing loss has a much less important role in tinnitus severity. For both men and women, the changes in depressive symptoms were predictive of tinnitus severity.

It is clear from our study that changes in depression and tinnitus scores are associated with each other and may be due to co-morbidity. It is important to note that this is a population study and not a self-selected sample of tinnitus or depressive patients. Therefore, the results can be broadly generalized on a population level. Future studies are needed to assess possible clinical relevance on an individual level. This study suggests that depressive symptoms should be assessed in tinnitus patients and vice versa. While it may be more common to assess depressive symptoms in tinnitus patients, assessing tinnitus in depressive patients is uncommon. Finally, this study highlights the importance of co-morbidity and its detrimental impact on tinnitus severity. Since the sound of tinnitus cannot be cured, our findings suggest that treating depressive symptoms, a significant tinnitus co-morbidity, should lead to a better quality of life by decreasing both depressive and tinnitus severity symptoms. Given the high prevalence of tinnitus, our study therefore is potentially a meaningful contribution to public health.

Author Contributions

Conceived and designed the experiments: BC DH SH TT. Analyzed the data: SH BC DH TT. Wrote the paper: SH BC DH HW LMH TT.

References

1. Hasson D, Theorell T, Westerlund H, Canlon B (2010) Prevalence and characteristics of hearing problems in a working and non-working Swedish population. J Epidemiol Community Health 64: 453–460.
2. Shargorodsky J, Curhan GC, Farwell WR (2010) Prevalence and characteristics of tinnitus among US adults. American Journal of Medicine 123: 711–718.
3. Bulbul SF, Muluk NB, Cakir EP, Tufan E (2009) Subjective tinnitus and hearing problems in adolescents. International Journal of Pediatric Otorhinolaryngology 73: 1124–1131.
4. Shargorodsky J, Curhan SG, Curhan GC, Eavey R (2010) Change in prevalence of hearing loss in US adolescents. JAMA 304: 772–778.
5. Agrawal Y, Platz EA, Niparko JK (2008) Prevalence of hearing loss and differences by demographic characteristics among US adults: data from the National Health and Nutrition Examination Survey, 1999–2004. Arch Intern Med 168: 1522–1530.
6. Saunders GH, Griest SE (2009) Hearing loss in veterans and the need for hearing loss prevention programs. Noise & Health 11: 14–21.
7. Hébert S, Canlon B, Hasson D (in press) Emotional exhaustion as a predictor of tinnitus. Psychother Psychosom.
8. Holgers KM, Erlandsson SI, Barrenas ML (2000) Predictive factors for the severity of tinnitus. Audiology 39: 284–291.
9. Weisz N, Hartmann T, Dohrmann K, Schlee W, Norena A (2006) High-frequency tinnitus without hearing loss does not mean absence of deafferentation. Hearing Research 222: 108–114.
10. Schaette R, McAlpine D (2011) Tinnitus with a normal audiogram: physiological evidence for hidden hearing loss and computational model. J Neurosci 31: 13452–13457.
11. Gopinath B, McMahon CM, Rochtchina E, Karpa MJ, Mitchell P (2010) Risk Factors and Impacts of Incident Tinnitus in Older Adults. Annals of Epidemiology 20: 129–135.
12. Hasson D, Theorell T, Wallen MB, Leineweber C, Canlon B (2011) Stress and prevalence of hearing problems in the Swedish working population. BMC Public Health 11: 130.
13. Rauschecker JP, Leaver AM, Mühlau M (2010) Tuning out the noise: limbic-auditory interactions in tinnitus. Neuron 66: 819–826.
14. Krog NH, Engdahl B, Tambs K (2010) The association between tinnitus and mental health in a general population sample: Results from the HUNT study. Journal of Psychosomatic Research 69: 289–298.
15. Martinez-Devesa P, Perera R, Theodoulou M, Waddell A (2010) Cognitive behavioural therapy for tinnitus. Cochrane Database of Systematic Reviews 9: CD005233.
16. Langguth B, Goodey R, Azevedo A, Bjorne A, Cacace A, et al. (2007) Consensus for tinnitus patient assessment and treatment outcome measurement: Tinnitus Research Initiative meeting, Regensburg, July 2006. In: B. Langguth GHTKAC, Mller AR, eds. Progress in Brain Research: Elsevier. pp 525–536.
17. Hesser H, Weise C, Westin VZ, Andersson G (2011) A systematic review and meta-analysis of randomized controlled trials of cognitive-behavioral therapy for tinnitus distress. Clin Psychol Rev 31: 545–553.
18. Magnusson Hanson LL, Theorell T, Oxenstierna G, Hyde M, Westerlund H (2008) Demand, control and social climate as predictors of emotional exhaustion symptoms in working Swedish men and women. Scand J Public Health 36: 737–743.
19. Davis AC (1989) The prevalence of hearing impairment and reported hearing disability among adults in Great Britain. Int J Epidemiol 18: 911–917.
20. Palmer KT, Griffin MJ, Syddall HE, Davis A, Pannett B, et al. (2002) Occupational exposure to noise and the attributable burden of hearing difficulties in Great Britain. Occup Environ Med 59: 634–639.
21. Lipmann R (1986) Depression scales derived from Hopkins Symptom Checklist. In: Sartorius N, Ban TA, eds. Assessment of depression. Berlin: Springer-Verlag. pp 232–248.
22. Magnusson Hanson LL, Theorell T, Bech P, Rugulies R, Burr M, et al. (2009) Psychosocial working conditions and depressive symptoms among Swedish employees. Int Arch Occup Environ Health 82: 951–960.
23. Langguth B, Landgrebe M, Kleinjung T, Sand GP, Hajak G (2011) Tinnitus and depression. World J Biol Psychiatry.
24. Bartels H, Middel B, Pedersen SS, Staal MJ, Albers FW (2010) The distressed (Type D) personality is independently associated with tinnitus: a case-control study. Psychosomatics 51: 29–38.
25. Bartels H, Pedersen SS, van der Laan BF, Staal MJ, Albers FW, et al. (2010) The impact of Type D personality on health-related quality of life in tinnitus patients is mainly mediated by anxiety and depression. Otol Neurotol 31: 11–18.
26. Ooms E, Meganck R, Vanheule S, Vinck B, Watelet JB, et al. (2011) Tinnitus severity and the relation to depressive symptoms: a critical study. Otolaryngol Head Neck Surg 145: 276–281.
27. Beck AT, Steer RA, Brown GK (1996) BDI-II, Beck depression inventory : manual. San Antonio, Tex. Boston: Psychological Corp.; Harcourt Brace. vi, 38.
28. Schlee W, Kleinjung T, Hiller W, Goebel G, Kolassa IT, et al. (2011) Does tinnitus distress depend on age of onset? PLoS ONE [Electronic Resource] 6: e27379.

14

Does Tinnitus Distress Depend on Age of Onset?

Winfried Schlee[1]*, Tobias Kleinjung[2,3], Wolfgang Hiller[4], Gerhard Goebel[5], Iris-Tatjana Kolassa[1], Berthold Langguth[3,6]

1 Department of Clinical and Biological Psychology, University of Ulm, Ulm, Germany, 2 Department of Otorhinolaryngology, University of Zurich, Zurich, Switzerland, 3 Interdisciplinary Tinnitus Clinic, University of Regensburg, Regensburg, Germany, 4 Department of Clinical Psychology, University of Mainz, Regensburg, Germany, 5 Medical-Psychomatic Hospital, Schoen Clinic Roseneck, Prien, Germany, 6 Department of Psychiatry and Psychotherapy, University of Regensburg, Regensburg, Germany

Abstract

Objectives: Tinnitus is the perception of a sound in the absence of any physical source of it. About 5–15% of the population report hearing such a tinnitus and about 1–2% suffer from their tinnitus leading to anxiety, sleep disorders or depression. It is currently not completely understood why some people feel distressed by their tinnitus, while others don't. Several studies indicate that the amount of tinnitus distress is associated with many factors including comorbid anxiety, comorbid depression, personality, the psychosocial situation, the amount of the related hearing loss and the loudness of the tinnitus. Furthermore, theoretical considerations suggest an impact of the age at tinnitus onset influencing tinnitus distress.

Methods: Based on a sample of 755 normal hearing tinnitus patients we tested this assumption. All participants answered a questionnaire on the amount of tinnitus distress together with a large variety of clinical and demographic data.

Results: Patients with an earlier onset of tinnitus suffer significantly less than patients with an onset later in life. Furthermore, patients with a later onset of tinnitus describe their course of tinnitus distress as more abrupt and distressing right from the beginning.

Conclusion: We argue that a decline of compensatory brain plasticity in older age accounts for this age-dependent tinnitus decompensation.

Editor: Li I. Zhang, University of Southern California, United States of America

Funding: The authors have no support or funding to report.

Competing Interests: The authors have declared that no competing interests exist.

* E-mail: Winfried.Schlee@uni-ulm.de

Introduction

Tinnitus is the perception of sound in the absence of an auditory stimulus. Averaged over all age groups 5–15% of the western population experience some form of tinnitus. Many people can cope with chronic tinnitus, but about 1–2% of the population experience significant impairments in their quality of life due to their tinnitus.

The prevalence of chronic tinnitus increases with increasing age, peaking at 14.3% in people between 60 and 69 years of age [1]. The increase in tinnitus prevalence with age is at least partly explained by the fact that hearing loss is an important risk factor for tinnitus and hearing loss prevalence also increases with age [2].

Neuroplastic processes play a crucial role both in the generation of tinnitus [3] and in the amount of suffering [4]. Imaging studies reveal that neuroplastic changes in the central auditory system are generating the tinnitus percept [5] and that coactivation of nonauditory structures in the frontal cortex and the limbic system are involved in tinnitus related distress [6,7].

Studies in animals and humans have shown that the mechanisms of cortical plasticity change over the lifetime with a tendency of decreased and less efficient neuroplastic potential as demonstrated by decreased induction and maintenance of long-term-potentiation (LTP) [8] and reduced long-term depression (LTD)-like effects with advancing age [9].

With these changes in the neuroplastic potential across the life span, age may not only have an influence on the incidence of tinnitus, but also on tinnitus related distress. A first hint for such a relation is given by a large epidemiological study demonstrating that people with bothersome tinnitus are elder than those with non-bothersome tinnitus (mean age 42 vs 38; p<0.001) [10]. Considering that tinnitus duration also influences its annoyance [11] we focused here especially on the role of tinnitus onset. In detail we hypothesized that the age of tinnitus onset may influence the perceived tinnitus related distress. More specifically, we assumed that early tinnitus onset is associated with less distress than later tinnitus onset.

Methods

Sample Description

The database of the German Tinnitus League [11,12] provides a large sample of data from tinnitus patients with a broad age distribution to test this hypothesis. It was collected by a mail survey that was conducted among the members of the German Tinnitus League (Deutsche Tinnitus Liga, DTL). The questionnaires contained a large variety of clinical and demographic data and also included the Mini Tinnitus Questionnaire (Mini-TQ, [13]). Out of the database we selected 3'878 questionnaires where data about the following items were complete and valid: age at assessment, age at tinnitus onset, report of hearing impairment and all items of the Mini-Tinnitus Questionnaire. In this sample, the mean age was 56.1 years (SD 12.1), ranging from 16 to 95 years, 41.1% of the sample were women. Data were collected by the Psychological Institute of the University of Mainz and the Roseneck Center of Behavioral Medicine in Prien, Germany.

Material

The data analysis is based on the questionnaire items asking for age at assessment, tinnitus duration, type of tinnitus onset (gradually versus abrupt), subjective hearing impairment, tinnitus distress after tinnitus onset and on the Mini-TQ total score. The questionnaire also assessed some more tinnitus-related variables, which are not subject of this data analysis [12]. All participants were informed that the storage of the data will be completely anonymized. The study was in accordance with the declaration of Helsinki and was approved by the ethical committee at the University of Regensburg. The ethics committee waived the need for consent from the participants for the analysis of the anonymized dataset.

The Mini-TQ is a short and psychometrically validated version of the Tinnitus Questionnaire [14,15], which assesses the tinnitus distress on a one-dimensional scale with scores ranging from 0 (no annoyance) to 24 (maximum annoyance).

Statistical Analysis

The influence of the age of tinnitus onset on the perceived tinnitus distress was tested by means of regression analysis. In order to exclude the complex confounding role of hearing loss only subjects who reported no hearing impairment were included in this analysis. Statistical analysis was done using the statistical software package R (www.r-project.org, version 2.7.2).

Results

Prevalence of hearing impairment among tinnitus patients

Overall, 80.5% of participants (3,123 out of 3,878) complained about some form of hearing impairment. The prevalence of subjective hearing impairment increased with the age of the tinnitus patients. In the lowest quartile of the sample (16–48 years), 66.7% patients reported an impairment of their hearing, which increased to 85.9% in the oldest quartile (64–95 years, see figure 1a).

Age at tinnitus onset influences tinnitus distress

In the investigation of the relationship between tinnitus onset and tinnitus severity, hearing loss is an important confounding factor, which interacts in a complex way with age and tinnitus severity. First the prevalence of hearing loss increases with age, second hearing loss increases the risk for developing tinnitus [10], and third the amount of tinnitus distress is influenced by the distress the participant experiences because of the hearing loss accompanying the tinnitus. Thus, the following analysis concentrated on tinnitus patients that report a normal level of hearing ($n = 755$). Among those patients, the mean age of tinnitus onset was 42.4 years (SD = 13.5 years, see also the histogram in figure 1b). The mean total score of tinnitus distress according to the Mini-TQ was 11.5 (SD = 7.4). A stepwise regression analysis was calculated to investigate the association between the amount of tinnitus

distress and the age at tinnitus onset. We started with a regression model explaining tinnitus distress by the age of the participant, the duration of tinnitus, the age at tinnitus onset, and the type of tinnitus onset (sudden onset vs. gradually increasing). Backward elimination based on Akaike's Information Criterion (AIC) was used to identify and exclude variables that do not improve the regression model significantly. Following this procedure, participant's age, duration of tinnitus, and type of tinnitus onset were eliminated and only the age at tinnitus onset remained in the model. In the final regression model, we found that tinnitus distress was associated with the age of the participant at the onset of the tinnitus ($\beta = .05$, $t = 2.32$, $p = .02$) demonstrating that patients with an earlier onset of tinnitus suffer less from their tinnitus (figure 1c).

Furthermore, a non-linear analysis was calculated and compared with the above described linear model. The comparison of the two models based on the AIC-criterion, however, revealed that the linear model is superior to the non-linear model suggesting a continuous increase of tinnitus distress with the participant's age at tinnitus onset.

Age at onset of tinnitus influences the course of tinnitus distress

Additionally, the participants were asked if their tinnitus was distressing from the beginning or whether the tinnitus distress increased later on. Again, only participants without any subjective hearing impairment were included in the analysis. A logistic regression was calculated showing that the age at tinnitus onset predicts the probability that the tinnitus is perceived as stressful right from the beginning of tinnitus onset ($z = 2.185$, $p = 0.029$).

Discussion

The main finding of our analysis is an influence of the age at tinnitus onset on tinnitus related distress. Higher age at tinnitus onset is associated with higher tinnitus related distress. To our knowledge this is the first report about an influence of age of tinnitus onset on tinnitus severity. This effect is independent from the age at tinnitus assessment, the duration of tinnitus and the type of tinnitus onset (gradual versus abrupt).

A large variety of different variables have been identified in the past as contributing factors to tinnitus distress, among them tinnitus loudness, hearing loss, vertigo/dizziness, hyperacusis, depression, anxiety and personality factors [11,12,16,17]. Our study adds "age of onset" as an additional influencing factor underscoring the relevance of time related aspects in the pathophysiology of tinnitus. Earlier studies identified age and tinnitus duration as relevant factors. Age is strongly influencing tinnitus prevalence [1] and tinnitus duration plays an important role for response to treatment [18–21]. Though the effect of age of onset is statistically highly significant, it is rather small. However, considering the many variables, which exert a known influence on tinnitus related distress, this is not surprising.

Even though we cannot derive direct implications of our results on the clinical management of tinnitus patients, they may be relevant for a better understanding of both physiologic changes of brain function with increasing age and the pathophysiologic mechanisms involved in the generation of tinnitus distress. Many aspects of brain structure, brain function and brain plasticity are changing with age in a complex way [22]. These changes also involve adaptive and compensatory neural mechanisms [23]. Both the generation of tinnitus and the amount of tinnitus distress are thought to depend on adaptive and compensatory brain mechanisms [4]. In this context higher tinnitus distress at higher age of onset suggests an age-related decline in the efficiency of this

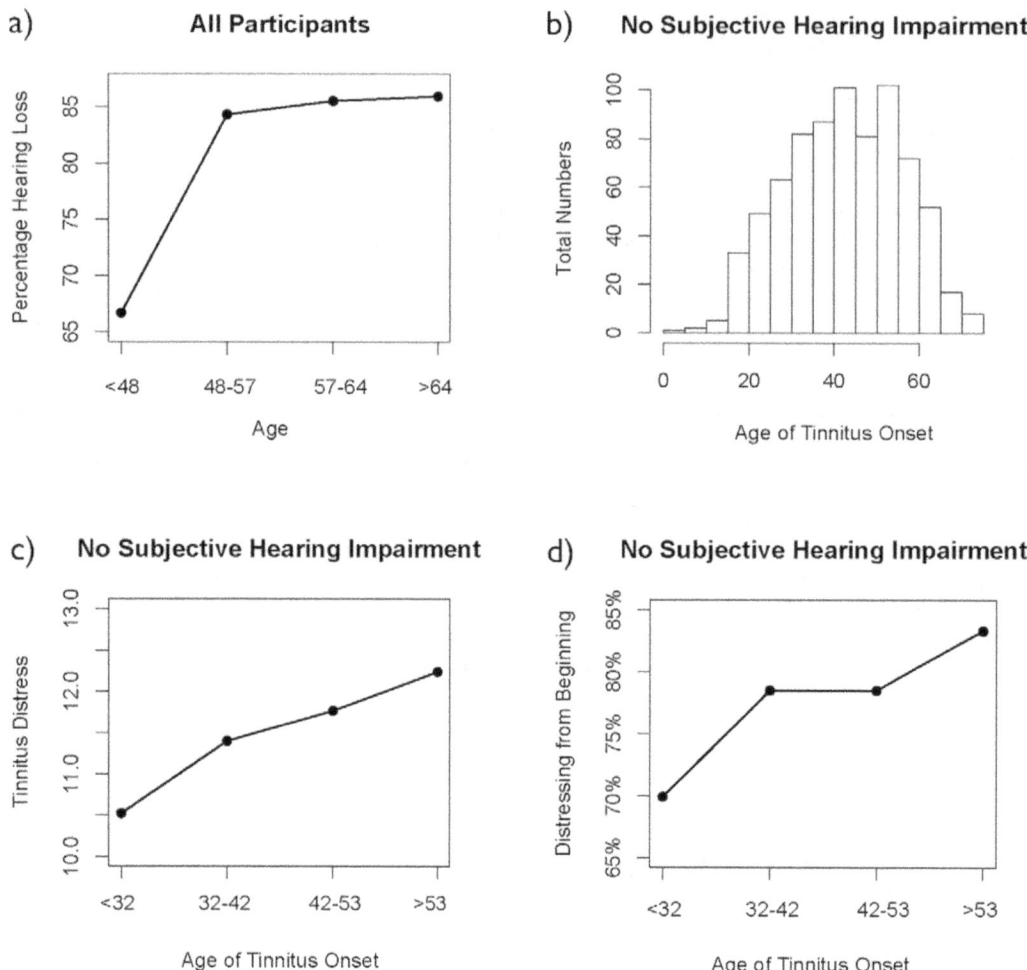

Figure 1. Graphical illustration of the sample data and results. a) The prevalence of hearing impairment increases with the participant's age. Prevalence data were aggregated with respect to age quantiles (Q1: 16–48 years, Q2: 48–57 years, Q3: 57–64 years, Q4: 64–95 years). Figures b) and c) report data from the group of subjects without subjectively reported hearing impairment. b) Histogram of the participant's age at tinnitus onset. c) Tinnitus distress increases with the age of tinnitus onset. The data were aggregated with respect to the age of onset quartiles (Q1: <32 years, Q2: 32–42 years, Q3: 42–53 years, Q4: 53–72 years). d) The percentage of patients that describe their tinnitus as "distressing from the beginning" increase for older age of onset. For illustration purposes, the sample was stratified as quartiles from early (1st quartile: tinnitus onset before the age of 32) to later tinnitus onset (2nd quartile: age 32–42; 3rd quartile: age 42–53; 4th quartile: over age 53). We found that the percentage of patients describing their tinnitus as distressing from the beginning augments with the tinnitus onset age 69.9 in the first quartile) up to 83.3% in the oldest quartile.

compensatory mechanism for tinnitus. Thus our finding is in line with the observation that a decrease of cognition is related to higher tinnitus related distress [24]. Future studies are invited to further characterize the interactions between age related changes in neuroplastic potential, cognitive function and their influence on tinnitus distress.

Some limitations on the data analysis need to be noted here: The presented analysis is based on data from self report questionnaires of individuals with tinnitus and subjectively normal hearing. This selected sample may not be representative for all patients with tinnitus [25]. Also, the sample is restricted to active members of the German tinnitus patient association, which implies first a local selection and second a selection to people who are impaired by their tinnitus. Therefore, we are aware that our conclusions can only be preliminary as long as these data are not replicated in further independent samples. However, earlier analyses based on the same sample have provided results [8,9], which are in line with the literature, indicating that the dataset is representative.

Tinnitus related distress is influenced by many variables such as tinnitus loudness, hearing loss, vertigo/dizziness, hyperacusis, depression, anxiety and personality factors. Here we suggest that the age at tinnitus onset might be an additional factor. Patients with a later onset of tinnitus in their life report greater distress than patients with an early tinnitus onset. The decline of neuroplasticity with advancing age might be an underlying mechanism for this observation.

Acknowledgments

We want to thank the German Tinnitus League for giving us the opportunity to analyse their dataset.

Author Contributions

Conceived and designed the experiments: WH GG. Performed the experiments: WH GG. Analyzed the data: WS BL TK. Wrote the paper: WS TK WH GG IK BL.

References

1. Shargorodsky J, Curhan SG, Curhan GC, Eavey R (2010) Change in prevalence of hearing loss in US adolescents. JAMA 304: 772–778.
2. Pilgramm M, Rychlick R, Lebisch H, Siedentrop H, Goebel G, et al. (1999) Tinnitus in the Federal Republic of Germany: a representative epidemological study. In Hazell JWP, ed. Proceedings of the Sixth International Tinnitus Seminar. London: The Tinnitus and Hyperacusis Centre. pp 64–67.
3. Eggermont JJ, Roberts LE (2004) The neuroscience of tinnitus. Trends Neurosci 27: 676–682.
4. Moller AR (2007) The role of neural plasticity in tinnitus. Prog Brain Res 166: 37–45.
5. Weisz N, Dohrmann K, Elbert T (2007) The relevance of spontaneous activity for the coding of the tinnitus sensation. Prog Brain Res 166: 61–70.
6. Schlee W, Hartmann T, Langguth B, Weisz N (2009) Abnormal resting-state cortical coupling in chronic tinnitus. BMC Neurosci 10: 11.
7. Vanneste S, Plazier M, van der Loo E, Van de Heyning P, De Ridder D (2011) The difference between uni- and bilateral auditory phantom percept. Clin Neurophysiol 122(3): 578–87.
8. Rosenzweig ES, Barnes CA (2003) Impact of aging on hippocampal function: plasticity, network dynamics, and cognition. Prog Neurobiol 69(3): 143–179.
9. Freitas C, Perez J, Knobel M, Tormos JM, Oberman L, et al. (2011) Changes in cortical plasticity across the lifespan. Front Aging Neurosci 9: 3–5.
10. Hoffman HJ, Reed GW (2004) Epidemiology of tinnitus. In: Snow JB, ed. Tinnitus: Theory and Management. Lewiston, NY: BC Decker Inc. pp 16–41.
11. Hiller W, Goebel G (2006) Factors influencing tinnitus loudness and annoyance. Arch Otolaryngol Head Neck Surg 132: 1323–1330.
12. Hiller W, Goebel G (2007) When tinnitus loudness and annoyance are discrepant: audiological characteristics and psychological profile. Audiol Neurootol 12: 391–400.
13. Hiller W, Goebel G (2004) Rapid assessment of tinnitus-related psychological distress using the Mini-TQ. Int J Audiol 43: 600–604.
14. Goebel G, Hiller W (1994) The tinnitus questionnaire. A standard instrument for grading the degree of tinnitus. Results of a multicenter study with the tinnitus questionnaire. HNO 42: 166–172.
15. Hallam R (1986) Psychological approaches to the evaluation and management of tinnitus distress. In: Hazell J, ed. Tinnitus. London: Churchill and Livingston. pp 1–50.
16. Crocetti A, Forti S, Ambrosetti U, Bo LD (2009) Questionnaires to evaluate anxiety and depressive levels in tinnitus patients. Otolaryngol Head Neck Surg 140: 403–405.
17. Langguth B, Kleinjung T, Fischer B, Hajak G, Eichhammer P, et al. (2007) Tinnitus severity, depression, and the big five personality traits. Prog Brain Res 166: 221–225.
18. De Ridder D, Vanneste S, Adriaenssens I, Lee AP, Plazier M, et al. (2010) Microvascular decompression for tinnitus: significant improvement for tinnitus intensity without improvement for distress. A 4-year limit. Neurosurgery 66: 656–660.
19. De Ridder D, Verstraeten E, Van der Kelen K, De Mulder G, Sunaert S, et al. (2005) Transcranial magnetic stimulation for tinnitus: influence of tinnitus duration on stimulation parameter choice and maximal tinnitus suppression. Otol Neurotol 26: 616–619.
20. Khedr EM, Rothwell JC, Ahmed MA, El-Atar A (2008) Effect of daily repetitive transcranial magnetic stimulation for treatment of tinnitus: comparison of different stimulus frequencies. Journal of neurology, neurosurgery, and psychiatry 79: 212–215.
21. Kleinjung T, Steffens T, Sand P, Murthum T, Hajak G, et al. (2007) Which tinnitus patients benefit from transcranial magnetic stimulation? Otolaryngol Head Neck Surg 137: 589–595.
22. Goh JO, Park DC (2009) Neuroplasticity and cognitive aging: the scaffolding theory of aging and cognition. Restor Neurol Neurosci 27: 391–403.
23. Zollig J, Eschen A (2009) Measuring compensation and its plasticity across the lifespan. Restor Neurol Neurosci 27: 421–433.
24. Andersson G, McKenna L (2006) The role of cognition in tinnitus. Acta Otolaryngol Suppl 556: 39–43.
25. Savastano M (2008) Tinnitus with or without hearing loss: are its characteristics different? Eur Arch Otorhinolaryngol 265(11): 1295–300.

15

Altered Neuronal Intrinsic Properties and Reduced Synaptic Transmission of the Rat's Medial Geniculate Body in Salicylate-Induced Tinnitus

Yan-Yan Su[1,2⌕], Bin Luo[1,2⌕], Yan Jin[1,2], Shu-Hui Wu[3], Edward Lobarinas[4], Richard J. Salvi[4], Lin Chen[1,2]*

1 CAS Key Laboratory of Brain Function and Disease, School of Life Sciences, University of Science and Technology of China, Hefei, China, 2 Auditory Research Laboratory, University of Science and Technology of China, Hefei, China, 3 Department of Neuroscience, Carleton University, Ottawa, Ontario, Canada, 4 Center for Hearing and Deafness, State University of New York at Buffalo, Buffalo, New York, United States of America

Abstract

Sodium salicylate (NaSal), an aspirin metabolite, can cause tinnitus in animals and human subjects. To explore neural mechanisms underlying salicylate-induced tinnitus, we examined effects of NaSal on neural activities of the medial geniculate body (MGB), an auditory thalamic nucleus that provides the primary and immediate inputs to the auditory cortex, by using the whole-cell patch-clamp recording technique in MGB slices. Rats treated with NaSal (350 mg/kg) showed tinnitus-like behavior as revealed by the gap prepulse inhibition of acoustic startle (GPIAS) paradigm. NaSal (1.4 mM) decreased the membrane input resistance, hyperpolarized the resting membrane potential, suppressed current-evoked firing, changed the action potential, and depressed rebound depolarization in MGB neurons. NaSal also reduced the excitatory and inhibitory postsynaptic response in the MGB evoked by stimulating the brachium of the inferior colliculus. Our results demonstrate that NaSal alters neuronal intrinsic properties and reduces the synaptic transmission of the MGB, which may cause abnormal thalamic outputs to the auditory cortex and contribute to NaSal-induced tinnitus.

Editor: Manuel S. Malmierca, University of Salamanca- Institute for Neuroscience of Castille and Leon and Medical School, Spain

Funding: This work was supported by the National Basic Research Program of China (Grant 2011CB504506) and the National Natural Science Foundation of China (Grants 30730041 and 30970977). The funders had no role in study design, data collection and analysis, decision to publish, or preparation of the manuscript.

Competing Interests: The authors have declared that no competing interests exist.

* E-mail: linchen@ustc.edu.cn

⌕ These authors contributed equally to this work.

Introduction

Sodium salicylate (NaSal), an active metabolite of aspirin, is one of the most widely used analgesic, anti-inflammatory, and antipyretic drugs. High doses of NaSal have long been known to cause reversible tinnitus in patients [1,2] and in animals [3,4,5,6]. Because the clinical presentation of tinnitus is subjective, of unknown etiology, and variable, exploring the underlying mechanism of tinnitus in humans is difficult. To examine its biological bases, researchers frequently use NaSal to induce transient tinnitus in animal models [3,5,6,7].

NaSal is believed to depress the neural output of the cochlea while cause hyperexcitability in some regions along the central auditory pathways [6,8]. There is growing evidence that NaSal raises the excitability of the auditory cortex. For example, *in vivo* studies have shown that NaSal significantly increases both the sound-evoked [6,9,10] and spontaneous [11] neural activity in auditory cortex region. Fluorine-18 fluoro-2-deoxyglucose activity, a measure of metabolic/neuronal activation, increases in the rat auditory cortex after NaSal treatment [12]. Hyperexcitability in the auditory cortex is also reflected by increased numbers of c-Fos immunoreactive neurons after NaSal treatment [13]. Our previous work on slices of the auditory cortex demonstrated that NaSal reduced the inhibitory postsynaptic current (IPSC) [14] and selectively suppressed the current-evoked firing of GABAergic

interneurons without affecting glutamatergic pyramidal neurons [15]. Both of these effects increase the excitability of the auditory cortex by altering the balance between excitation and inhibition. Collectively, these results suggest that increased neural excitability in the auditory cortex may be a key mechanism underlying NaSal-induced tinnitus [16,17]. NaSal also increases neuronal excitability in the rat hippocampus. It does so by reducing GABAergic inhibition without affecting intrinsic membrane excitability in CA1 pyramidal neurons [18]. The NaSal-induced increase in hippocampal excitability may contribute to non-auditory aspects of tinnitus because the limbic system has been implicated in tinnitus perception [17,19,20,21]. The ability of NaSal to elevate the excitability in the cerebral cortex (e.g., the auditory cortex and the hippocampus) raises a question of whether NaSal exerts the same effect in subcortical brain structures, which may be part of a neural network involved in the perception of tinnitus.

The medial geniculate body (MGB) is the part of the classical auditory pathway, which provides the primary and immediate inputs to the auditory cortex. The MGB has extensive afferent and efferent connections with the auditory cortex and plays a key role in auditory perception [22,23]. In this way, it makes an appropriate candidate for the study of the neural mechanisms underlying tinnitus. To date, only a few studies have examined the effect of NaSal on neural activity in the MGB [12,24], and the data are limited at the cellular level. To address this issue, we investigated how NaSal modulates the intrinsic membrane properties and synaptic responses of MGB neurons using whole-cell patch-clamp recordings from brain slices. In addition, we used the gap prepulse inhibition of acoustic startle (GPIAS) paradigm to confirm that salicylate induces tinnitus-like behavior in rats [6,25].

Results

NaSal induced tinnitus-like behavior in rats

Tinnitus was evaluated in 6 rats following treatment with saline and a 350 mg/kg dose of NaSal. NaSal caused a statistically significant decrease in GPIAS values relative to baseline across multiple frequencies (Fig. 1). This indicated that these rats were experiencing tinnitus. A two-way repeated measures analysis of variance (RM-ANOVA) with main effect treatment (factor 1) and frequency (factor 2) indicated a significant difference between NaSal treatment and baseline ($P<0.001$) and a significant difference between NaSal treatment and saline ($P<0.001$). However, there was no difference between baseline and saline treatments ($P>0.05$) indicating that saline treatment had no effect on GPIAS at these frequencies. The post hoc Tukey's test revealed a statistically significant frequency effect between NaSal treatment and baseline GPIAS values at 12, 16, 20 and 24 kHz, demonstrating that NaSal induces tinnitus over a broad range of high frequencies.

NaSal decreased membrane input resistance and hyperpolarized MGB neurons

To determine how NaSal affects the membrane excitability of MGB neurons, we applied NaSal in the bath solution during current-clamp recording. Fig. 2A shows sample traces of membrane potentials recorded from a MGB neuron following step current injections from which the membrane input resistance was derived. Group data show that NaSal significantly decreased the membrane input resistance from 248.8 ± 18.1 MΩ to 188.8 ± 15.4 MΩ ($n=23$, $P<0.001$) (Fig. 2B). This decrease in the membrane input resistance was reversible following washout ($P>0.05$). NaSal also significantly hyperpolarized the resting

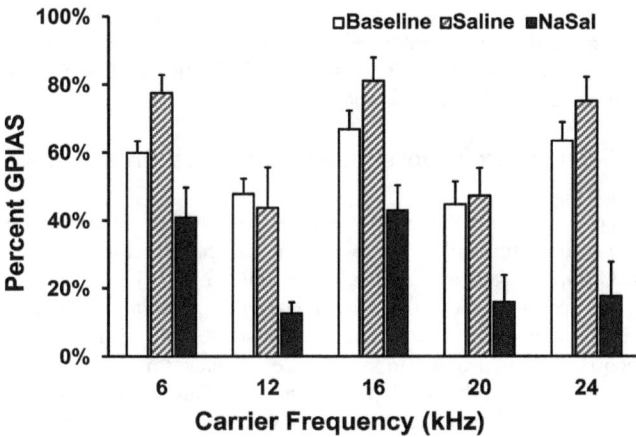

Figure 1. Gap prepulse inhibition of acoustic startle (GPIAS) as a function of carrier frequency for saline and sodium salicylate (NaSal) treatments relative to baseline. Saline treatment had no effect on GPIAS performance ($n=6$, $P>0.05$). In contrast, treatment of NaSal at a dose of 350 mg/kg caused a significant reduction in GPIAS performance ($n=6$, $P<0.001$). Data are the mean ± SEM. (two-way repeated measures analysis of variance, two way RM-ANOVA).

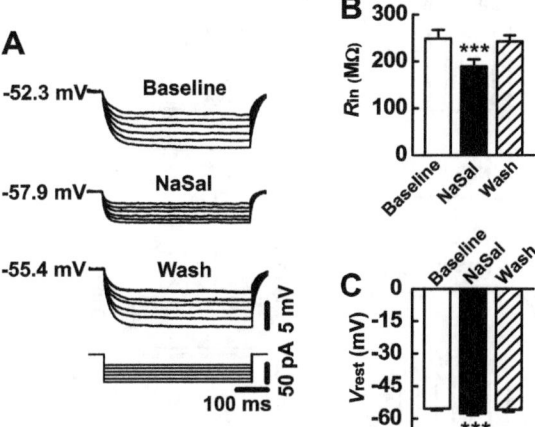

Figure 2. Effects of NaSal on membrane input resistance (R_{in}) and resting membrane potential (V_{rest}) of neurons in the medial geniculate body (MGB). (A) A series of hyperpolarizing current ranging from -30 to -80 pA (-10 pA/step) was injected into a MGB neuron for 500 ms before (Baseline), during (NaSal), and after (Wash) application of 1.4 mM NaSal. The V_{rest} is indicated beside the traces. (B) Mean R_{in} ($n=23$) and (C) V_{rest} ($n=28$) before (Baseline), during (NaSal), and after (Wash) application of 1.4 mM NaSal in the MGB neuron. Data are the mean ± SEM. ***$P<0.001$ relative to baseline (one-way ANOVA with Bonferroni correction, 3 pairwise comparisons).

membrane potential from -55.3 ± 0.8 mV to -57.5 ± 0.7 mV ($n=28$, $P<0.001$) (Fig. 2A and C). This hyperpolarizing effect was also reversible following washout ($P>0.05$).

NaSal suppressed the current-evoked firing and changed the action potential in MGB neurons

Electrical currents at various levels up to 70 pA above the threshold level were injected into MGB neurons to evoke action potential firing. NaSal reversibly decreased the firing rates in all 23 neurons tested (Fig. 3). Among these neurons, firing of 13 neurons evoked by current injections at these various levels was completely blocked by NaSal (Fig. 3A, upper two traces). Two-way ANOVA revealed that NaSal significantly decreased the evoked firing rate of the neurons at current levels up to 70 pA above the threshold current ($n=9$–23 for different current levels, $P<0.001$) (Fig. 3C). To rule out the possibility that the suppression of firing was due to the membrane hyperpolarization caused by NaSal, we adjusted the resting membrane potential equal to the level before drug application in 4 neurons during their exposure to NaSal to determine whether the depression persisted. The firing remained suppressed after the adjustment, as illustrated in Fig. 3A (third trace from the top). Neither the change in resting membrane potential ($n=19$, $P=0.089$, $r^2=0.16$) nor the change in membrane input resistance ($n=19$, $P=0.067$, $r^2=0.183$) was correlated with the change in firing rate (at 40 pA re threshold level), indicating that other mechanisms rather than resting membrane potential or membrane input resistance are involved in the effects of NaSal on the evoked firing.

The action potential properties of the 10 neurons that generated spikes during NaSal treatment were also affected. Fig. 3C shows sample action potentials in the presence and absence of NaSal. For this neuron, the action potential threshold was increased by ≈2 mV and the threshold current was increased by 20 pA (Before NaSal, 80 pA induced one action potential, and after NaSal, 100 pA induced one action potential) (Fig. 3C, top and middle traces). The amplitude, rise and decay time, and half-width of action potential were all affected by NaSal (Fig. 3C, bottom trace). Table 1 shows that,

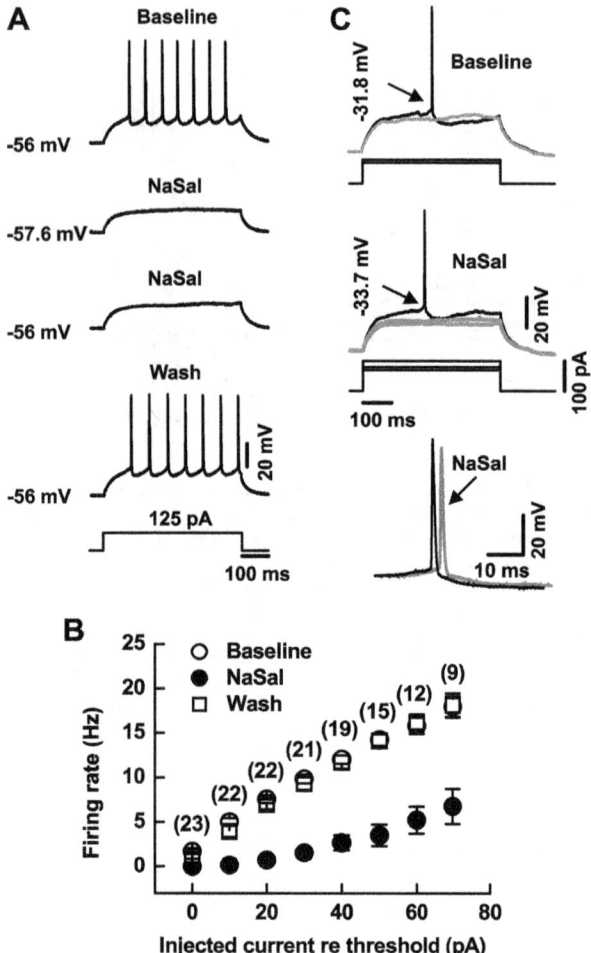

Figure 3. Effects of NaSal on current evoked firing and the action potential properties of MGB neurons. (A) A 125 pA current was injected into a MGB neuron for 500 ms before (Baseline), during (NaSal), and after (Wash) application of 1.4 mM NaSal. Note that the neuron's resting membrane potential was adjusted to the baseline levels during NaSal exposure (third trace from the top). (B) Mean evoked firing rate at all superthreshold levels before (Baseline), during (NaSal), and after (Wash) application of 1.4 mM NaSal in MGB neurons. Treatment with NaSal caused a significant reduction in evoked firing rate ($P<0.001$). Sample sizes are indicated in parentheses (two-way ANOVA). (C) Upper traces: responses of a MGB neuron to 70 pA (gray) and 80 pA (black) current injections for 500 ms before NaSal. Middle traces: responses of the same neuron to 80 and 90 pA (gray) and 100 pA (black) current injections for 500 ms during NaSal. Lower traces: action potential waveforms shown in upper (black) and middle (gray) traces are overlapped. The thresholds for generation of action potentials are indicated by arrows.

during NaSal treatment, the action potential amplitude ($n=10$, $P<0.01$), rise slope ($n=10$, $P<0.05$), and decay slope ($n=10$, $P<0.01$) were all reduced significantly, and the action potential threshold ($n=10$, $P<0.05$), half-width ($n=10$, $P<0.05$), and the threshold current ($n=10$, $P<0.001$) increased significantly. However, the afterhyperpolarization (AHP) remained unchanged ($n=10$, $P>0.05$).

NaSal depressed the rebound depolarization in MGB neurons

Almost all of the MGB neurons tested had a rebound depolarization (Fig. 4A), which consisted of depolarization

Table 1. Effects of 1.4 mM sodium salicylate (NaSal) on action potential properties ($n=10$).

Measurements	Before NaSal perfusion			After NaSal perfusion		
Threshold (mV)[1]	−31.3	±	1.4	−29.3	±	1.6*
Amplitude (mV)[2]	68.0	±	2.7	63.4	±	2.8**
Rise slope (mV/ms)	83.4	±	11.9	72.4	±	11.9*
Decay slope (mV/ms)	−32.6	±	3.1	−29.0	±	2.7**
Half-width (ms)	1.5	±	0.1	1.6	±	0.1*
Threshold current (pA)[3]	44.5	±	6.7	77.5	±	11.8***

All data are expressed as means ± SEM. *, ** and *** indicate $P<0.05$, $P<0.01$ and $P<0.001$, respectively (paired Student's t-test).
[1]The action potential threshold was defined as the membrane potential at which the potential of the membrane began to rise rapidly and the neuron generated only one or two spikes.
[2]The action potential amplitude was calculated by subtracting the threshold from the peak value of the action potential.
[3]The threshold current was defined as the minimum current that is required to elicit one or two spikes.

immediately following membrane hyperpolarization [26,27,28]. NaSal reversibly reduced the rebound in all 10 neurons tested. Fig. 4A shows sample traces of rebound potentials recorded from a MGB neuron in the presence and absence of NaSal. The amplitude of rebound depolarization was gradually and drastically decreased from 23.9 ± 1.6 mV to 6.5 ± 2.8 mV by NaSal ($n=10$, $P<0.001$) (Fig. 4B).

Note that the membrane input resistance was also decreased by NaSal (Fig. 4A middle panel). Because the amplitude of the rebound depolarization would decrease if the magnitude of the preceding hyperpolarization were smaller [29], the reduction in the rebound might be due to smaller pre-hyperpolarization induced by NaSal. To rule out this possibility, we injected larger negative currents into 3 neurons during NaSal treatment in order to match the hyperpolarization to the level observed in the absence of NaSal. Under these conditions, NaSal still suppressed the rebound (Fig. 4C). No correlation was observed between the change in rebound amplitude and the change in membrane input resistance ($n=10$, $P=0.384$, $r^2=0.096$), indicating that NaSal had a direct action on the rebound.

NaSal depressed evoked postsynaptic responses in MGB neurons

To evoke postsynaptic responses in MGB neurons, we electrically stimulated the brachium of the inferior colliculus (BIC), which contains colliculogeniculate axons (Fig. 5A). The evoked postsynaptic activity was recorded in current-clamp mode without application of receptor antagonists. Among 11 neurons we recorded, 6 neurons had a mixture of excitatory postsynaptic responses and inhibitory postsynaptic responses (Fig. 5B) [26] whereas the others either had a unitary excitatory response (3 out of 11 neurons) or had a unitary inhibitory response (2 out of 11 neurons). Fig. 5C shows sample traces of mixed postsynaptic responses recorded from a MGB neuron in the absence and presence of NaSal. There is no significant difference in the peak amplitude of postsynaptic responses with excitatory components (i.e., the mixed responses together with the unitary excitatory responses) before and after application of NaSal (8.9 ± 1.8 vs. 7.7 ± 1.1 mV, $n=9$, $P>0.05$) (Fig. 5D). However, NaSal signifi-

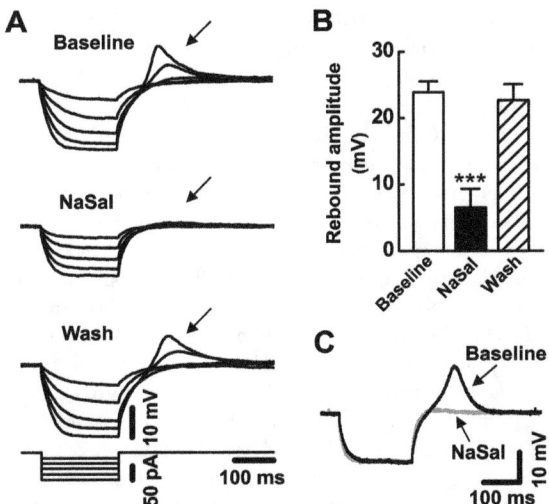

Figure 4. Effects of NaSal on rebound depolarization in MGB neurons. (A) A series of hyperpolarizing current ranging from −20 pA to −100 pA (20 pA/step) was injected into a MGB neuron before (Baseline), during (NaSal), and after (Wash) application of 1.4 mM NaSal. The rebound depolarization following membrane hyperpolarization is indicated with an arrow. (B) The mean amplitude of rebound depolarization before (Baseline), during (NaSal), and after (Wash) application of 1.4 mM NaSal in the MGB neurons ($n = 10$). Data are the mean ± SEM. ***$P < 0.001$ relative to baseline (one-way ANOVA with Bonferroni correction, 3 pairwise comparisons). (C) Response of another neuron to −80 pA current injection in ACSF (black trace) and to −100 pA current injection in 1.4 mM NaSal (gray trace).

cantly and reversibly decreased the response area above the resting membrane potential from 1965.6 ± 264.6 to 1428.1 ± 194.5 mV•ms ($n = 9$, $P < 0.05$) (Fig. 5E).

NaSal depressed the postsynaptic responses mediated by GABA$_A$ or NMDA receptors, but not AMPA receptors in MGB neurons

The fast postsynaptic responses recorded from MGB neurons are mediated mainly by GABA$_A$, NMDA, and AMPA receptors [26,28]. We were interested in which receptors NaSal acts on for the reduction of the postsynaptic responses. To address this issue, we took voltage-clamp recordings of MGB neurons with specific antagonists added to ACSF or the pipette solution. We also clamped the membrane potentials to specific levels in order to distinguish the postsynaptic responses mediated by different receptors.

To determine the IPSC mediated by GABA$_A$ receptors, we blocked ionotropic glutamatergic receptors by adding 4 mM of kynurenic acid to the bath solution and maintained the membrane potential at 0 mV. NaSal gradually and reversibly decreased the amplitude of GABA$_A$ receptor-mediated IPSCs by $31.8 \pm 8.9\%$ of the control ($n = 22$, $P < 0.001$) (Fig. 6A). To determine the excitatory postsynaptic current (EPSC) mediated by NMDA receptors, we blocked GABA$_A$ receptors and AMPA receptors by adding picrotoxin (100 μmol/L) and CNQX (10 μmol/L) to the bath solution and held the membrane potential at +40 mV to relieve the voltage-dependent Mg^{2+} blockade on the NMDA receptor channels. NaSal gradually and reversibly decreased the amplitude of NMDA receptor-mediated EPSCs by $21.3 \pm 6.7\%$ of the control ($n = 18$, $P < 0.001$) (Fig. 6B). To determine the EPSC mediated by AMPA receptors, we blocked GABA$_A$ receptors by adding picrotoxin (100 μmol/L) to the bath solution and

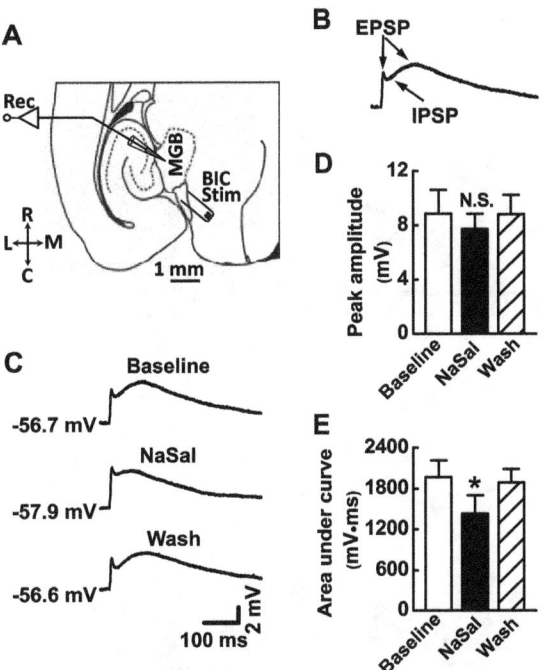

Figure 5. Effects of NaSal on postsynaptic responses of MGB neurons evoked by stimulating the brachium of the inferior colliculus (BIC). (A) A schematic drawing of a brain slice with horizontal section of the MGB. Locations of recording (Rec) and electrical stimulation (Stim) are illustrated. R, rostral; C, caudal; L, lateral; M, middle. (B) Sample trace of the typical postsynaptic potential (PSP) recorded. The PSP had two components: excitatory postsynaptic potential (EPSP) and inhibitory postsynaptic potential (IPSP). The trace was averaged from 6 consecutive sweeps. (C) Representative traces of PSP before (Baseline), during (NaSal), and after (Wash) application of 1.4 mM NaSal in a MGB neuron. Each trace was averaged from 6 consecutive sweeps. The resting membrane potential is indicated beside the traces. (D) Mean peak amplitude of the PSP ($n = 9$) and (E) area under PSP curve ($n = 9$) before (Baseline), during (NaSal), and after (Wash) application of 1.4 mM NaSal in the MGB neuron. Data are the mean ± SEM. *$P < 0.05$, $^{N.S.}P > 0.05$ relative to baseline (one-way ANOVA with Bonferroni correction, 3 pairwise comparisons).

minimized NMDA receptor-mediated components by maintaining the membrane potential at −80 mV. NaSal did not significantly change the amplitude of AMPA receptor-mediated EPSCs (Fig. 6C) ($n = 15$, $P > 0.05$).

Discussion

Using a GPIAS paradigm, we successfully demonstrated that a high dose of NaSal (350 mg/kg) can reliably induce tinnitus-like behavior in Wistar rats (Fig. 1). This is consistent with previous reports using other strains [3,6,25,30,31]. To explore the underlying neural mechanisms of this tinnitus-like behavior in rats, we examined effects of NaSal on the neuronal and synaptic responses in rat MGB *in vitro*. The neurons we recorded were likely from two main subdivisions of the MGB, the dorsal and ventral MGB because of their characteristic electrophysiological properties (i.e., the monophasic AHPs and rebound bursts, data not shown) [32]. We have found that (1) NaSal changed the intrinsic properties of MGB neurons, such as the membrane input resistance (Fig. 2), the resting membrane potential (Fig. 2), the current-evoked firing (Fig. 3), the shape of the action potential (Fig. 3, Table 1) and the rebound depolarization (Fig. 4); (2) NaSal

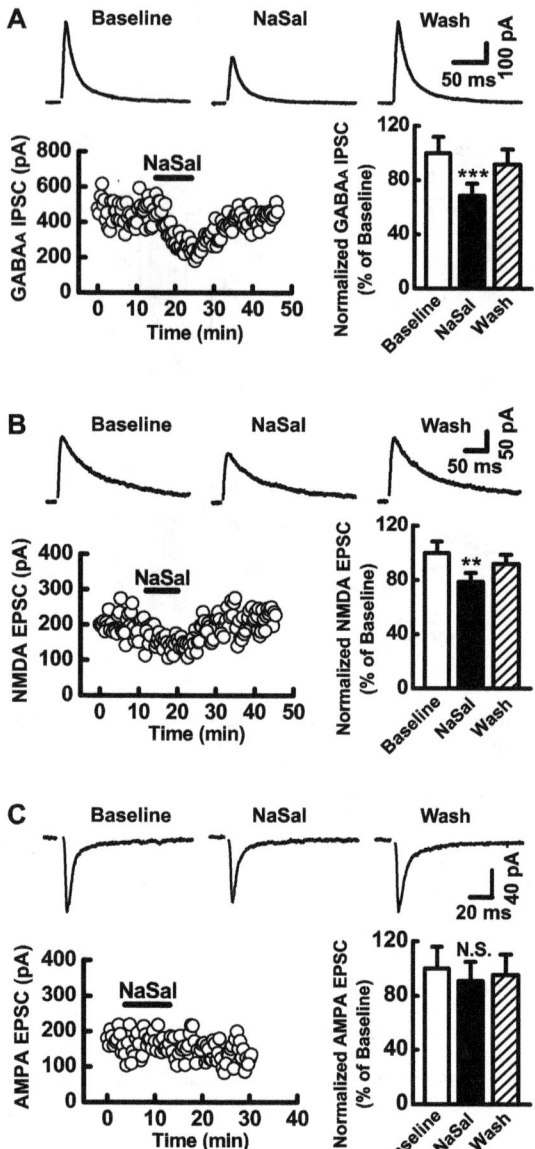

NaSal may alter the intrinsic properties of MGB neurons by targeting membrane ion channels

It is likely that NaSal alters the intrinsic properties of MGB neurons through its actions on the membrane ion channels expressed in the MGB neurons. In the present study, NaSal significantly reduces the membrane input resistance of MGB neurons and hyperpolarizes their resting membrane potentials (Fig. 2). This suggests that NaSal influences the ion channels that maintain the resting membrane potential, such as the KCNK channels [33,34]. Although the detailed mechanisms are not fully understood, one possibility is that NaSal causes more K^+ ions to leak out of the cell, thereby reducing the membrane resistance and hyperpolarizing the membrane potential. NaSal was demonstrated in inferior colliculus neurons to modulate the function of voltage-gated Na^+ channels [35], which mediate the rapidly rising phase and initial component of the falling phase of an action potential [36,37]. By blocking the voltage-gated Na^+ channels in the MGB neurons, NaSal could reduce the evoked firing rate, elevate action potential threshold, decrease action potential amplitude, reduce the action potential's rise and decay slopes, and prolong the action potential half-width as we observed in the present study (Fig. 3, Table 1). In the MGB, rebound depolarization is mediated by the low-threshold Ca^{2+} channels [26,27,28]. The present study shows that NaSal directly depresses the rebound depolarization (Fig. 4), suggesting that NaSal may also have a depressive effect on these low-threshold Ca^{2+} channels. The notion that NaSal changes the intrinsic properties of MGB neurons through its actions on the membrane ion channels needs to be confirmed using voltage-clamp recordings.

How does NaSal reduce the afferent synaptic transmission in the MGB?

The present study shows that NaSal depressed postsynpatic responses in MGB neurons to the stimulation of the BIC. Because the BIC contains colliculogeniculate axons, the evoked postsynaptic responses recorded in the MGB neurons simulated the afferent synaptic inputs from the inferior colliculus. These fast postsynaptic responses are mediated mainly by $GABA_A$, NMDA, and AMPA receptors [26,28]. In the present study, the IPSC mediated by $GABA_A$ receptors was depressed significantly by NaSal. In addition, the EPSC mediated by NMDA receptors, but not by AMPA receptors, was depressed by NaSal (Fig. 6). These results indicate that NaSal reduces both inhibitory and excitatory postsynaptic responses mainly through its actions on $GABA_A$ and NMDA receptors.

Although NaSal suppressed both inhibitory and excitatory postsynaptic responses in the MGB, the inhibitory component of postsynaptic currents was suppressed to a more pronounced degree (Fig. 6A) than the excitatory component (Fig. 6B). However, the summed postsynaptic response consisting of inhibitory and excitatory components was not potentiated by NaSal as a net effect (Fig. 5E). This is probably because there was a difference in the number between excitatory and inhibitory fibers of the BIC that were recruited by electrical stimulation. If more excitatory fibers are activated, NaSal would suppress EPSCs more than IPSCs, resulting in less excitation than inhibition. In this way, no potentiation of the overall synaptic responses would take place. In addition, the decreased membrane input resistance, hyperpolarized resting membrane potential, and cross-talk between NMDA and $GABA_A$ receptors [38] may also contribute to the suppressive effect of NaSal on the synaptic response.

Figure 6. Effects of NaSal on the GABA$_A$, the NMDA, and the AMPA receptor-mediated postsynaptic current of MGB neurons evoked by stimulating the BIC. Upper panels in (A), (B) and (C): representative traces of GABA$_A$ receptor-mediated inhibitory postsynaptic current (IPSC), NMDA, and AMPA receptor-mediated excitatory postsynaptic current (EPSC) before (Baseline), during (NaSal), and after (Wash) application of 1.4 mM NaSal in a MGB neuron, respectively. Each trace was averaged from 6 consecutive sweeps. Lower left panels in (A), (B) and (C): time course of the amplitude of IPSCs and the EPSCs recorded in the same neuron as in each upper panel with application of 1.4 mM NaSal (horizontal bar). Lower right panels in (A), (B) and (C): mean amplitude of GABA$_A$ receptor-mediated IPSCs ($n=22$), NMDA receptor-mediated EPSCs ($n=18$) and AMPA receptor-mediated EPSC ($n=15$) before (Baseline), during (NaSal), and after (Wash) application of 1.4 mM NaSal in the MGB neurons. Data are the mean ± SEM. ***$P<0.001$, **$P<0.01$, $^{N.S.}P>0.05$ relative to baseline (one-way ANOVA with Bonferroni correction, 3 pairwise comparisons).

reduced the postsynaptic response evoked by stimulating the BIC. The altered intrinsic neuronal properties and reduced synaptic transmission by NaSal suggest a possible role of the MGB in NaSal-induced tinnitus.

NaSal likely lowers the excitability of the MGB

The altered neuronal intrinsic properties (Figs. 2, 3, 4) as well as reduced synaptic transmission (Figs. 5 and 6) by NaSal suggests reduced neuronal excitability of the MGB in rats following treatment of NaSal. The specific evidence supporting this notion includes: (1) the decrease in the membrane input resistance together with the hyperpolarized resting membrane potential caused by NaSal would lower neuronal excitability; (2) the suppressed probability of generating action potentials by NaSal is a reflection of the reduced membrane excitability of MGB neurons after NaSal perfusion; (3) rebound depolarization is believed to enhance membrane excitability and promote the production of action potentials [29,39]. If this is correct, then the depression of the rebound by NaSal may acts as another mechanism by which NaSal suppresses neuronal excitability; (4) the reduction in postsynaptic responses evoked by BIC stimulation as a net effect after NaSal perfusion indicates that NaSal reduces the efficacy of synaptic transmission from the inferior colliculus to MGB neurons (Fig. 5). In rat MGB, GABAergic neurons are in low abundance (<1%) [40,41] although there are morphologically different cell types [42,43]. Thus, most neurons we recorded in the MGB were likely glutamatergic and the reduced neuronal excitability of these presumably glutamatergic neurons by NaSal suggests lowered excitability of the MGB.

NaSal can penetrate the blood-brain barrier and reach concentrations up to 310 mg/L (1.94 mM) in the cerebrospinal fluid of animals treated with high doses of NaSal [44]. Consequently, when it is systemically applied, NaSal not only affects the cochlea but can directly affect the excitability of broad brain regions within and outside of the central auditory system including the MGB to generate tinnitus. We have previously demonstrated that NaSal (1.4 mM) selectively depressed the firing rate of GABAergic fast-spiking interneurons without affecting the firing rate of pyramidal neurons in the auditory cortex [15]. In other areas of the forebrain, such as the hippocampus, NaSal also exerted an excitatory effect [18]. In the inferior colliculus, NaSal induces an increase of the spontaneous activity [45,46]. However, in the dorsal cochlear nucleus, NaSal suppresses spontaneous and evoked firing in fusiform cells but has little effect on the firing of glycinergic cartwheel cells [47]. In the MGB, the neural excitability is likely lowered by NaSal as illustrated in the present study. Taken together, these results indicate that the effects of NaSal on neural activity are remarkably dependent on brain region. Why NaSal has such widely varied effects on different auditory structures remains largely a mystery at this point. Discovering the reasons for the brain-region-dependent actions of NaSal may have important implications for our understanding of the neural mechanisms underlying tinnitus.

Role of the MGB in NaSal-induced tinnitus

The MGB provides the primary and immediate inputs to the auditory cortex. Paradoxically, we found that NaSal likely lowers the excitability of the MGB but increases the excitability of neurons in the auditory cortex [9,15]. If the context of the neural networks mediates the perception of tinnitus, then there is a question as to how NaSal-induced decreases in MGB excitability contribute to the generation of tinnitus-like behavior in rats. We speculate that the decreased excitability of the MGB will lead to reduced thalamic inputs to the auditory cortex. Because these inputs have been shown to activate inhibitory interneurons more strongly than excitatory neurons in the neocortex [48], the reduced inputs by NaSal would presumably change the inhibition-excitation balance towards excitatory side, resulting in an increase in excitability in the neural networks of the auditory cortex. In this

sense, the MGB plays a role in generation of NaSal-induced tinnitus.

Difference in the age between animals used in behavior and *in vitro* experiments

One of limitations of the present study is that young animals (15.8±0.2 postnatal days) were used for the patch-clamp experiment whereas adult animals (3–5 months old) were used in the behavioral experiment. Although there is evidence to show that the intrinsic properties (e.g. the resting membrane potential and the membrane input resistance) of MGB neurons do not change very much from 16 to 21 postnatal days in rats [49,50], caution should still be taken when the results obtained in the patch-clamp experiment are used to interpret those in the behaviral experiment.

Materials and Methods

Subjects

Adult male Wistar rats (3–5 months old, 325–450 g) were used to assess NaSal-induced tinnitus using GPIAS. Young Wistar rats of both sexes (13–21 postnatal days; average age slices were recorded from is 15.8±0.2 postnatal days) were used for patch-clamp experiments. The behavioral experimental procedures used in the present study were approved by the University at Buffalo Institutional Animal Care and Use Committee. The experimental procedures for the patch-clamp experiments were in accordance with the protocols approved by the Institutional Animal Care and Use Committee of University of Science and Technology of China. All efforts were made to minimize the number of animals used and their suffering.

Behavioral measures of NaSal-induced tinnitus

Tinnitus was assessed using the GPIAS paradigm as described in detail in previous reports [6,25]. This procedure utilized the acoustic startle reflex test in animals treated with NaSal. Baseline measures of GPIAS were collected first, followed by treatment with saline (2.2–3.2 ml i.p.). Following a 5 day washout period, rats were treated with NaSal (350 mg/kg, 2.2–3.2 ml saline vehicle, 50 mg/ml concentration, i.p.). GPIAS testing began 1 hour after administration of either saline or NaSal. Each rat was placed in an acoustically transparent wire-mesh cage mounted on Plexiglas base which rested on a sensitive piezoelectric transducer that generated a voltage proportional to the magnitude of the startle response evoked by sound stimuli generated digitally by digital signal processor (Tucker Davis, TDT RX6, U.S.). The output of the startle platform was amplified, sampled, and stored on a computer for offline analysis.

GPIAS sessions were composed of 100 gap trials and 100 no-gap trials. Twenty measurements were taken at each noise-band center frequency (narrow band noise centered at 6, 12, 16, 20, or 24 kHz). Gap and no-gap trials were presented in random pairs. Trials were separated by a variable intertrial interval of 7–15 s. A 2 minute acclimation period occurred at the beginning of each session during which no stimuli were presented. Gap trials started with a background of narrow band noise centered at 6, 12, 16, 20, or 24 kHz (≈60 dB SPL, BW = 100–5000 Hz). During each gap trial, a brief, silent 75 ms gap was inserted 100 ms prior to the startling stimulus (5–10 kHz bandpass noise, 105 dB SPL). No-gap trials were identical to gap trials except that the silent gaps were omitted from the trials.

Preparation of brain slices

On the day of patch-clamp experiment, the brain slices of MGB were prepared as described previously [51]. Briefly, the animal was decapitated and the brain was carefully taken out. Using a vibrating microtome (VT-1000S; Leica, Germany), three or four 290–390 µm thick horizontal slices including MGB were obtained from the brain. After at least 1 hour of incubation in oxygenated (95% O_2 and 5% CO_2) artificial cerebrospinal fluid (ACSF) at 26°C, one slice was transferred to a submerged recording chamber that was continuously perfused (3 ml/min) with oxygenated ACSF. The temperature of the bath solution was monitored and maintained at 25–26°C.

Solutions and drugs used for patch-clamp recording

The composition of the standard ACSF was (in mM): NaCl 124; KCl 5; $MgSO_4$ 1.3; KH_2PO_4 1.2; glucose 10; $NaHCO_3$ 24; $CaCl_2$ 2.4 (pH: 7.4, osmolarity: 290–300 mOsm/L). The composition of the pipette solution was (in mM): K-gluconate 130; $MgCl_2$ 2; KCl 5; EGTA 0.6; HEPES 10; Na-GTP 0.3; Mg-ATP 2 (pH: 7.2, osmolarity: 280 mOsm/L) for current-clamp recording and (in mM): Cs-methanesulfonate 130; $CaCl_2$ 0.15; $MgCl_2$ 2.0; EGTA 2.0; HEPES 10; Na_2-ATP 2.0; Na_3-GTP 0.25; QX-314 10 (pH: 7.2, osmolarity: 282 mOsm/L) for voltage-clamp recording. NaSal was dissolved in ACSF just before use and the concentration of NaSal we used was 1.4 mM, the typical concentration found in the cerebrospinal fluid of animal models with NaSal-induced tinnitus [52,53]. After stable baseline responses were acquired, NaSal was normally administrated for 7–10 min when the reactions to the drug were most prominent. All drugs used in this study were purchased from Sigma Aldrich, Co. (St. Louis, MO, U.S.).

Whole-cell patch-clamp recording and electrical stimulation

Patch pipettes were pulled from glass capillaries with an outer diameter of 1.5 mm on a two-stage puller (PC-10; Narishige, Tokyo, Japan). The resistance of the recording electrode filled with pipette solution was 3–5 MΩ. A patch-clamp amplifier (EPC9; HEKA Electronics, Germany) and a built-in PCI-16 interface board were used for whole-cell patch-clamp recordings. The MGB neurons were visualized under a 40× water immersion objective on an upright microscope (E-600-FN; Nikon, Japan) equipped with an infrared camera. Data were sampled using a computer installed with Pulse software (Version 8.80; HEKA Electronics, Germany). Only those neurons with series resistance <30 MΩ and input resistance >100 MΩ were included in this study. If the series resistance changed by more than 20% of the initial value during the recording, the data was discarded.

To evoke postsynaptic responses, we placed a bipolar stimulating electrode consisted of two tungsten wires separated by ~500 µm on the BIC just caudal to the MGB (Fig. 5A). A single 100–200 µs rectangular electrical pulse was generated by a stimulator (SEN-7203; Hikon Kohden, Japan) and delivered at 0.05 Hz through an isolation unit (SS-202J; Hikon Kohden, Japan). The electrical stimulation to the BIC, which contains the colliculogeniculate axons, simulated the neural inputs from the inferior colliculus to the MGB. The strength of stimulation was set to a level at which the EPSC or IPSC amplitude was about 50–70% of the maximum amplitude evoked.

Data analysis

GPIAS was calculated by computing the average ratio of trials with a gap versus trials with no-gaps for each frequency using the formula: $GPIAS = (1-(AvgT_{gap}/AvgT_{nogap}))\times100\%$; where $AvgT_{gap}$ is the average amplitude during gap trials, and $AvgT_{nogap}$ is the average amplitude of trials with no gap. The data were analyzed using a two-way RM-ANOVA to determine the main effects of treatment and the interaction between treatment and frequency, and post-hoc Tukey's tests were performed to make multiple comparison on different frequencies (SigmaStat 3.5 software).

For patch-clamp experiments, all the measurements were made from the recordings at least 5–10 min after establishing a whole-cell configuration and showing a stable resting membrane potential. The methods for data analysis of intrinsic membrane properties and synaptic responses were similar to those described previously [54]. Changes in membrane potential elicited by intracellular current injection (−30 to −80 pA) were measured between the baseline membrane potential and the peak hyperpolarization. The current-voltage (I–V) curve was plotted and then the slope was calculated from the linear range of the curve. The value of the I–V curve slope was defined as the input resistance of the cell membrane. The action potential threshold was defined as the membrane potential at which the potential of the membrane began to rise rapidly and the neuron generated only one or two spikes. The threshold current for firing was defined as the minimum amplitude of current injection required to elicit at least one or two spikes. The amplitude of an action potential was defined as the difference between the action potential threshold and the peak voltage of the action potential. The amplitude of the rebound depolarization following membrane hyperpolarization was defined as the difference between the resting membrane potential and the peak of the rebound.

Off-line data analysis for patch-clamp experiments was carried out using Pulse software version 8.80 (HEKA Electronic, Germany), Clampfit software version 9.2 (Axon Instruments Inc, U.S.), and MiniAnalysis software version 6.03 (Synaptosoft Inc, U.S.). For the purpose of statistical analysis, the data from the same neuron were averaged samples within a 2 min time window and collected before (baseline recording), during (NaSal exposure), and after (wash) NaSal application. The processed data were imported into Origin software version 7.5 (OriginLab Corporation, U.S.) for generating graphs. The statistical significance of differences between two groups was determined using paired Student's t-tests. For multiple group comparisons, statistical significance was determined using one-way analysis of variance (ANOVA) with Bonferroni correction or two-way ANOVA. All data are expressed as means ± SEM, where n represents the number of neurons. Two-sided $P\leq0.05$ was regarded as statistically significant.

Acknowledgments

The authors thank Yi-Na Huang and Ke-Qing Zhou for their technical support.

Author Contributions

Conceived and designed the experiments: LC SHW RJS YYS. Performed the experiments: EL YYS BL YJ. Analyzed the data: YYS EL. Wrote the paper: LC SHW RJS YYS.

References

1. Day RO, Graham GG, Bieri D, Brown M, Cairns D, et al. (1989) Concentration-response relationships for salicylate-induced ototoxicity in normal volunteers. Br J Clin Pharmacol 28: 695–702.

2. Mongan E, Kelly P, Nies K, Porter WW, Paulus HE (1973) Tinnitus as an indication of therapeutic serum salicylate levels. JAMA 226: 142–145.

3. Guitton MJ, Caston J, Ruel J, Johnson RM, Pujol R, et al. (2003) Salicylate induces tinnitus through activation of cochlear NMDA receptors. J Neurosci 23: 3944–3952.

4. Jastreboff PJ, Brennan JF, Coleman JK, Sasaki CT (1988) Phantom auditory sensation in rats: an animal model for tinnitus. Behav Neurosci 102: 811–822.

5. Kizawa K, Kitahara T, Horii A, Maekawa C, Kuramasu T, et al. (2010) Behavioral assessment and identification of a molecular marker in a salicylate-induced tinnitus in rats. Neuroscience 165: 1323–1332.

6. Yang G, Lobarinas E, Zhang L, Turner J, Stolzberg D, et al. (2007) Salicylate induced tinnitus: behavioral measures and neural activity in auditory cortex of awake rats. Hear Res 226: 244–253.

7. Liu XP, Chen L (2012) Auditory brainstem response as a possible objective indicator for salicylate-induced tinnitus in rats. Brain Res. In press.

8. Cazals Y (2000) Auditory sensori-neural alterations induced by salicylate. Prog Neurobiol 62: 583–631.

9. Sun W, Lu J, Stolzberg D, Gray L, Deng A, et al. (2009) Salicylate increases the gain of the central auditory system. Neuroscience 159: 325–334.

10. Zhang X, Yang P, Cao Y, Qin L, Sato Y (2011) Salicylate induced neural changes in the primary auditory cortex of awake cats. Neuroscience 172: 232–245.

11. Eggermont JJ, Kenmochi M (1998) Salicylate and quinine selectively increase spontaneous firing rates in secondary auditory cortex. Hear Res 117: 149–160.

12. Paul AK, Lobarinas E, Simmons R, Wack D, Luisi JC, et al. (2009) Metabolic imaging of rat brain during pharmacologically-induced tinnitus. Neuroimage 44: 312–318.

13. Wallhausser-Franke E, Mahlke C, Oliva R, Braun S, Wenz G, et al. (2003) Expression of c-fos in auditory and non-auditory brain regions of the gerbil after manipulations that induce tinnitus. Exp Brain Res 153: 649–654.

14. Wang HT, Luo B, Zhou KQ, Xu TL, Chen L (2006) Sodium salicylate reduces inhibitory postsynaptic currents in neurons of rat auditory cortex. Hear Res 215: 77–83.

15. Su YY, Luo B, Wang HT, Chen L (2009) Differential effects of sodium salicylate on current-evoked firing of pyramidal neurons and fast-spiking interneurons in slices of rat auditory cortex. Hear Res 253: 60–66.

16. Eggermont JJ (2008) Role of auditory cortex in noise- and drug-induced tinnitus. Am J Audiol 17: S162–169.

17. Leaver AM, Renier L, Chevillet MA, Morgan S, Kim HJ, et al. (2011) Dysregulation of limbic and auditory networks in tinnitus. Neuron 69: 33–43.

18. Gong N, Zhang M, Zhang XB, Chen L, Sun GC, et al. (2008) The aspirin metabolite salicylate enhances neuronal excitation in rat hippocampal CA1 area through reducing GABAergic inhibition. Neuropharmacology 54: 454–463.

19. Landgrebe M, Langguth B, Rosengarth K, Braun S, Koch A, et al. (2009) Structural brain changes in tinnitus: grey matter decrease in auditory and non-auditory brain areas. Neuroimage 46: 213–218.

20. Lockwood AH, Salvi RJ, Coad ML, Towsley ML, Wack DS, et al. (1998) The functional neuroanatomy of tinnitus: evidence for limbic system links and neural plasticity. Neurology 50: 114–120.

21. Mahlke C, Wallhausser-Franke E (2004) Evidence for tinnitus-related plasticity in the auditory and limbic system, demonstrated by arg3.1 and c-fos immunocytochemistry. Hear Res 195: 17–34.

22. Lanting CP, de Kleine E, van Dijk P (2009) Neural activity underlying tinnitus generation: results from PET and fMRI. Hear Res 255: 1–13.

23. Malmierca MS (2003) The structure and physiology of the rat auditory system: an overview. Int Rev Neurobiol 56: 147–211.

24. Basta D, Goetze R, Ernst A (2008) Effects of salicylate application on the spontaneous activity in brain slices of the mouse cochlear nucleus, medial geniculate body and primary auditory cortex. Hear Res 240: 42–51.

25. Ralli M, Lobarinas E, Fetoni AR, Stolzberg D, Paludetti G, et al. (2010) Comparison of salicylate- and quinine-induced tinnitus in rats: development, time course, and evaluation of audiologic correlates. Otol Neurotol 31: 823–831.

26. Bartlett EL, Smith PH (1999) Anatomic, intrinsic, and synaptic properties of dorsal and ventral division neurons in rat medial geniculate body. J Neurophysiol 81: 1999–2016.

27. Hu B (1995) Cellular basis of temporal synaptic signalling: an in vitro electrophysiological study in rat auditory thalamus. J Physiol 483 (Pt 1): 167–182.

28. Peruzzi D, Bartlett E, Smith PH, Oliver DL (1997) A monosynaptic GABAergic input from the inferior colliculus to the medial geniculate body in rat. J Neurosci 17: 3766–3777.

29. Sun H, Wu SH (2008) Physiological characteristics of postinhibitory rebound depolarization in neurons of the rat's dorsal cortex of the inferior colliculus studied in vitro. Brain Res 1226: 70–81.

30. Lobarinas E, Sun W, Cushing R, Salvi R (2004) A novel behavioral paradigm for assessing tinnitus using schedule-induced polydipsia avoidance conditioning (SIP-AC). Hear Res 190: 109–114.

31. Ruttiger L, Ciuffani J, Zenner HP, Knipper M (2003) A behavioral paradigm to judge acute sodium salicylate-induced sound experience in rats: a new approach for an animal model on tinnitus. Hear Res 180: 39–50.

32. Smith PH, Bartlett EL, Kowalkowski A (2006) Unique combination of anatomy and physiology in cells of the rat paralaminar thalamic nuclei adjacent to the medial geniculate body. J Comp Neurol 496: 314–334.

33. Goldstein SA, Bockenhauer D, O'Kelly I, Zilberberg N (2001) Potassium leak channels and the KCNK family of two-P-domain subunits. Nat Rev Neurosci 2: 175–184.

34. Meuth SG, Kanyshkova T, Meuth P, Landgraf P, Munsch T, et al. (2006) Membrane resting potential of thalamocortical relay neurons is shaped by the interaction among TASK3 and HCN2 channels. J Neurophysiol 96: 1517–1529.

35. Liu Y, Li X (2004) Effects of salicylate on voltage-gated sodium channels in rat inferior colliculus neurons. Hear Res 193: 68–74.

36. Hodgkin AL, Huxley AF (1952) Currents carried by sodium and potassium ions through the membrane of the giant axon of Loligo. J Physiol 116: 449–472.

37. Jung HY, Mickus T, Spruston N (1997) Prolonged sodium channel inactivation contributes to dendritic action potential attenuation in hippocampal pyramidal neurons. J Neurosci 17: 6639–6646.

38. Cong D, Tang Z, Li L, Huang Y, Wang J, et al. (2011) Cross-talk between NMDA and GABA(A) receptors in cultured neurons of the rat inferior colliculus. Sci China Life Sci 54: 560–566.

39. Surges R, Sarvari M, Steffens M, Els T (2006) Characterization of rebound depolarization in hippocampal neurons. Biochem Biophys Res Commun 348: 1343–1349.

40. Winer JA, Larue DT (1988) Anatomy of glutamic acid decarboxylase immunoreactive neurons and axons in the rat medial geniculate body. J Comp Neurol 278: 47–68.

41. Winer JA, Larue DT (1996) Evolution of GABAergic circuitry in the mammalian medial geniculate body. Proc Natl Acad Sci U S A 93: 3083–3087.

42. Clerici WJ, Coleman JR (1990) Anatomy of the rat medial geniculate body: I. Cytoarchitecture, myeloarchitecture, and neocortical connectivity. J Comp Neurol 297: 14–31.

43. Clerici WJ, McDonald AJ, Thompson R, Coleman JR (1990) Anatomy of the rat medial geniculate body: II. Dendritic morphology. J Comp Neurol 297: 32–54.

44. Silverstein H, Bernstein JM, Davies DG (1967) Salicylate ototoxicity. A biochemical and electrophysiological study. Ann Otol Rhinol Laryngol 76: 118–128.

45. Basta D, Ernst A (2004) Effects of salicylate on spontaneous activity in inferior colliculus brain slices. Neurosci Res 50: 237–243.

46. Chen GD, Jastreboff PJ (1995) Salicylate-induced abnormal activity in the inferior colliculus of rats. Hear Res 82: 158–178.

47. Wei L, Ding D, Sun W, Xu-Friedman MA, Salvi R (2010) Effects of sodium salicylate on spontaneous and evoked spike rate in the dorsal cochlear nucleus. Hear Res 267: 54–60.

48. Cruikshank SJ, Lewis TJ, Connors BW (2007) Synaptic basis for intense thalamocortical activation of feedforward inhibitory cells in neocortex. Nat Neurosci 10: 462–468.

49. Tennigkeit F, Schwarz DW, Puil E (1998) Postnatal development of signal generation in auditory thalamic neurons. Brain Res Dev Brain Res 109: 255–263.

50. Hsieh CY, Chen Y, Leslie FM, Metherate R (2002) Postnatal development of NR2A and NR2B mRNA expression in rat auditory cortex and thalamus. J Assoc Res Otolaryngol 3: 479–487.

51. Luo B, Wang HT, Su YY, Wu SH, Chen L (2011) Activation of presynaptic GABA(B) receptors modulates GABAergic and glutamatergic inputs to the medial geniculate body. Hear Res 280: 157–165.

52. Deer BC, Hunter-Duvar I (1982) Salicylate ototoxicity in the chinchilla: a behavioral and electron microscope study. J Otolaryngol 11: 260–264.

53. Jastreboff PJ, Hansen R, Sasaki PG, Sasaki CT (1986) Differential uptake of salicylate in serum, cerebrospinal fluid, and perilymph. Arch Otolaryngol Head Neck Surg 112: 1050–1053.

54. Sun H, Wu SH (2009) The physiological role of pre- and postsynaptic GABA(B) receptors in membrane excitability and synaptic transmission of neurons in the rat's dorsal cortex of the inferior colliculus. Neuroscience 160: 198–211.

16

Prefrontal Cortex based Sex Differences in Tinnitus Perception: Same Tinnitus Intensity, Same Tinnitus Distress, Different Mood

Sven Vanneste*, Kathleen Joos, Dirk De Ridder

Brai²n, TRI & Department of Neurosurgery, University Hospital Antwerp, Belgium

Abstract

Background: Tinnitus refers to auditory phantom sensation. It is estimated that for 2% of the population this auditory phantom percept severely affects the quality of life, due to tinnitus related distress. Although the overall distress levels do not differ between sexes in tinnitus, females are more influenced by distress than males. Typically, pain, sleep, and depression are perceived as significantly more severe by female tinnitus patients. Studies on gender differences in emotional regulation indicate that females with high depressive symptoms show greater attention to emotion, and use less anti-rumination emotional repair strategies than males.

Methodology: The objective of this study was to verify whether the activity and connectivity of the resting brain is different for male and female tinnitus patients using resting-state EEG.

Conclusions: Females had a higher mean score than male tinnitus patients on the BDI–II. Female tinnitus patients differ from male tinnitus patients in the orbitofrontal cortex (OFC) extending to the frontopolar cortex in beta1 and beta2. The OFC is important for emotional processing of sounds. Increased functional alpha connectivity is found between the OFC, insula, subgenual anterior cingulate (sgACC), parahippocampal (PHC) areas and the auditory cortex in females. Our data suggest increased functional connectivity that binds tinnitus-related auditory cortex activity to auditory emotion-related areas via the PHC-sgACC connections resulting in a more depressive state even though the tinnitus intensity and tinnitus-related distress are not different from men. Comparing male tinnitus patients to a control group of males significant differences could be found for beta3 in the posterior cingulate cortex (PCC). The PCC might be related to cognitive and memory-related aspects of the tinnitus percept. Our results propose that sex influences in tinnitus research cannot be ignored and should be taken into account in functional imaging studies related to tinnitus.

Editor: Thomas Koenig, University of Bern, Switzerland

Funding: These authors have no support or funding to report.

Competing Interests: The authors have declared that no competing interests exist.

* E-mail: sven.vanneste@ua.ac.be

Introduction

Subjective tinnitus is a condition in which a patient perceives an auditory phantom sound that can take the form of ringing, buzzing, roaring or hissing in the absence of an external sound [1]. This is also referred to as a phantom auditory sensation. In 5 to 15% of the population, this tinnitus sensation is unremitting and it is estimated that for 2–3 in 100 this auditory phantom percept severely affects the quality of life as tinnitus causes a considerable amount of distress [2].

Studying the affective dimension of tinnitus, distress has been considered as an aversive state in which a person is unable to adapt completely to stressors (i.e. tinnitus) and shows maladaptive behaviors [3,4]. It has been suggested that females are more influenced by distress in comparison to males, as different assessment instruments capture females and male reactions to the stressor in a different way. Typically, pain, sleep, and energy, are perceived to be significantly more severe by female tinnitus patients [5]. However, these symptoms can also have an influence

on tinnitus perception. As such, tinnitus distress and other severe problems might influence each other in both directions. In addition, women tend to show more hypersensitivity to aversive musical stimuli [6]. Females also tend to respond to distress more with rumination, a coping method that focuses on internal feelings rather than by externally oriented direct actions for stress reliefs [7]. Further studies on gender differences in emotional regulation indicate that females with high depressive symptoms show greater attention to emotion, with less anti-rumination emotional repair strategies than males [8].

Several neuroimaging studies have reported gender differences in brain locations involved both in perception [9], subjective experience of emotion [10] and emotion regulation [11]. Particularly, neural activity in the orbitofrontal cortex, the anterior cingulate cortex, the insula and the amygdala [11,12] have shown to differ between sexes during emotional processing and emotional regulation. These brain areas are also important in tinnitus perception and tinnitus-related distress [13–16]. Furthermore, functional differences in the neural mechanism between sexes in auditory processing have been demonstrated [17]. For example, differences in the primary auditory cortex activation exist between males and females in silent lip reading [18] as well as in processing of noise stimuli [19]. In addition, women demonstrate a greater overall structural connectivity of the underlying organization of their cortical networks than men [20]. Sex-related functional connectivity differences were found in the amygdala as well during an eyes closed, "resting" condition [21].

Given the different prevalence's of affective disturbances based on tinnitus perception and tinnitus-related distress, we hypothesized that male and female tinnitus patients might show different patterns of neural activity and connectivity. We therefore focus on the differences in cortical sources of the resting-state EEG (eyes closed) between male and female tinnitus patients using continuous scalp EEG recordings and Low Resolution Electromagnetic Tomography (sLORETA), a tomographic inverse solution imaging technique [22].

Results

Tinnitus Questionnaire and Beck Depression Inventory

A comparison between males ($M = 54.51$, $Sd = 14.91$) and females (52.60, $Sd = 15.43$) with tinnitus on the TQ showed no significant effect ($F(1,34) = .16$, $p = .70$), while the BDI–II revealed that females had a higher mean score ($M = 14.56$, $Sd = 13.20$) than males ($M = 7.83$, $Sd = 5.40$) ($F(1,34) = 4.10$, $p<.05$). In addition, we further explore whether males and females differ on the different subscales of the TQ, namely emotional and cognitive distress, intrusiveness, auditory perceptual difficulties, sleep disturbances and somatic complaints. However, no significant gender differences were obtained ($p>.40$).

Source localization

A comparison was made between tinnitus patients and a control group. This analysis revealed a significant difference for the beta1 and beta2 frequency band demonstrating that tinnitus patients have an increased activity in the posterior cingulate cortex (see Figure 1; $P<.05$). No significant differences could be retrieved in the delta, theta, alpha1, alpha2, beta3 and gamma frequency bands.

A similar analysis comparing females (control+tinnitus patients) and males (control+tinnitus patients) did not obtain significant effects for delta, theta, alpha1, alpha2, beta1, beta2, beta3 and gamma frequency bands.

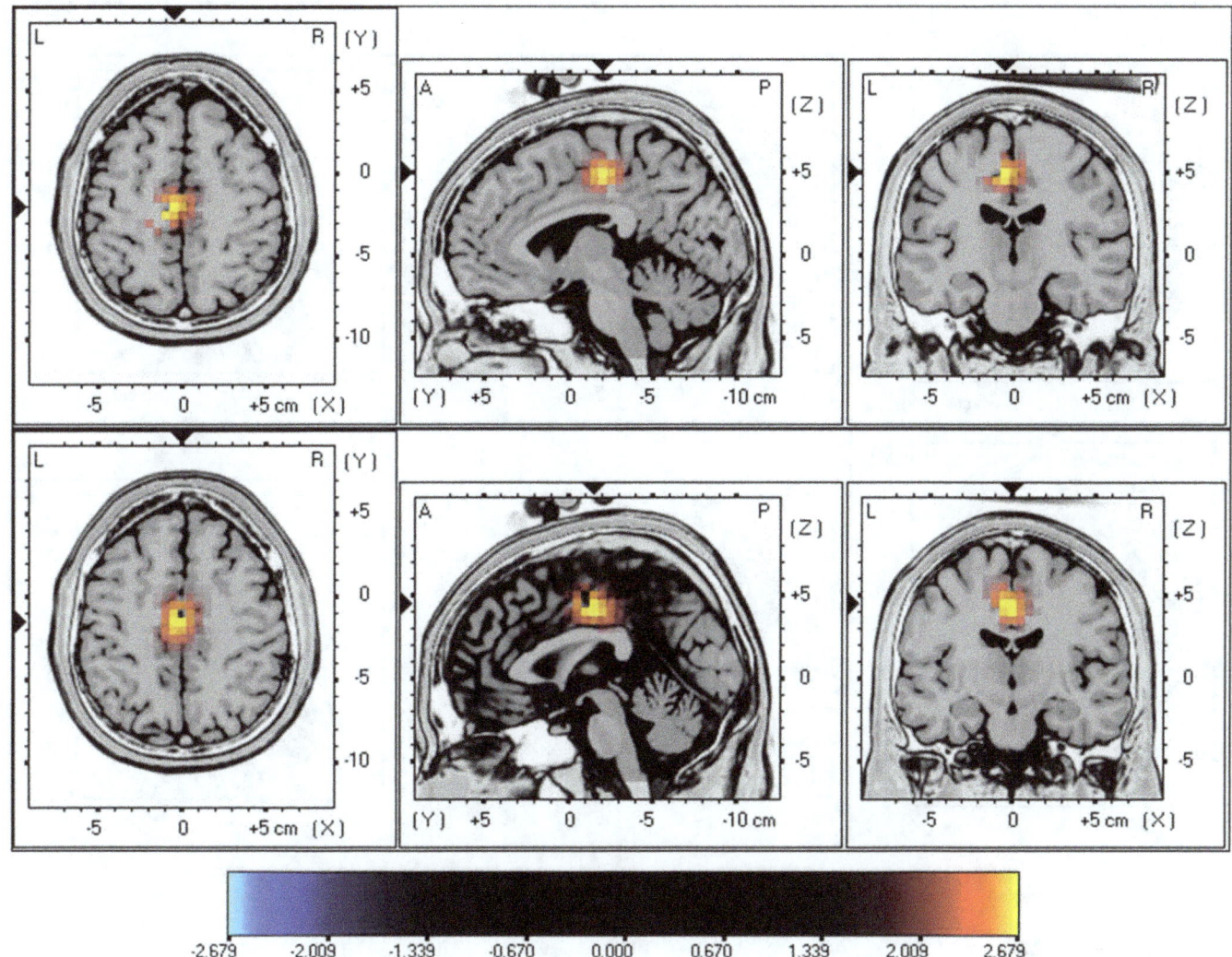

Figure 1. sLoreta constrast analysis between tinnitus versus control ($p<.05$). Increased neural synchonization within Beta1 (13–18 Hz; Top Panel) and Beta2 (18.5–21 Hz; Bottom Panel) in the posterior cingulate cortex (BA23).

sLORETA showed significant differences between female and male tinnitus patients. Increased synchronized beta1 and beta2 activity could be revealed in the orbitofrontal (BA11) extending to frontopolar (BA10) cortex for females in comparison to males (see Figure 2; $P < .05$). No significant differences could be retrieved in the delta, theta, alpha1, alpha2, beta3 and gamma frequency bands.

A comparison between males and females control subjects did not obtain significant effects for delta, theta, alpha1, alpha2, beta1, beta2, beta3 and gamma frequency bands.

Next the tinnitus patients are compared with gender and age-matched control group for beta1 and beta2 activity. Analysis revealed again increased synchronized beta1 and beta2 activity in the frontopolar and orbitofrontal cortex (BA10 & BA11) for females with tinnitus in comparison to female controls (see Figure 3; $P < .05$). No significant differences could be retrieved in the delta, theta, alpha1, alpha2, beta1, beta3 and gamma frequency bands.

A similar analysis for males with tinnitus in comparison to male controls did obtain a significant effect for beta3 (see Figure 4; $P < .05$) demonstrating increased activity in the posterior cingulate cortex (PCC; BA23) for male tinnitus patients. No significant differences could be retrieved in the delta, theta, alpha1, alpha2, beta1, beta2 and gamma frequency bands.

Correlations

Pearson correlation revealed that the BDI correlates with the Orbitofrontal cortex beta1 ($r = .34$, $p < .05$) and beta2 ($r = .39$, $p < .05$), respectively (see Figure 5). In addition, a similar analysis was conducted excluding outliers, i.e. based on visual inspection one could argue that 3 females score higher on the BDI in comparison to the other males and females. However, after excluding these possible outliers still a positive correlation was obtained between the BDI correlates with the orbitofrontal cortex beta1 ($r = .46$, $p < .05$) and beta2 ($r = .35$, $p < .05$).

Region of interest analysis

1. Orbitofrontal cortex. A two-way MANOVA with gender (males vs. females)×group (tinnitus vs. control) as independent variables and log-transformed current density for the different groups on the orbitofrontal cortex (left and right) for the beta1 and beta2 frequency band was conducted (see Figure 6). Analysis

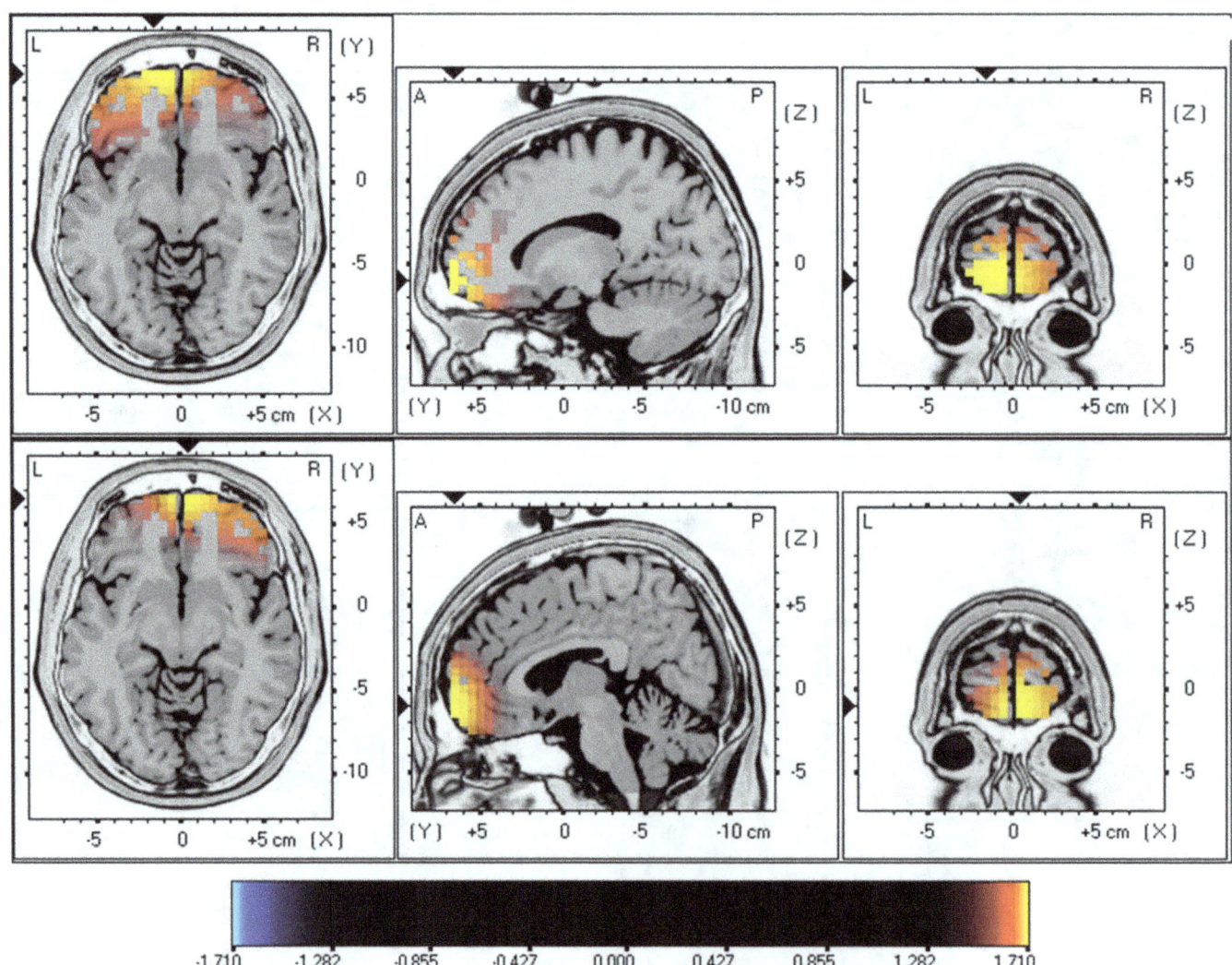

Figure 2. sLORETA contrast analysis between female versus male tinnitus patients ($p < .05$). Increased neural synchronization within Beta1 (13–18 Hz; Top Panel) and Beta2 (18.5–21 Hz; Bottom Panel) in the orbitofrontal cortex (OFC; BA10 and BA11).

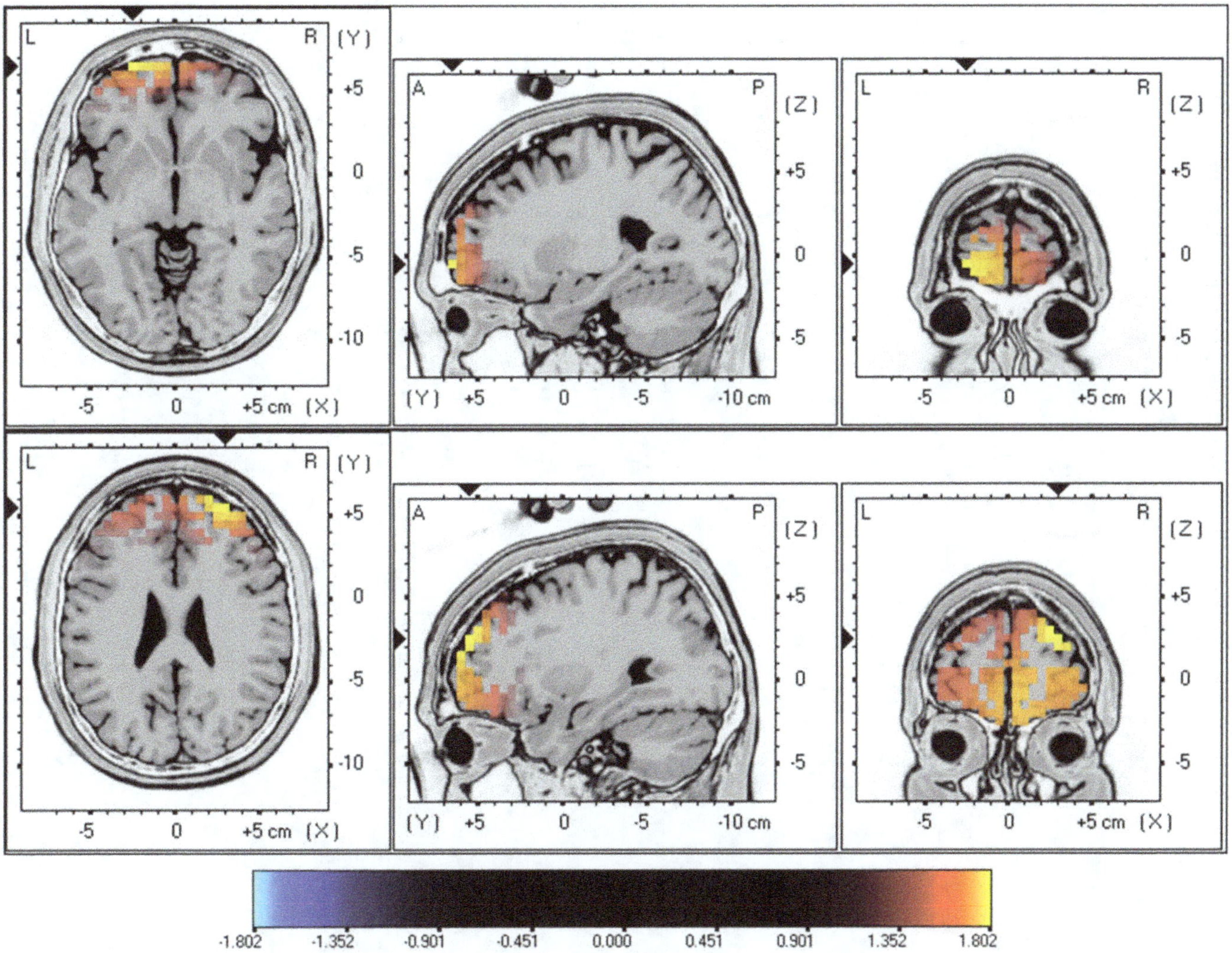

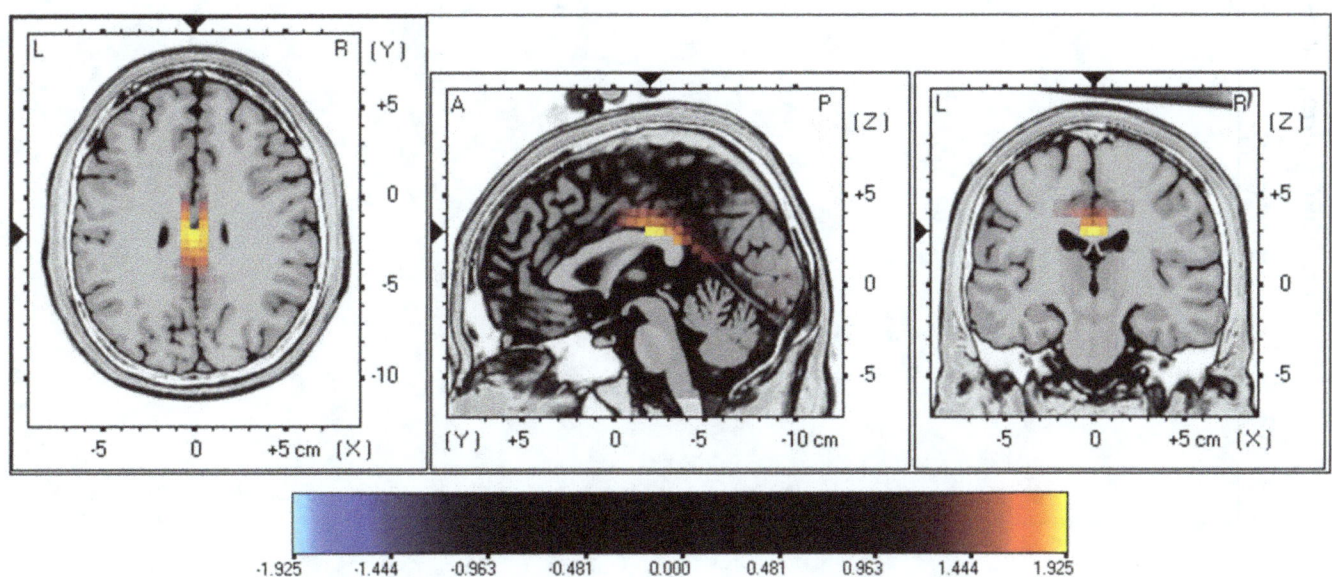

Figure 3. sLORETA contrast analysis between Females with tinnitus versus Female controls (*p*<.05). Increased neural synchronization within Beta1 (13–18 Hz; Top Panel) and Beta2 (18.5–21 Hz; Bottom Panel) in the orbitofrontal cortex (OFC; BA10 and BA11).

Figure 4. sLoreta constrast analysis between tinnitus versus control males (*p*<.05). Increased neural synchronization within Beta3 (21.5–30 Hz; Top Panel) in the posterior cingulate cortex (BA23).

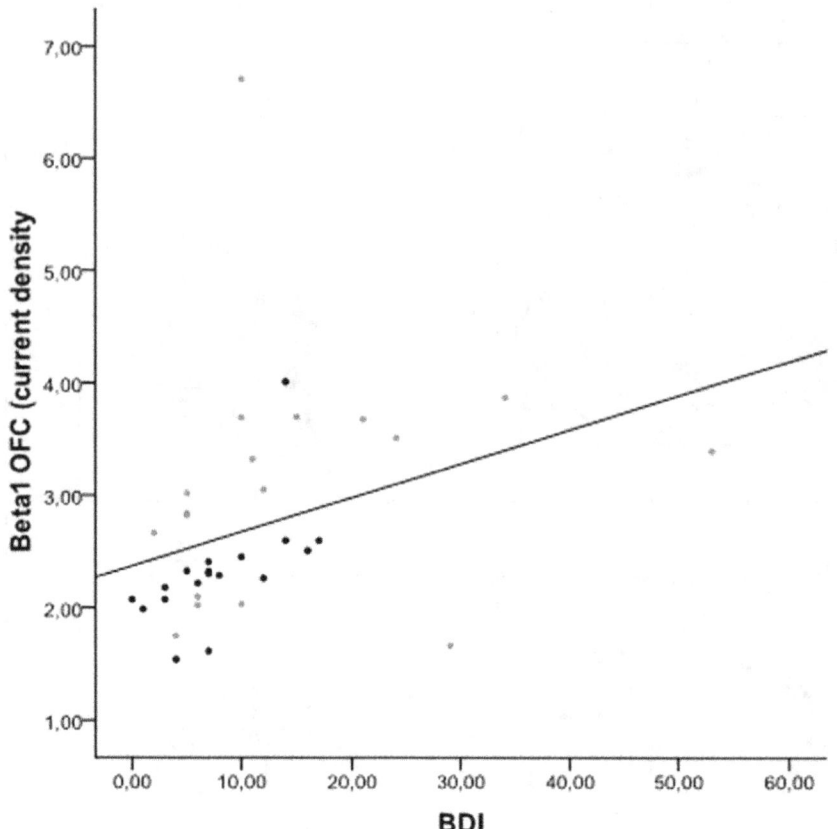

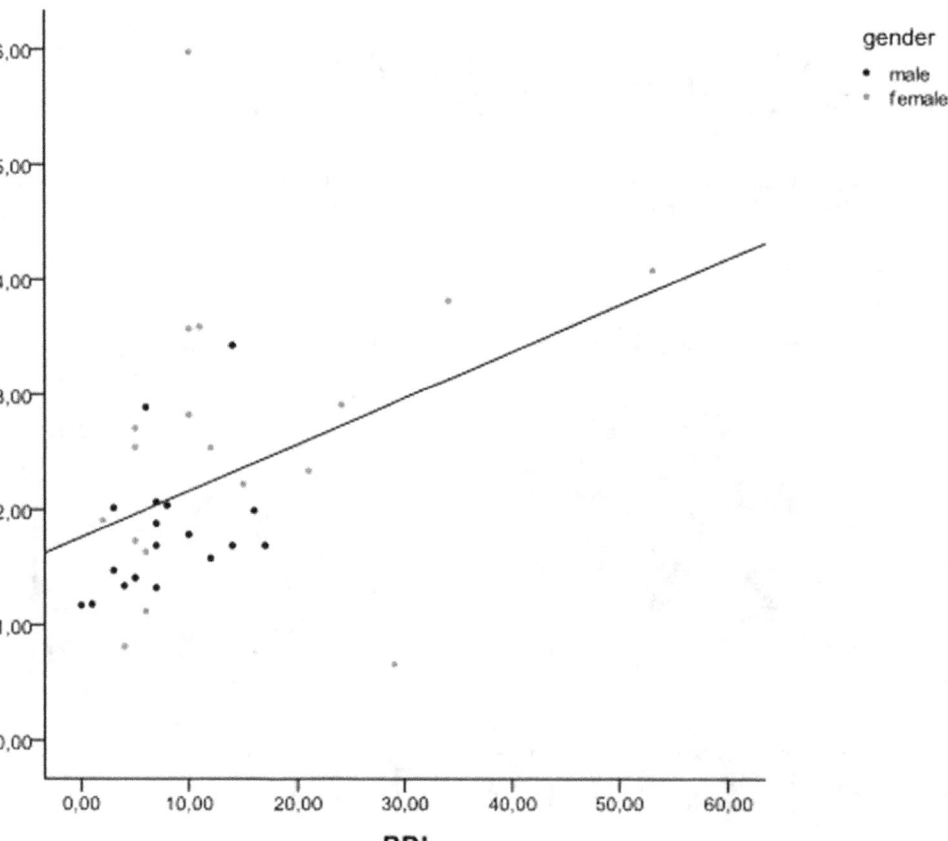

Figure 5. Pearson correlation between BDI and respectively Beta1 Orbifrontal cortex and Beta2 Orbitofrontal cortex.

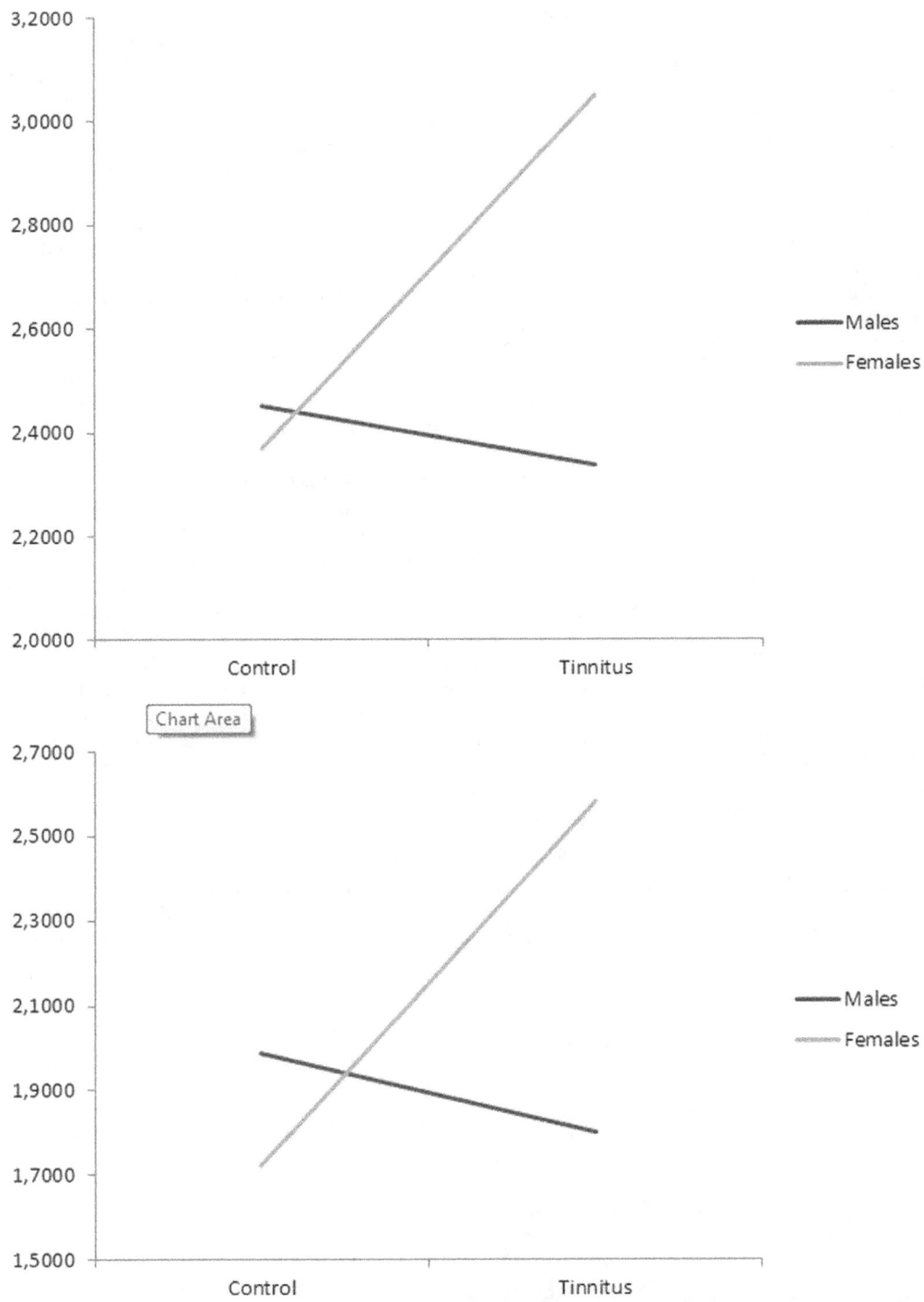

Figure 6. Region of interest analysis for the Orbitofrontal cortex for respectively beta1 and beta2 frequency band (log-transformed current density).

revealed no significant main effect for respectively gender $F(2,67) = 1.39$, $p = .26$ and group $F(2,67) = 1.37$, $p = .26$. However an interaction effect was obtained for gender (males vs. females)×group (tinnitus vs. control), $F(2,67) = 3.14$, $p<.05$. An univariate ANOVA further showed that for both beta1 $(F(1,68) = 4.48$, $p<.05)$ and beta2 $(F(1,68) = 5.78$, $p<.05)$ frequency bands a significant interaction effect was obtained. For both beta1 $(F(1,68) = 7.20$, $p<.01)$ and beta2 $(F(1,68) = 6.43$,

$p<.05)$ contrast analysis revealed that females with tinnitus have an increased log-transformed current density in comparison to female control subjects. In addition, a contrast analysis for beta1 $(F(1,68) = 6.75$, $p<.05)$ and beta2 $(F(1,68) = 8.08$, $p<.01)$ demonstrated increased log-transformed current density for female tinnitus patients in comparison to male tinnitus patient. For both beta1 and beta2 no significant effects were obtained when comparing males with tinnitus and male control subjects as well as a comparison between female and male control subjects.

2. Auditory cortex. A significant effect was found for the log-transformed current density for the different groups on the region of interest (auditory cortex) for the gamma frequency band, $F(4,65) = 5.38$, $p < .001$ (see Figure 7). Univariate ANOVA further yielded a significant effect for respectively left primary auditory cortex ($F(1, 68) = 19.34$, $p < .001$), right primary auditory cortex ($F(1,68) = 11.37$, $p < .001$), left secondary auditory cortex ($F(1, 68) = 17.83$, $p < .001$), right secondary auditory cortex ($F(1, 68) = 5.79$, $p < .05$) indicating that the control subjects had significant lower log averaged current density in comparison to tinnitus patients. No significant effect was obtained for the comparison of females and males ($F(4,65) = 1.55$, $p = .22$) and no interaction effect (gender (males vs. females)×group (tinnitus vs. control)) ($F(4,65) = 1.08$, $p = .37$) was obtained as well. No significant differences were found for delta, theta, alpha2, beta1, beta2, and beta3 bands.

Hierarchical regression analyses

In order to investigate the relative importance of both gender and BDI on the OFC for respectively beta1 and beta2, hierarchical regression analyses with OFC for respectively beta1 and beta2 as the dependent variable and BDI and gender as independent variables were conducted. First we compared BDI and gender by alternatively including the variables in the first and second block. A first analysis revealed a significant effect for BDI on OFC Beta1 ($F = 4.12$, $p < .05$, $R^2 = .11$). After including gender to the modal a significant effect was obtained ($F = 4.44$, $p < .05$, $R^2 = .21$) revealing that gender significantly contributed to the model ($F_{change} = 4.34$, $p < .05$, $\Delta R^2 = 10\%$). A similar analysis for the OFC in Beta2 revealed a significant effect for BDI on OFC Beta2 ($F = 6.24$, $p < .05$, $R^2 = .15$). After including gender to the modal a significant effect was obtained ($F = 4.49$, $p < .05$, $R^2 = .23$) demonstrating that gender significantly, however marginal, contributed to the model ($F_{change} = 2.96$, $p < .10$, $\Delta R^2 = 8\%$).

Functional connectivity

Functional connectivity analysis yielded a significant difference between female and male tinnitus patients in the alpha1 frequency band ($P < .05$). Females demonstrated increased functional connectivity in comparison to males between both left and right parahippocampus and subgenual anterior cingulate cortex (sgACC), and from the sgACC connectivity to the left insula (see Figure 8). From the left insula also increased functional connectivity was found to the left OFC. Furthermore, a functional connection for alpha1 was shown between the left OFC and left secondary auditory cortex (lA2) as well as between the left parahippocampal area and the right primary auditory cortex (rA1). No significant differences were found for delta, theta, alpha2, beta1, beta2, beta3 and gamma bands.

Functional connectivity analysis between female and male control patients yielded no significant effects for respectively delta, theta, alpha1, alpha2, beta1, beta2, beta3 and gamma bands.

Brain topography and Power Spectra

To verify whether the obtained results in the OFC are not artifact related both brain topographies and a power spectrum analysis was conducted. The topographies demonstrate that most power was retrieved occipitally and not frontally for male and female control subjects as well as male and female tinnitus patients (see Figure 9). The distribution for the frontal electrodes was similar across the different groups over the different frequency bands. For the beta band female tinnitus patients have an increased power from 14 to 22 Hz. However, these differences were not significant in comparison to the other group (see Figure 10).

Discussion

This study investigated gender-specific neural correlates of tinnitus. It was demonstrated that tinnitus patients had an increased activity for beta1 and beta2 in the PCC compared to a control group. In addition, the tinnitus revealed differences in

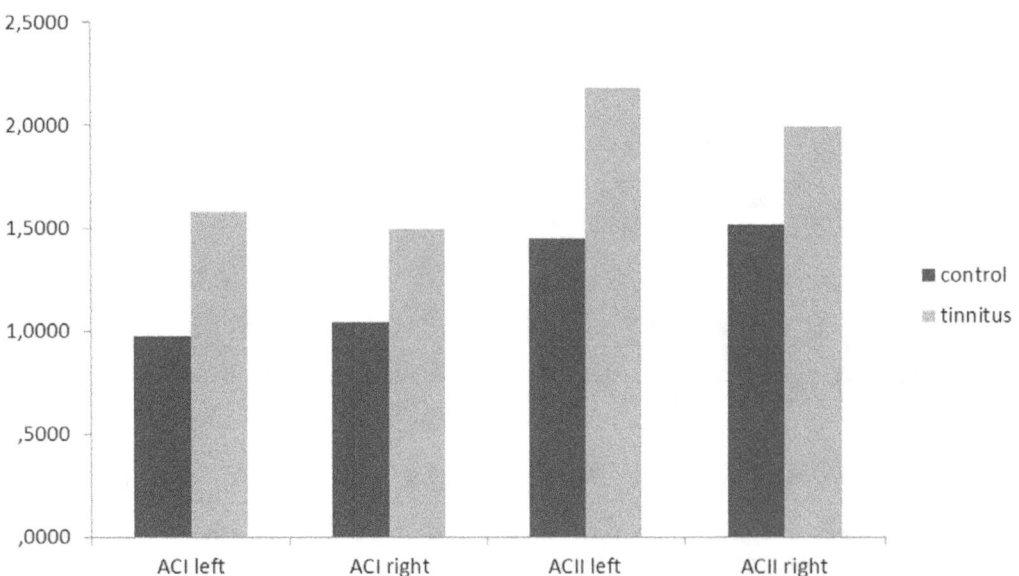

Figure 7. Region of interest analysis for the left and right primary and secondary auditory cortex for gamma band frequency (log-transformed current density).

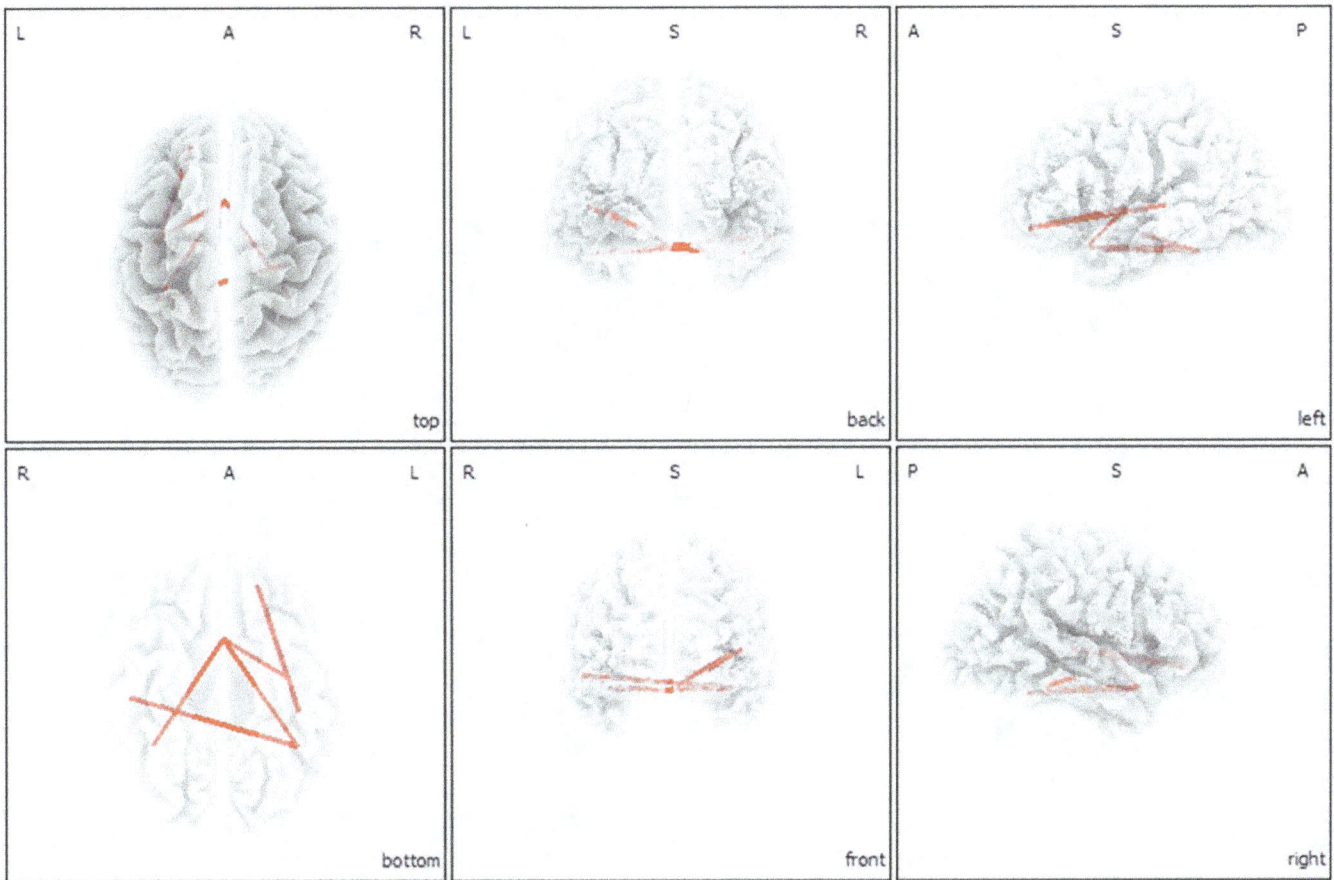

Figure 8. Connectivity contrast analysis between female and males tinnitus patients ($p<.05$). Increased neural synchronization within alpha 1 (8–10 Hz) connectivity for female tinnitus patients.

comparison to the control group for gamma activity in primary and secondary auditory cortex. Female tinnitus patients further demonstrated differences from male tinnitus patients in the OFC (BA11) extending to the frontopolar (BA10) for beta1 and beta2 oscillatory activity. These results confirm a recent bifrontal tDCS study where females showed better responses than males on their tinnitus [23].

In addition, when comparing to a control group of females, female tinnitus patients showed more frontopolar OFC for beta1 and beta2 oscillatory activity, These findings were further confirmed by a interaction effect indicating that specifically female tinnitus patients had an increased beta1 and beta2 activity in the frontopolar and OFC in comparison to male tinnitus patients, as well as to a male and female control group. Also a correlation was obtained between activity in beta1 and beta2 frequency bands in the OFC and mood measured with the BDI. But even when controlling for mood, the OFC beta activity correlated with gender, suggesting that the OFC beta activity does differentiate female from male patients. Comparing male tinnitus patients to a control group of males significant differences could be found for beta3 oscillatory activity in the PCC. In addition, we established differences in functional connectivity between the different regions of interest for alpha1 band. Female tinnitus patients yielded increased connectivity between left and right parahippocampus and sgACC, and from the sgACC connectivity to the left insula (see Fig. 3). From the left insula also increased connectivity was found to the left OFC. Furthermore, a functional connection for

alpha1 was shown between the left OFC and left secondary auditory cortex (lA2) as well as between the left parahippocampal area and the right primary auditory cortex (rA1).

A main concern might be that the difference found in the frontopolar and OFC might be artefact related. However, our results firstly demonstrated that there was a clear correlation between OFC and BDI. In addition, brain topography analyses showed that most power was located occipital for all groups. If frontopolar and OFC differences were artefact related one would expect more activity frontally, as muscle related activity is usually broader and generates more power [24]. A specific analysis on the frontal electrodes (FP1, FP2, F7, F8) showed an increased power from female tinnitus patients within the 14–22 Hz window, however these results were not significant. The power spectra show a typical distribution for the different groups on the specific electrodes indicating that the activity measured might be not artefact related.

This study demonstrated that female tinnitus patients had a higher score on the BDI–II than male tinnitus patients for the same amount of tinnitus related distress and the same tinnitus intensity. Differences on BDI–II between males and females have already been described in previous literature, showing that women in general have significant higher depression severity scores than men [25,26]. In this study the BDI scores are low in comparison to the depression literature [25,26], but similar to other tinnitus studies [27].

The posterior cingulate cortex might be related to cognitive and memory related aspects of the tinnitus percept, as the PCC is

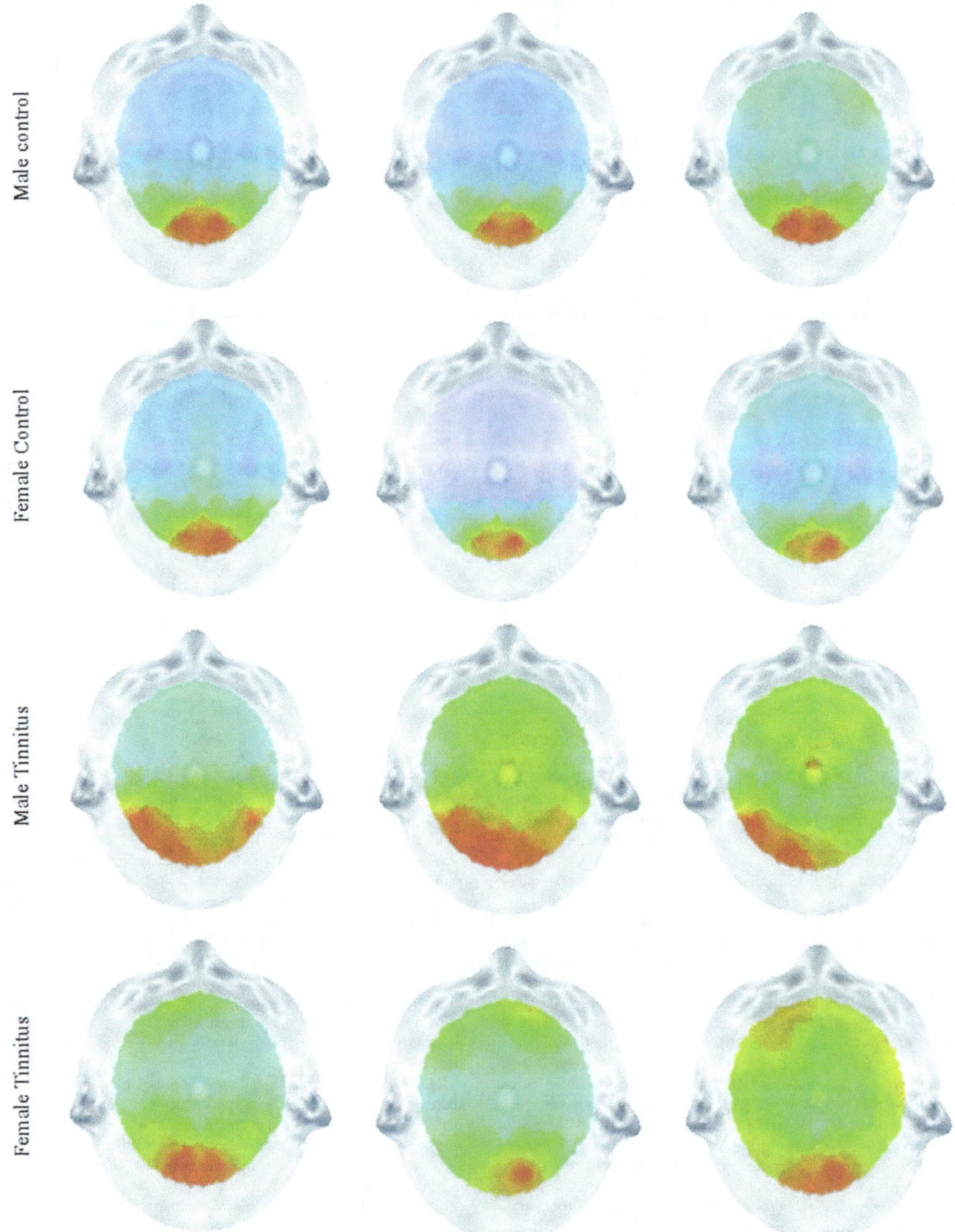

Figure 9. Scalp topography for Beta1, Beta2 and Beta3 for respectively Male Controls, Female Controls, Males Tinnitus patients and Female Tinnitus Patients.

involved in cognitive aspects of auditory processing [28]. Activity in the posterior cingulate cortex has indeed been linked to successful retrieval from auditory (and visual) memory [29,30]. The PCC has been proposed to exert a salience based cognitive auditory comparator function [28]. When the PCC component is deficient or less active, such as in tinnitus distress [31], this could reflect an incapacity of the PCC/precuneus to exert its salience based comparator function, pulling irrelevant auditory (tinnitus) sound from hippocampal memory [32], via dysfunctional para-hippocampal auditory sensory gating [33], analogous to what has been proposed for auditory hallucinations [34].

Previous research has already shown that the OFC is important for emotional processing of sounds [35–38]. For example, patients with OFC lesions had reduced self-evaluated perception of the unpleasantness of the acoustic probe stimulus [39]. Koch et al. also found that an interaction between negative emotion and working memory in females involved activation in the OFC, suggesting that during the control of emotion, females mainly recruit the emotion-associated areas [40]. Furthermore, the OFC is known to serve as a store of implicitly acquired linkages between factual knowledge and bio-regulatory states, including those that constitute feelings and emotions [41]. Female tinnitus patients have been found to be more emotionally responsive to tinnitus-related distress [42] as well as in physiological responses to negative emotional stimuli than males [43]. We found similar results, as both males and females had a similar score on the tinnitus questionnaire which measure tinnitus related distress, but scored differently on the BDI.

The OFC together with the insula plays a key role in the top-down modulation of automatic or peripheral physiological responses to emotional experiences [44,45]. The increased

synchronized alpha connectivity between the OFC and the insula for females might represent a modulation of the autonomic physiological responses evoked by tinnitus. The OFC connects with other limbic areas important for processing of emotion [46].

This study also finds an indirect increased functional connectivity between the OFC and the sgACC. The sgACC has previously been associated with negative affect [47], processing of aversive sounds [48] and unpleasant music [38] as well as tinnitus [16] and tinnitus related distress. As such, tinnitus and tinnitus-related distress might have stronger impact on OFC in females.

An increased functional connectivity between the parahippocampal areas and the sgACC for females is demonstrated in our study. The parahippocampal area has strong functional connections with the sgACC [31,49] which changes under distress [50]. It also has strong functional connections with the amygdala [49], involved in emotional auditory memory [51,52]. The role of the parahippocampal areas in the network might be related to a constant updating of the tinnitus sound from emotional memory, preventing habituation [32]. The hippocampal involvement in auditory habituation is already demonstrated in auditory sensory gating studies [33]. Gender differences in auditory sensory gating have been described: females had less inhibitory mechanisms acting on the generator substrates [53], which might also be present in our study.

Tinnitus is characterized by an ongoing abnormal spontaneous activity [54] and reorganization [55] of the auditory cortex. The auditory cortex encodes tinnitus intensity [56]. Sex differences were already detected in processing noise, indicating that females activate their auditory cortex significantly more than males [19].

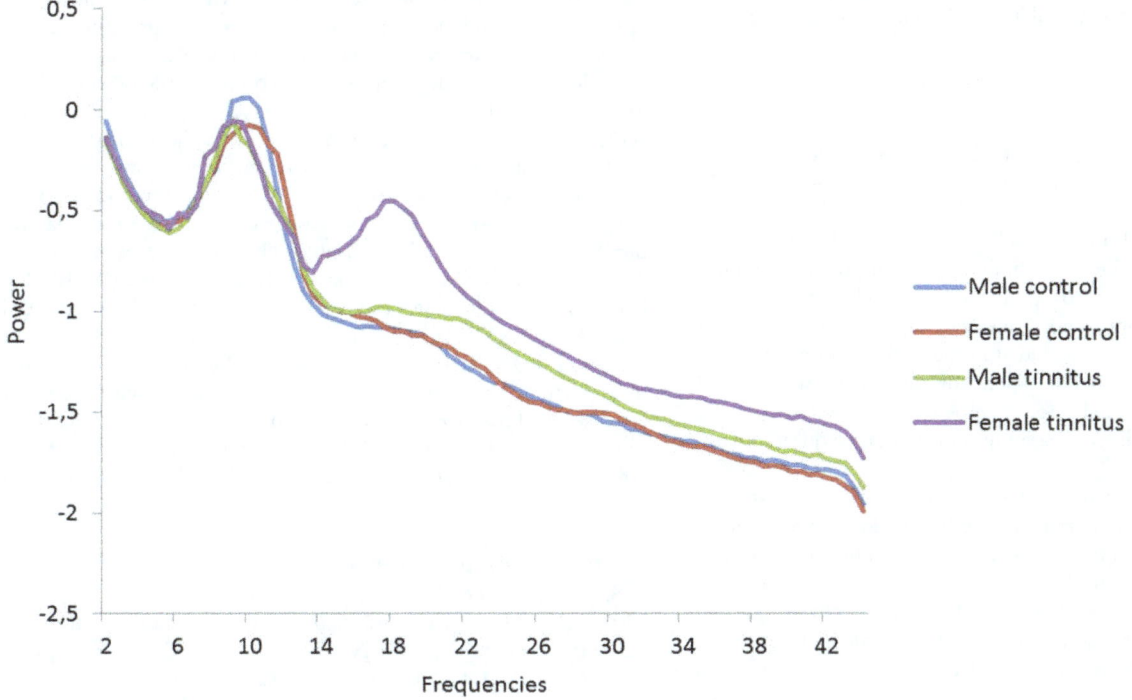

Figure 10. Power spectrum analysis for respectively Male Controls, Female Controls, Males Tinnitus patients and Female Tinnitus patients.

However, this study did not reveal any activity differences in the auditory cortex. This fits with the fact that tinnitus intensity was not significantly different between females and males. But females demonstrated increased functional connectivity between the auditory cortex and the OFC. As the auditory cortex is important in tinnitus and more specifically in the tinnitus intensity [56], a direct functional connection with the OFC might further enforce emotional reactivity to the phantom sound.

Gender differences were found in the OFC that might explain why in females the same tinnitus related distress and the same tinnitus intensity induces more depressive feelings than in males, as was found on the BDI. Yet, since depression is more frequent in women, the higher depression scores in the female tinnitus group could be completely unrelated to the presence of tinnitus.

Additional research is needed to further explore the differences between male and female tinnitus patients. The strength of this study is that we conducted our analyses on a very homogeneous group of tinnitus patients, namely patients with narrow band noise bilateral tinnitus. However, previous research already showed that there are cortical differences between unilateral and bilateral tinnitus [57], as well as pure tone and narrow band noise tinnitus [58]. Based on these findings additional research is needed to further explore gender effects in tinnitus type and mood to generalize the results.

In summary, the increased beta activity in the prefrontal cortex (BA11-10) with its increased functional alpha connectivity between the OFC, insula, sACC, parahippocampal areas and the auditory cortex in females explains that tinnitus related auditory cortex activity is functionally connected to auditory emotion related areas resulting in more a depressive state even though the tinnitus intensity and tinnitus related distress are not different from men. Male tinnitus patients have more beta activity in the PCC which might be related to cognitive and memory related aspects of the tinnitus percept. As such, our results clearly show that sex influences in tinnitus research cannot be ignored and should be taken into account in functional imaging studies related to tinnitus.

Methods

Participants

Thirty-six patients with narrow band noise bilateral tinnitus (N = 36; 18 males and 18 females) with a mean age of 51.47 (SD = 12.95 years) were selected from the multidisciplinary Tinnitus Research Initiative (TRI) Clinic of the University Hospital of Antwerp, Belgium. Individuals with pulsatile tinnitus, Ménière disease, otosclerosis, chronic headache, neurological disorders such as brain tumors, and individuals being treated for mental disorders were not included in the study in order to obtain a homogeneous sample. No significant differences were found between males and females for tinnitus duration, VAS intensity, and tinnitus related distress based upon the tinnitus questionnaire (see Table 1).

All patients were investigated for the extent of hearing loss using audiograms. Tinnitus matching was performed looking for tinnitus pitch (frequency) and tinnitus intensity. No significant differences were found for hearing loss between males and females, as measured by the loss in decibels (dB HL) at the tinnitus frequency.

Participants were requested to refrain from alcohol consumption 24 hours prior to recording and from caffeinated beverages on the day of recording.

Subjective depression was assessed with the Beck Depression Inventory-revised (BDI–II), a 21-item self-report instrument with good psychometric properties [59].

Table 1. Patients' characteristics.

	Gender		
	Females	**Males**	*p-values*
Age	50.82	52.12	.70
Tinnitus duration	4.96	5.23	.72
VAS intensity	6.54	6.87	.53
Hearing Loss (HL)	26.94	23.98	.68
Tinnitus pitch	26.94	23.89	.44

This study was approved by the local ethical committee (Antwerp University Hospital) and was in accordance with the declaration of Helsinki. Patients gave oral informed consent before the procedure. The EEG was obtained as a standard procedure for diagnostic and neuromodulation treatment purposes.

EEG recording

EEG recordings were obtained in a fully lighted room with each participant sitting upright on comfortable chair. The actual recording lasted approximately 5 min. The EEG was sampled with 19 electrodes (Fp1, Fp2, F7, F3, Fz, F4, F8, T7, C3, Cz, C4, T8, P7, P3, Pz, P4, P8, O1 O2) in the standard 10–20 International placement referenced to linked ears and impedances were checked to remain below 5 kΩ. Data were collected eyes-closed (sampling rate = 1024 Hz, band passed 0.15–200 Hz). Data were resampled to 128 Hz, band-pass filtered (fast Fourier transform filter) to 2–44 Hz and subsequently transposed into Eureka! Software [60], plotted and carefully inspected for manual artifact-rejection. All episodic artifacts including eye blinks, eye movements, teeth clenching, body movement, or ECG artifact were removed from the stream of the EEG. In addition, an independent component analysis (ICA) was conducted to further verify if all artifacts were excluded. To investigate the effect of possible ICA component rejection we compared the power spectra in two approaches: (1) after visual artifact rejection only (before ICA) and (2) after additional ICA component rejection (after ICA). To test for significant differences between the two approaches we performed a repeated-measure ANOVA, considering mean band power as within-subject variable and groups (unilateral vs. bilateral tinnitus) as between-subject variable. The mean power in delta (2–3.5 Hz), theta (4–7.5 Hz), alpha1 (8–10 Hz), alpha2 (10–12 Hz), beta1 (13–18 Hz), beta2 (18.5–21 Hz), beta3 (21.5–30 Hz) and gamma (30.5–45 Hz) did not show a statistically significant difference between the two approaches. Therefore, we continue by reporting the results of ICA corrected data. Average Fourier cross-spectral matrices were computed for bands delta (2–3.5 Hz), theta (4–7.5 Hz), alpha1 (8–10 Hz), alpha2 (10–12 Hz), beta1 (13–18 Hz), beta2 (18.5–21 Hz), beta3 (21.5–30 Hz) and gamma (30.5–44 Hz).

Control database subjects

Similarly to the tinnitus patients, EEGs (Mitsar, Nova Tech EEG, Inc, Mesa) were selected from an in-house normative database as a control group (N = 36; 18 males and 18 females) with a mean age of 51.47 (SD = 12.95 years). Recordings were made in similar circumstances, i.e.e in a fully lighted room with each participant sitting upright in a comfortable chair. None of these subjects were known to suffer from tinnitus or hearing loss. Exclusion criteria for the control subjects were known psychiatric or neurological illness, drug/alcohol abuse, current psychotropic/ CNS active medications, history of head injury (with loss of consciousness) or seizures. The EEG was sampled with 19 electrodes (Fp1, Fp2, F7, F3, Fz, F4, F8, T7, C3, Cz, C4, T8, P7, P3, Pz, P4, P8, O1 O2) in the standard 10–20 International placement referenced to linked lobes and impedances were checked to remain below 5 kΩ. Data were collected for 100 2-s epochs eyes closed, sampling rate = 1024 Hz, and band passed from 0.15 to 200 Hz. Data were resampled to 128 Hz, band-pass filtered (fast Fourier transform filter) to 2–44 Hz. The data were cleaned-up in a similar way to the tinnitus patients by manual artifact rejection and ICA. Again to investigate the effect of possible ICA component rejection we compared the power spectra in two approaches: (1) after visual artifact rejection only (before ICA) and (2) after additional ICA component rejection (after ICA). To test for significant differences between the two approaches we performed a repeated-measure ANOVA, considering mean band power as within-subject variable.

Source localization

Standardized low-resolution brain electromagnetic tomography (sLORETA) was used to estimate the intracerebral electrical sources that generated the scalp-recorded activity in each of the eight frequency bands [61]. sLORETA computes electric neuronal activity as current density (A/m^2) without assuming a predefined number of active sources. The sLORETA solution space consists of 6,239 voxels (voxel size: 5×5×5 mm) and is restricted to cortical gray matter and hippocampi, as defined by digitized MNI152 template [62]. Scalp electrode coordinates on the MNI brain are derived from the international 5% system [63]. The tomography sLORETA has received considerable validation from studies combining LORETA with other more established localization methods, such as functional Magnetic Resonance Imaging (fMRI) [64,65], structural MRI [66], Positron Emission Tomography (PET) [67–69]. Further sLORETA validation has been based on accepting as ground truth the localization findings obtained from invasive, implanted depth electrodes, in which case there are several studies in epilepsy [70,71] and cognitive ERPs [72]. It is worth emphasizing that deep structures such as the anterior cingulate cortex [73], and mesial temporal lobes [74] can be correctly localized with this method.

Functional connectivity

Coherence and phase synchronization between time series corresponding to different spatial locations are usually interpreted as indicators of the "functional connectivity". However, any measure of dependence is highly contaminated with an instantaneous, non-physiological contribution due to volume conduction and low spatial resolution (Pascual-Marqui, 2007a). Therefore Pascual-Marqui, (2007b) introduced a new technique (i.e. Hermitian covariance matrices) that removes this confounding factor considerably. As such, this measure of dependence can be applied to any number of brain areas jointly, i.e. distributed cortical networks, whose activity can be estimated with sLORETA. Measures of linear dependence (coherence) between the multivariate time series are defined. The measures are expressed as the sum of lagged dependence and instantaneous dependence. The measures are non-negative, and take the value zero only when there is independence of the pertinent type and are defined in the frequency domain: delta (1–3.5 Hz), theta (4–7.5 Hz), alpha1 (8–10 Hz), alpha2 (10–12 Hz), beta1 (13–18 Hz), beta2 (18.5–21 Hz), beta3 (21.5–30 Hz) and gamma (30.5–45 Hz). Based on this principle lagged linear connectivity was calculated. Regions of interest were defined based on previous brain research on tinnitus

(see table 2 for overview) and the present findings based on the source analysis (e.g. orbitofrontal cortex and posterior cingulate cortex).

Statistical analysis

In order to identify potential differences in brain electrical activity between groups, sLORETA was then used to perform voxel-by-voxel between-condition comparisons of the current density distribution. Nonparametric statistical analyses of functional sLORETA images (statistical non-parametric mapping; SnPM) were performed for each contrast employing a t-statistic for unpaired groups and a corrected ($P<0.05$). As explained by Nichols and Holmes, the SnPM methodology does not require any assumption of Gaussianity and corrects for all multiple comparisons [75]. We performed one voxel-by-voxel test (comprising 6,239 voxels each) for the different frequency bands.

Region of interest analysis

The log-transformed electric current density was averaged across all voxels belonging to the region of interest, respectively left and right primary auditory cortex (BA40 and BA41) and left and right secondary auditory cortex(BA21 and BA22) separately for the gamma frequency band. Also the region of interest analysis was performed for the frontopolar and orbitofrontal cortex (BA10 & BA11).

A multivariate ANOVA (i.e. Wilks' Lambda) for the frequency bands was used with the respective region of interest (i.e. left and right primary auditory cortex (BA40 and BA41) and left and right secondary auditory cortex (BA21 and BA22) as dependent variables and different groups (pure tone, narrow band noise and control subjects) as independent variable. A Bonferroni correction was applied for multiple comparisons.

A Pearson correlation was calculated between BDI and frontopolar and orbitofrontal cortex (BA10 & BA11). Also a hierarchical regression analysis was conducted with BDI and gender as independent variables and frontopolar and orbitofrontal cortex (BA10 & BA11) as dependent variable. The aim was to verify whether gender significantly contributed to the model.

Brain topography and Power Spectra

A digital FFT-based power spectrum analysis (Time Domain Tapering: Hamming, Frequency Domain Smoothing: Blackman, Overlapping FFT Windows Advancement Factor: 8) computed the power density of EEG rhythms with 0.5 Hz frequency resolution.

Table 2. Regions of Interest.

		Authors
Anterior Cingulate Cortex	Dorsal	[14]
		[13]
	Subgenual	[16]
Auditory Cortex		[55]
		[76]
		[15]
		[54]
Dorsal Lateral Prefrontal Cortex		[77]
Insula		[15]
		[31]
Parahippocampus		[78]

In order to verify whether the findings obtained are not related to artifacts (i.e. eye movements and muscle activity) we verified the power spectral analysis for the 4 frontal electrodes (FP1, FP2, F7, F8). To summarize the data and because spectra from all electrodes demonstrated similar shape and scale, we averaged the log transformed spectra of all 4 scalp electrodes for each subject. We then averaged these individual spectra to one spectrum for respectively male controls, female controls, male tinnitus patients and female tinnitus patients. In addition also the brain topographies for beta 1, beta2, and beta3 were calculated to further detect possible artifacts.

Acknowledgments

The authors thank Jan Ost, Bram Van Achteren, Bjorn Devree and Pieter van Looy for their help in preparing this manuscript.

Author Contributions

Conceived and designed the experiments: SV DDR. Performed the experiments: SV KJ. Analyzed the data: SV DDR. Contributed reagents/materials/analysis tools: SV. Wrote the paper: SV KJ DDR.

References

1. Eggermont JJ, Roberts LE (2004) The neuroscience of tinnitus. Trends Neurosci 27: 676–682.
2. Heller AJ (2003) Classification and epidemiology of tinnitus. Otolaryngol Clin North Am 36: 239–248.
3. Brown GW, Harris TO (1989) Depression. New York: Guilford.
4. Lazarus RS, Folkman S (1984) Stress, appraisal, and coping. New York: Springer.
5. Erlandsson SI, Holgers KM (2001) The impact of perceived tinnitus severity on health-related quality of life with aspects of gender. Noise Health 3: 39–51.
6. Nater UM, Abbruzzese E, Krebs M, Ehlert U (2006) Sex differences in emotional and psychophysiological responses to musical stimuli. Int J Psychophysiol 62: 300–308.
7. Nolen-Hoeksema S, Girgus JS (1994) The emergence of gender differences in depression during adolescence. Psychol Bull 115: 424–443.
8. Thayer JF, Rossy LA, Ruiz-PAdial E, Johnsen BH (2003) Gender differences in the relationship between emotional regulation and depressive symptoms. Cognitive Therapy and Research. pp 349–364.
9. Lee TM, Liu HL, Hoosain R, Liao WT, Wu CT, et al. (2002) Gender differences in neural correlates of recognition of happy and sad faces in humans assessed by functional magnetic resonance imaging. Neurosci Lett 333: 13–16.
10. Canli T, Desmond JE, Zhao Z, Gabrieli JD (2002) Sex differences in the neural basis of emotional memories. Proc Natl Acad Sci U S A 99: 10789–10794.
11. Mak AK, Hu ZG, Zhang JX, Xiao Z, Lee TM (2009) Sex-related differences in neural activity during emotion regulation. Neuropsychologia 47: 2900–2908.
12. Butler T, Imperato-McGinley J, Pan H, Voyer D, Cunningham-Bussel AC, et al. (2007) Sex specificity of ventral anterior cingulate cortex suppression during a cognitive task. Hum Brain Mapp 28: 1206–1212.
13. Schlee W, Hartmann T, Langguth B, Weisz N (2009) Abnormal resting-state cortical coupling in chronic tinnitus. BMC Neurosci 10: 11.
14. Plewnia C, Reimold M, Najib A, Reischl G, Plontke SK, et al. (2007) Moderate therapeutic efficacy of positron emission tomography-navigated repetitive transcranial magnetic stimulation for chronic tinnitus: a randomised, controlled pilot study. J Neurol Neurosurg Psychiatry 78: 152–156.
15. Smits M, Kovacs S, de Ridder D, Peeters RR, van Hecke P, et al. (2007) Lateralization of functional magnetic resonance imaging (fMRI) activation in the auditory pathway of patients with lateralized tinnitus. Neuroradiology 49: 669–679.
16. Muhlau M, Rauschecker JP, Oestreicher E, Gaser C, Rottinger M, et al. (2006) Structural brain changes in tinnitus. Cereb Cortex 16: 1283–1288.
17. Kaiser A, Kuenzli E, Zappatore D, Nitsch C (2007) On females' lateral and males' bilateral activation during language production: a fMRI study. Int J Psychophysiol 63: 192–198.
18. Ruytjens L, Albers F, van Dijk P, Wit H, Willemsen A (2007) Activation in primary auditory cortex during silent lipreading is determined by sex. Audiol Neurootol 12: 371–377.
19. Ruytjens L, Georgiadis JR, Holstege G, Wit HP, Albers FW, et al. (2007) Functional sex differences in human primary auditory cortex. Eur J Nucl Med Mol Imaging 34: 2073–2081.
20. Gong G, Rosa-Neto P, Carbonell F, Chen ZJ, He Y, et al. (2009) Age- and gender-related differences in the cortical anatomical network. J Neurosci 29: 15684–15693.
21. Kilpatrick LA, Zald DH, Pardo JV, Cahill LF (2006) Sex-related differences in amygdala functional connectivity during resting conditions. Neuroimage 30: 452–461.
22. Pascual-Marqui RD, Michel CM, Lehmann D (1994) Low resolution electromagnetic tomography: a new method for localizing electrical activity in the brain. Int J Psychophysiol 18: 49–65.
23. Frank E, Schecklmann M, Landgrebe M, Burger J, Kreuzer P, et al. (2011) Treatment of chronic tinnitus with repeated sessions of prefrontal transcranial direct current stimulation: outcomes from an open-label pilot study. J Neurol.
24. Kropotov JD (2009) Quantitative EEG, event-related potentials and neurotherapy. San Diego: Academic Press.
25. van Noorden MS, Giltay EJ, den Hollander-Gijsman ME, der Wee NJ, van Veen T, et al. (2010) Gender differences in clinical characteristics in a naturalistic sample of depressive outpatients: The Leiden Routine Outcome Monitoring Study. J Affect Disord 125: 116–123.
26. Verhagen M, van der Meij A, van Deurzen PA, Janzing JG, Arias-Vasquez A, et al. (2010) Meta-analysis of the BDNF Val66Met polymorphism in major depressive disorder: effects of gender and ethnicity. Mol Psychiatry 15: 260–271.
27. Frank G, Kleinjung T, Landgrebe M, Vielsmeier V, Steffenhagen C, et al. (2010) Left temporal low-frequency rTMS for the treatment of tinnitus: clinical predictors of treatment outcome - a retrospective study. Eur J Neurol 17: 951–956.
28. Laufer I, Negishi M, Constable RT (2009) Comparator and non-comparator mechanisms of change detection in the context of speech–an ERP study. Neuroimage 44: 546–562.
29. Shannon BJ, Buckner RL (2004) Functional-anatomic correlates of memory retrieval that suggest nontraditional processing roles for multiple distinct regions within posterior parietal cortex. J Neurosci 24: 10084–10092.
30. Sadaghiani S, Hesselmann G, Kleinschmidt A (2009) Distributed and antagonistic contributions of ongoing activity fluctuations to auditory stimulus detection. J Neurosci 29: 13410–13417.
31. Vanneste S, Plazier M, der Loo E, de Heyning PV, Congedo M, et al. (2010) The neural correlates of tinnitus-related distress. Neuroimage 52: 470–480.
32. De Ridder D, Fransen H, Francois O, Sunaert S, Kovacs S, et al. (2006) Amygdalohippocampal involvement in tinnitus and auditory memory. Acta Otolaryngol Suppl: 50–53.
33. Boutros NN, Mears R, Pflieger ME, Moxon KA, Ludowig E, et al. (2008) Sensory gating in the human hippocampal and rhinal regions: regional differences. Hippocampus 18: 310–316.
34. Diederen KM, Neggers SF, Daalman K, Blom JD, Goekoop R, et al. (2010) Deactivation of the parahippocampal gyrus preceding auditory hallucinations in schizophrenia. Am J Psychiatry 167: 427–435.
35. Dias R, Robbins TW, Roberts AC (1996) Dissociation in prefrontal cortex of affective and attentional shifts. Nature 380: 69–72.
36. Wheeler RE, Davidson RJ, Tomarken AJ (1993) Frontal brain asymmetry and emotional reactivity: a biological substrate of affective style. Psychophysiology 30: 82–89.
37. Damasio AR (1996) The somatic marker hypothesis and the possible functions of the prefrontal cortex. Philos Trans R Soc Lond B Biol Sci 351: 1413–1420.
38. Blood AJ, Zatorre RJ, Bermudez P, Evans AC (1999) Emotional responses to pleasant and unpleasant music correlate with activity in paralimbic brain regions. Nat Neurosci 2: 382–387.
39. Angrilli A, Bianchin M, Radaelli S, Bertagnoni G, Pertile M (2008) Reduced startle reflex and aversive noise perception in patients with orbitofrontal cortex lesions. Neuropsychologia 46: 1179–1184.
40. Koch K, Pauly K, Kellermann T, Seiferth NY, Reske M, et al. (2007) Gender differences in the cognitive control of emotion: An fMRI study. Neuropsychologia 45: 2744–2754.
41. Volz KG, von Cramon DY (2009) How the orbitofrontal cortex contributes to decision making - a view from neuroscience. Prog Brain Res 174: 61–71.
42. Dineen R, Doyle J, Bench J (1997) Audiological and psychological characteristics of a group of tinnitus sufferers, prior to tinnitus management training. Br J Audiol 31: 27–38.
43. Gard MG, Kring AM (2007) Sex differences in the time course of emotion. Emotion 7: 429–437.
44. Craig AD (2003) Interoception: the sense of the physiological condition of the body. Curr Opin Neurobiol 13: 500–505.
45. Critchley HD, Wiens S, Rotshtein P, Ohman A, Dolan RJ (2004) Neural systems supporting interoceptive awareness. Nat Neurosci 7: 189–195.
46. Beauregard M (2007) Mind does really matter: evidence from neuroimaging studies of emotional self-regulation, psychotherapy, and placebo effect. Prog Neurobiol 81: 218–236.
47. Zald DH, Mattson DL, Pardo JV (2002) Brain activity in ventromedial prefrontal cortex correlates with individual differences in negative affect. Proc Natl Acad Sci U S A 99: 2450–2454.
48. Zald DH, Pardo JV (2002) The neural correlates of aversive auditory stimulation. Neuroimage 16: 746–753.
49. Kahn I, Andrews-Hanna JR, Vincent JL, Snyder AZ, Buckner RL (2008) Distinct cortical anatomy linked to subregions of the medial temporal lobe revealed by intrinsic functional connectivity. J Neurophysiol 100: 129–139.

50. Daniels JK, McFarlane AC, Bluhm RL, Moores KA, Clark CR, et al. (2010) Switching between executive and default mode networks in posttraumatic stress disorder: alterations in functional connectivity. J Psychiatry Neurosci 35: 258–266.

51. LeDoux JE (1993) Emotional memory systems in the brain. Behav Brain Res 58: 69–79.

52. Ledoux JE, Muller J (1997) Emotional memory and psychopathology. Philos Trans R Soc Lond B Biol Sci 352: 1719–1726.

53. Hetrick WP, Sandman CA, Bunney WE, Jr., Jin Y, Potkin SG, et al. (1996) Gender differences in gating of the auditory evoked potential in normal subjects. Biol Psychiatry 39: 51–58.

54. Weisz N, Muller S, Schlee W, Dohrmann K, Hartmann T, et al. (2007) The neural code of auditory phantom perception. J Neurosci 27: 1479–1484.

55. Muhlnickel W, Elbert T, Taub E, Flor H (1998) Reorganization of auditory cortex in tinnitus. Proc Natl Acad Sci U S A 95: 10340–10343.

56. van der Loo E, Gais S, Congedo M, Vanneste S, Plazier M, et al. (2009) Tinnitus intensity dependent gamma oscillations of the contralateral auditory cortex. PLoS One 4: e7396.

57. Vanneste S, Plazier M, van der Loo E, Van de Heyning P, De Ridder D (2011) The difference between uni- and bilateral auditory phantom percept. Clin Neurophysiol 122: 578–587.

58. Vanneste S, Plazier M, van der Loo E, Van de Heyning P, De Ridder D (2010) The Differences in Brain Activity between Narrow Band Noise and Pure Tone Tinnitus. PLoS One 5: e13618.

59. Beck AT, Steer RA, Carbin MG (1988) Psychometric properties of the Beck Depression Inventory: twenty-five years of evaluation. Clinical Psychology Review 8: 77–100.

60. Congedo M (2002) EureKa! (Version 3.0) [Computer Software]. Knoxville, TN: NovaTech EEG Inc, Freeware available at www.NovaTechEEG.

61. Pascual-Marqui RD (2002) Standardized low-resolution brain electromagnetic tomography (sLORETA): technical details. Methods Find Exp Clin Pharmacol 24 Suppl D: 5–12.

62. Fuchs M, Kastner J, Wagner M, Hawes S, Ebersole JS (2002) A standardized boundary element method volume conductor model. Clin Neurophysiol 113: 702–712.

63. Jurcak V, Tsuzuki D, Dan I (2007) 10/20, 10/10, and 10/5 systems revisited: their validity as relative head-surface-based positioning systems. Neuroimage 34: 1600–1611.

64. Mulert C, Jager L, Schmitt R, Bussfeld P, Pogarell O, et al. (2004) Integration of fMRI and simultaneous EEG: towards a comprehensive understanding of localization and time-course of brain activity in target detection. Neuroimage 22: 83–94.

65. Vitacco D, Brandeis D, Pascual-Marqui R, Martin E (2002) Correspondence of event-related potential tomography and functional magnetic resonance imaging during language processing. Hum Brain Mapp 17: 4–12.

66. Worrell GA, Lagerlund TD, Sharbrough FW, Brinkmann BH, Busacker NE, et al. (2000) Localization of the epileptic focus by low-resolution electromagnetic tomography in patients with a lesion demonstrated by MRI. Brain Topogr 12: 273–282.

67. Dierks T, Jelic V, Pascual-Marqui RD, Wahlund L, Julin P, et al. (2000) Spatial pattern of cerebral glucose metabolism (PET) correlates with localization of intracerebral EEG-generators in Alzheimer's disease. Clin Neurophysiol 111: 1817–1824.

68. Pizzagalli DA, Oakes TR, Fox AS, Chung MK, Larson CL, et al. (2004) Functional but not structural subgenual prefrontal cortex abnormalities in melancholia. Mol Psychiatry 9: 325, 393–405.

69. Zumsteg D, Wennberg RA, Treyer V, Buck A, Wieser HG (2005) H2(15)O or 13NH3 PET and electromagnetic tomography (LORETA) during partial status epilepticus. Neurology 65: 1657–1660.

70. Zumsteg D, Lozano AM, Wennberg RA (2006) Depth electrode recorded cerebral responses with deep brain stimulation of the anterior thalamus for epilepsy. Clin Neurophysiol 117: 1602–1609.

71. Zumsteg D, Lozano AM, Wieser HG, Wennberg RA (2006) Cortical activation with deep brain stimulation of the anterior thalamus for epilepsy. Clin Neurophysiol 117: 192–207.

72. Volpe U, Mucci A, Bucci P, Merlotti E, Galderisi S, et al. (2007) The cortical generators of P3a and P3b: a LORETA study. Brain Res Bull 73: 220–230.

73. Pizzagalli D, Pascual-Marqui RD, Nitschke JB, Oakes TR, Larson CL, et al. (2001) Anterior cingulate activity as a predictor of degree of treatment response in major depression: evidence from brain electrical tomography analysis. Am J Psychiatry 158: 405–415.

74. Zumsteg D, Lozano AM, Wennberg RA (2006) Mesial temporal inhibition in a patient with deep brain stimulation of the anterior thalamus for epilepsy. Epilepsia 47: 1958–1962.

75. Nichols TE, Holmes AP (2002) Nonparametric permutation tests for functional neuroimaging: a primer with examples. Hum Brain Mapp 15: 1–25.

76. Schneider P, Andermann M, Wengenroth M, Goebel R, Flor H, et al. (2009) Reduced volume of Heschl's gyrus in tinnitus. Neuroimage 45: 927–939.

77. Mirz F, Gjedde A, Ishizu K, Pedersen CB (2000) Cortical networks subserving the perception of tinnitus–a PET study. Acta Otolaryngol Suppl 543: 241–243.

78. Landgrebe M, Langguth B, Rosengarth K, Braun S, Koch A, et al. (2009) Structural brain changes in tinnitus: grey matter decrease in auditory and non-auditory brain areas. Neuroimage 46: 213–218.

17

Effects of *C-phycocyanin* and *Spirulina* on Salicylate-Induced Tinnitus, Expression of NMDA Receptor and Inflammatory Genes

Juen-Haur Hwang[1,2], Jin-Cherng Chen[2,3], Yin-Ching Chan[4]*

1 Department of Otolaryngology, Buddhist Dalin Tzu-Chi General Hospital, Dalin, Chiayi, Taiwan, **2** School of Medicine, Tzu Chi University, Hualien, Taiwan, **3** Department of Neurosurgery, Buddhist Dalin Tzu-Chi General Hospital, Dalin, Chiayi, Taiwan, **4** Department of Food and Nutrition, Providence University, Shalu, Taichung, Taiwan

Abstract

Effects of C-phycocyanin (C-PC), the active component of *Spirulina platensis* water extract on the expressions of N-methyl D-aspartate receptor subunit 2B (NR2B), tumor necrosis factor–α (TNF-α), interleukin-1β (IL-1β), and cyclooxygenase type 2 (COX-2) genes in the cochlea and inferior colliculus (IC) of mice were evaluated after tinnitus was induced by intraperitoneal injection of salicylate. The results showed that 4-day salicylate treatment (unlike 4-day saline treatment) caused a significant increase in NR2B, TNF-α, and IL-1β mRNAs expression in the cochlea and IC. On the other hand, dietary supplementation with C-PC or *Spirulina platensis* water extract significantly reduced the salicylate-induced tinnitus and down-regulated the mRNAs expression of NR2B, TNF-α, IL-1β mRNAs, and COX-2 genes in the cochlea and IC of mice. The changes of protein expression levels were generally correlated with those of mRNAs expression levels in the IC for above genes.

Editor: Alfred Lewin, University of Florida, United States of America

Funding: This study was supported by grants from the National Science Council, Taiwan (NSC-95-231693-B-126-008 and NSC-99-2314-B-303-001-MY3). The funders had no roles in study design, data collection and analysis, decision to publish, or preparation of the manuscript.

Competing Interests: The authors have declared that no competing interests exist.

* E-mail: ycchan@pu.edu.tw

Introduction

Tinnitus can be perceived in one or both ears or in the head in the absence of acoustic stimulation. The prevalence of chronic tinnitus is estimated between 10.1% to 14.5% in adult population [1], and increased with age [2]. Salicylate-induced tinnitus in mice has been a popular animal model for the study of tinnitus [3]. High doses of salicylate (250–300 mg/kg sodium Salicylate, i.p.) are known to reduce otoacoustic emissions, elevate hearing thresholds, and reliably induce tinnitus [3–6].

Some mechanisms were proposed to explain the causes of tinnitus. For example, tinnitus may arise from an increase in excitatory neurotransmission, and was associated with *N*-methyl *D*-aspartate receptor (NMDA receptor, NR) activity [4]. Recently, our study group found that mRNA expression levels of the NR subtype 2B (NR2B) gene, tumor necrosis factor –α (TNF-α) and interleukine-1β (IL-1β) genes were elevated significantly in the cochlea and in the inferior colliculus (IC) in salicylate-induced tinnitus [5,6]. And, we suggested that the proinflammatory cytokines might lead to tinnitus directly or via modulating NR gene expression [5,6].

Although some medications appeared to be effective for tinnitus, the results were still not so satisfactory and/or their adverse side effects prevent them as a regular treatment for mice and/or humans [7–9]. Therefore, it is still worth searching for more "safe and effective" medications for tinnitus.

Spirulina is a microscopic blue-green algae living both in sea and fresh water. It is composed of high quality protein, iron, gamma-linolenic fatty acid, carotenoids, vitamins B_1 and B_2, minerals, and its active component: C-phycocyanin(*C-PC*), etc [10]. It has been reported that *Spirulina platensis* water extract or *C-PC* exerts anti-oxidative, anti-inflammatory activities and neuroprotective effects via inhibition of COX [11] and/or nicotinamide adenine dinucleotide phosphate (NADPH) oxidase enzymes [12]. Meanwhile, as we mentioned above, tinnitus were associated with up-regulation of the NR2B and proinflammatory genes [5,6]. So, *Spirulina* might be also a good candidate for prevention or treatment of tinnitus.

In this study, we aim to investigated whether *C-PC* or *spirulina platensis* water extract could reduce the tinnitus score and expression levels of NR2B, TNF-α, IL-1β, and COX-2 genes in the cochlea and IC in response to intraperitoneal injections of salicylate.

Results

Figure 1 showed the tinnitus score was elevated day-by-day after intraperitoneal injection of 300 mg/kg sodium salicylate (tinnitus group) but not after injection of saline (control group). The mean tinnitus score at day 4 was 0.5 ± 0.5 for the control group, 8.0 ± 1.5 for the salicylate group, 7.0 ± 1.3 for the *Spirulina* group, and 6.8 ± 1.1 for the *C-PC* group. The differences in tinnitus score among the four groups were significant on each day (one-way ANOVA, p<0.0001). Post-hoc analysis showed that the tinnitus scores of the *Spirulina* group and *C-PC* group were significantly lower than those of the salicylate (tinnitus) group on each day (p<0.001 at days 1, 2, and 3 for both groups; p = 0.037 and 0.005 on day 4, respectively).

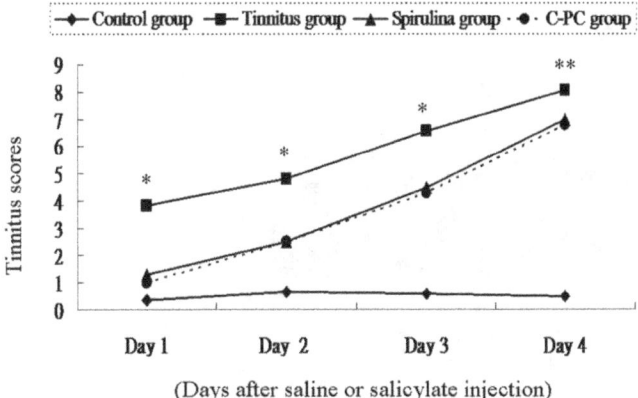

(Days after saline or salicylate injection)

Figure 1. The tinnitus scores of four groups after intraperitoneal saline or salicylate injection. The tinnitus scores were significantly higher in the salicylate group than the control group on each day. In addition, the tinnitus scores of the *Spirulina* group and C-PC group were significantly lower than those of the salicylate group on each day (*p<0.001 at days 1, 2, and 3 for both groups; **p=0.037 and 0.005 on day 4, respectively).

Figures 2, 3, 4 and 5 showed the mRNA expression levels of NR2B, TNF-α, IL-1β, and COX-2 in the four groups. The respective differences in NR2B, TNF-α, IL-1β, and COX-2 mRNA level among the four groups were significant (one-way ANOVA, p<0.001).

Post-hoc analysis showed that, compared to the control group, the tinnitus group had significantly increased NR2B mRNA levels in the cochlea (3.7±0.5 *versus* 2.3±0.1, p<0.001) and IC (1.6±0.6 *versus* 1.0±0.4, p=0.003). However, NR2B mRNA levels were significantly decreased in the cochlea (2.8±0.3 *versus* 3.7±0.5, p<0.001) and IC (1.0±0.7 *versus* 1.6±0.6, p=0.001) of the *Spirulina* group and the *C-PC* group (cochlea: 2.5±0.3 *versus* 3.7±0.5, p<0.001; IC: 0.8±0.2 *versus* 1.6±0.6, p<0.001) compared to the tinnitus group (Figure 2).

Post-hoc analysis showed that, compared to the control group, the tinnitus group had significantly increased TNF-α mRNA levels in the cochlea (1.9±0.2 *versus* 0.9±0.1, p<0.001) and IC (2.1±0.2 *versus* 1.7±0.2, p<0.001). However, TNF-α mRNA levels were significantly decreased in the cochlea (1.3±0.1 *versus* 1.9±0.2, p<0.001) and IC (1.4±0.2 *versus* 2.1±0.2, p<0.001) of the *Spirulina* group and *C-PC* group (cochlea: 1.0±0.1 *versus* 1.9±0.2, p<0.001; IC: 1.0±0.1 *versus* 2.1±0.2, p<0.001), compared with the tinnitus group (Figure 3).

(a) NR2B versus β-actin

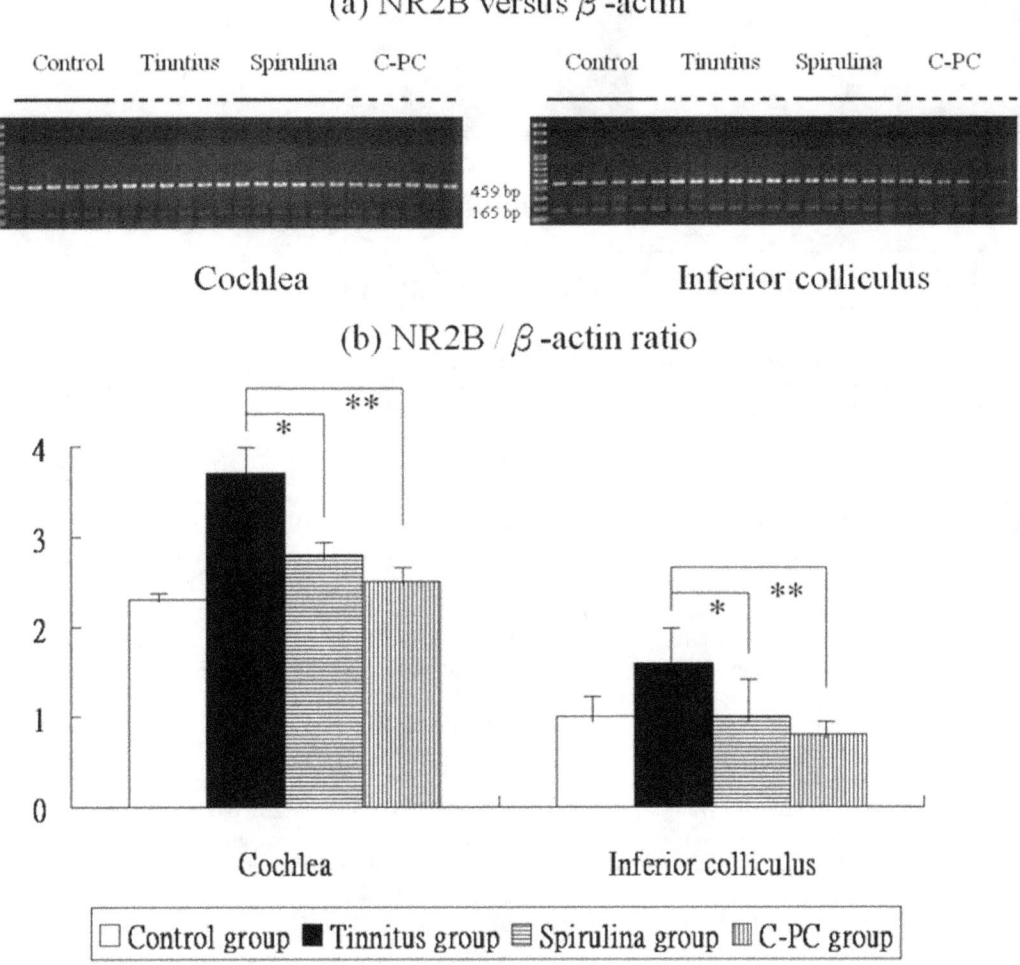

(b) NR2B / β-actin ratio

Figure 2. The levels of NR2B mRNA expression in the four groups (a,b). There are significant differences in these levels among the four groups. The NR2B mRNA expression were significantly higher in the salicylate group than the control group. Compared to the tinnitus group, the *Spirulina* group (*) or *C-PC* group (**) exhibits significantly reduced NR2B mRNA levels in the cochlea and IC.

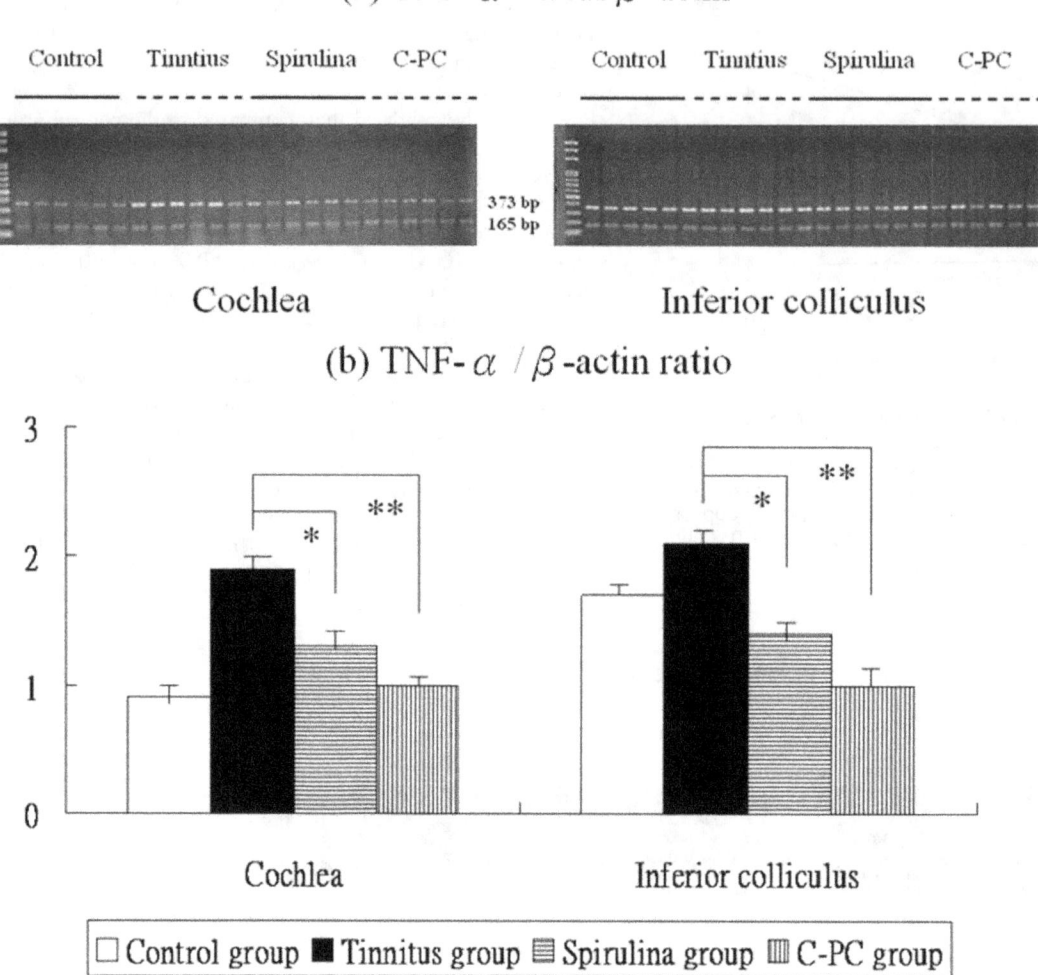

Figure 3. The levels of TNF-α mRNA expression in the four groups (a,b). There are significant differences in these levels among the four groups. The TNF-α mRNA expression were significantly higher in the salicylate group than the control group. Compared to the tinnitus group, the *Spirulina* group (*) or *C-PC* group (**) exhibits significantly reduced TNF-α mRNA levels in the cochlea and IC.

Post-hoc analysis showed that, compared to the control group, the tinnitus group had significantly increased the IL-1β mRNA levels in the cochlea (3.5±1.1 *versus* 2.8±0.3, p=0.031) and IC (2.9±0.5 *versus* 1.2±0.5, p<0.001). However, IL-1β mRNA level was significantly decreased in the IC (2.3±0.7 *versus* 2.9±0.5, p=0.002) but not in the cochlea (3.1±1.1 *versus* 3.5±1.1, p=0.473) of the *Spirulina* group, and significantly decreased in the cochlea (2.2±0.7 *versus* 3.5±1.1, p<0.001) and IC (1.9±0.6 *versus* 2.9±0.5, p<0.001) of the *C-PC* group (Figure 4).

Post-hoc analysis showed that, compared to the control group, the tinnitus group had similar COX-2 mRNA level in the cochlea (1.1±0.3 *versus* 1.3±0.5, p=0.205) and IC (0.9±0.1 *versus* 1.0±0.4, p=0.188). Nonetheless, COX-2 mRNA level was significantly decreased in the cochlea (0.8±0.4 *versus* 1.1±0.3, p=0.034) and IC (0.7±0.3 *versus* 0.9±0.1, p=0.021) of the *Spirulina* group and *C-PC* group (cochlear: 0.8±0.1 *versus* 1.1±0.3, p=0.009; IC: 0.5±0.2 *versus* 0.9±0.1, p<0.001) compared with the tinnitus group (Figure 5).

Figure 6, 7, 8 and 9 showed the protein expression levels of NR2B, TNF-α, IL-1β, and COX-2 in the IC. The respective differences in NR2B, TNF-α, and IL-1β protein level (one-way

ANOVA, p<0.001) among the four groups were significant, but not in COX-2 (one-way ANOVA, p=0.056).

Post-hoc analysis showed that, compared to the control group, the tinnitus group had not significantly increased NR2B protein levels in the IC (1.30±0.17 *versus* 1.18±0.12, p=1.000). However, NR2B protein levels in the IC were significantly decreased in the *Spirulina* group (0.89±0.08 *versus* 1.30±0.17, p=0.014) and in the *C-PC* group (0.66±0.04 *versus* 1.30±0.17, p=0.001), compared with the tinnitus group (Figure 6).

Post-hoc analysis showed that, compared to the control group, the tinnitus group had not significantly increased TNF-α protein levels in the IC (1.51±0.19 *versus* 1.20±0.02, p=0.085). However, TNF-α protein levels in the IC were significantly decreased in the *Spirulina* group (0.59±0.13 *versus* 1.51±0.19, p<0.001) and in the *C-PC* group (0.53±0.04 *versus* 1.51±0.19, p<0.001), compared with the tinnitus group (Figure 7).

Post-hoc analysis showed that, compared to the control group, the tinnitus group had not significantly increased IL-1β protein levels in the IC (1.45±0.18 *versus* 1.16±0.08, p=0.057). However, IL-1β protein levels in the IC were significantly decreased in the *Spirulina* group (0.91±0.07 *versus* 1.45±0.18, p=0.001) and in the

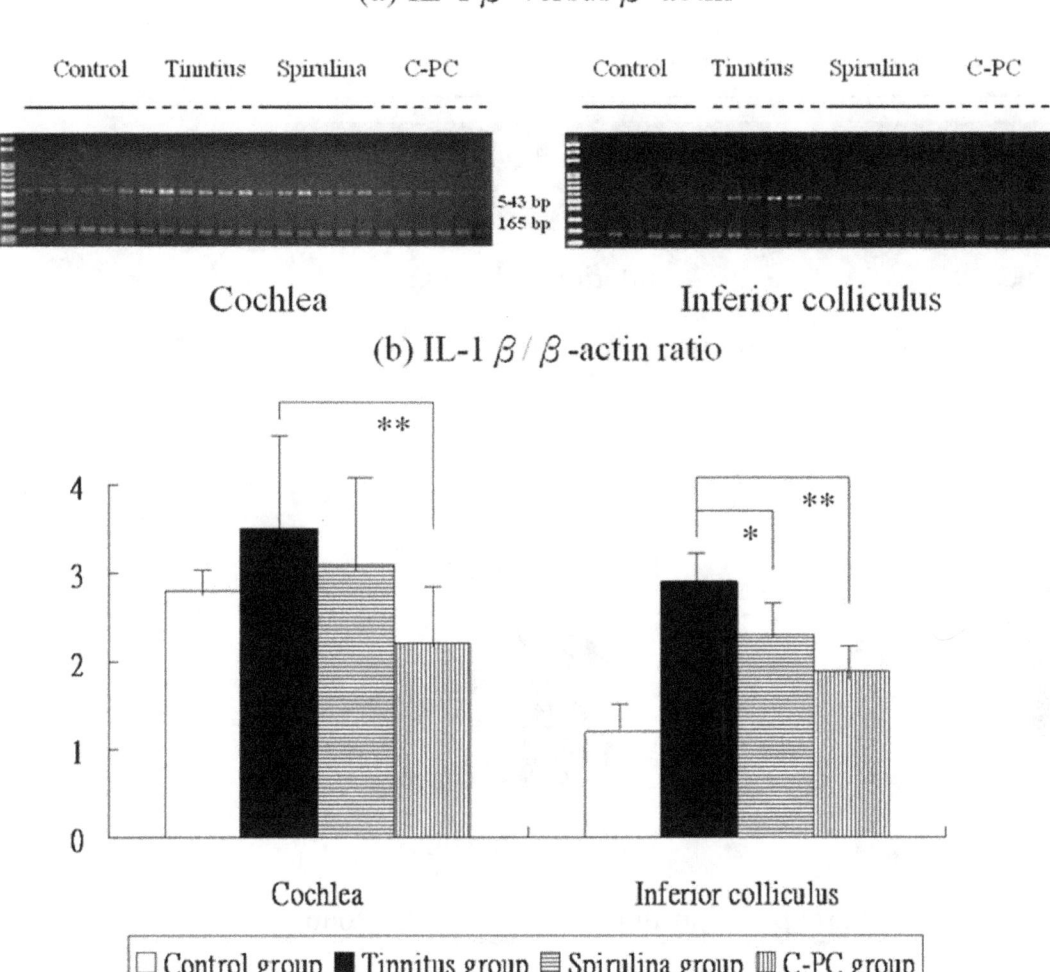

(a) IL-1 β versus β-actin

(b) IL-1 β / β-actin ratio

Figure 4. The levels of IL-1β mRNA expression in the four groups (a,b). There are significant differences in these levels among four groups. The IL-1β mRNA expression were significantly higher in the salicylate group than the control group. Compared to the tinnitus group, the *Spirulina* group (*) exhibits significantly reduced IL-1β mRNA level in the IC, whereas the *C-PC* group (**) exhibits significantly reduced IL-1β mRNA level in the cochlea and IC.

C-PC group (0.56±0.01 *versus* 1.45±0.18, p<0.001), compared with the tinnitus group (Figure 8).

Compared to the control group (1.12±0.10), the tinnitus group (0.97±0.17, p = 1.000), *Spirulina* group (0.82±0.08, p = 0.401), and C-PC group (0.66±0.28, p = 0.071) had decreased COX-2 protein levels in the IC, but the differences were not significant (Figure 9).

Discussion

This experimental study showed that the both of *spirulina platensis* water extract and its active component (*C-PC*) could reduce salicylate-induced tinnitus and reduce expression of NR2B, TNF-α, IL-1β, and COX-2 genes in the cochlea and IC. As we mentioned above, salicylate-induced tinnitus was associated with up-expression of NR2B, TNF-α, and IL-1β genes [5,6] and with enzymatic inhibition of COX [4]. But, this study found that expression of COX-2 gene was not altered significantly by salicylate. Therefore, we suggested that the beneficial effects of *spirulina* or *C-PC* on tinnitus mainly via inhibiting mRNA expression of NR2B, TNF-α, IL-1β, and/or COX-2 genes.

Inflammation is associated with many neurodegenerative diseases, including Alzheimer's disease [13], Parkinson's disease [14], and many types of hearing impairment. For example, noise-induced cochlear damage [15], and cisplatin-induced ototoxicity [16]. Also, previous studies showed that TNF-α and IL-1β might interact with the NR [17], for example, in inflammatory hyperalgesia [18], and in spinal cord injury [19]. Recently, proinflammatory cytokines were linked to tinnitus [20]. We also found that the proinflammatory cytokines might lead to tinnitus directly or via modulating NR gene expression [5,6].

Spirulina might be helpful for the neuroinflammatory and/or neurodegenerative diseases [11,12]. *C-PC* has been shown to be a potent inhibitor of nicotinamide adenine dinucleotide phosphate (NADPH) oxidase [12]. On the other hand, the elevated cellular NADPH oxidase activity might contribute to their pathogenic impact, collaborating with increased iNOS activity to generate the cytotoxic oxidant peroxynitrite [12]. Wang et al. [21]reported that *Spirulina* can reduce the ischemia/reperfusion-induced apoptosis and cerebral infarction in mice with focal ischemia. Spirulina can also enhance striatal dopamine recovery and induce rapid, transient microglia activation after injury of the rat nigrostriatal

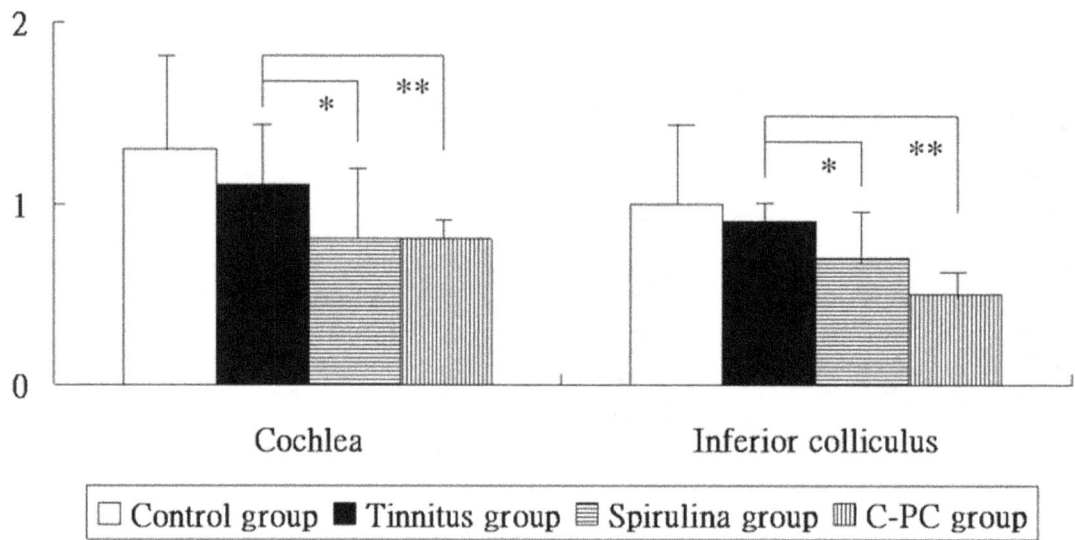

(a) COX-2 versus β-actin

(b) COX-2/ β-actin ratio

Figure 5. The levels of COX-2 mRNA expression in the four groups (a,b). There are significant differences in these levels among the four groups. The COX-2 mRNA expression were significantly higher in the salicylate group than the control group. Compared to the tinnitus group, the *Spirulina* group (*) or *C-PC* group (**) exhibits significantly reduced COX-2 mRNA levels in the cochlea and IC.

dopamine system [22]. Our study group also found that *spirulina* could prevent memory dysfunction, reduce oxidative stress damage and augment catalase activity in senescence-accelerated mice [23]. Now, this study showed that *spirulina* or *C-PC* could significantly inhibit salicylate-induced over-expression of NR2B and proinflammatory genes.

As for the role of COX on tinnitus, Guitton et al. [4] hypothesized that the accumulation of arachidonic acid (AA) caused by inhibition of COX, could potentiate NR currents at the synapses between the inner hair cells and the dendrites of the cochlear spiral ganglion neuron in salicylate-induced tinnitus. Meanwhile, inhibition of COX could reduce inflammatory responses and prevent neural damages [11]. With these two contradictory or opposite sequelae, the point is that which pathways or mechanisms were more dominant for tinnitus production. In this study, we found that mRNA and protein expression levels of COX-2 gene were not inhibited significantly by salicylate injection, although COX could be inhibited at enzymatic level, but could be inhibited significantly by *spirulina* or *C-PC*. Thus, we supposed that anti-inflammation effect by COX inhibition could overcome the harmful effect of AA accumulation

on NR activity, and was the dominant mechanism underlying the beneficial effect of *spirulina* or *C-PC* on salicylate-induced tinnitus.

Although this study showed significant results, there were still some weak points. According to our previous study, we found that the hearing thresholds elevated about 10 to 20 dB four days after salicylate injection, but elevated about 5–10 dB four days after salicylate injection plus spirulina water extract treatment. Thus, we had increased sound level of stimulation just for the salicylate-alone group, but not for salicylate plus spirulina and salicylate plus C-PC groups. Even though, we are not sure whether the sound level would need to be increased to maintain perceptual level for the salicylate group. And, we are also not sure whether the results would be violated by the increased sound levels in the salicylate group. Second, we could not document any potential changes in the expression levels of NR2B, TNF-alpha, IL-1beta, and COX-2 genes under spirulina or C-PC treatment in the absence of salicylate.

In conclusion, we suggested that *spirulina platensis* water extract and its active component (*C-PC*) could reduce salicylate-induced tinnitus. The beneficial role of *spirulina* mainly via inhibiting expression of NR, COX-2 and proinflammatory genes.

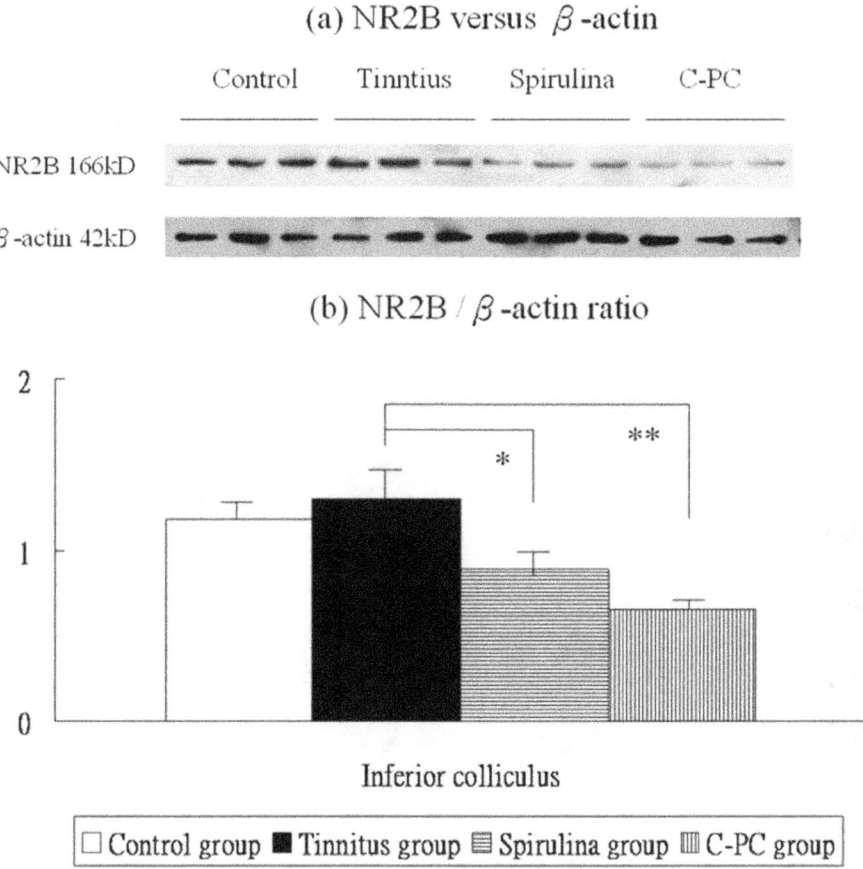

Figure 6. The levels of NR2B protein expression in the IC (a,b). There are significant differences in these levels among the four groups. The NR2B mRNA expression were not significantly higher in the salicylate group than the control group. Compared to the tinnitus group, the *Spirulina* group (*) or *C-PC* group (**) exhibits significantly reduced NR2B protein levels in the IC.

Materials and Methods

Animals

Three-month-old male SAMP8 mice (n = 96) weighing between 22.5 and 32.8 gm were randomly divided into four groups (n = 24 each) to receive saline (control group), salicylate treatment (tinnitus group), salicylate treatment plus *Spirulina platensis* water extract supplementation (*Spirulina* group), and salicylate treatment plus *C-PC* supplementation (*C-PC* group). The "control" and "tinnitus" groups were fed a normal diet, whereas the *Spirulina* group was fed a daily dietary supplement of *Spirulina platensis* water extract (1000 mg/kg body weight [BW]) and the *C-PC* group was fed *C-PC* (130 mg/kg BW) beginning on the first day of behavioral conditioning for tinnitus. Institutional Animal Care and Use Committee of Buddhist Dalin Tzu Chi General hospital had approved the protocol used in this study.

The *Spirulina platensis* water extract or *C-PC* were supplied by Far East Bio-Tec Co., Ltd. (Taipei, Taiwan). In brief, *Spirulina platensis* water extract was prepared as follows:

Spirulina platensis powder and pure water were mixed to form a suspension; the cells of *Spirulina platensis* in suspension were disrupted at a temperature lower than room temperature for 24 hours (patent pending) and centrifuged; the extract (supernatant) was collected and lyophilized. The lyophilized *Spirulina platensis* water extract contained 15–25% phycobiliproteins (C-phycocyanin and allophycocyanin), 35–45% polysaccharides, 10–20% proteins other than phycobiliproteins, 5–8% water, and 10–12%

ash. The well-known active compounds in the extract are sulfated polysaccharides and phycobiliproteins.

Behavioral Measurement of Tinnitus Score

All mice were trained in an active avoidance task, which was performed in a conditioning box with a climbing pole and a floor that could deliver an electric shock, according to the design of Guitton et al. [4] and Hwang et al. [5,6].

Conditioning to the Task

The conditioning paradigm consisted of 6 sessions per day (each lasting 15–20 min) with 10 trials per session performed for 5 days (day 1~5). Inter-trial intervals were at least 1 minute. For each trial, the conditioning stimulus was a 50-dB sound pressure level (SPL) pure tone signal with a frequency of 10 kHz and a 3-second duration, and the unconditioned stimulus was a 3.7 mA electric foot-shock presented for up to 30 seconds, as described in Guitton's protocol [4], by adjusting the voltage to the copper wire grid fixed to the floor.

The time between the conditioned stimulus and the unconditioned stimulus was 1 second. The mice would climb up the pole to reach a safe area after the coupled conditioned and unconditioned stimuli. Delivery of the electrical shocks was stopped by the experimenter when the animal climbed correctly. The "true-positive" score was the level of performance assessed by the number of times mice climbed correctly in response to sound. Mice were considered to be conditioned when the level of

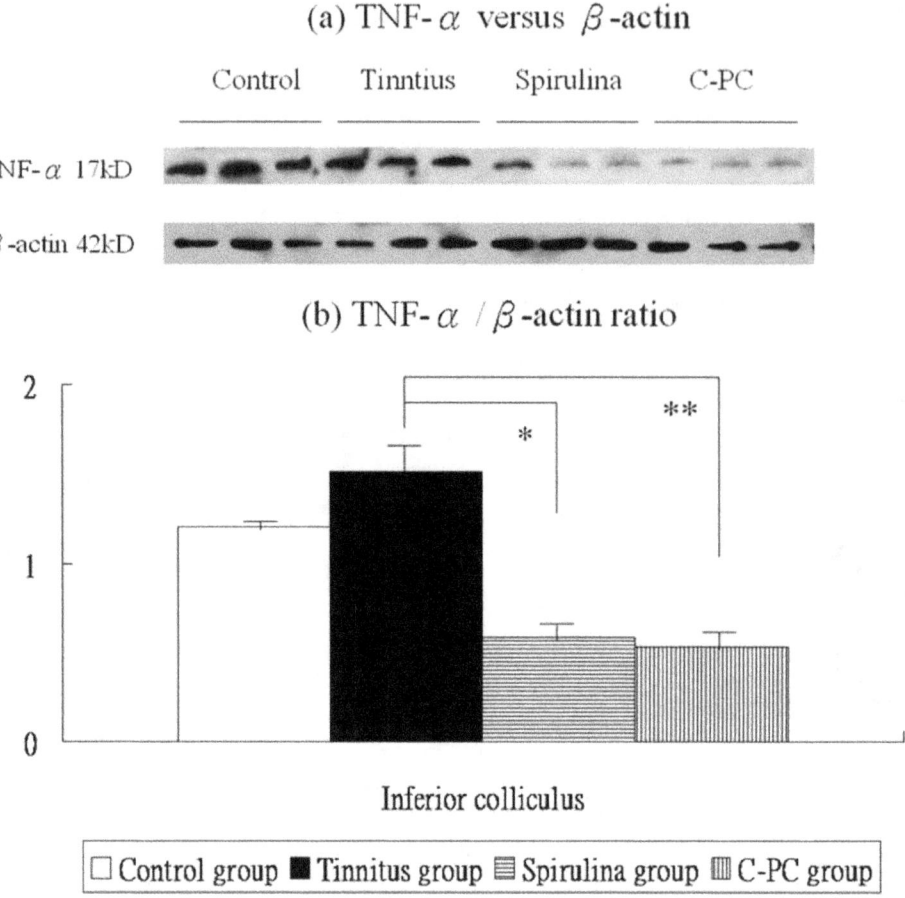

(a) TNF-α versus β-actin

(b) TNF-α / β-actin ratio

Inferior colliculus

☐ Control group ■ Tinnitus group ▤ Spirulina group ▥ C-PC group

Figure 7. The levels of TNF-α protein expression in the IC (a,b). There are significant differences in these levels among the four groups. The TNF-α mRNA expression were not significantly higher in the salicylate group than the control group. Compared to the tinnitus group, the *Spirulina* group (*) or *C-PC* group (**) exhibits significantly reduced TNF-α protein levels in the IC.

performance reached at least 80% in three consecutive sessions. Only conditioned mice were used the tinnitus experiments.

Induction and Testing of Tinnitus

When conditioned, the mice rested for 1 day (day 6). Then, one session (10 trials) of an active avoidance task of was performed 2 hours after intraperitoneal injections of saline either alone or containing 300 mg/kg sodium salicylate (Sigma, St. Louis, MO) for 4 days (day 7~10). To avoid changes attributable to hearing loss induced by salicylate (about 10–20 dB during 4 days of injections) [5,6], the intensity of sound that elicited the behavioral responses was adjusted by increasing the sound intensity to 70 dB (SPL) for salicylate-treated group only. By doing so, the perceived level of sound in all mice in both groups was similar.

During testing, a sound of 3-second duration was given first in each trial, and the mice were observed for another 5 seconds to see whether they would perform the task correctly. If so (true-positive), the mice were put down on the floor for ongoing observation. If animals did not go to the safe area and stay >10 sec, an electrical shock was given by the experimenter to remind them to climb up. The mice were also put down on the floor for ongoing observation, if they stayed in the safe area >10 sec. Finally, the experimenter observed the total number (false-positive score or tinnitus score) of times that mice climbed during the inter-trial silent periods of 1 minute of 10 trials.

Sample Isolation and RNA Extraction from the Cochlea and IC

The pairs of cochlea and IC were immediately dissected under a Zeiss stereomicroscope and stored at –80°C until use. Tissue was homogenized with a tissue homogenizer, and RNA was isolated using RNA-Bee isolation reagent (Friendswood, TX, USA) according to the manufacturer's protocol. The RNA quality was assessed on the Agilent Bioanalyzer 2100 (Agilent Technologies, Palo Alto, CA, USA) and the ratio of absorbance measurements at 260 and 280 nm was obtained using a Nanodrop Spectro-photomer (NanoDrop, Wilmington, DE, USA).

Reverse Transcription-polymerase Chain Reaction (RT-PCR)

cDNA was synthesized from total RNA by reverse transcription using a MasterAmp™ High Fidelity RT-PCR Kit (Epicentre Biotechnologies, Madison, WI, USA) in a P×2 Thermal cycler (Thermo Electron Corporation Bioscience Technologies Division, San Jose, CA, USA). For each RT reaction, a positive control (1 μg of total RNA) was included. RT was carried out at 37°C for 1 hour. For PCR amplification, 7.5 μL cDNA and primers were used according to the kit supplier's instructions. To allow comparison of mRNA levels, we used β-actin as a loading control during quantitation of target mRNAs by RT-PCR. The primers were: NR2B-F, 5'-TCC GCC GAG AGT CCT CCG T-3',

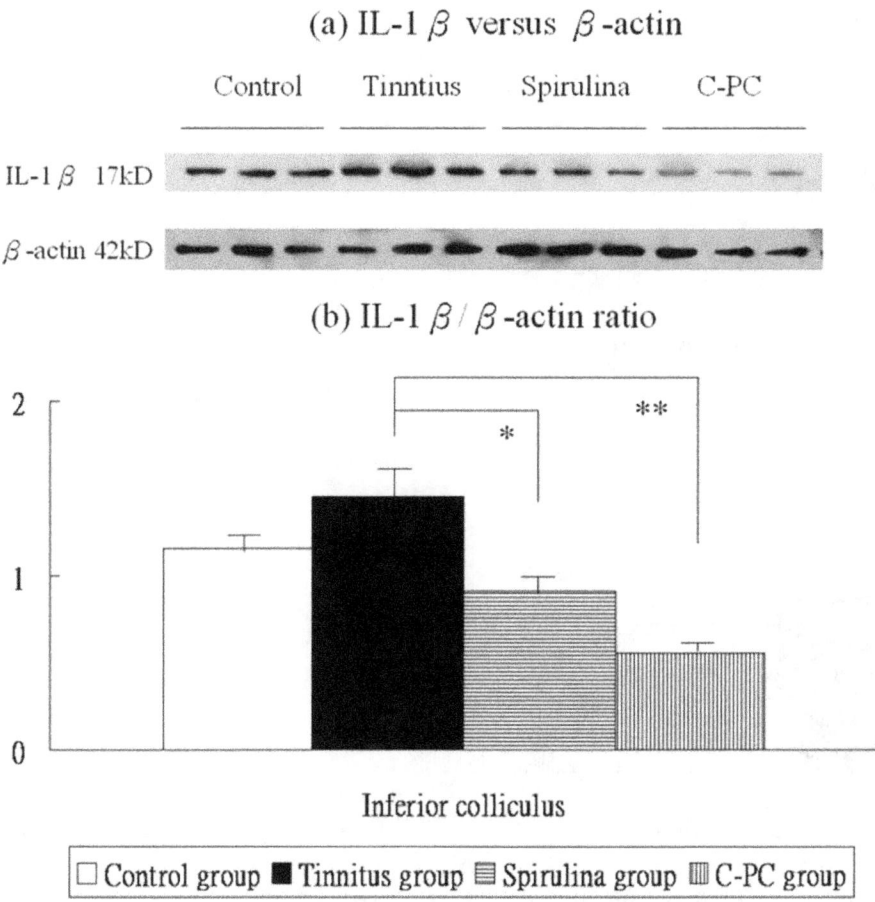

(a) IL-1 β versus β-actin

Control   Tinntius   Spirulina   C-PC

IL-1β 17kD

β-actin 42kD

(b) IL-1 β / β-actin ratio

Inferior colliculus

☐ Control group ■ Tinnitus group ▤ Spirulina group ▥ C-PC group

Figure 8. The levels of IL-1β protein expression in the IC (a,b). There are significant differences in these levels among four groups. The IL-1β protein expression were not significantly higher in the salicylate group than the control group. Compared to the tinnitus group, the *Spirulina* group (*) or *C-PC* group (**) exhibits significantly reduced TNF-α protein levels in the IC.

NR2B-R, 5′-CTG CGT TGC CCT CGA TGT T-3′; TNF-α-F, 5′-CCCCTCAGCAAACCACCAAG-3′, TNF-α-R, 5′-CTTGGCAGATTGACCTCAGC-3′; IL-1β-F, 5′-GAGTGTG-GATCCCAAGCAAT-3′, IL-1β-R, 5′-CTCAGTGCAGGC-TATGACCA-3′; COX-2-F, 5′-CTG AAG CCC ACC CCA AAC A-3′, COX-2-R, 5′-AGT ATT CGC TCC TGG ACC CAA-3′; β-actin-F, 5′-CCACACCCGCCACCAGTTCG-3′, and β-actin-R, 5′-CCCATTCCCACCATCACACC-3′ (Protech-Taiwan, Taipei, Taiwan).

The thermal cycling conditions for PCR were as follows: 3 min initial set-up at 95°C; followed by 50 cycles, each of which consisted of 45 s of denaturation at 95°C, 45 s of annealing at 53°C, and 72 s of extension at 72°C for the TNF-α genes; of 45 s of denaturation at 95°C, 45 s of annealing at 52°C, and 72 s of extension at 72°C for the IL-1β gene; of 45 s of denaturation at 95°C, 45 s of annealing at 54°C, and 72 s of extension at 72°C for the NR2B gene; and of 45 s of denaturation at 95°C, 45 s of annealing at 50°C, and 72 s of extension at 72°C for the β-actin gene. A final 10 min extension at 72°C was performed for all the above genes.

Quantitation of PCR Products

The DNA products were separated by the Mini Horizontal Electrophoresis System (MJ-105/MP-100; Major Science, Taipei,

Taiwan) and analyzed using a E-Box-1000/26M Inspection Certificate & Analysis System (E-Box Spp-010 E-capt Software, Pharr, TX, USA). The expression levels of NR2B, TNF-α, IL-1β, and COX-2 genes are presented as relative ratios to that of β-actin.

Western Blot Analysis

Equal amounts of the total protein in the IC were separated by 10% SDS–PAGE and transferred to nitrocellulose membranes, the membranes were soaked in blocking buffer (1% Bovine serum albumin). Proteins were detected using polyclonal antibodies against NR2B, TNF-α, IL-1β, or COX-2, and then visualized using goat-anti-rabbit or goat-anti-mouse IgG conjugated with peroxidase (HRP) as the HRP substrate. The expression level of above protein was presented as relative ratios in comparison to β-actin.

Statistical Analysis

The data are presented as the mean ± standard deviation (SD), unless indicated otherwise. The expression levels of NR2B, TNF-α, IL-1β, or COX-2 genes were compared separately between four study groups by one-way ANOVA with post-hoc Bonferroni correction. All the above analyses were performed using the commercially available program STATA10, and p values <0.05 were considered statistically significant.

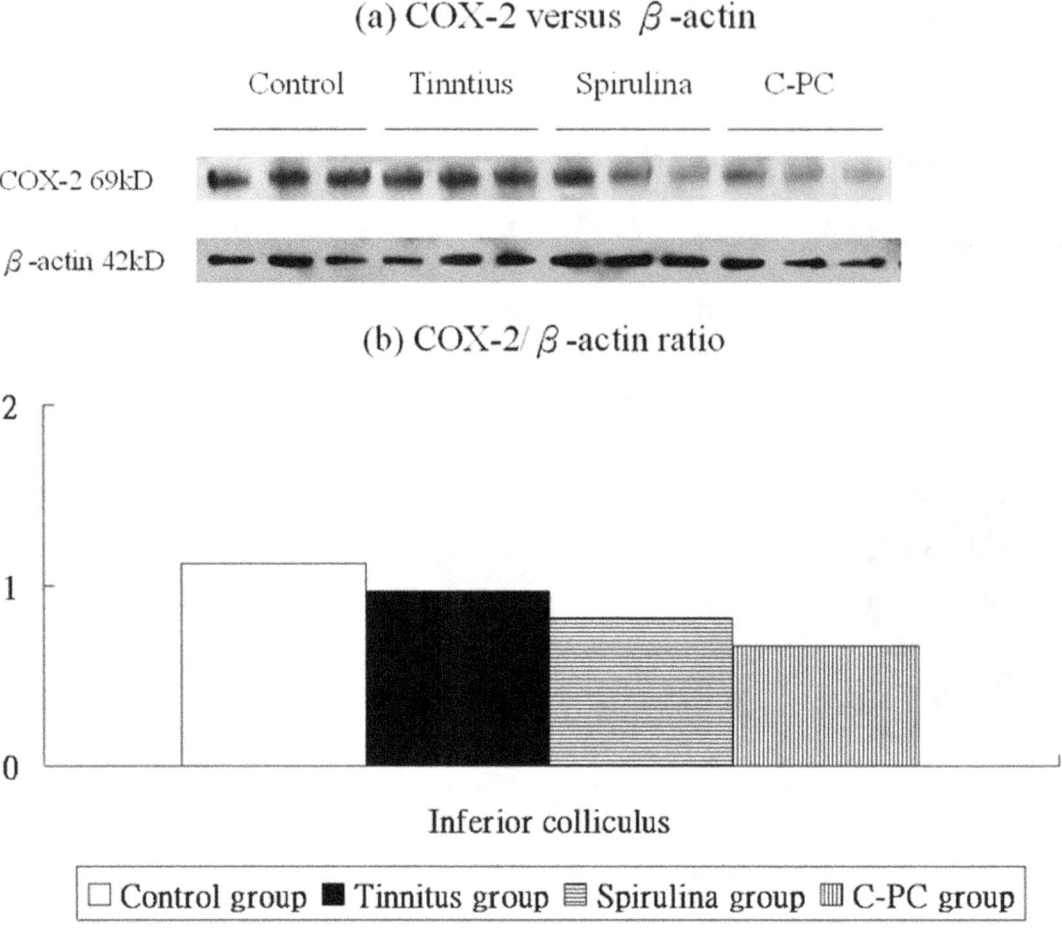

Figure 9. The levels of COX-2 protein expression in the IC (a,b). There are not significant differences in these levels among the four groups.

Author Contributions

Conceived and designed the experiments: J-HH. Performed the experiments: J-HH. Analyzed the data: J-HH. Contributed reagents/materials/analysis tools: J-CC Y-CC. Wrote the paper: J-HH.

References

1. Cooper JC Jr (1994) Health and Nutrition Examination Survey of 1971–75: Part II. Tinnitus, subjective hearing loss, and well-being. J Am Acad Audiol. 5(1): 37–43.
2. Phoon WH, Lee HS, Chia SE (1993) Tinnitus in noise-exposed workers. Occup Med (Lond). 43(1): 35–3.
3. Jastreboff PJ, Brennan J, Coleman JK, Sasaki CT (1988) Phantom auditory sensation in rats: an animal model for tinnitus. Behav. Neurosci. 102: 811–822.
4. Guitton MJ, Caston J, Ruel J, Johnson RM, Pujol R, et al. (2003) Salicylate induces tinnitus through activation of cochlear NMDA receptors. J Neurosci 23: 3944–3952.
5. Hwang JH, Chen JC, Yang SY, Wang MF, Chan YC (2011a) Expression of TNF-alpha and IL-1beta genes in the cochlea and midbrain in salicylate-induced tinnitus. J Neuroinflammation 8: 30–36.
6. Hwang JH, Chen JC, Yang SY, Wang MF, Liu TC, et al. (2011b) Expression of COX-2 and NMDA receptor genes at the cochlea and midbrain in salicylate-induced tinnitus. Laryngoscope 121: 361–364.
7. Megwalu UC, Finnell JE, Piccirillo JF (2006) The effects of melatonin on tinnitus and sleep. Otolaryngol Head Neck Surg. 134(2): 210–213.
8. Smith PF, Darlington CL (2005) Drug treatments for subjective tinnitus: serendipitous discovery versus rational drug design. Curr Opin Investig Drugs. 6(7): 712–716.
9. Wallhäusser-Franke E, Cuautle-Heck B, Wenz G, Langner G, Mahlke C (2006) Scopolamine attenuates tinnitus-related plasticity in the auditory cortex. Neuroreport. 17(14): 1487–1491.
10. Sanghvi AM, Lo YM (2010) Present and potential industrial applications of macro- and microalgae. Recent Pat Food Nutr Agric 2: 187–194.
11. Romay C, Ledon N, Gonzalez R (1999) Phycocyanin extract reduces leukoltriene B4 levels in arachidonic acid-induced mouse ear inflammation test. Journal of Pharmacy & Pharmacology 51: 641–642.
12. McCarty MF, Barroso-Aranda J, Contreras F (2010) Oral phycocyanobilin may diminish the pathogenicity of activated brain microglia in neurodegenerative disorders. Medical Hypotheses 74: 601–605.
13. Kreutzberg GW (1996) Microglia: a sensor for pathological events in the CNS. Trends Neurosci 19: 312–318.
14. McGuire SO, Ling ZD, Lipton JW, Sortwell CE, Collier TJ, et al. (2001) Tumor necrosis factor alpha is toxic to embryonic mesencephalic dopamine neurons. Experimental Neurology 169: 219–230.
15. Wakabayashi K, Fujioka M, Kanzaki S, Okano HJ, Shibata S (2010) Blockade of interleukin-6 signaling suppressed cochlear inflammatory response and improved hearing impairment in noise-damaged mice cochlea. Neurosci Res. 66: 345–352.
16. Park HJ, Kim HJ, Bae GS, Seo SW, Kim DY (2009) Selective GSK-3beta inhibitors attenuate the cisplatin-induced cytotoxicity of auditory cells. Hear Res. 257: 53–62.
17. Wheeler D, Knapp E, Bandaru VV, Wang Y, Knorr D (2009) Tumor necrosis factor-alpha-induced neutral sphingomyelinase-2 modulates synaptic plasticity by controlling the membrane insertion of NMDA receptors. J Neurochem. 109: 1237–1249.
18. Zhang RX, Li A, Liu B, Wang L, Ren K (2008) IL-1ra alleviates inflammatory hyperalgesia through preventing phosphorylation of NMDA receptor NR-1 subunit in rats. Pain. 135: 232–239.

19. Han P, Whelan PJ (2010) Tumor necrosis factor alpha enhances glutamatergic transmission onto spinal motoneurons. J Neurotrauma 27: 287–292.

20. Weber C, Arck P, Mazurek B, Klapp BF (2002) Impact of a relaxation training on psychometric and immunologic parameters in tinnitus sufferers. J Psychosom Res. 52: 29–33.

21. Wang Y, Chang CF, Chou J, Chen HL, Deng X (2005) Dietary supplementation with blueberries, spinach, or Spirulina reduces ischemic brain damage. Exp Neurol 193: 75–84.

22. Strömberg I, Gemma C, Vila J, Bickford PC (2005) Blueberry- and Spirulina-enriched diets enhance striatal dopamine recovery and induce a rapid, transient microglia activation after injury of the rat nigrostriatal dopamine system. Exp Neurol 196: 298–307.

23. Hwang JH, Lee IT, Jeng KC, Wang MF, Hou RC (2011c) Spirulina prevents memory dysfunction, reduces oxidative stress damage and augments antioxidant activity in senescence-accelerated mice. J Nutri Sci Vitaminol 57: 186–191.

18

Combining Transcranial Direct Current Stimulation and Tailor-Made Notched Music Training to Decrease Tinnitus-Related Distress

Henning Teismann[1,2]*, Andreas Wollbrink[1], Hidehiko Okamoto[3], Gottfried Schlaug[4], Claudia Rudack[5], Christo Pantev[1]

1 Institute for Biomagnetism and Biosignalanalysis, University Hospital, Münster, Germany, 2 Institute for Epidemiology and Social Medicine, University Hospital, Münster, Germany, 3 Department of Integrative Physiology, National Institute for Physiological Sciences, Okazaki, Japan, 4 Department of Neurology, Beth Israel Deaconess Medical Center and Harvard Medical School, Boston, Massachusetts, United States of America, 5 Department of Otorhinolaryngology, University Hospital, Münster, Germany

Abstract

The central auditory system has a crucial role in tinnitus generation and maintenance. Curative treatments for tinnitus do not yet exist. However, recent attempts in the therapeutic application of both acoustic stimulation/training procedures and electric/magnetic brain stimulation techniques have yielded promising results. Here, for the first time we combined tailor-made notched music training (TMNMT) with transcranial direct current stimulation (tDCS) in an effort to modulate TMNMT efficacy in the treatment of 32 patients with tonal tinnitus and without severe hearing loss. TMNMT is characterized by regular listening to so-called notched music, which is generated by digitally removing the frequency band of one octave width centered at the individual tinnitus frequency. TMNMT was applied for 10 subsequent days (2.5 hours of daily treatment). During the initial 5 days of treatment and the initial 30 minutes of TMNMT sessions, tDCS (current strength: 2 mA; anodal (N = 10) vs. cathodal (N = 11) vs. sham (N = 11) groups) was applied simultaneously. The active electrode was placed on the head surface over left auditory cortex; the reference electrode was put over right supra-orbital cortex. To evaluate treatment outcome, tinnitus-related distress and perceived tinnitus loudness were assessed using standardized tinnitus questionnaires and a visual analogue scale. The results showed a significant treatment effect reflected in the Tinnitus Handicap Questionnaire that was largest after 5 days of treatment. This effect remained significant at the end of follow-up 31 days after treatment cessation. Crucially, tDCS did not significantly modulate treatment efficacy - it did not make a difference whether anodal, cathodal, or sham tDCS was applied. Possible explanations for the findings and functional modifications of the experimental design for future studies (e.g. the selection of control conditions) are discussed.

Editor: Andrea Antal, University Medical Center Goettingen, Germany

Funding: This work was supported by the "Interdisziplinäre Zentrum für Klinische Forschung Münster" (CRA05) and the "Japan Society for the Promotion of Science for Young Scientists" (23689070). We acknowledge support by the "Deutsche Forschungsgemeinschaft" and the "Open Access Publication Fund of the University of Münster". The funders had no role in study design, data collection and analysis, decision to publish, or preparation of the manuscript.

Competing Interests: Gottfried Schlaug owns shares in Tinnix, Inc. No relationship exists between Tinnix, Inc. and the results reported in this manuscript, and Tinnix, Inc. did not provide any support, material, or technology to this project.

* E-mail: h.teismann@uni-muenster.de

Introduction

Chronic tinnitus (i.e. permanent and lasting ringing sensation in the ear(s) in the absence of a physical sound source) is a significant public health concern that impairs the quality of life for millions of patients around the world. Tinnitus incidence and prevalence rates appear to be increasing not only in older people, but also in younger adults, probably due to the exposure to occupational and recreational sounds such as amplified music [1,2].

In the majority of cases, tinnitus is probably triggered by inner ear hair cell injury. Nonetheless, the neural generators of tinnitus are most likely located in the *central* auditory pathway. One possible consequence of injury to hair cells (and the subsequently decreased input to tonotopic maps in auditory cortex) is a loss of lateral inhibition from cortical neural populations which would normally code activity from the now damaged and silent receptors. As a result of such and other disturbances of the balance of excitatory and inhibitory neural transmissions, activations of neural plasticity in the central auditory system lead to alterations of neuronal activity. Among them are (i) hyperactivity, (ii) increased synchrony, and (iii) increased burst firing [3,4]. Moreover, in many if not all cases of chronic tinnitus, also non-auditory brain structures are part of the tinnitus generating and tinnitus sustaining networks [5].

Traditional and also the more recently developed tinnitus treatment programs use management strategies like cognitive behavior therapy or sound masking which are aimed at the successful habituation of the effects caused by the tinnitus. However, most patients with tinnitus want more of a relief or a cure [6,7]. Unfortunately, chronic tinnitus has proven to be difficult to treat - presently, there are no curative treatments [1]. One important problem is that chronic tinnitus is most likely a systemic disorder, affecting different parts of the auditory system and other related systems [8]. Another problem is that there are many different treatment targets in the tinnitus network (e.g. auditory cortex, thalamus, dorsal/ventral cochlear nuclei, inferior colliculus, cochlear nerve, and the limbic system [9]). Among those different targets, the auditory cortex might be the most important one, since alterations in its excitatory/inhibitory networks seem to correlate with the subjective tinnitus percept [10]. A non-invasive means to modulate the activity of auditory cortical neural populations contributing to tinnitus perception is acoustic input. Acoustic neuromodulation can be precise and specific by targeting defined auditory neural populations through passive sound stimulation [11] or auditory training [12] using the natural sensory pathway. A recent acoustic neuromodulation strategy is the "tailor-made notched music training (TMNMT)" for chronic tonal tinnitus [13]. TMNMT uses enjoyable, individually modified acoustic input (i.e. patient-selected music notched to exclude the individual tinnitus frequency) to specifically target auditory cortex neuronal populations which code the tinnitus frequency. Both long-term (12 months) and short-term (5 days) TMNMT studies [14–16] have yielded results which indicate that TMNMT is a specific treatment holding the potential to reduce tinnitus-related cortical activity along with perceived tinnitus loudness (measured by visual analogue scale) and distress. At this stage of research, it is assumed that TMNMT is suitable for patients with tinnitus frequencies below approximately 8 kHz and without severe hearing losses. We presume that notching out the specific tinnitus frequency (and surrounding frequencies) may confer added benefit compared to other, reportedly effective acoustic neurostimulation approaches, which for instance use complex sounds covering the tinnitus frequency [17], or sequences of pure tones with a distance of one or two octaves to the tinnitus frequency [18]. We assume that the beneficial effects of TMNMT are due to the de-synchronization of tinnitus-related neural activity by lateral inhibition distributed into the notched region [19,20]. However, another possibility is that listening to notched music for extended periods might rescale auditory sensitivity, leading to a reduction of both the perceived loudness of sound in the notched frequency region and corresponding brain activity [13].

Other forms of non-invasive brain-stimulation have also been used to influence perceived tinnitus loudness and/or tinnitus-related distress. Methods such as transcranial magnetic stimulation (TMS) and transcranial direct current stimulation (tDCS) become increasingly popular to examine causal contributions of particular neural structures to defined cognitive processes (e.g. perception, working memory, or attention) and as neuromodulatory tools to treat patients with psychiatric or neurologic diseases (e.g. depression, schizophrenia, obsessive-compulsive disorder, stroke, Parkinson's, epilepsy, neuropathic pain, or dysphagia) [21]. Both TMS and tDCS have almost no side-effects if the limits of safe stimulation are met. Compared to TMS, tDCS has the advantages that (i) it does not generate any acoustic noise, and that (ii) effective sham stimulation can be delivered [22]. However, tDCS has the disadvantage of being comparably less focal; the current flow between the cathodal and anodal scalp surface electrodes (i.e. the exact "path" that the current takes through the brain) is not always easy to predict or model [23]. A considerable amount of current can also be shunted through the skin and subcutaneous tissue and does not enter the brain [24]; however, various studies have shown that physiological processes in the brain can be altered by tDCS [25]. Several studies have shown that tDCS does not directly trigger action potentials; rather, neuronal excitability and activity are modulated by tonic de- or hyper-polarization of the resting membrane potential. Thereby, spontaneous neural activity is indirectly manipulated. As a function of stimulation polarity, tDCS can either up- or down-regulate cortical excitability - anodal

stimulation leads to cortical excitability increment, while cathodal tDCS causes a decrement [26].

On grounds of studies in animals, it has been proposed that three neuronal mechanisms might underlie tinnitus perception: (i) spontaneous firing rate alterations of central auditory system neurons, (ii) changes in temporal activity patterns of such neurons (increased synchrony), and (iii) plastic reorganization of tonotopic maps [27]. In accordance with this assumption, several $[^{15}O]H_2O$ PET studies [28–34] have yielded results indicating tinnitus-related elevated blood flow in auditory structures. Noteworthy, studies using $[^{18}F]$deoxyglucose PET found increased *left* auditory cortex activation in tinnitus patients compared to controls, independent of perceived tinnitus laterality [35–37]. Based on these findings, the treatment potential of tDCS over left temporo-parietal cortex has been explored in patients with chronic tinnitus [38,39]. In both studies, single sessions of anodal or cathodal tDCS were applied. The reference electrode was placed over the right supra-orbital area. Both studies reported significant, transient reductions in perceived tinnitus intensity ([38]: rating scale; [39]: visual analogue scale) under anodal tDCS; no effects were found under cathodal stimulation. Evidently, these effects persisted for several days in some patients [39]. Noteworthy, these findings are counter-intuitive, because anodal tDCS is assumed to increase cortical excitability. So far, there are no studies with repeated applications of tDCS over auditory brain areas in tinnitus patients [40].

However, even though the auditory cortex appears to be an obvious treatment target in tinnitus, it should be noted that the dorsolateral prefrontal cortex (DLPFC) has also been postulated as a possible target for non-invasive brain stimulation, considering that it is important for the integration of sensory and emotional aspects of tinnitus [41]. tDCS over DLPFC was successful in reducing depression, impulsiveness, and pain [42], and some studies have shown that bifrontal tDCS is also effective in alleviating perceived tinnitus intensity (measured by rating scales) and/or perceived tinnitus-related distress (measured by tinnitus questionnaires) to some degree [41–46]. Presumably, perceived tinnitus intensity/distress could be modulated directly by targeting both auditory and/or frontal cortices [43]; however, tDCS could also indirectly influence functionally connected brain areas relevant for tinnitus distress and tinnitus intensity [44].

In the recent past, it has become more and more obvious that tinnitus is a system-wide problem [8], which is sustained by a complex and wide-spread tinnitus network [47]. The complexity of the phenomenon needs to be considered when it comes to the development and application of treatment approaches. While effective systemic treatments are not yet available, it appears promising to combine established neuromodulation strategies in order to possibly achieve additive effects. In the present study, we combined two complementary neuromodulation strategies in an explorative manner: (i) TMNMT, and (ii) tDCS over the left auditory cortex. Previous studies [14,16] have shown that TMNMT is able to specifically reduce potentially tinnitus-related auditory cortex activity, possibly through the activation of neural plasticity; it is assumed that TMNMT attracts lateral inhibition to auditory neurons coding the tinnitus frequency. tDCS, on the other hand, has the potential to either up- or down-regulate neuronal activity and possibly promote plastic reorganization by simultaneously combining tDCS with another sensory stimulation technique [48–51]. Moreover, previous studies in healthy subjects have shown that tDCS over auditory cortex is able to modulate both auditory evoked potentials [52] and auditory perception [53]. Furthermore, initial studies in patients demonstrated that tDCS over left auditory cortex *alone* could alleviate perceived tinnitus intensity [38,39]. Thus, both anodal and cathodal tDCS could theoretically reinforce or facilitate effects of TMNMT. However, due to potentially complex interactions between tDCS polarity and effects induced by the TMNMT treatment sounds, it is hard to predict if and how anodal and/or cathodal tDCS combined with TMNMT would shape perceived tinnitus loudness/distress.

Based on these considerations, we investigated whether tDCS polarity over left auditory cortex would *modulate* the efficacy of short-term combined tDCS + TMNMT treatment for not severely hearing impaired patients suffering from chronic tonal tinnitus. TMNMT (2.5 hours of training per day over 10 subsequent days) and tDCS (30 min of – depending on treatment group membership - either anodal (N = 10), cathodal (N = 11), or sham (N = 11) stimulation) were applied simultaneously - the direct current was delivered while the patients were listening to their individually modified training music. Given that TMNMT is a re-training strategy, requiring repeated and regular "exercise", we decided to also apply tDCS repeatedly (5 subsequent days) (Figure 1). Iterative tDCS appears promising also against the background of lasting stimulation after effects, which seem to represent transient modulations of synaptic transmission efficacy [22], and which might permit effect accumulation.

Materials and Methods

Ethics Statement

The study was performed in accordance with the Declaration of Helsinki and was approved by the Ethics Commission of the Medical Faculty, University of Münster, Germany. The patients gave written informed consent for the participation in the study.

Participants

We recruited 34 patients who had (i) chronic (≥3 months) tonal tinnitus, (ii) dominant tinnitus frequencies below 9 kHz, and (iii) reported to have no history of psychiatric or neurologic diseases. All patients reported hearing one single tinnitus percept. Tinnitus could be either uni- or bilateral. In case of bilateral tinnitus, the dominant tinnitus frequency did not differ between ears according to patient's reports.

Two patients dropped out during treatment (patient 1 (cathodal tDCS treatment) due to an inability to comply with the study requirements; patient 2 (anodal tDCS treatment) due to novel tinnitus percepts arising in the treatment phase). 32 patients (94.1%) completed the study. Table 1 displays average patient characteristics. Figure 2 displays average hearing thresholds of the patients.

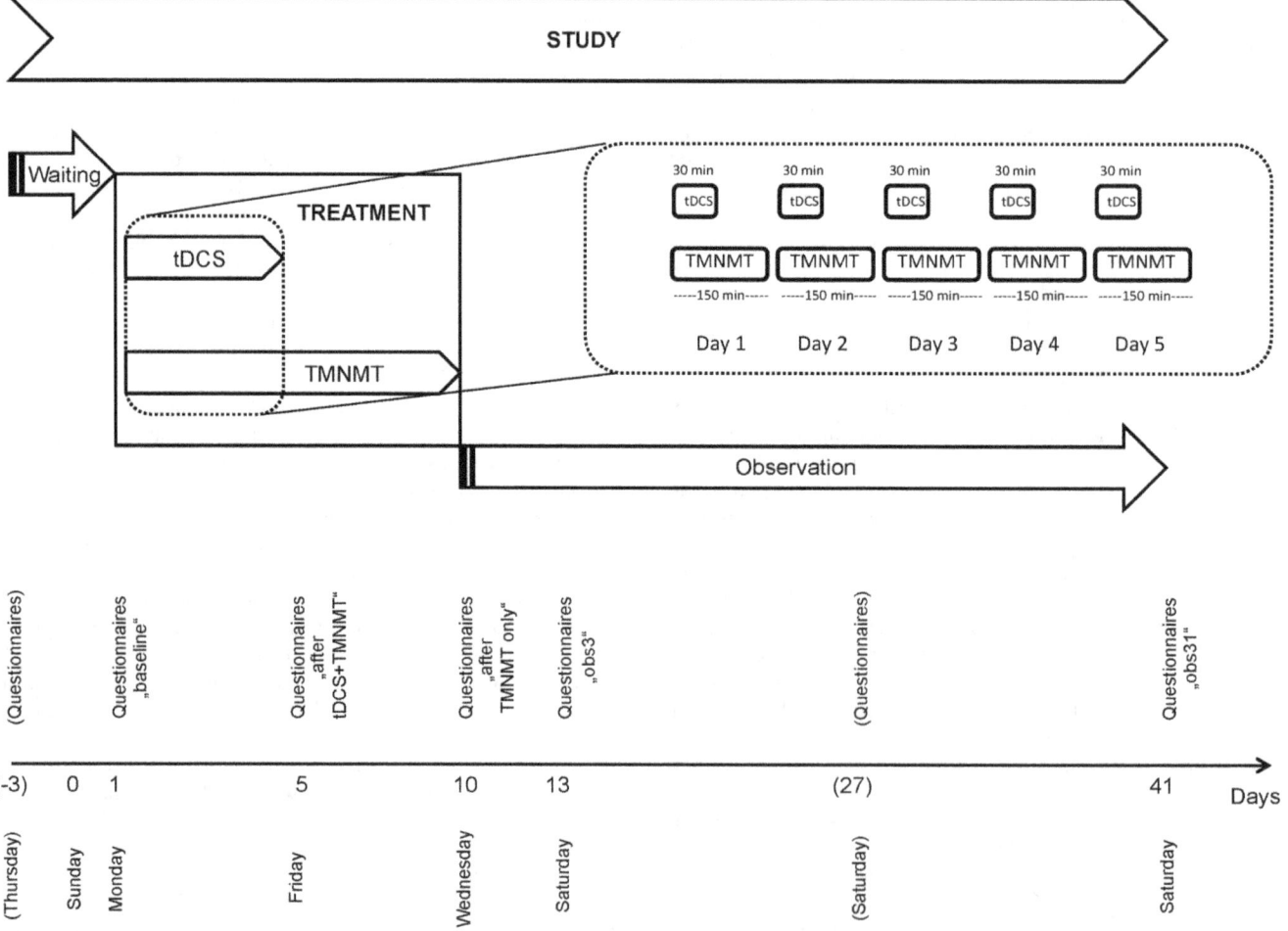

Figure 1. Study design. For each participant, the study took 45 days (4 days of pre-treatment waiting, 10 days of treatment, and 31 days of post-treatment observation). During the initial 5 days of treatment, transcranial direct current stimulation (tDCS) and the tailor-made notched music training (TMNMT) were applied simultaneously; during the remaining 5 days of treatment, only TMNMT was applied. Throughout the study, perceived tinnitus-related distress data were sampled repeatedly.

Table 1. Patient characteristics.

Groups	Age[1] [years]	Tinnitus frequency[2] [Hz]	Tinnitus duration[1] [years]	General psychopathological distress[1] [SCL-90-R[3]]	Depression[1] [ADS-L[4]]	State anxiety[1] [STAI[5]]
Anodal tDCS[6] (N = 10)	42.90 (6.87)	4440.28 (1.78)	10.70 (7.26)	36.90 (39.84)	8.00 (5.85)	36.50 (11.37)
Cathodal tDCS (N = 11)	44.45 (13.29)	4654.66 (1.34)	10.27 (11.33)	30.91 (25.11)	12.09 (7.46)	35.82 (8.53)
Sham tDCS (N = 11)	44.91 (9.92)	4119.98 (1.69)	5.82 (6.15)	28.27 (25.75)	7.45 (6.67)	37.18 (10.45)

[1]Arithmetic mean (standard deviation).
[2]Geometric mean (standard deviation in octaves).
[3]Symptom Checklist 90 Revisited [57];
[4]Allgemeine Depressionsskala, Langform [58];
[5]State-Trait Anxiety Inventory [59].
[6]Transcranial direct current stimulation.

Study Design

The participants were randomly assigned to one out of three tDCS treatment conditions: (i) anodal group (N = 10), (ii) cathodal group (N = 11), (iii) or sham group (N = 11). Retrospectively, there were no significant differences between groups regarding relevant patient characteristics (cf. Table 1 and section "Patient characteristics" below). All patients received a combined tDCS + TMNMT treatment. The study was performed double-blindly. Prior to the

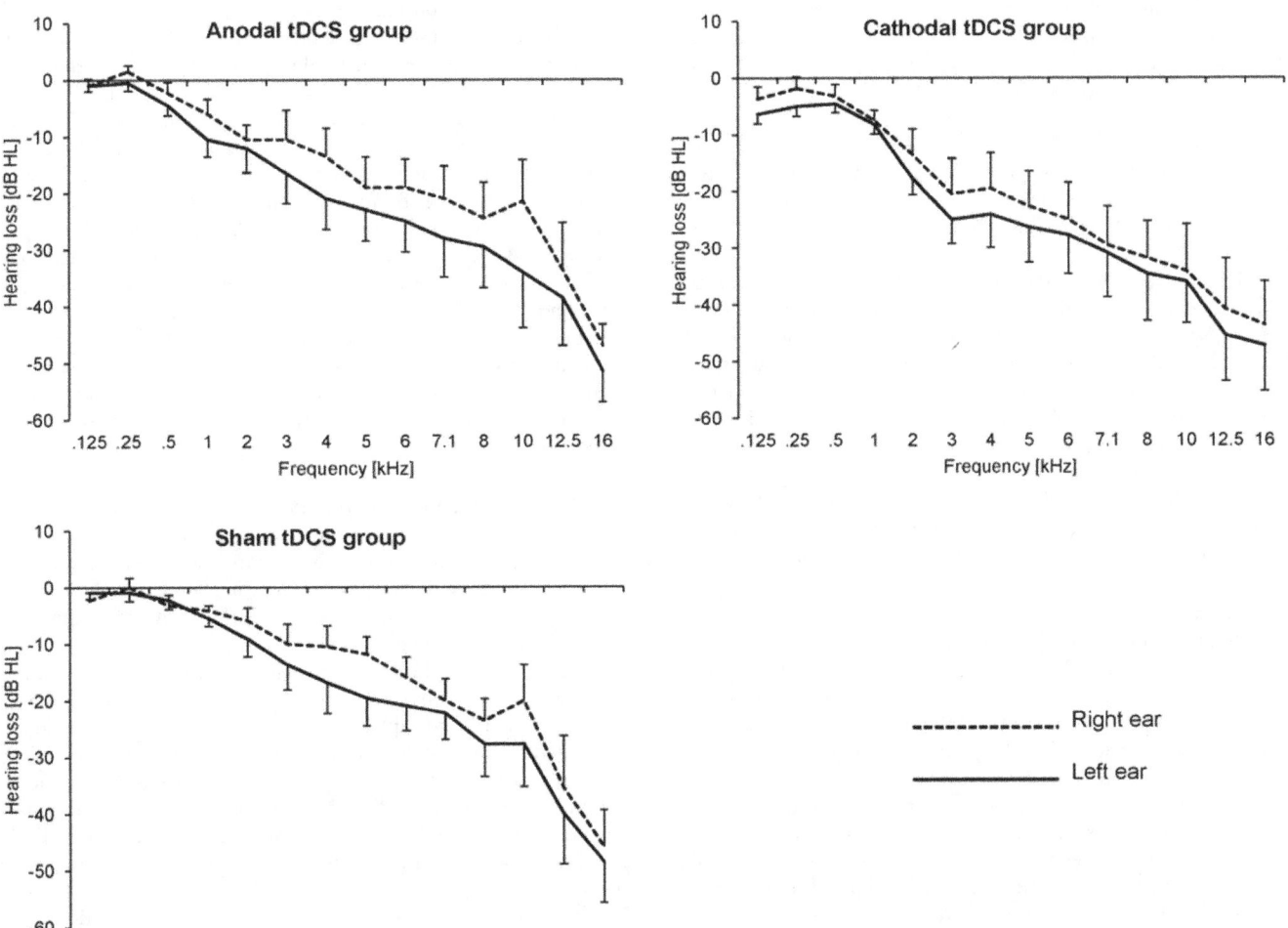

Figure 2. Average hearing thresholds. Thresholds from 0.125 to 16 kHz as functions of transcranial direct current stimulation (tDCS) condition (anodal group vs. cathodal group vs. sham group) and ear (left vs. right). The error bars denote standard error of the mean. Negative values reflect hearing loss.

study, the patients were informed that they would receive target (i.e. anodal or cathodal) tDCS treatment with a likelihood of 66.67%, and placebo (i.e. sham) tDCS treatment with a likelihood of 33.33%. Moreover, in order to reduce potential unspecific treatment effects, the patients were also told that they would receive target or placebo TMNMT with a likelihood of 50%. In fact, all patients were treated with target TMNMT; placebo TMNMT was not administered [16]. After the study, the patients were de-briefed.

The treatment phase took 10 subsequent days (1–10; Monday to Wednesday). The tDCS treatment was administered for 5 consecutive days (1–5; Monday to Friday); the TMNMT was administered for 10 consecutive days (1–10; Monday to Wednesday). During the initial 5 days (1–5; Monday to Friday), both treatments were administered simultaneously. In this phase, the patients received tDCS during the initial 30 min of music listening (which took 2.5 hours per day without interruptions). During the last 5 days (6–10; Saturday to Wednesday), only the TMNMT was administered. A waiting phase of 4 days (-3 to 0; Thursday to Sunday) preceded treatment onset. Treatment offset was followed by an observation phase of 31 days (11–41; Thursday to Saturday) (Figure 1).

tDCS Specifics

tDCS was applied using the "DC-STIMULATOR PLUS" (neuroConn GmbH, Ilmenau, Germany). Independent of tinnitus laterality, the active electrode (area = 35 cm^2) was horizontally placed over the skull surface representation of left Heschl's Gyrus (1 cm inferior to the halfway point between C3 and T3 of the 10–20 system of EEG [53]). The reference electrode (area = 100 cm^2) was placed contra-laterally to the active electrode in the supra-orbital region, just above the right eyebrow. The current strength was set to 2 mA. Stimulation duration was 30 min per training day.

In the anodal and cathodal (i.e. the "real") tDCS conditions, the direct current was faded in to 2 mA over the course of 30 sec. After 29.5 min of stimulation, the current was faded out to 0 mA. Total stimulation duration was 30 min. In the sham tDCS condition, the direct current was faded in to 2.0 mA and then directly faded out to 0 mA, in each case over the course of 30 sec. The same procedure was repeated 29 min after stimulation onset (Figure 3). Thus, in both the "real" and the sham stimulation conditions, the patients felt the tingling sensation of stimulation, but in the sham condition basically no current was delivered for the duration (= 30 min) of the "stimulation" session.

TMNMT Specifics

Each patient provided up to 10 hours of their favorite music in CD quality (44100 Hz, 16 bit, stereo). The music was modified in two successive steps. First, the energy spectrum of the music was "flattened" by the re-distribution of energy from low to high frequency ranges. Second, the frequency band of one octave width centered at the individual tinnitus frequency (i.e. the most prominent pitch match frequency) was removed from the music energy spectrum using a Butterworth notch filter (order = 150; low notch edge = tinnitus frequency · $2^{-1/2}$; high notch edge = tinnitus frequency · $2^{1/2}$) [16] (Figure 4). The modified training music (44100 Hz, 16 bit, stereo,.wav) was re-played with supplied portable music players ("TrekStor i.Beat move S 2.0 8 GB", TrekStor GmbH, Lorsch, Germany) and via supplied headphones ("Sennheiser HD 201", Sennheiser electronic GmbH & Co. KG, Wedemark Wennebostel, Germany), which are characterized by a sufficiently flat frequency response across the relevant frequency range. Patients listened to their training music in a quiet environment and were instructed to relax. It was not mandatory to focus on the training music, and patients were allowed to read or surf the internet during listening. Listening duration was 2.5 hours (without interruptions) per training day; during the first 30 min of music listening, tDCS was applied simultaneously. Patients were told not to listen to normal, non-modified music during the treatment phase.

Tinnitus Frequency Determination

The dominant tinnitus frequency (i.e. the dominant tinnitus pitch) was matched once prior to study onset. The matching was performed by audiometrists using a clinical audiometer (Madsen Astera, GN Otometrics, Taastrup, Denmark) and a closed headphone ("Sennheiser HDA200", Sennheiser electronic GmbH & Co. KG, Wedemark Wennebostel, Germany) following a structured protocol. The frequency resolution was 1/12 octave. In case of unilateral tinnitus, the tinnitus ear was tested. In case of bilateral tinnitus, the ear in which tinnitus was perceived as being louder was tested. In case of identical tinnitus loudness in both ears, the better hearing ear was tested.

In a first step, seven "tinnitus frequency candidates" were collected. During this procedure, the tinnitus frequency and loudness were matched seven times, starting from seven different anchor frequencies (in given order: 1000, 12500, 2000, 10000, 4000, 8000, and 6000 Hz).

In a second step, the "winner tinnitus frequency candidate" was determined. During this procedure, in each case two of the previously determined tinnitus frequency candidates (with matched tinnitus loudness) were directly compared in a two-forced-choice procedure, starting with the lowest candidate. The winner of each comparison was tested against the lowest remaining candidate frequency. This procedure was repeated until the winner tinnitus frequency candidate was found.

In a third step, an octave confusion test was performed. First, the octaves of the winner tinnitus frequency candidate between 1000 and 16000 Hz were calculated. Second, the tinnitus loudness was matched for each of these octaves. Third, the winner tinnitus frequency candidate and its octaves (with matched tinnitus loudness) were directly compared in a two-forced-choice procedure, according to step two, until the tinnitus frequency was finally determined.

Treatment Outcome Measures

To assess treatment outcome, (i) perceived tinnitus-related distress and (ii) perceived tinnitus loudness were monitored throughout the study, i.e. prior to training onset (waiting phase), during training (treatment phase), and after training completion (observation phase) (Figure 1).

Tinnitus-related distress was assessed with (i) the Tinnitus Handicap Questionnaire (THQ; focus at perceived degree of tinnitus-related handicap) [54] as the (a priori defined) primary outcome measure, and the (ii) Tinnitus Handicap Inventory (THI; focus at perceived functioning) [55] and the German version of the Tinnitus Questionnaire (TQ; focus at tinnitus-related emotional/cognitive distress) [56] as secondary outcome measures. The THQ was defined as the primary outcome measure due to its presumed short-term change sensitivity (any number between 0 and 100 can be given as an answer to each of the items). The questionnaires were given (i) before the waiting phase, (ii) before the treatment phase, (iii) after completion of the tDCS treatment, (iv) after the treatment phase, and (v–vii) 3, 17, and 31 days after treatment completion (Figure 1). For statistical analyses, the questionnaire total scores were used. In case of the TQ, the E+C subscale (TQ$_{E+C}$) was analyzed [16] in addition to the total score (TQ$_{total}$).

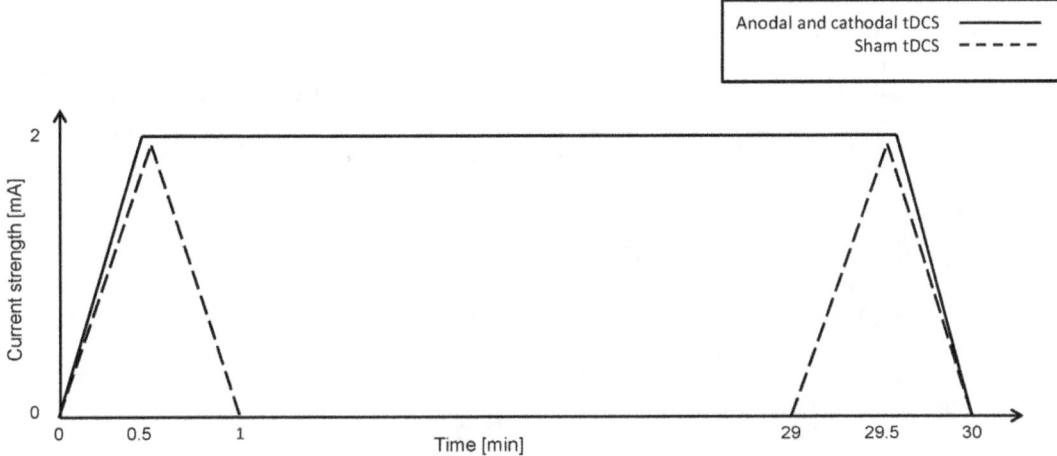

Figure 3. Transcranial direct current stimulation (tDCS). Time course of direct current strength in the different tDCS conditions.

Tinnitus loudness was estimated by visual analog scale (VAS) twice per day (scale poles: 0 (=tinnitus gone) vs. 100 (=personal tinnitus loudness maximum experienced so far) [16]). In the treatment phase, the loudness estimations were made directly before the beginning of the training session and 15 min after the end of the training session. During the waiting and observation phases, the loudness estimations were made with at least 4 hours in between estimations. For statistical analyses, averages across the two daily loudness estimates were used.

Results

The data were analyzed with "Statistica 9". The significance level was set to $\alpha = .05$ (two-tailed). If the sphericity assumption of repeated measures was violated, degrees of freedom were Greenhouse-Geisser corrected. Significant main effects or interactions were further explored by means of least significant difference (Fisher LSD) post-hoc tests (family-wise error rate controlled).

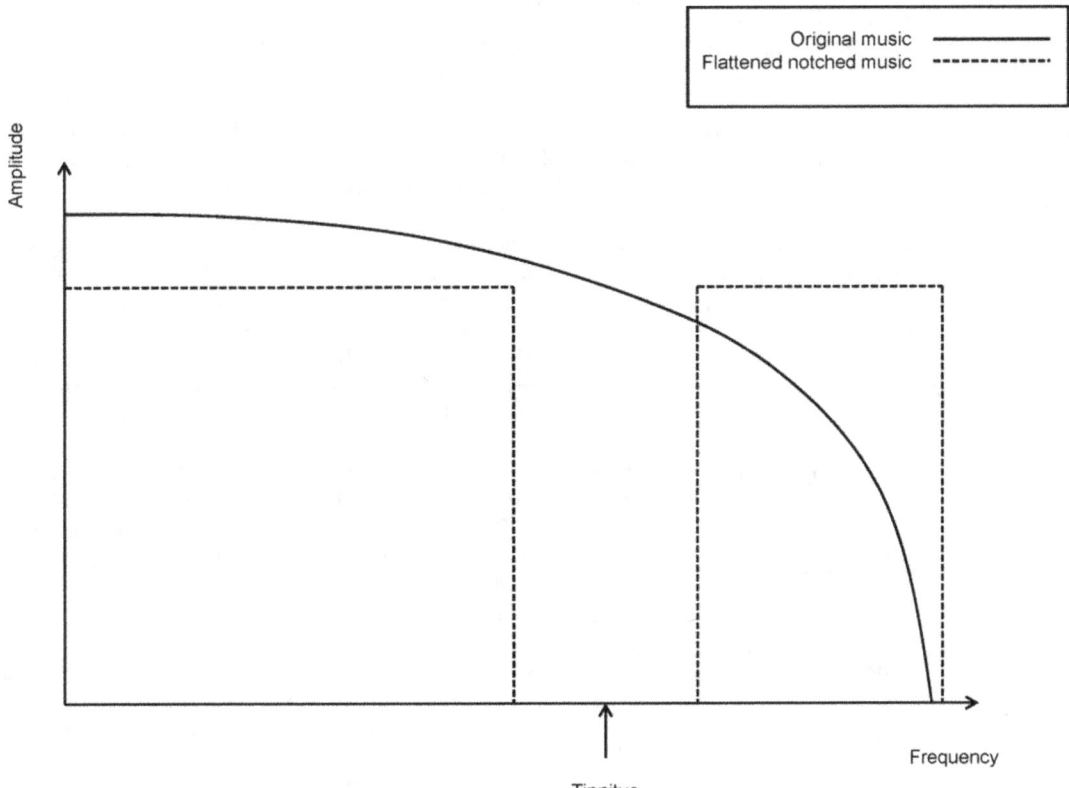

Figure 4. Music spectra. Schematic frequency spectra of original music (solid line) and flattened notched music (dashed dotted line).

Patient Characteristics

The hearing thresholds of the patients of the three different tDCS conditions did not significantly differ (the ANOVA results showed neither a significant main effect of tDCS-CONDITION (anodal vs. cathodal vs. sham) ($F_{(2,28)} = 0.38$, p = 0.69) nor were there significant interactions tDCS-CONDITION×EAR (left vs. right) ($F_{(2,28)} = 0.29$,   p = 0.75),   tDCS-CONDITION×FRE-QUENCY (.125 vs.25 vs.5 vs. 1 vs. 2 vs. 3 vs. 4 vs. 5 vs. 6 vs. 7.1 vs. 8 vs. 10 vs. 12.5 vs. 16 kHz) ($F_{(26,364)} = 0.31$, p = 0.91), or tDCS-CONDITION×EAR×FREQUENCY   ($F_{(26,364)} = 0.71$, p = 0.73)) (Figure 2). Moreover, age ($F_{(2,29)} = 0.11$, p = 0.90), (logarithmized) tinnitus frequency ($F_{(2,29)} = 0.18$, p = 0.84), and tinnitus duration ($F_{(2,29)} = 1.07$, p = 0.36) did not significantly differ between tDCS conditions (Table 1). Furthermore, at treatment onset (i.e. at baseline, see below) there were no significant differences in general psychopathological distress ("SCL-90-R") [57] ($F_{(2,29)} = 0.22$, p = 0.81), depression ("ADS-L") [58] ($F_{(2,29)} = 1.55$, p = 0.23), and state anxiety ("STAI") [59] ($F_{(2,29)} = 0.05$, p = 0.95) between tDCS conditions (Table 1).

Music Enjoyment

Enjoyment of the training music ($F_{(2,29)} = 0.996$, p = 0.381) as well as degree of relaxation experienced during listening to the training music ($F_{(2,29)} = 0.112$, p = 0.895) did not significantly differ between tDCS conditions (Table 2).

Treatment Outcome

In order to assess treatment outcome, we calculated relative change values for the time points (i) after the tDCS treatment offset at day 5 ("after tDCS + TMNMT"), (ii) after the TMNMT treatment offset at day 10 ("after TMNMT only"), (iii) three days after treatment completion at day 13 ("obs3"), and (iv) 31 days after treatment completion at day 41 ("obs31"). The baseline values were sampled directly before treatment onset. The following formula was used to calculate relative change values: $[(V_{(i, ii, iii, iv)}/V_{baseline}) - 1]$.

Separately for each outcome measure (i.e. THQ change, tinnitus loudness change, TQ_total change, TQ_E+C change, and THI change), the data were analyzed by ANOVA including TIME (baseline vs. after tDCS + TMNMT vs. after TMNMT only vs. obs3 vs. obs31) as repeated measure, and tDCS-CONDITION (anodal vs. cathodal vs. sham) as between subjects measure. There was a significant main effect of TIME ($F_{(4,116)} = 3.44$, p = 0.042) for THQ change. Post-hoc tests revealed significant differences between "baseline" and "after tDCS + TMNMT" (p = 0.0007), "baseline" and "TMNMT only" (p = 0.009), "baseline" and "obs3" (p = 0.007), and "baseline" and "obs31" (p = 0.017) (Figure 5). There were no significant main effects or interactions for tinnitus loudness change, TQ_total change,

Table 2. Subjective music perception.

Groups	Music perception	
	Enjoyment[1]	Relaxation[1]
Anodal tDCS[2] (N = 10)	66.1 (21.2)	63.1 (22.98)
Cathodal tDCS (N = 11)	66.45 (20.51)	66.64 (17.25)
Sham tDCS (N = 11)	76.36 (15.58)	67.09 (22.51)

[1]Arithmetic mean (standard deviation); range: 0–100.
[2]Transcranial direct current stimulation.

Table 3. Treatment outcome.

Outcome measures	ANOVA[1]: Main effects and interaction		
	Time	tDCS[2] condition	Time×tDCS condition
Tinnitus loudness	p = .10	p = .45	p = .76
TQ_total[3]	p = .56	p = .83	p = .37
TQ_E+C[4]	p = .16	p = .50	p = .60
THQ[5]	p = .04*	p = .81	p = .93
THI[6]	p = .06	p = .98	p = .91

[1]Analysis of variance.
[2]Transcranial direct current stimulation.
[3]Tinnitus Questionnaire, total score.
[4]Tinnitus Questionnaire, subscale emotional + cognitive distress.
[5]Tinnitus Handicap Questionnaire, total score.
[6]Tinnitus Handicap Inventory, total score.
*Statistically significant.

TQ_E+C change, and THI change. The p-values for all calculated statistical tests are summarized in Table 3.

Given that longer lasting treatment effects would be most relevant for the efficacy of the intervention, we calculated one additional, explorative statistical test at the last time point of measurement (i.e. obs31). The one-way ANOVA using tDCS-CONDITION (anodal vs. cathodal vs. sham) as between-subjects factor did not show a significant main effect ($F_{(2,29)} = 0.071$, p = 0.932).

Discussion

This study investigated whether tDCS polarity (anodal vs. cathodal) over left auditory cortex would modulate the efficacy of a combined tDCS + TMNMT short-term treatment for not severely hearing impaired patients suffering from chronic tonal tinnitus. To the best of our knowledge, this study was the first to repeatedly apply tDCS over auditory cortex in chronic tinnitus patients, and it was also the first study to combine tDCS with an acoustic neuromodulation strategy. The results indicate that, under the prevailing circumstances, there was no significant modulating effect of tDCS polarity: significant main effects or interactions of tDCS condition were neither found in the primary outcome measure (THQ; Figure 5; Table 3) nor in any of the secondary outcome measures (THI, TQ, or loudness VAS; Table 3), indicating that tDCS polarity did not influence perceived tinnitus-related distress or tinnitus loudness. However, the significant main effect of time observed in the main outcome measure (THQ; Figure 5; Table 3) implies that the combined tDCS + TMNMT short-term treatment (independently of tDCS condition) may have effectively reduced tinnitus-related distress. Alternatively, the parsimonious conclusion to draw is that this result could reflect an unspecific treatment/placebo effect. Moreover, the results of the calculated post-hoc tests, which revealed significant differences between baseline values and values at all other time points during and after treatment, but not between values at different time points during and after treatment, indicate (i) that the major efficacy component was triggered during the initial 5 days of treatment (where tDCS and TMNMT had been applied simultaneously), and (ii) that the induced reduction of tinnitus-related tinnitus distress was longer lasting, persisting

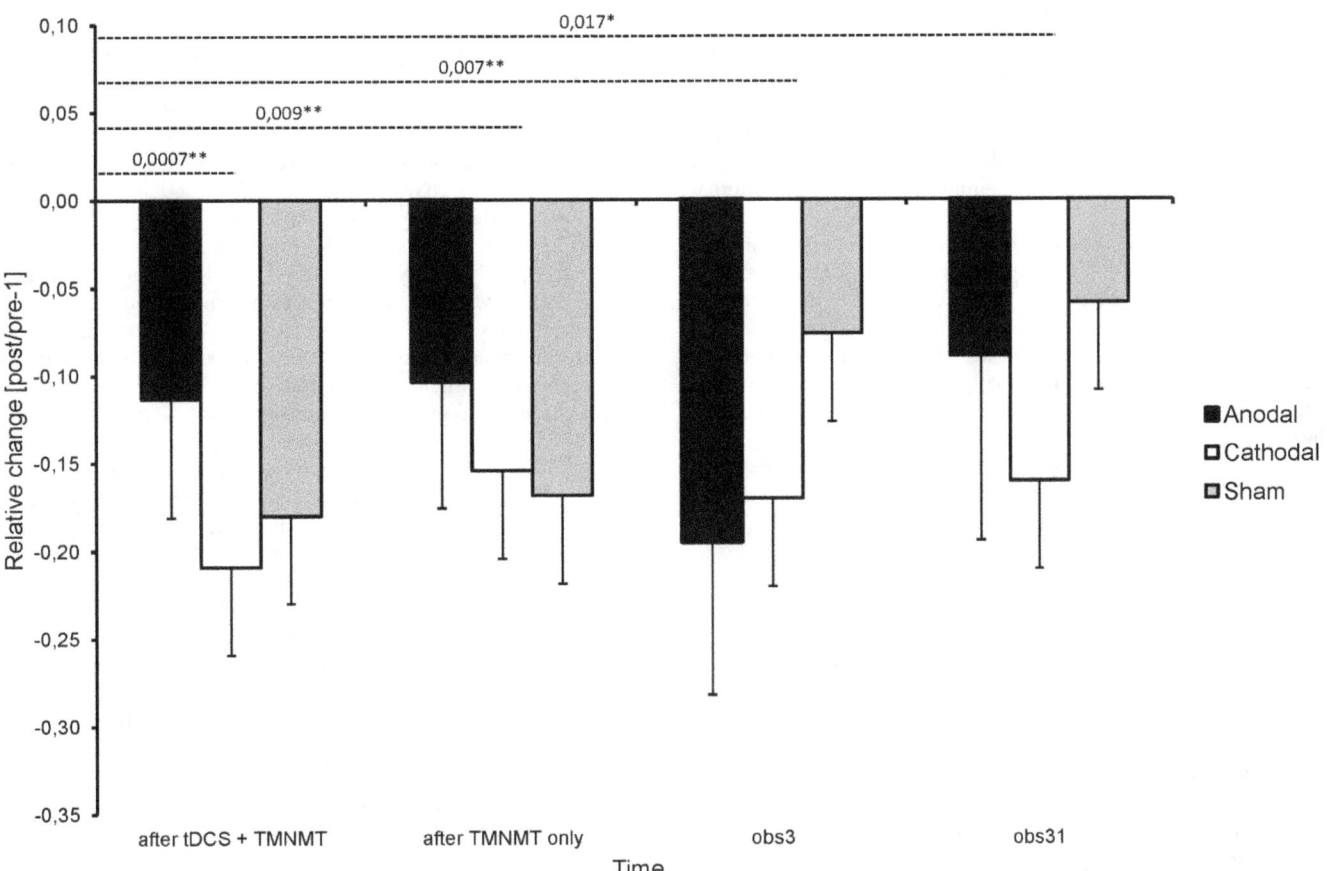

Figure 5. Changes in Tinnitus Handicap Questionnaire (THQ) values during and after treatment. Changes in THQ total scores relative to the baseline scores as functions of time (after tDCS[1] + TMNMT[2] vs. after TMNMT only vs. obs3 vs. obs31) and tDCS condition (anodal group vs. cathodal group vs. sham group). Bars represent means, error bars denote standard errors of the mean. Negative values reflect improvement. Dashed black lines indicate significant post-hoc tests. *p<.05, **p<.01; [1]Transcranial direct current stimulation; [2]Tailor-made notched music training.

beyond the end of the treatment and probably even beyond the end of the study.

tDCS appears to be a promising tinnitus treatment strategy, because this technique allows to modulate cortical excitability through anodal and cathodal stimulation, and the combination of external sensory stimulation with non-invasive brain-stimulation might enhance the effect of each stimulation by itself and increase the possibility of synaptic plasticity to occur [60]. Through tDCS, spontaneous cortical activity can be indirectly down-regulated or up-regulated, and it is assumed that synaptic transmission efficacy can be transiently altered, presumably promoting activations of neural plasticity. Thus, cathodal tDCS over auditory cortex could possibly reduce tinnitus-related hyperactivity, while anodal tDCS might either (i) boost adaptive changes triggered by treatment agents, or might (ii) change the likelihood for plastic changes to occur in the presence of other sensory input.

A study in healthy probands showed that auditory discrimination abilities can indeed decline when cathodal tDCS is applied over the surface representation of auditory cortex [53]. Surprisingly however, previous studies in chronic tinnitus patients implied that single sessions of cathodal tDCS over left temporo-parietal cortex were ineffective, while anodal stimulation could decrease perceived tinnitus intensity [38,39]. This somewhat unexpected finding indicates that the relationship between tDCS-induced changes in cortical excitability and perceived tinnitus perception is probably more complex than theoretically predicted.

The absence of significant tDCS effects in the present study should be evaluated in the context of the specific tDCS settings that were applied. One aspect to consider is the potentially functional role of the reference electrode over right supraorbital cortex. Interactions between auditory and orbitofrontal regions could have been modulated by stimulation at either nodal point and could have had an effect on tinnitus perception. Nevertheless, there were large differences in the electrode size, making it less likely that there was a biologically meaningful effect over the orbito-frontal region. A second aspect to consider is the functional anatomy of the auditory cortex, more precisely the tonotopic organization of Heschl's gyrus; given the usually high tinnitus frequencies, it appears conceivable that the tinnitus percept is elicited more medial than lateral on Heschl's gyrus. A more medial location would make it harder for tDCS to have an effect on the corresponding cortex. Further, it is possible and likely that tDCS effects were not limited to the auditory cortex; rather, neural activity in associated and more remote nodes of the tinnitus network could have been enhanced or suppressed. The effects of such modulations on treatment efficacy are difficult to assess. Obviously, these points should be carefully considered in subsequent studies combining tDCS and TMNMT. Crucially, a (for instance electrophysiological) measure of cortical activity should be included in order to assess whether intended modulations of neural activity are actually achieved.

Relevant tDCS settings include for instance DC strength, stimulation duration, repetition scheme, electrode locations, and electrode sizes. In this context it appears at least unlikely that current strength (2 mA) and/or stimulation duration (30 min) were too weak or too short to evoke effects; on the contrary, compared to previous studies these parameters were rather exhausted to the limits of safe stimulation. However, optimal electrode positioning is an important point in transcranial stimulation designs. On the one hand, there are electrode location differences between different studies targeting identical cortex regions, including auditory cortex. On the other hand, modeling studies indicate that traditional electrode positioning schemes (i.e. active electrode with rather small area over the cortex region of interest, and reference electrode with rather large area far away, e.g. on the other side of the head) are probably amendable when the goal is to maximize current density in the region of interest. Moreover, differential conductivities of different brain tissues (skin, skull compacta/spongiosa, gray/white matter and in particular CSF) and corresponding local current flow differences might play an important role [23].

It is an interesting question whether and how tDCS polarity would modulate the efficacy of TMNMT. Unfortunately, the present study does not allow us to draw firm conclusions, since tDCS and TMNMT were applied simultaneously and no separate anodal or cathodal over sham effect evolved. Theoretically, tDCS and TMNMT treatments could have had interactions on different time scales. *First*, during the initial 5 days and in each case the initial 30 min of treatment, tDCS and TMNMT were applied simultaneously (Figure 1); beyond that, the TMNMT treatment was continued for another 120 min, while the tDCS treatment (which could have had lasting after-effects) was stopped. During the initial 30 min of simultaneous application, potential tDCS and TMNMT effects could have been independent from each other, complementary, or diametrical to each other, and the net effect of the combined tDCS and TMNMT treatments on tinnitus-related cortical activity could have been beneficial, detrimental, or neutral. *Secondly*, during the initial 5 days of treatment, both strategies (tDCS and TMNMT) were applied; beyond that, the TMNMT treatment was continued for another 5 days, while the tDCS treatment (which could have had lasting and accumulative effects) was stopped (Figure 1). Again, the net effect of the combined tDCS and TMNMT treatments on tinnitus-related cortical activity during the first 5 days could have been beneficial, detrimental, or neutral.

However, although it remains unresolved whether and how tDCS and TMNMT effects may have interacted, the significant post-hoc test in the main outcome measure (THQ; Figure 5; Table 3) implies that the combined tDCS + TMNMT treatment could effectively reduce tinnitus-related distress during the initial 5 days of training; this effect was independent of tDCS conditions (anodal, cathodal, and sham). Such a finding would be predicted under the following assumptions: (i) tinnitus-related cortical activity is increased for neurons coding the tinnitus frequency ("tinnitus-related peak") compared to all other frequencies ("baseline"). (ii) TMNMT specifically reduces activity in the neurons coding the tinnitus frequency *and* increases activity in neurons coding notch edge frequencies. (iii) tDCS globally decreases/increases (depending on polarity) overall neural activity in an additive manner. (iv) The activity difference/ratio between involved ("tinnitus-related peak") and non-involved ("baseline") neurons would be critical for per-

ceived tinnitus intensity, while the magnitude of baseline neural activity (i.e. activity of neurons, which are not involved into tinnitus perception) does not influence tinnitus perception. Under these conditions, a tDCS polarity-independent reduction in tinnitus intensity under combined tDCS and TMNMT treatments would be expected. In future studies, sequential combination of TMNMT and anodal/cathodal tDCS would possibly be a valuable option to treat tinnitus.

The present findings should be reviewed in the context of our previous, "pure" TMNMT studies [14–16], which indicated specific TMNMT efficacy. However, the present and the previous studies are difficult to compare, because there are several relevant differences between studies. Aside from parameters such as treatment duration and total listening time, which mainly differ between [14] on the one hand, and [16] and the present study on the other hand, there are also differences between [16] and the present study, such as the treatment time per day, the treatment schedule, and the treatment location. One important aspect for TMNMT efficacy may exactly be influenced by parameters such as the latter three: the patient's perceived degrees of freedom in TMNMT execution. Degrees of freedom were maximal in [14] and [16], as patients were allowed to listen to their music whenever and wherever they wished, making it likely that the treatment was experienced as relaxing and enjoyable. Enjoyment of music is an important key factor for the activation of the reward system of the brain and for cortical plasticity [61]. In the present study however, patients had almost no degrees of freedom. Due to the intended application of tDCS, patients had to spend most of their treatment time at our institute, following a strict time schedule. The combined tDCS + TMNMT procedure may have been straining for the patients, and the load may have counteracted the positive effects of TMNMT.

Conclusion

The present pilot study is the first attempt to simultaneously apply TMNMT and tDCS in order to treat chronic tinnitus. Our results are difficult to understand, since (i) we do not know how and where in the brain TMNMT and tDCS interact, and since (ii) the study design could have been further optimized by including additional control conditions (e.g. placebo TMNMT, wait list controls). Nevertheless, the effects in our primary outcome measure, THQ, suggest that a short-term combined treatment of tDCS + TMNMT may have reduced tinnitus-related distress. Thus, the stimulation and treatment parameters of combined tDCS + TMNMT treatment for chronic tinnitus should be further explored in future studies.

Acknowledgments

We are grateful to Karin Berning, Ute Trompeter, Hildegard Deitermann, Noelle Bernstein, and Lea Waasem for their support in patient scheduling and treatment application.

Author Contributions

Conceived and designed the experiments: HT CP GS. Performed the experiments: HT AW. Analyzed the data: HT. Wrote the paper: HT. Made substantial contributions to analysis and interpretation of the data: HT AW HO GS CR CP. Revised the article critically for important intellectual content: HT AW HO GS CR CP. Approved the final version of the article to be published: HT AW HO GS CR CP.

References

1. Eggermont JJ, Roberts LE (2012) The neuroscience of tinnitus: understanding abnormal and normal auditory perception. Front Syst Neurosci 6: 53. Available: http://www.pubmedcentral.nih.gov/articlerender.fcgi?artid = 3394370&tool = pmcentrez&rendertype = abstract. Accessed 2013 March 28 March.

2. Okamoto H, Teismann H, Kakigi R, Pantev C (2011) Broadened population-level frequency tuning in human auditory cortex of portable music player users. PLoS One 6: e17022. Available: http://www.pubmedcentral.nih.gov/articlerender.fcgi?artid = 3047532&tool = pmcentrez&rendertype = abstract. Accessed 2012 May 3.

3. Kaltenbach JA (2011) Tinnitus: Models and mechanisms. Hear Res 276: 52–60. Available: http://www.pubmedcentral.nih.gov/articlerender.fcgi?artid = 310 9239&tool = pmcentrez&rendertype = abstract. Accessed 2012 March 1.

4. Preece J, Tyler R, Noble W (2003) The management of tinnitus. Geriatr Ageing 6. Available: http://onlinelibrary.wiley.com/doi/10.1288/00005537-195005000-00002/abstract. Accessed 2013 Dec 11.

5. De Ridder D, Elgoyhen AB, Romo R, Langguth B (2011) Phantom percepts: tinnitus and pain as persisting aversive memory networks. Proc Natl Acad Sci U S A 108: 8075–8080. Available: http://www.pubmedcentral.nih.gov/articlerender.fcgi?artid = 3100980&tool = pmcentrez&rendertype = abstract. Accessed 2013 March 1.

6. Langguth B (2012) Tinnitus: the end of therapeutic nihilism. Lancet 379: 1926–1928. Available: http://www.ncbi.nlm.nih.gov/pubmed/22633023. Accessed 2013 March 14.

7. Tyler RS (2012) Patient preferences and willingness to pay for tinnitus treatments. J Am Acad Audiol 23: 115–125. Available: http://www.ncbi.nlm.nih.gov/pubmed/22353680. Accessed 2013 Dec 11.

8. Kaltenbach JA (2011) The Neuroscientist. In: Moller A, Langguth B, DeRidder D, Kleinjung T, editors. Textbook of Tinnitus. Springer. 259–269.

9. Langguth B (2009) Emerging pharmacotherapy of tinnitus. Expert Opin Emerg Drugs 14: 687–702. Available: http://informahealthcare.com/doi/abs/10.1517/14728210903206975. Accessed 2013 March 28.

10. Eggermont JJ (2006) Cortical tonotopic map reorganization and its implications for treatment of tinnitus. Acta Otolaryngol Suppl: 9–12. Available: http://www.ncbi.nlm.nih.gov/pubmed/17114136. Accessed Accessed 2013 March 1.

11. Del Bo L, Baracca G, Forti S, Norena A (2011) Sound stimulation. In: Moller A, Langguth B, DeRidder D, Kleinjung T, editors. Textbook of Tinnitus. Springer. 597–604.

12. Roberts LE, Bosnyak DJ (2011) Auditory training. In: Moller A, Langguth B, DeRidder D, Kleinjung T, editors. Textbook of Tinnitus. Springer. 563–573.

13. Pantev C, Okamoto H, Teismann H (2012) Music-induced cortical plasticity and lateral inhibition in the human auditory cortex as foundations for tonal tinnitus treatment. Front Syst Neurosci 6: 1–19. Available: http://www.ncbi.nlm.nih.gov/pmc/articles/PMC3384223/. Accessed 2013 March 28.

14. Okamoto H, Stracke H, Stoll W, Pantev C (2010) Listening to tailor-made notched music reduces tinnitus loudness and tinnitus-related auditory cortex activity. Proc Natl Acad Sci U S A 107: 1207–1210. Available: http://www.pubmedcentral.nih.gov/articlerender.fcgi?artid = 2824261&tool = pmcentrez&rendertype = abstract. Accessed 2012 March 6.

15. Stracke H, Okamoto H, Pantev C (2010) Customized notched music training reduces tinnitus loudness. Commun Integr Biol 3: 274–277. Available: http://www.landesbioscience.com/journals/27/article/11558/. Accessed 2013 April 16.

16. Teismann H, Okamoto H, Pantev C (2011) Short and intense tailor-made notched music training against tinnitus: the tinnitus frequency matters. PLoS One 6: e24685. Available: http://www.pubmedcentral.nih.gov/articlerender.fcgi?artid = 3174191&tool = pmcentrez&rendertype = abstract. Accessed 2012 April 14.

17. Davis PB, Paki B, Hanley PJ (2007) Neuromonics Tinnitus Treatment: Third Clinical Trial. Ear Hear 28: 242–259. Available: http://content.wkhealth.com/linkback/openurl?sid = WKPTLP: landingpage&an = 00003446-200704000-00010.

18. Tass PA, Adamchic I, Freund HJ, von Stackelberg T, Hauptmann C (2012) Counteracting tinnitus by acoustic coordinated reset neuromodulation. Restor Neurol Neurosci 30: 137–159. Available: http://www.ncbi.nlm.nih.gov/pubmed/22414611. Accessed 21 March 2012.

19. Pantev C, Wollbrink A, Roberts LE, Engelien A, Lütkenhöner B (1999) Short-term plasticity of the human auditory cortex. Brain Res 842: 192–199. Available: http://www.ncbi.nlm.nih.gov/pubmed/10526109.

20. Okamoto H, Kakigi R, Gunji a, Kubo T, Pantev C (2005) The dependence of the auditory evoked N1m decrement on the bandwidth of preceding notch-filtered noise. Eur J Neurosci 21: 1957–1961. Available: http://www.ncbi.nlm.nih.gov/pubmed/15869488. Accessed 2013 May 3.

21. Fregni F, Pascual-Leone A (2007) Technology insight: noninvasive brain stimulation in neurology-perspectives on the therapeutic potential of rTMS and tDCS. Nat Clin Pract Neurol 3: 383–393. Available: http://www.ncbi.nlm.nih.gov/pubmed/17611487. Accessed 2013 March 5.

22. Nitsche MA, Paulus W (2007) Transkranielle Gleichstromstimulation. In: Siebner HR, Ziemann U, editors. Das TMS-Buch. Heidelberg: Springer. 533–542.

23. Neuling T, Wagner S, Wolters CH, Zaehle T, Herrmann CS (2012) Finite-Element Model Predicts Current Density Distribution for Clinical Applications of tDCS and tACS. Front Psychiatry 3: 83. Available: http://www.pubmedcentral.nih.gov/articlerender.fcgi?artid = 3449241&tool = pmcentrez&rendertype = abstract. Accessed 2013 March 11.

24. Dymond AM, Coger RW, Serafetinides EA (1975) Intracerebral current levels in man during electrosleep therapy. Biol Psychiatry 10: 101–104. Available: http://www.ncbi.nlm.nih.gov/pubmed/1120172. Accessed Accessed 2013 March 28.

25. Zheng Y, Hamilton E, McNamara E, Smith PF, Darlington CL (2011) The effects of chronic tinnitus caused by acoustic trauma on social behaviour and anxiety in rats. Neuroscience 193: 143–153. Available: http://www.ncbi.nlm.nih.gov/pubmed/21782007. Accessed 2012 March 1.

26. Nitsche MA, Cohen LG, Wassermann EM (2008) Transcranial direct current stimulation: State of the art 2008. Brain Stimul 1: 206–223. Available: http://www.sciencedirect.com/science/article/pii/S1935861X08000405. Accessed 2013 April 8.

27. Eggermont JJ, Roberts LE (2004) The neuroscience of tinnitus. Trends Neurosci 27: 676–682. Available: http://www.ncbi.nlm.nih.gov/pubmed/15474168. Accessed 2012 March 20.

28. Lockwood AH, Salvi RJ, Coad ML (1998) The functional neuroanatomy of tinnitus: evidence for limbic system links and neural plasticity. Neurology 50: 114–120. Available: http://www.neurology.org/content/50/1/114.short. Accessed 2013 April 18.

29. Giraud AL, Chéry-Croze S, Fischer G, Fischer C, Vighetto A, et al. (1999) A selective imaging of tinnitus. Neuroreport 10: 1–5. Available: http://www.ncbi.nlm.nih.gov/pubmed/10094123.

30. Mirz F, Pedersen CB, Ishizu K (1999) Positron emission tomography of cortical centers of tinnitus. Hear Res 134: 133–144. Available: http://www.sciencedirect.com/science/article/pii/S0378595599000751. Accessed 2013 April 8.

31. Mirz F, Gjedde A, Sødkilde-Jrgensen H, Pedersen CB (2000) Functional brain imaging of tinnitus-like perception induced by aversive auditory stimuli. Neuroreport 11: 633–637. Available: http://www.ncbi.nlm.nih.gov/pubmed/10718327.

32. Lockwood AH, Wack DS, Burkard RF, Coad ML, Reyes SA, et al. (2001) The functional anatomy of gaze-evoked tinnitus and sustained lateral gaze. Neurology 56: 472–480. Available: http://www.neurology.org/cgi/doi/10.1212/WNL.56.4.472. Accessed 2013 March 28.

33. Reyes SA, Salvi RJ, Burkard RF, Coad ML (2002) Brain imaging of the effects of lidocaine on tinnitus. Hear Res 171: 43–50. Available: http://www.sciencedirect.com/science/article/pii/S0378595502003465. Accessed 2013 March 28.

34. Plewnia C, Reimold M, Najib A, Brehm B, Reischl G, et al. (2007) Dose-dependent attenuation of auditory phantom perception (tinnitus) by PET-guided repetitive transcranial magnetic stimulation. Hum Brain Mapp 28: 238–246. Available: http://www.ncbi.nlm.nih.gov/pubmed/16773635. Accessed 2013 March 28.

35. Arnold W, Bartenstein P, Oestreicher E (1996) Focal metabolic activation in the predominant left auditory cortex in patients suffering from tinnitus: a PET study with deoxyglucose. ORL J Otorhinolaryngol Relat Spec 58: 195–199. Available: http://www.karger.com/Article/Abstract/276835. Accessed 8 April 2013.

36. Langguth B, Eichhammer P (2006) The impact of auditory cortex activity on characterizing and treating patients with chronic tinnitus-first results from a PET study. Acta oto-laryngologica Suppl 556: 84–88. Available: http://informahealthcare.com/doi/abs/10.1080/03655230600895317. Accessed 2013 April 8.

37. Wang H, Tian J, Yin D, Jiang S, Yang W (2001) Regional glucose metabolic increases in left auditory cortex in tinnitus patients: a preliminary study with positron emission tomography. Chin Med J (Engl) 114: 848–851. Available: http://www.cmj.org/Periodical/paperlist.asp?id = LW8738&linkintype = pubmed. Accessed 2013 April 8.

38. Fregni F, Marcondes R, Boggio PS, Marcolin MA, Rigonatti SP, et al. (2006) Transient tinnitus suppression induced by repetitive transcranial magnetic stimulation and transcranial direct current stimulation. Eur J Neurol 13: 996–1001. Available: http://www.ncbi.nlm.nih.gov/pubmed/16930367. Accessed 2013 March 5.

39. Garin P, Gilain C, Van Damme JP, de Fays K, Jamart J, et al. (2011) Short- and long-lasting tinnitus relief induced by transcranial direct current stimulation. J Neurol 258: 1940–1948. Available: http://www.pubmedcentral.nih.gov/articlerender.fcgi?artid = 3214608&tool = pmcentrez&rendertype = abstract. Accessed 2013 March 28.

40. Langguth B, Schecklmann M, Lehner A, Landgrebe M, Poeppl TB, et al. (2012) Neuroimaging and neuromodulation: complementary approaches for identifying the neuronal correlates of tinnitus. Front Syst Neurosci 6: 15. Available: http://www.pubmedcentral.nih.gov/articlerender.fcgi?artid = 3321434&tool = pmcentrez&rendertype = abstract. Accessed 2013 March 28.

41. Faber M, Vanneste S, Fregni F, De Ridder D (2012) Top down prefrontal affective modulation of tinnitus with multiple sessions of tDCS of dorsolateral prefrontal cortex. Brain Stimul 5: 492–498. Available: http://www.ncbi.nlm.nih.gov/pubmed/22019079. Accessed 2013 March 28.

42. Vanneste S, Plazier M, Ost J, van der Loo E, Van de Heyning P, et al. (2010) Bilateral dorsolateral prefrontal cortex modulation for tinnitus by transcranial direct current stimulation: a preliminary clinical study. Exp brain Res 202: 779–

785. Available: http://www.ncbi.nlm.nih.gov/pubmed/20186404. Accessed 2013 March 8.

43. Vanneste S, Langguth B, De Ridder D (2011) Do tDCS and TMS influence tinnitus transiently via a direct cortical and indirect somatosensory modulating effect? A combined TMS-tDCS and TENS study. Brain Stimul 4: 242–252. Available: http://www.ncbi.nlm.nih.gov/pubmed/22032739. Accessed 2013 March 15.

44. Vanneste S, De Ridder D (2011) Bifrontal transcranial direct current stimulation modulates tinnitus intensity and tinnitus-distress-related brain activity. Eur J Neurosci 34: 605–614. Available: http://www.ncbi.nlm.nih.gov/pubmed/21790807. Accessed 2013 March 28.

45. Vanneste S, Focquaert F, Van de Heyning P, De Ridder D (2011) Different resting state brain activity and functional connectivity in patients who respond and not respond to bifrontal tDCS for tinnitus suppression. Exp brain Res 210: 217–227. Available: http://www.ncbi.nlm.nih.gov/pubmed/21437634. Accessed 2012 March 1.

46. Frank E, Schecklmann M, Landgrebe M, Burger J, Kreuzer P, et al. (2012) Treatment of chronic tinnitus with repeated sessions of prefrontal transcranial direct current stimulation: outcomes from an open-label pilot study. J Neurol 259: 327–333. Available: http://www.ncbi.nlm.nih.gov/pubmed/21808984. Accessed 2013 March 28.

47. Schlee W, Weisz N, Bertrand O, Hartmann T, Elbert T (2008) Using auditory steady state responses to outline the functional connectivity in the tinnitus brain. PLoS One 3: e3720. Available: http://www.pubmedcentral.nih.gov/articlerender.fcgi?artid = 2579484&tool = pmcentrez&rendertype = abstract. Accessed 2013 March 26.

48. Schlaug G, Renga V, Nair D (2008) Transcranial direct current stimulation in stroke recovery. Arch Neurol 65: 1571–1576. Available: http://www.ncbi.nlm.nih.gov/pubmed/22964028.

49. Vines BW, Norton AC, Schlaug G (2011) Non-invasive brain stimulation enhances the effects of melodic intonation therapy. Front Psychol 2: 230. Available: http://www.pubmedcentral.nih.gov/articlerender.fcgi?artid = 3180169&tool = pmcentrez&rendertype = abstract. Accessed 2013 March 7.

50. Schlaug G, Marchina S, Wan CY (2011) The use of non-invasive brain stimulation techniques to facilitate recovery from post-stroke aphasia. Neuropsychol Rev 21: 288–301. Available: http://www.pubmedcentral.nih.gov/articlerender.fcgi?artid = 3176334&tool = pmcentrez&rendertype = abstract. Accessed 2013 March 28.

51. Lindenberg R, Zhu LL, Schlaug G (2012) Combined central and peripheral stimulation to facilitate motor recovery after stroke: the effect of number of sessions on outcome. Neurorehabil Neural Repair 26: 479–483. Available: http://www.ncbi.nlm.nih.gov/pubmed/22258156. Accessed 2013 March 1.

52. Zaehle T, Beretta M, Jäncke L, Herrmann CS, Sandmann P (2011) Excitability changes induced in the human auditory cortex by transcranial direct current stimulation: direct electrophysiological evidence. Exp brain Res 215: 135–140. Available: http://www.ncbi.nlm.nih.gov/pubmed/21964868. Accessed 2013 March 7.

53. Mathys C, Loui P, Zheng X, Schlaug G (2010) Non-invasive brain stimulation applied to Heschl's gyrus modulates pitch discrimination. Front Psychol 1: 193. Available: http://www.pubmedcentral.nih.gov/articlerender.fcgi?artid = 3028589&tool = pmcentrez&rendertype = abstract. Accessed 2013 March 24.

54. Kuk FK, Tyler RS, Russell D, Jordan H (1990) The psychometric properties of a tinnitus handicap questionnaire. Ear Hear 11: 434–445. Available: http://www.ncbi.nlm.nih.gov/pubmed/21208381.

55. Newman CW, Jacobson GP, Spitzer JB (1996) Development of the tinnitus handicap inventory. Arch Otolaryngol - Head Neck Surg 122: 143–148.

56. Hallam R (1988) Cognitive variables in tinnitus annoyance. Br J Clin Psychol: 213–222. Available: http://onlinelibrary.wiley.com/doi/10.1111/j.2044-8260.1988.tb00778.x/abstract. Accessed 2013 April 18.

57. Schmitz N, Hartkamp N, Kiuse J (2000) The symptom check-list-90-R (SCL-90-R): a German validation study. Qual Life Res 9: 185–193. Available: http://link.springer.com/article/10.1023/A: 1008931926181. Accessed 2013 April 8.

58. Hautzinger M, Bailer M (2012) Allgemeine Depressions-Skala: ADS; Manual. Psychiatr Prax 39: 302–304. Available: https://www.thieme-connect.com/ejournals/abstract/10.1055/s-0032-1326702. Accessed 2013 April 18.

59. Spielberger CD, Gorsuch RL, Lushene RE (1970) Manual for the state-trait anxiety inventory. Palo Alto, CA: Consulting Psychologists Press. Available: http://ubir.buffalo.edu/xmlui/handle/10477/2895. Accessed 2013 April 8.

60. Fritsch B, Reis J, Martinowich K, Schambra HM, Ji Y, et al. (2010) Direct current stimulation promotes BDNF-dependent synaptic plasticity: potential implications for motor learning. Neuron 66: 198–204. Available: http://www.pubmedcentral.nih.gov/articlerender.fcgi?artid = 2864780&tool = pmcentrez&rendertype = abstract. Accessed 2013 Feb 28.

61. Blood AJ, Zatorre RJ (2001) Intensely pleasurable responses to music correlate with activity in brain regions implicated in reward and emotion. Proc Natl Acad Sci U S A 98: 11818–11823. Available: http://www.pubmedcentral.nih.gov/articlerender.fcgi?artid = 58814&tool = pmcentrez&rendertype = abstract.

19

Costs of Suppressing Emotional Sound and Countereffects of a Mindfulness Induction: An Experimental Analog of Tinnitus Impact

Hugo Hesser[1]*, Peter Molander[1], Mikael Jungermann[2], Gerhard Andersson[1,3]

1 Department of Behavioural Sciences and Learning, Swedish Institute for Disability Research, Linköping University, Linköping, Sweden, **2** Department of Behavioural Sciences and Learning, Linköping University, Linköping, Sweden, **3** Psychiatry Section, Department of Clinical Neuroscience, Karolinska Institutet, Stockholm, Sweden

Abstract

Tinnitus is the experience of sounds without an appropriate external auditory source. These auditory sensations are intertwined with emotional and attentional processing. Drawing on theories of mental control, we predicted that suppressing an affectively negative sound mimicking the psychoacoustic features of tinnitus would result in decreased persistence in a mentally challenging task (mental arithmetic) that required participants to ignore the same sound, but that receiving a mindfulness exercise would reduce this effect. Normal hearing participants ($N = 119$) were instructed to suppress an affectively negative sound under cognitive load or were given no such instructions. Next, participants received either a mindfulness induction or an attention control task. Finally, all participants worked with mental arithmetic while exposed to the same sound. The length of time participants could persist in the second task served as the dependent variable. As hypothesized, results indicated that an auditory suppression rationale reduced time of persistence relative to no such rationale, and that a mindfulness induction counteracted this detrimental effect. The study may offer new insights into the mechanisms involved in the development of tinnitus interference. Implications are also discussed in the broader context of attention control strategies and the effects of emotional sound on task performance. The ironic processes of mental control may have an analog in the experience of sounds.

Editor: Jan de Fockert, Goldsmiths, University of London, United Kingdom

Funding: The study was sponsored in part by a grant from the Swedish Research Council (HEAD Linneaus grant). The authors report no financial relationships with commercial interests. The funders had no role in study design, data collection and analysis, decision to publish, or preparation of the manuscript. No additional external funding was received for this study.

Competing Interests: The authors have declared that no competing interests exist.

* E-mail: hugo.hesser@liu.se

Introduction

Despite our best efforts to engage in mental activities (e.g., reading, writing), sounds of relatively low intensity can force themselves on our awareness and interrupt what we are doing (c.f., irrelevant-sound effect; [1]). Unwanted and uncontrollable sounds may be particularly interfering when they evoke strong negative emotional reactions. At such moments, an individual may resort to mental control strategies, such as trying to avoid thinking about the sound, in an attempt to control behavior and minimize interference. Yet, as an analog to theories on mental control such strategies may backfire [2]. That is, suppression as effortful regulation strategy may prolong and intensify the experience of the sound, creating more interference over time. Drawing on theories of mental control [3,4], the present study examined attentional strategies in the context of emotional sound that mimicked the psychoacoustic characteristics of tinnitus.

Tinnitus is the experience of sounds without any external auditory source [5]. The sounds may vary greatly but are generally conceived as ringing, hizzing or buzzing. These auditory sensations are often accompanied by hearing loss, and there is considerable overlap between tinnitus and other auditory-related problems, including hyperacusis (noise sensitivity) and dizziness/vertigo [5]. Tinnitus is common with prevalence rates of 10 to 15% in the general adult population [6,7], and the incidence seems to be rising as due to increasing noise exposure and an aging population in the western part of the world [8]. The majority of those affected, however, do no conceive tinnitus as a source of great distress, but for a subsample of individuals, tinnitus sounds can trigger strong emotional reactions and seriously impact daily functioning [8,9]. In particular, individuals who find tinnitus to be annoying often report concentration difficulties, an observation that parallel recent findings showing that cognitive ability is generally compromised in individuals with tinnitus [10,11].

The role of psychological variables as a mediating link between sound perception and interference/distress was noted early [12]. Given this, psychological approaches were developed and tested at an early stage, and over the years behavioral and cognitive treatment techniques targeting the consequences of tinnitus have gained empirical support [13,14]. More recently, neuroscience research has provided evidence suggesting that non-auditory brain regions subserving emotions and attention play an essential role in both tinnitus perception and interference [15,16]. Thus, tinnitus is intertwined with emotional and attentional processing. However, to date the mechanisms by which tinnitus causes distress and interference are largely unknown. Still, certain theories posit that the ways in which the auditory stimuli is appraised, processed and attended to may play a pivotal role in the development and maintenance of tinnitus distress [16,17,18]. For example, Hallam et al. [18] suggested that a preoccupation with tinnitus would slow down the natural process of habituating to tinnitus. Unfortunately, Hallam el al. offered little details of the psychological processes that would produce such a preoccupation with tinnitus in the first place. In fact, there is a paucity of research on psychological processes involved in tinnitus perception and interference.

Theories on mental control, such as the Ironic Process Theory [2,19], may provide a useful explanation for the underlying processes involved in the development and maintenance of tinnitus interference, in particular why certain individuals may become preoccupied with the sensation. The Ironic Process Theory suggests that efforts to control mental states to achieve a particular desired state of mind often result in effects diametrically opposite of the original intent. For example, the theory predicts that efforts aimed at suppressing a particular thought will ultimately fail and will give rise to increased occurrence of the target thought. Indeed, suppression – a term associated with expressive suppression, thought suppression, and experiential avoidance – is one of the most widely studied regulation-strategies of mental and emotional events [20,21]. There is considerable evidence to suggest that these strategies are counterproductive when applied to emotions or thoughts, as they tend to maintain, or even paradoxically increase, the internal sensations that they are suppose to regulate, especially under mental load [2,22].

More recent empirical studies have shown that this phenomenon has an analog in the domain of physical sensations, in particular in relation to pain [23,24]. For example, Cioffi and Holloway [23] found that subjects instructed to suppress the experience of pain experienced slower recovery from a cold-pressor pain induction and rated a second somatic induction as more unpleasant as compared with subjects who were instructed to monitor physical sensations or to use distraction. Thus, it appears that attentional strategies specifically designed to remove a "forbidden" sensation or mental event from mind can produce negative consequences over time, exacerbating the very sensation that one was trying to avoid. Moreover, such a strategy may deplete mental resources and compromise goal-direct behavior. Indeed, mental and emotional control strategies have consistently shown to impact performance negatively in subsequent task requiring self-control (c.f., ego-depletion; [25,26]). Studies have shown maladaptive behavioral consequences of suppression, including decreased persistence [25], behavioral control [27], and willingness to approach emotionally evocative tasks [28]. It is important to note that these effects are not observed directly when the suppression strategy is employed, but show up later, for example, when individuals abandon the attempt to suppress, are asked to revisit the suppressed target at a later time [22], or when they are engaged in subsequent tasks that require high-degree of self-control [25].

Counterintuitively, strategies that increase attention to interfering or aversive stimuli may in fact be a better way of facilitating adaptive responding. Sensory monitoring – which is to attend, in a neutral way, to discrete sensory aspects of a sensation – has in series of laboratory experiments shown to be an effective strategy to increase pain tolerance and reduce discomfort during noxious stimulation [29,30]. However, the effect of monitoring is often moderated by length and intensity of the stimulus. That is, distraction often works better when the stressor is acute, whereas monitoring works better when the stimulus is persistent [29,31].

Mindfulness is "a process of regulating attention in order to bring a quality of non-elaborative awareness to current experience and a quality of relating to one's experience within an orientation of curiosity, experiential openness, and acceptance." ([32] p. 234).

Defined in this way, mindfulness bares many similarities with sensory monitoring. Indeed, it has been associated with similar beneficial outcomes in laboratory settings [33,34]. Mindfulness is often utilized in treatments as means to promote psychological acceptance, which connotes an active process of allowing internal reactions (physiological, emotional, or cognitive) to be experienced as they are without defense or control [3,35]. Recent theories posit that such a stance undermines maladaptive strategies (e.g., suppression), and, thereby, reduces the harmful effects associated with control strategies (see, [36], for a review of different treatments promoting similar processes; see also [22]). A growing body of experimental work suggests that, when compared to approaches such as suppression, acceptance can be an adaptive strategy to increase tolerance of aversive stimuli and reduce negative affect (e.g., induced pain or anxiety; [28,37,38]). There is also tentative evidence to support that acceptance of emotions requires fewer resources than suppression and that it may therefore improve performance in tasks requiring self-control [39]. To sum, attending mindfully to sensations rather than suppressing them may, at least in certain circumstances, be a better approach to reduce distress and facilitate adaptive responding during aversive stimulation.

Despite its potential relevance for the effects of sound on performance in general and for tinnitus interference in particular, little experimental work has been conducted to examine the effects of the above-mentioned attentional strategies in the context of auditory stimuli. However, there is growing evidence for that these strategies are in fact of importance in the development and maintenance of tinnitus interference and distress. That is, correlational studies have provided initial support to the beneficial consequences of acceptance on the experience of tinnitus [40,41,42], and avoidance-based coping has found to be associated with increased tinnitus-related distress [43,44]. Furthermore, psychological treatments that have incorporated mindfulness/acceptance related-techniques have recently been shown to be effective in treating distress and impact of tinnitus [45,46,47].

Yet, only a few experimental studies have been carried out on related processes and they have provided mixed findings. For example, Andersson et al. [48] compared instructions to suppress or to attend to thoughts about tinnitus with a control condition in participants with tinnitus. They found that, immediately following manipulation, instructions to suppress decreased thoughts about tinnitus whereas instructions to attend to tinnitus increased such thoughts. In another tinnitus study the effects of suppression and acceptance strategies on ability to attend to a mental imagery were examined [49]. Participants who were instructed to accept tinnitus were able to focus for a longer period of time on the imagery than participants in a control condition (no instructions), but no significant difference was observed between the suppression and acceptance condition.

To indirectly test control strategies in tinnitus perception, Hesser et al. [50] manipulated ability to control background sounds in participants with tinnitus. Control was associated with a rebound effect over time, that is, participants who were instructed to control the background sounds (an active choice of type and loudness) exhibited an increase in self-rated tinnitus interference and a slower rate of improvement on cognitive performance measures over repeated trials when compared with participants who had no control of the backgrounds sounds (i.e., they were not able to chose background sound). Interestingly, control was initially (the first trial after manipulation) associated with lower rating of tinnitus interference, suggesting the importance of examining temporal aspects of the effects of different control strategies. Indeed, this finding parallel that people can in fact successfully suppress thoughts, but the detrimental effects of suppression often occur over an extended period when the thoughts rebound [2]. Furthermore, as noted earlier, findings suggest differential advantages of certain mental strategies (monitoring, distraction) depending on the length of stimulus presentation [31]. This may be one explanation to discrepancy in findings observed in experimental studies that have examined the effects of control or suppression in participants with tinnitus. That is, given that suppression may cause effects of significant magnitude over time (i.e., postsuppression rebound effect), future experiments on suppression (or related strategies) need to employ a design that will allow to examine the delayed effects of such mental control efforts.

In the present study, we used an emotional sound to simulate tinnitus and associated affective reactions in participants without auditory deficits. Tinnitus can be qualitatively similar to externally generated sounds [8]. In other words, the tinnitus sound can at least partly be described by using audiological equipment and synthesizers. Given this, a few studies [51,52] have simulated the experience of tinnitus in laboratory settings. Simulating tinnitus allows for experimental control of the auditory stimuli and eliminates influence of extraneous factors commonly encountered in experiments with participants with significant tinnitus (i.e., individual differences in affective, cognitive or audiological problems).

In the current laboratory study, we developed a model to test the unique effects of different strategies (suppression and mindfulness) that represent the opposite of two theorized aspects of mental control [3,4]. Specifically, we examined a) the potential delayed costs of suppressing an affectively negative sound that mimicked the characteristics of tinnitus. We also examined whether b) a mindfulness induction could counteract the hypothesized detrimental effects associated with auditory suppression. To examine behavioral consequences over time, the experiment was divided into two distinct phases. Given prior research on the effects of suppression of thoughts and emotion and initial work on attentional strategies in the auditory domain (i.e., tinnitus), we predicted that the effects of suppression of an affectively negative sound would be observed in subsequent rather than concurrent task performance. In accordance with theory and research reviewed above, we also predicted that these delayed effects of suppression would be attenuated with a brief mindfulness exercise.

Methods

Ethics Statement

The experiment followed the ethical principles as outlined in the Declaration of Helsinki for human studies. Signed informed consent was obtained from all participants. Data were stored anonymously. The study protocol was approved by the institutional review board at Linköping University, Sweden.

Participants

One hundred twenty-one volunteers (73 women, 48 men) were recruited from a Swedish student population. Participants age range from 18 to 37 years ($M = 24.9$, $SD = 3.3$). Prior to taking part of the experiment, participants reported that they had no problems with tinnitus, vision, hearing, or sensitivity to noise. After completing the experiment, which lasted for approximately 20 minutes, participants were thanked, debriefed, and compensated with an USB-flash drive (cost ≈ $15 each). We excluded one participant who acknowledged that she did not comply with experimental instructions, and one participant who had clear problems with communication/comprehension, resulting in a total sample of 119 participants.

Overall Design

To address the specific hypotheses posed in the current study, we adopted the dual-task paradigm, an experimental paradigm commonly used to test delayed effects of suppression of thoughts and feelings [25,26]. That is, adopting this paradigm, studies have consistently shown that deliberate attempts to suppress thoughts or feelings impair performance on subsequent tasks requiring high-degree of self-control. The current experiment was designed to test the delayed effects of suppressing an affectively negative sound on persistence behavior, and to examine whether the specific effects of suppression could be reduced following a brief mindfulness induction. We used suppression of the sound, defined as a deliberate attempt to put it "out of mind" [21,23], as the experimental manipulation.

Participants were randomly assigned to conditions of a 2 (suppression manipulation: suppression instructions vs. no instructions) ×2 (counterinduction manipulation: mindfulness vs. attention control) design. All participants performed two mental tasks in a fixed order while exposed to the auditory stimulus: They completed a memory test and then performed mental arithmetic. Manipulation of suppression was done prior to the memory test and was intended to direct participants to use the mental strategy during the first task. Manipulation of the counterinduction was done prior to the mental arithmetic task (the second mental task). After both tasks, participants responded to a trial demand questionnaire. The time participants could persist in working with mental arithmetic while being exposed to the affectively negative sound in the second task was recorded and served as the dependent variable in the experiment.

Materials

Auditory stimulus. An artificial high frequency, high pitched sound (a sinusoidal tone, amplitude modulated at approximately 100 Hz, with a center frequency of 4.5 kHz) was used in the experiment. The sound was presented binaurally in the headphones (Telephonics TDH 39P) using an AD 229e diagnostic audiometer with a loudness level at ear level of 65 dB HL (hearing level). The sound has been used in a previous study in which 12 tinnitus-like sounds were developed to simulate the psychoacoustics of tinnitus [53]. These sounds have shown to elicit physiological and subjective stress responses in normal hearing participants and in participants with tinnitus [53]. To further validate the stimulus used in the present study, 10 participants not involved in the study rated the sound and 12 sounds selected from the International Affective Digitized Sounds system (IADS-2 [54]). Participants rated a total of 16 sounds: 4 tinnitus-like sounds, 4 affectively negative sounds from the IADS-2 (normative mean valence ratings below 4; sound no. 106, 115, 380, 709), 4 affectively positive sounds from the IADS-2 (normative mean valence ratings above 6; sound no. 151, 226, 251, 360), and 4 affectively neutral sounds from the IADS-2 (normative mean valence ratings between 4 and 6; sound no. 322, 403, 700, 708). Using the normative rating methods (see, [54], for a thorough description of rating procedures), these participants rated each sound based on two separate dimensions (the Valence and the Arousal dimension; each dimension rated on 9-point scale, with high ratings indicating high pleasure and high arousal, respectively). We selected 8 sounds on the endpoints of the valence dimension: 4 were affectively negative (normative mean valence ratings of 4 or lower) and 4 were affectively positive (normative mean valence ratings of 6 or higher). Sounds were presented in a random order. The auditory stimulus used in the present study was rated as significantly more unpleasant ($M = 2.4$, $SD = 1.7$) and arousing ($M = 7.0$, $SD = 1.9$) compared with ratings for 4 affectively positive sounds (Cohen's d range $= 1.72$ to 2.10, and Cohen's d range $= 0.59$ to 1.39, respectively). In addition, the sound was rated as significantly more unpleasant compared with 3 out of 4 affectively negative sounds (all Cohen's $d > 0.77$).

Serial recall test. To induce cognitive load during the suppression manipulation, participants completed the serial recall test (adapted from Jones & Macken [1]). The serial recall test consisted of seven letters (R, H, L, K, F, M, Q). Each letter was displayed at the center of the computer screen for 1 second. After all seven letters had been displayed, participants were asked to repeat the letter sequence in the order they were presented using a keyboard. Participants had 1 minute to recall the letter sequence, after which a new trial began. After completing one practice trial, participants completed 7 trials of the test.

Attentional strategy manipulation. Participants randomly assigned to the suppression condition were given instructions to suppress the auditory stimulus prior to engaging in the first cognitive task. Instruction were adapted from instructions used in previous experiments on suppression of pain and thoughts [23,55]:

"Your task is to use all your mental power to suppress the sound you're about to hear. We know this can be hard but you should still try as hard as you can to not think about the sound. If you still notice the sound then mentally block it as quickly as possible. Suppress it. Distract yourself. Fight against it and retake control!"

To further reinforce the manipulation, participants were also told to press a red button on the desk in front of them each time they noticed the sound (c.f., thought suppression; [56]). In contrast, participants in the control condition were given no such instructions.

Counterinduction manipulation. Following the first mental task, participants listened to a 300 seconds audio recording. Participants randomly assigned to the mindfulness induction condition listened to a brief mindfulness exercise, informed by interventions in treatments [57] and rationales used in experimental settings [3,28,33]. The aim of the exercise was to have participants to direct their attention towards inner experiences, in particular their breathing. Participants were asked to notice, observe and accept feelings, thoughts and sensations in the moment. Participants were also instructed to notice discomforting sensations and actively explore such sensations without struggling with them; they were, for example, told "to make room for difficult sensations" and that "Thoughts are thoughts. Physical sensations are physical sensations, and feelings are feelings. Nothing more, nothing less. Don't struggle with the discomfort, let it be there".

Participants randomly assigned to the attention control listened to a documentary on an unrelated topic in a foreign language, but fairly similar to participants' native tongue (i.e., a Danish documentary). Participants were instructed to listen carefully as they might have to answer questions on the subject later on. Listening to Danish is demanding for most Swedish persons and hence the task could be described as being difficult. The task was used to control for attention and experimental demand (c.f., [28,34]).

Trial demand questionnaire. Following the mental tasks, participants responded to four questions on trial demand characteristics concerning the following aspects: fatigue, task demand, distress caused by sound, and interference of sound.

Each question was rated on a 7-point scale, with high ratings indicating greater endorsement of effect on the specific item (i.e., high fatigue, high task demand, high distress, and high interference). Due to a technical error, responses on trial demand questions were not recorded in seven instances. In those instances, responses were omitted from the analysis.

Dependent variable: Persistence in the context of affectively negative sound. The length of time participants worked with mental arithmetic in the presence of the affectively negative sound in the second part of the experiment served as measure of persistence in goal-directed behavior. The disruption of mental performance by task-irrelevant sound is a well-established phenomenon [1,58]. Thus, we presumed that ignoring an affectively negative sound in this context would require high amount of effortful persistence. Mental arithmetic was used to create a laboratory analog of a series of daily mental activities/stressors that people with tinnitus often complain about (e.g., reading or writing; e.g., [9]). Furthermore, time of persistence in mentally challenging or unsolvable tasks has been frequently used as a dependent variable in studies that have experimentally manipulated self-control in dual-task paradigms [26], including studies that have employed suppression of emotion or thought to impair later attempts of self-control [25,59,60]. In addition, persistence at mentally challenging tasks has been used as a measure of frustration tolerance in experiments designed to examine the adverse postadaptive effects following repeatedly presented aversive noise [61].

Procedure

Two male experimenters conducted the experiment. Participants were asked to take part in two different studies; the first examining the relationship between interfering sound and memory, and the second examining the relationship between interfering sound and mental arithmetic.

After receiving general instructions by the experimenter and completing the consent form, participants were asked to take a seat in front of a 17 inch LCD computer screen, put on a pair of headphones, and to watch the screen for further instructions. From that point on, the experimental procedures were fully automated. All instructions and visual stimuli were presented with E-prime (Version 2.0); responses and duration (ms) were automatically recorded.

Next, participants completed the serial recall test. Participants completed 7 trials of the test while being exposed to the sound presented binaurally in the headphones. Participants in the suppression condition were additionally instructed to actively suppress the sound while performing the task. Once the serial recall test finished, the sound stopped, and all participants responded to the questionnaire on trial demand characteristics. Next, all participants listened to an audio recording (300 s). Half of the participants listened to a brief mindfulness exercise (counterinduction condition), whereas the rest of the participants listened to the documentary (attention control condition).

Following the mindfulness induction or the control task, all participants completed math assignments (1-by-1, 2-by-2, and 3-by-3 digit multiplication tasks presented in a fixed order) while exposed to the same affectively negative sound used during the serial recall test. Each assignment was displayed at the center of the screen and participants used the keyboard to answer. Participants were told that there were an infinite number of math assignments and that they were to solve as many math assignments as possible, but to stop when they wanted to give up. After each assignment, participants responded by pushing a marked key to either continue to the next assignment or stop. No participant was, however, allowed to exceed 20 minutes on this task. After giving up, participants answered the questionnaire on trial demand characteristics. The length of time (ms) from the first stimulus (i.e., first math assignment) until the participant voluntarily ended the task was recorded.

Statistical Analysis

Before conducting the primary analysis, data were checked for significant outliers, missing cases, data analytical and distributional assumptions. The main dependent variable in the experiment (i.e., time of persistence in the second task) was analyzed using a 2 (suppression manipulation: suppression instructions vs. no instructions) ×2 (counterinduction manipulation: mindfulness vs. attention control) analysis of variance (ANOVA). Congruent with the hypothesis that the delayed effects of suppression would differ as a function of counterinduction manipulation, we predicted to observe a significant two-way interaction between suppression and counterinduction manipulation. Specifically, we expected to observe a pattern of results to support that, in the attention control, participants who were instructed to suppress the sound in the first task (the serial recall task) would on average persist for a shorter amount of time than participants who did not receive such instructions. In contrast, we expected that, in the mindfulness condition, participants who were instructed to suppress would on average persist for a similar amount of time as participants who did not receive such instructions. To further examine the interaction, simple planned comparisons (uncorrected t-tests) were made between suppression and no suppression instructions within each induction (i.e., mindfulness and attention control). Assuming an alpha level of .05, the current sample size provided the primary analysis with sufficient statistical power $(1 - \beta = .80)$ to detect a moderate effect size.

Results

Immediate Effects of Auditory Suppression

Participants made an average of 29.3 ($SD = 8.1$) correct responses on the serial recall test across the seven trials. However, participants in the two conditions (suppression instruction vs. no instruction) did not significantly differ on the mean number of accurate responses on the serial recall test across trials, $t(117) = 1.14$, $p = .25$. Similar, average subjective ratings of trial demand characteristics did not differ as a function of condition (all t's <1.34; all p's >.19). Means (with standard deviations in parentheses) for experimental demand questions fatigue, task demand, distress of sound, and interference of sound were 3.2 (1.4), 3.6 (1.6), 4.6 (1.4), and 3.9 (1.7), respectively.

Delayed Effects: Persistence in the Context of Interfering Emotional Sound

The length of time spent attempting to solve math assignments in the subsequent task served as measure of persistence in goal-directed behavior in the presence of the affectively negative sound. Participants could on average persist in the task for 260 seconds ($SD = 140$). Our hypotheses predicted that suppression of the sound during the first task would produce reduced persistence, but that a mindfulness induction between tasks will attenuate this effect. Figure 1 depicts means as a function of manipulations. A 2 (suppression manipulation: suppression instructions vs. no instructions) ×2 (counterinduction manipulation: mindfulness vs. attention control) analysis of variance (ANOVA) revealed neither a main effect of suppression, $F(1, 115) = 0.68$, $p = .41$, $\eta^2 = .01$, nor of counterinduction, $F(1, 115) = 0.16$, $p = .69$, $\eta^2 = .00$. However, as predicted, there was a statistically significant interaction effect of

suppression × counterinduction, $F(1, 115) = 5.12$, $p = .026$, $\eta^2 = .04$. In the attention control condition, participants who received instructions to suppress the sound in the first task (during the serial recall test) spent significantly less time persisting ($M = 216$ s, $SD = 95$, $n = 29$) than those who received no such instructions ($M = 294$ s, $SD = 168$, $n = 30$), $t(57) = 2.18$, $p = .01$ (one-tailed), $d = -0.57$. Thus, suppression was associated with a delayed cost. In contrast, in the mindfulness condition, participants who received instructions to suppress the sound in the first task did not spend significantly less time persisting ($M = 283$ s, $SD = 161$, $n = 30$) than those who received no suppression instructions ($M = 247$ s, $SD = 109$, $n = 30$), $t(58) = 0.31$, $p = .31$, $d = 0.26$. Thus, the mindfulness induction between tasks counteracted the detrimental effects of suppression (as illustrated in Figure 1).

Because the variances were not equal across conditions and there were some tendencies that time deviated from a normal distribution, we recalculated the main analysis with a robust estimation method (i.e., bootstrapping). The results remained the same. In addition, p-values corrected for homogeneity of variance violations did not differ substantially from those reported above.

Control Analyses

Demographic variables (age, gender) were unrelated to the dependent variable (i.e., time of effortful persistence) used in the study. To be sure that there were no time-accuracy trade-offs on the second task, such that, for example, no instruction participants in the attention control condition could persist for a longer time because they provided more correct responses on the math assignments, we included an individual's percentage of correct responses (correct response/number of assignment completed) as a covariate in the ANOVA. This did not alter the findings, that is, the interaction effect was still significant, $F(1, 114) = 4.96$, $p = .028$. It is plausible that differences observed are a function of perceived experimental demand in the first task (fatigue, task demand, distress of sound, and interference of sound). However, correlations between experimental demand ratings from the first task and time of persistence in the subsequent task were all

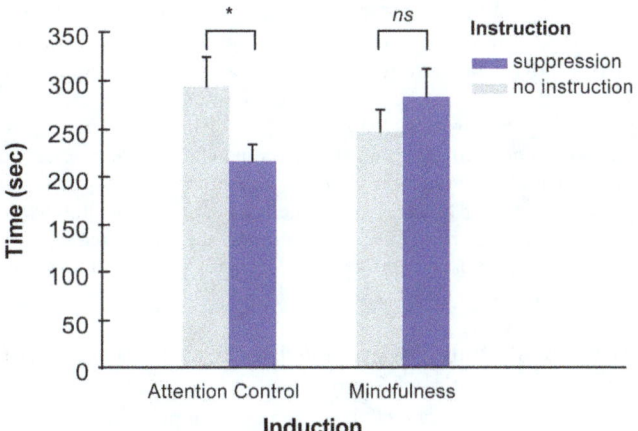

Figure 1. Time of effortful persistence as function of experimental manipulations (instruction and induction). Participants were required to ignore emotional task-irrelevant sound while performing a mentally challenging task (mental arithmetic). Induction manipulation (attention control vs. mindfulness induction) followed the suppression manipulation (suppression vs. no instructions) in the experiment; thus, these are the delayed effects of suppression. Error bar denotes standard error of mean. * = p<.05; ns = non-significant at specified alpha level (.05).

nonsignificant (all r's $<.17$; all p's $>.05$), with the exception for distress of sound that had a small negative correlation with the dependent variable ($r = -.27$, $p<.01$). Again, the interaction effect between suppression and counterinduction on time of persistence remained significant even when controlling for distress of sound, $F(1, 114) = 4.53$, $p = .035$.

Furthermore, a series of 2×2 ANOVAs revealed no significant interaction effect on any of the mean subjective ratings of experimental demand following the second task (all F's $<.51$, all p's $>.82$). Taken together, this indicated that the experimental effects were not simply due to trial demand characteristics. Means (with standard deviations in parentheses) for experimental demand questions fatigue, task demand, distress of sound, and interference of sound were 4.2 (1.5), 4.3 (1.8), 5.3 (1.1), and 4.1 (1.7), respectively. Noteworthy, is that participants on average rated the sound as significantly more distressing and interfering in the second task ($M = 4.3$, $SD = 1.8$, and $M = 5.3$, $SD = 1.1$, respectively) than in the first task ($M = 3.6$, $SD = 1.6$, and $M = 3.9$ $SD = 1.8$, respectively), t's >4.80, p's $<.001$. This suggested that participants had not habituated to the auditory stimulus that was used throughout the experiment.

Discussion

The present study examined the effects of attentional strategies in the context of an emotional interfering sound that mimicked the acoustic characteristics of tinnitus. We tested a model whereby we could study two strategies that represent the opposite of two theorized aspects of mental control. Specifically, we predicted that suppression of the auditory stimulus would result in delayed costs in the form of decreased persistence in a subsequent task that required participants to work with mental arithmetic while presented with the same sound. We also expected that a brief mindfulness induction between tasks would attenuate the delayed effects of suppression. As hypothesized, in the attention control, participants who were instructed to suppress the sound under mental load were less likely to persist in a subsequent task relative to participants who had received no such instructions. Furthermore, a mindfulness induction between tasks counteracted this effect. The significance of the latter finding is emphasized by the fact that the mindfulness exercise was brief (300 sec) and gave no specific advice on how to approach stimuli in the second task. Thus, the positive effects of the mindfulness induction are particularly noteworthy (c.f., [33,34]). Furthermore, there was little evidence to support that these effects were due to experimental demand. The findings are broadly consistent with the accumulating body of experimental work on the impact of suppression and mindfulness/acceptance on performance and affective responses in the context of aversive stimuli in non-auditory domains.

Attentional Strategies and Persistence in the Context of Interfering Emotional Sound

Why might deliberate efforts of trying to suppress an emotional interfering sound impair ability to persist in task-relevant behavior in the context of a subsequent presentation of the same sound, and why might mindfulness eliminate these impairments? Critical to any adaptive regulation is our ability to exert control over attention processes. Attempts to suppress a given stimulus may create paradoxical effects producing more of the suppressed targets. Suppressing an emotion stimulus (e.g., anxious thoughts) may even exacerbate the associated emotional responses [22]. Thus, deliberate efforts of keeping emotional sounds "out of mind" could potentially create a rebound effect with increased interference and negative affect over time. It is important to note that the effects of suppression were delayed rather than immediate. In fact, analyses revealed no evidence for any difference between suppression and no instruction on concurrent task performance (on the serial recall test). Indeed, these results parallel the findings from research on suppression in other domains (i.e., postsuppression rebound effect [2,22]). For example, in the physical domain, Cioffi and Holloway [23] in a study found no difference between suppression and other attentional strategies (monitoring, distraction) on tolerance time for acute pain experience (on a cold-pressor task). Differences were, however, observed on post pain recovery ratings and on the interpretation of a subsequent somatic stimulus. The current findings extend the evidence for such postsuppression rebound effects by suggesting divergent effects of auditory suppression depending on time of assessment (i.e., immediate vs. delayed).

Wegner's [2,22] theory on cognitive processes involved in thought suppression may provide a useful explanation for the delayed effects observed. The theory posits that there are two distinct processes that operate over different temporal periods: An intentional operating process that seeks to produce the desired mental state by using distractors, and an involuntary ironic process that actively searches for the to-be-suppressed target. First, during suppression, the ironic process works together with the operating process to achieve mental control, as the former signals the latter of the need to reactivate distraction efforts when conscious awareness of the unwanted mental event becomes imminent. In a later stage, however, when the operating process is voluntary terminated, the ironic process may continue to seek for the unwanted mental event, thereby creating a postsuppression rebound effect. Indeed, studies using functional magnetic resonance imaging have provided evidence that parallel the temporal aspects of the theory involved in attempts to suppress thoughts [62]. Accordingly, one explanation to impaired persistence among participants who initially engaged in suppression might be impaired attention control following an ineffective mental control strategy. That is, participants might have become more sensitive to the unwanted sound in the second task due to a lingering monitoring process of the sensation, making them less likely to continue with the task in the presence of the sound.

The mindfulness induction reversed the effects of suppression: Participants who initially were instructed to suppress the sound but later received a brief mindfulness exercise were able to persist to similar extent as those who had not received instructions to suppress. What is important to note is that mindfulness did not seem to promote a general ability to persist in the second task as no significant main effect of induction was found in the current experiment; rather, the effects of mindfulness seem to be specific. This finding is highly consistent with theories that posit that mindfulness and related processes such acceptance may undermine ineffective control strategies [35,36]. Wegner [4] has suggested that ironic processes involved in mental control might be prevented by paradoxical interventions, mindfulness and acceptance-based techniques. This may obstruct ironic processes by providing an incompatible mental approach to mental control strategies such as suppression. Thus, promoting people to attend mindfully to sensations may prevent them from using ineffective strategies (i.e., suppression). Furthermore, acceptance of an uncontrollable sound and associated emotional responses – noticing and embracing them without resisting them – may facilitate a context in which one's attention can be focused on the primary task irrespectively of interfering irrelevant stimuli, thereby, minimizing interference and demand. Indeed, preliminary evidence support that mindfulness training may achieve its positive effects through enhanced working memory capacity, response inhibition and executive control [63,64]. Furthermore, acceptance has been found to be more efficient in terms of resources than suppression when applied to emotions [39]. This may be a product of acceptance being a non-goal oriented process; unlike suppression where the goal is to have an "empty" mind in relation to the target-to-be suppressed sensation, acceptance as a mental strategy desires no specific mental end-state. As such, it may require fewer resources and therefore offer greater opportunities for flexible interactions with the environment [37,39]. Still, the discussion above is only speculative and future work should try to illuminate the processes involved in the phenomena that were observed here. Further investigations should focus on how suppression of auditory stimuli may disrupt mental activities and how mindfulness may work to undermine potentially negative effects of auditory suppression.

Implications for Tinnitus

Given that we simulated tinnitus in the current experiment, our results may only have limited relevance for the understanding of tinnitus. It could be argued, of course, that the very nature of the experiment (i.e., individuals exposed to an affectively negative sound) falls short of providing an explanation for tinnitus distress and interference. Notwithstanding this, our findings are broadly consistent with work showing that avoidance-based coping is associated with increased tinnitus-related distress [43] and that acceptance-based techniques, including mindfulness, can alleviate suffering caused by tinnitus [45]. It is plausible that specific mental efforts to control the experience of tinnitus can work temporarily, reducing thoughts about tinnitus [48] or interference of the sound [50]. However, such strategies may not work over time when it comes to an uncontrollable auditory perceptual phenomenon such as tinnitus [50]. Indeed, our results provide initial support to the notion that suppressing a tinnitus-like sound can be associated with delayed costs.

How an individual attend, process and evaluate tinnitus may play an important part in determining degree of tinnitus impact [18]. Yet, the mechanisms involved in tinnitus distress are still poorly understood. It has been suggested that cognitive interference may act as starting point for later evaluative emotional processes in tinnitus [17]. The present results extend such a theoretical model by focusing on how a specific attentional control strategy may influence the ability to engage in mental activities over time in the context of emotional interfering sound. That is, individuals who engage in suppression of tinnitus may experience problems with sustained mental control in everyday activities such as reading, writing or listening. This may cause a vicious circle in which tinnitus becomes associated with negative emotional reactions, which in turn, results in increased attention to tinnitus and cognitive interference. Approaching and paying attention in a non-evaluative way to tinnitus might be one way to undermine the natural tendency to suppress, and thus, preventing a preoccupation with the sensation. In fact, the ability to accept, notice and distance oneself from inner sensations associated with tinnitus has been related to improved long-term outcomes in acceptance-based treatment [42]. Yet, a considerable amount of more work is needed to explore the psychological underpinnings of such a cycle.

Limitations

Although the present results are promising, the study has limitations. First, the study relied on simulated tinnitus. Although previous research has been able to mimic the characteristics of tinnitus, both in terms of psychoacoustics and affective responses [51,52], the results of our study may only with caution be applied to tinnitus. That is, there might be significant differences between tinnitus, which is the experience of sound in the absence of any appropriate external source, and externally generated sounds with regard to the psychological processes involved in sound perception and interference. Nevertheless, we believe that simulated tinnitus in laboratory settings offers a unique opportunity to explore mechanisms involved in both development and treatment of tinnitus distress. Such experiments allow for greater experimental control of auditory stimuli and eliminate extraneous factors commonly encountered in experiments with participants with significant tinnitus (i.e., individual differences in affective, cognitive or audiological problems).

Second, participants were recruited from a student population. Thus, the findings may not generalize to other non-clinical and clinical populations. Third, we do not know the extent to which participants followed the scripted instructions to suppress the sound. On the other hand, it is difficult to conduct appropriate manipulation checks of mental control strategies and most studies that have examined suppression in other domains have relied on self-report to assess compliance with the mental strategy employed [19]. Still, future studies should develop and include objective measures to assess both compliance with mental instructions and cognitive accessibility of the avoided sensation, similar to the work that has been done on thought suppression [22].

Fourth, it is, of course, important to remember that the effects of the suppression manipulation cannot be interpreted in isolation from the second manipulation in the experiment (i.e., induction manipulation). Thus, future studies should examine the effects of auditory suppression in other experimental paradigms (e.g., without using any induction between tasks) and extend the work by systematically varying cognitive load, emotional valence of the sound, and by using other dependent measures of relevance to the phenomenon (subjective loudness of the sound, physiological states, behavioral avoidance in the context of aversive auditory stimuli, cognitive performance measures etc.).

Fifth, the ability to generalize effects of the intervention to a clinical setting is limited given the short mindfulness exercise that was used in the current experiment. Indeed, it has been argued that a "true" mindfulness induction requires extensive training [33] and in clinical practice, mindfulness is often promoted over weeks of training. On the other hand, positive effects of brief laboratory manipulations of mindfulness-related processes have been shown. For example, Erisman and Roemer [34] demonstrated that a brief mindfulness-type intervention (10 minute) could positively influence affective reactions.

Conclusions

Our work developed and tested a theoretical model based on how mental approaches may affect ability in the context of task-irrelevant emotional sound. To our knowledge, it is the first study of its kind. We demonstrate a novel phenomenon in which effortful suppression of an emotional sound can be associated with delayed costs on performance in the context of task-irrelevant sound, and that experimentally induced mindfulness can reduce the detrimental effect of auditory suppression. We encourage further investigations to continue this line of research. Such research efforts may not only have implications for tinnitus, but more broadly be relevant to situations in which unchangeable sound intrudes and disrupts performance, a common phenomenon in everyday life [58].

Acknowledgments

We wish to thank Cornelia Weise, Mathias Hällgren, and Daniel Västfjäll for valuable assistance with the experimental procedures and the stimuli materials.

Author Contributions

Revised and approved the final version of the paper: HH PM MJ GA. Conceived and designed the experiments: HH PM MJ GA. Performed the experiments: PM MJ. Analyzed the data: HH. Wrote the paper: HH.

References

1. Jones DM, Macken WJ (1993) Irrelevant tones produce an irrelevant speech effect: Implications for phonological coding in working memory. J Exp Psychol Learn Mem Cogn 19: 369–381.
2. Wegner DM (1994) Ironic processes of mental control. Psychol Rev 101: 34–52.
3. Hayes SC, Bissett RT, Korn Z, Zettle RD, Rosenfarb IS, et al. (1999) The impact of acceptance versus control rationales on pain tolerance. Psychological Record 49: 33–47.
4. Wegner DM (2011) Setting free the bears: escape from thought suppression. Am Psychol 66: 671–680.
5. Lockwood AH, Salvi RJ, Burkard RF (2002) Tinnitus. N Engl J Med 347: 904–910.
6. Shargorodsky J, Curhan GC, Farwell WR (2010) Prevalence and characteristics of tinnitus among US adults. Am J Med 123: 711–718.
7. Hasson D, Theorell T, Westerlund H, Canlon B (2010) Prevalence and characteristics of hearing problems in a working and non-working Swedish population. J Epidemiol Community Health 64: 453–460.
8. Henry J, Dennis K, Schechter M (2005) General review of tinnitus: Prevalence, mechanisms, effects, and management. J Speech Lang Hear Res 48: 1204–1235.
9. Tyler R, Baker L (1983) Difficulties experienced by tinnitus sufferers. J Speech Hear Disord 48: 150–154.
10. Andersson G, Eriksson J, Lundh LG, Lyttkens L (2000) Tinnitus and Cognitive Interference: A Stroop Paradigm Study. J Speech Lang Hear Res 43: 1168–1173.
11. Rossiter S, Stevens C, Walker G (2006) Tinnitus and its effect on working memory and attention. J Speech Lang Hear Res 49: 150–160.
12. Fowler EP, Fowler EP (1955) Somatopsychic and psychosomatic factors in tinnitus, deafness and vertigo. Ann Otol Rhinol Laryngol 64: 29–37.
13. Andersson G (2002) Psychological aspects of tinnitus and the application of cognitive-behavioral therapy. Clin Psychol Rev 22: 977–990.
14. Hesser H, Weise C, Westin VZ, Andersson G (2011) A systematic review and meta-analysis of randomized controlled trials of cognitive-behavioral therapy for tinnitus distress. Clin Psychol Rev 31: 545–553.
15. Rauschecker JP, Leaver AM, Mühlau M (2010) Tuning out the noise: Limbic-auditory interactions in tinnitus. Neuron 66: 819–826.
16. Jastreboff PJ (1990) Phantom auditory perception (tinnitus): Mechanisms of generation and perception. Neurosci Res 8: 221–254.
17. Andersson G, McKenna L (2006) The role of cognition in tinnitus. Acta Otolaryngol (Stockh) 126: 39–43.
18. Hallam R, Rachman S, Hinchcliffe R (1984) Psychological aspects of tinnitus. In: Rachman S, editor. Contributions to Medical Psychology. Oxford, England: Pergaman. 31–53.
19. Wenzlaff RM, Wegner DM (2000) Thought suppression. Annu Rev Psychol 51: 59–91.
20. Werner K, Gross, J J (2010) Emotion regulation and psychopathology: A conceptual framework. In: Kring AM, Sloan, D M, editor. Emotion regulation and psychopathology: A transdiagnostic approach to etiology and treatment New York: Guilford Press. 13–37.
21. Salters-Pedneault K, Steenkamp M, Litz BT (2010) Suppression. In: Kring AM, Sloan DM, editors. Emotion regulation and psychopathology: A transdiagnostic approach to etiology and treatment New York: Guilford Press. 137–156.
22. Wegner DM (2009) How to think, say, or do precisely the worst thing for any occasion. Science 325: 48–50.
23. Cioffi D, Holloway J (1993) Delayed costs of suppressed pain. J Pers Soc Psychol 64: 274–282.
24. Masedo A, Rosa Esteve M (2007) Effects of suppression, acceptance and spontaneous coping on pain tolerance, pain intensity and distress. Behav Res Ther 45: 199–209.
25. Muraven M, Tice DM, Baumeister RF (1998) Self-control as limited resource: regulatory depletion patterns. J Pers Soc Psychol 74: 774–789.
26. Hagger MS, Wood C, Stiff C, Chatzisarantis NL (2010) Ego depletion and the strength model of self-control: a meta-analysis. Psychol Bull 136: 495–525.
27. Erskine JAK, Georgiou GJ, Kvavilashvili L (2010) I suppress, therefore I smoke: Effects of thought suppression on smoking behavior. Psychol Sci 21: 1225–1230.
28. Levitt JT, Brown TA, Orsillo SM, Barlow SH (2004) The effects of acceptance versus suppression of emotion on subjective and psychophysiological response to carbon dioxide challange in patients with panic disorder. Behav Ther 35: 746–766.
29. Ahles T, Blanchard E, Leventhal H (1983) Cognitive control of pain: Attention to the sensory aspects of the cold pressor stimulus. Cognitive Ther Res 7: 159–177.
30. Blitz B, Dinnerstein A (1977) Role of attentional focus in pain perception: Manipulation of response to noxious stimulation by instructions. J Abnorm Psychol 77: 42–45.
31. Cioffi D (1991) Beyond attentional strategies: cognitive-perceptual model of somatic interpretation. Psychol Bull 109: 25–41.
32. Bishop SR, Lau M, Shapiro S, Carlson L, Anderson ND, et al. (2004) Mindfulness: A proposed operational definition. Clin Psychol-Sci Pr 11: 230–241.
33. Arch JJ, Craske MG (2006) Mechanisms of mindfulness: emotion regulation following a focused breathing induction. Behav Res Ther 44: 1849–1858.
34. Erisman SM, Roemer L (2010) A preliminary investigation of the effects of experimentally induced mindfulness on emotional responding to film clips. Emotion 10: 72–82.
35. Roemer L, Orsillo SM (2002) Expanding our conceptualization of and treatment for generalized anxiety disorder: Integrating mindfulness/acceptance-based approaches with existing cognitive-behavioral models. Clin Psychol-Sci Pr 9: 54–68.
36. Hayes SC, Villatte M, Levin M, Hildebrandt M (2011) Open, aware, and active: contextual approaches as an emerging trend in the behavioral and cognitive therapies. Annu Rev Clin Psychol 7: 141–168.
37. Hayes S, Bissett R, Korn Z, Zettle R, Rosenfarb I, et al. (1999) The impact of acceptance versus control rationales on pain tolerance. Psychological Record 49: 33–47.
38. Masedo AI, Esteve MR (2007) Effects of suppression, acceptance and spontaneous coping on pain tolerance, pain intensity and distress. Behav Res Ther 45: 199–209.
39. Alberts HJ, Schneider F, Martijn C (2012) Dealing efficiently with emotions: acceptance-based coping with negative emotions requires fewer resources than suppression. Cogn Emot 26: 863–870.
40. Davis C, Morgan M (2008) Finding meaning, perceiving growth, and acceptance of tinnitus. Rehabil Psychol 53: 128–138.
41. Westin V, Hayes SC, Andersson G (2008) Is it the sound or your relationship to it? The role of acceptance in predicting tinnitus impact. Behav Res Ther 46: 1259–1265.
42. Hesser H, Westin V, Hayes SC, Andersson G (2009) Clients' in-session acceptance and cognitive defusion behaviors in acceptance-based treatment of tinnitus distress. Behav Res Ther 47: 523–528.
43. Budd R, Pugh R (1996) Tinnitus coping style and its relationship to tinnitus severity and emotional distress. JPsychosomRes 41: 327–335.
44. Hesser H, Andersson G (2009) The role of anxiety sensitivity and behavioral avoidance in tinnitus disability. Int J Audiol 48: 295–299.
45. Hesser H, Gustafsson T, Lunden C, Henrikson O, Fattahi K, et al. (2012) A randomized controlled trial of internet-delivered cognitive behavior therapy and acceptance and commitment therapy in the treatment of tinnitus. J Consult Clin Psychol 80: 649–661.
46. Philippot P, Nef F, Clauw L, de Romree M, Segal Z (2012) A randomized controlled trial of mindfulness-based cognitive therapy for treating tinnitus. Clin Psychol Psychother 19: 411–419.
47. Westin VZ, Schulin M, Hesser H, Karlsson M, Noe RZ, et al. (2011) Acceptance and commitment therapy versus tinnitus retraining therapy in the treatment of tinnitus: a randomised controlled trial. Behav Res Ther 49: 737–747.
48. Andersson G, Juris L, Classon E, Fredrikson M, Furmark T (2006) Consequences of suppressing thoughts about tinnitus and the effects of cognitive distraction on brain activity in tinnitus patients. Audiol Neurootol 11: 301–309.
49. Westin V, Östergren R, Andersson G (2008) The effects of acceptance versus thought suppression for dealing with the intrusiveness of tinnitus. Int J Audiol 47 Suppl 2: S112–118.
50. Hesser H, Pereswetoff-Morath CE, Andersson G (2009) Consequences of controlling background sounds: the effect of experiential avoidance on tinnitus interference. Rehabil Psychol 54: 381–389.
51. Mirz F, Gjedde A, Sodkilde-Jrgensen H, Pedersen CB (2000) Functional brain imaging of tinnitus-like perception induced by aversive auditory stimuli. Neuroreport 11: 633–637.
52. Penner MJ (1996) Rating the annoyance of synthesized tinnitus. Int Tinnitus J 2: 3–7.
53. Heinecke K, Weise C, Schwarz K, Rief W (2008) Physiological and psychological stress reactivity in chronic tinnitus. J Behav Med 31: 179–188.
54. Bradley MM, Lang PJ (2007) The International Affective Digitized Sounds (IADS-2): Affective ratings of sounds and instruction manual (Technical report B-3): University of Florida, Gainesville, Fl.
55. Wegner DM, Quillian F, Houston CE (1996) Memories out of order: thought suppression and the disturbance of sequence memory. J Pers Soc Psychol 71: 680–691.
56. Wegner DM, Schneider DJ, Carter SR 3rd, White TL (1987) Paradoxical effects of thought suppression. J Pers Soc Psychol 53: 5–13.
57. Eifert GH, Forsyth JP (2005) Acceptance and Commitment Therapy for Anxiety Disorders: A Practitioner's Treatment Guide to Using Mindfulness, Acceptance, and Values-based Behavior Change Strategies. Oakland, CA: New Harbinger Publications.

58. Banbury SP, Macken WJ, Tremblay S, Jones DM (2001) Auditory distraction and short-term memory: Phenomena and practical implications. Hum Factors 43: 12–29.

59. Tyler JM, Burns KC (2008) After depletion: The replenishment of the self's regulatory resources. Self Identity 7: 305–321.

60. Gailliot MT, Baumeister RF, DeWall CN, Maner JK, Plant EA, et al. (2007) Self-control relies on glucose as a limited energy source: Willpower is more than a metaphor. J Pers Soc Psychol 92: 325–336.

61. Glass DC, Siger JE, Friedman LN (1969) Psychic cost of adaptation to an environmental stressor. J Pers Soc Psychol 12: 200–210.

62. Mitchell JP, Heatherton TF, Kelley WM, Wyland CL, Wegner DM, et al. (2007) Separating sustained from transient aspects of cognitive control during thought suppression. Psychol Sci 18: 292–297.

63. Jha AP, Krompinger J, Baime MJ (2007) Mindfulness training modifies subsystems of attention. Cogn Affect Behav Neurosci 7: 109–119.

64. Jha AP, Stanley EA, Kiyonaga A, Wong L, Gelfand L (2010) Examining the protective effects of mindfulness training on working memory capacity and affective experience. Emotion 10: 54–64.

20

Memory Networks in Tinnitus: A Functional Brain Image Study

Maura Regina Laureano[1], Ektor Tsuneo Onishi[2]*, Rodrigo Affonseca Bressan[1,4], Mario Luiz Vieira Castiglioni[3], Ilza Rosa Batista[1,4], Marilia Alves Reis[1,4], Michele Vargas Garcia[5], Adriana Neves de Andrade[5], Roberta Ribeiro de Almeida[1], Griselda J. Garrido[6], Andrea Parolin Jackowski[1]

1 Laboratório Interdisciplinar de Neurociências Clínicas (LiNC), Departamento de Psiquiatria, Universidade Federal de São Paulo, São Paulo, Brasil, **2** Departamento de Otorrinolaringologia e Cirurgia de Cabeça e Pescoço, Universidade Federal de São Paulo, São Paulo, Brasil, **3** Seção de Medicina Nuclear, Departamento de Radiologia, Universidade Federal de São Paulo, São Paulo, Brasil, **4** Instituto do Cérebro – Hospital Israelita Albert Einstein, São Paulo, Brasil, **5** Departamento de Fonoaudiologia, Universidade Federal de São Paulo, São Paulo, Brasil, **6** Western Australian Centre for Health and Ageing, Centre for Medical Research, University of Western Australia, Perth, Australia

Abstract

Tinnitus is characterized by the perception of sound in the absence of an external auditory stimulus. The network connectivity of auditory and non-auditory brain structures associated with emotion, memory and attention are functionally altered in debilitating tinnitus. Current studies suggest that tinnitus results from neuroplastic changes in the frontal and limbic temporal regions. The objective of this study was to use Single-Photon Emission Computed Tomography (SPECT) to evaluate changes in the cerebral blood flow in tinnitus patients with normal hearing compared with healthy controls. Methods: Twenty tinnitus patients with normal hearing and 17 healthy controls, matched for sex, age and years of education, were subjected to Single Photon Emission Computed Tomography using the radiotracer ethylenedicysteine diethyl ester, labeled with Technetium 99 m (99 mTc-ECD SPECT). The severity of tinnitus was assessed using the "Tinnitus Handicap Inventory" (THI). The images were processed and analyzed using "Statistical Parametric Mapping" (SPM8). Results: A significant increase in cerebral perfusion in the left parahippocampal gyrus (pFWE <0.05) was observed in patients with tinnitus compared with healthy controls. The average total THI score was 50.8+18.24, classified as moderate tinnitus. Conclusion: It was possible to identify significant changes in the limbic system of the brain perfusion in tinnitus patients with normal hearing, suggesting that central mechanisms, not specific to the auditory pathway, are involved in the pathophysiology of symptoms, even in the absence of clinically diagnosed peripheral changes.

Editor: Berthold Langguth, University of Regensburg, Germany

Funding: Financial support was received from Fundação de Amparo à Pesquisa do Estado de São Paulo (FAPESP-2010/14804-6). The funders had no role in study design, data collection and analysis, decision to publish, or preparation of the manuscript.

Competing Interests: The authors have declared that no competing interests exist.

* E-mail: ektor_onishi@yahoo.com.br

Introduction

Tinnitus is an auditory phantom sensation, described as ringing or buzzing in one or both ears, in the absence of an external auditory stimulus. The prevalence of chronic tinnitus varies from 5–15%, and 1–3% of these cases severely affect the quality of life, resulting in anxiety and emotional disorders, sleep disturbance and work impairment [1].

Over 20 years, it has been suggested that tinnitus reflects peripheral pathology, primarily cochlear dysfunction or auditory nerve damage [2]. Recently, imaging and electrophysiological methods have suggested the involvement of central mechanisms in generation and perception of tinnitus symptoms. The central origin of tinnitus-related activity has replaced the peripheral hypothesis [3–6]. Increased spontaneous neural activity, synchrony or reorganized tonotopic maps have been proposed as neural substrates of tinnitus [7].

Groundbreaking imaging studies have shown structural and functional brain changes associated with tinnitus [8], although the exact location remains controversial [9]. Abnormal activity might

be interpreted and perceived as tinnitus in higher cortical centers and areas associated with auditory and emotional processing [3]. Recent studies using Magnetic Resonance Imaging (MRI), Positron-Emission Tomography (PET), and Single-Photon Emission Computed Tomography (SPECT) have demonstrated the involvement of non-auditory brain areas in a global network that encodes subjective tinnitus. These techniques provide evidence that structural and functional changes in temporal, prefrontal and limbic structures are the basis for tinnitus symptomatology [8,10]. Others studies using electrophysiological tests have demonstrated abnormal connectivity between auditory and non-auditory networks [11], and several concepts have been proposed to explain this involvement [12–13].

Conscious sound processing in auditory centers and the association of the signal with unpleasantness and distress might be responsible for the interpretation of the aberrant auditory signal as troublesome tinnitus [14]. These processes are influenced by the memory, attention and emotional state of the patient. It has been proposed that auditory centers play a major role in the generation of tinnitus-related activity, although tinnitus might be initially triggered through peripheral auditory deficits, even with a normal audiogram [5]. Schaette and McAlpine (2011) demonstrated that even in absence of elevated hearing thresholds, a fraction of auditory nerve fibers no longer respond to sound, and tinnitus could result from a homeostatic response of the central auditory system to reduced auditory nerve input [15]. Taken together, these observations suggest that tinnitus results from peripheral injury, the reorganization of central auditory pathways and changes in the encoding of the emotional content of sensory experiences in portions of limbic system.

Sataloff et al. (1996) demonstrated the diagnostic benefits of SPECT in assessing neurotological complaints. These researchers observed that among other techniques, including MRI, computed tomography (CT) and electroencephalography (EEG), SPECT is a more sensitive method for the analysis of neurotological conditions, such as dizziness, hearing loss and tinnitus. SPECT abnormalities were observed in 92% of tinnitus patients, while only 44% MRI and 22% computed tomography (CT) scan abnormalities were observed among these same patients [16]. Few studies have explored the use of SPECT for the investigation of dynamic and metabolic brain changes in tinnitus [16].

The purpose of the present study was to characterize the brain activity in patients with tinnitus and normal hearing using SPECT.

Methodology

Subjects

Twenty tinnitus patients and 17 control subjects, matched by age, sex, years of education and hearing, were enrolled in this study. The study participants were recruited among patients seeking treatment at the Tinnitus Center of the Federal University of São Paulo and through the website of the same institution.

The inclusion criteria were continuous uni- or bilateral tinnitus for longer than 3 months, between 18 and 60 years of age and normal hearing in both ears. All patients underwent complete otological and audiological examinations, including pure tone audiometry, tympanometry, stapedius reflex tests and otoscopy. Pure tone audiometry was performed using a clinical audiometer with 8 different octave frequencies (0.25, 0.5, 1, 2, 3, 4, 6 and 8 kHz). The exclusion criteria included thresholds >25 dB hearing level in any frequency, neurologic or psychiatric disorders, particularly epilepsy, migraine, or schizophrenia, pregnancy, and breastfeeding women. The Portuguese version [17] of the Tinnitus Handicap Inventory (THI) [18] was used to assess tinnitus severity, classified as none (0–16), mild (18–36), moderate (38–56) or severe (58–100) [19].

Ethics Statement

The local research ethics committee, "Comitê de Ética em Pesquisa da Universidade Federal de São Paulo/Hospital São Paulo", approved this study (protocol 2094/09). All participants provided written informed consent for clinical investigation and subsequent analysis after a comprehensive explanation of the procedures.

Assessment of Regional Brain Perfusion Using 99mTc-ECD SPECT in Tinnitus

SPECT was performed with an ethyl cysteinate dimer labeled with technetium-99 m (99mTc-ECD) using a double-head gamma camera (GE® Infinia - USA) equipped with a pair of low-energy fan-beam collimators.

The 99mTc-ECD was prepared from a lyophilized kit (IPEN ECD®) by adding from 3700 MBq/2 mL (100 mCi) freshly eluted 99mTc-pertechnetate from a 99Mo/99mTc generator (IPEN-

Tec®). Before labeling, the 99mTc must be freshly eluted (<2 hours) and the content of 99Mo must be determined. The radiochemical purity of the 99mTc-ECD (>90%) was determined through solvent extraction (3 mL of a 0.9% saline solution and 3 mL of chloroform).

All subjects rested with closed eyes in a dark quiet room for 30 min, followed by the intravenous injection of 25–30 mCi (925–1110 MBq) 99mTc-ECD and an additional 30 min of rest. Acquisition was achieved through 128 projections on a 128×128 matrix, with 40,000 counts per projection. The images were reconstructed as transaxial slices parallel to the orbitomeatal line, using filtered back projection with a Butterworth filter (cut-off frequency 0.48 cycles/pixel and order 10) and Chang's method for attenuation correction.

Data Analysis

For the analysis of the SPECT data, the reconstructed ECD images were exported to an NIfTI file format and processed using Statistical Parametric Mapping 8 [20] of the Wellcome Department of Imaging and Neuroscience, London (http://www.fil.ion.ucl.ac.uk/spm) using Matlab® 7.0 (Mathworks®, Sherborn, MA, USA). Morbelli et al (2008) showed that using the SPM8 standard HMPAO SPECT template for the spatial normalization of ECD SPECT images yields incorrect results [21]. To more closely match the template to the sample under investigation, the original images were linearly matched to a smoothed FWHM = 8 mm Gaussian kernel version of the MNI ECD SPECT template downloaded from the website according to Morbelli et al (2008) [21]. The resulting images were averaged and subsequently matched to a smoothed FWHM = 8 mm Gaussian kernel to create the study template. In a second phase, the original images were non-linearly deformed to the customized template yielding 2 mm×2 mm×2 mm images matched to a smoothed FWHM = 8 mm Gaussian kernel to account for interindividual brain anatomy differences and increase the signal-to-noise ratio. The images were globally normalized for signal intensity using proportional scaling to remove the confounding effects of global CBF changes, with a threshold of 0.8, and include only those voxels with intensities exceeded 80% of the global mean. Furthermore, a gray matter binary mask was used as an explicit mask to exclude white matter voxels from the statistical analysis.

Statistical Analysis

The demographic and baseline clinical characteristics between groups were compared using unpaired t-tests. We performed a descriptive analysis of the THI, considering emotional, functional, catastrophic, and final scores.

Voxel-based comparisons of the regional tracer uptake values between tinnitus patients and controls were performed using a two-sample t-test. The SPM results were displayed at $p<0.05$ uncorrected, with a cluster extent threshold = 50 voxels. The areas were identified using MRIcron (http://www.nitrc.org/projects/mricron) and xjview (http://www.alivelearn.net/xjview8).

The ROIs for SVC correction were created using MRIcron (http://www.mccauslandcenter.sc.edu/mricro/mricron/) version 6.6.2013 after one expansion of the temporal and limbic system regions extracted from the Automatic Anatomical Labeling (AAL) template [22]. After SVC correction, the results that survived at pFWE (Family-wise error) <0.05 at the peak level were accepted. The post hoc analyses showed that the pattern of the findings remained virtually unaltered after covarying for age and gender.

Results

No differences were observed between control individuals and tinnitus patients regarding age (42.95+9.03 years versus 41.41+ 9.98 years, respectively; p = 0.613), gender (6 males and 14 females versus 6 males and 11 females, respectively; p = 0.985), or years of education (11.2+3.87 versus 11.41+3.78, respectively; p = 0.860). The total mean score for disease severity was 50.8+18.24. The demographic and THI test scores (total, physical, emotional, and catastrophic domains) are presented in Table 1.

A comparison of the SPECT images revealed a significant increase in the metabolic activation of the left parahippocampal gyrus (pFWE<0.05, Table 2 and Figure 1) in patients compared with the controls. The stability of the results after covarying for age and gender suggested that the observed differences are associated with the effect of interest.

No unexpected findings survived at pFWE<0.005 at voxel level.

Discussion

Using 99mTc-ECD SPECT, the results obtained in the present study showed differences in the brain activation patterns in tinnitus patients with clinically normal hearing compared with healthy controls. The availability of an objective technique, whereby the location, extent and magnitude of neural activity can be measured, might greatly contribute to the understanding of tinnitus pathophysiology, as these processes are subjective and cannot be measured using laboratory tests. However, the use of SPECT to characterize tinnitus pathophysiology remains poorly described. There have only been 11 studies using SPECT for the investigation of these symptoms, with varying methodologies [3;14–15;23–30].

The functional brain abnormalities observed in the present study were evaluated in the presence of normal audiogram results, using carefully matched groups with respect to gender, age, years of education and hearing, to minimize or avoid the interference of these factors in the results shown. To date, only 3 SPECT studies

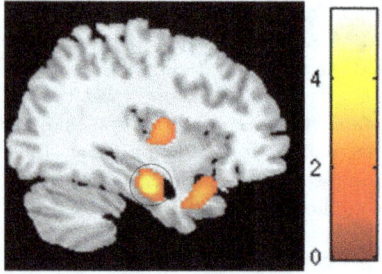

Figure 1. rCBF increase (pFWE <0.05 after SVC) in the left parahippocampal gyrus in tinnitus patients compared with control subjects.

have compared healthy controls with tinnitus patients; however, none of these studies matched the control group for the degree of hearing loss. Mahmoudiam et al (2012) examined 122 patients with subjective idiopathic tinnitus, and only 9 healthy controls were included in this study, and the hearing thresholds were not considered [30]. Farhadi et al (2010) also compared tinnitus patients with hearing loss to healthy controls, without pairing according to hearing thresholds [14]. Gardner et al (2002) compared depressed patients with and without tinnitus, but the sample of tinnitus patients only contained 3 individuals with normal hearing bilaterally, and these studies were not performed using healthy controls without depression [3].

It has recently been suggested that tinnitus without hearing loss does not necessarily indicate the absence of deafferentation [5;15;31–32]. It is possible that peripheral damage, particularly at high frequencies, could be present, but not detected through routine audiometry [32]. Even if patients with apparently normal audiograms show 'hidden hearing loss' due to damage to auditory nerve fibers [15], the control of the audiological symptoms reduces the difference between patients and controls and is a strategy that produces more consistent and reliable results associated with tinnitus. The stability of our results after covarying for age and gender suggests that the observed differences are directly associated with tinnitus.

Recent evidence on the neurobiology of tinnitus suggests that although auditory system dysfunction is necessary for tinnitus to occur, the neural changes in the presence of these symptoms are not only limited to the auditory pathway [3]. Studies have proposed that the limbic system might play a role in modulating or perpetuating tinnitus [33], and interactions between the limbic corticostriatal network and the primary auditory cortex might be the key to understanding chronic tinnitus. This limbic activation has been interpreted as a reflection of the emotional reaction of tinnitus patients to tinnitus sounds [34]. However, the precise involvement of the limbic system in tinnitus has yet to be elucidated [9].

Thus, the results obtained in the present study reinforce the current concepts. The increased cerebral perfusion in tinnitus patients was observed in the left parahippocampal gyrus, located in the medial temporal lobe, which is part of the limbic system and also considered as part of the neural circuitry associated with tinnitus [35].

It has been proposed that a fundamental function of para-hippocampal structures is the establishment of auditory memory for tinnitus [23]. The parahippocampal gyrus is involved in the maintenance of tinnitus, preventing the modification or elimination of hippocampal memory, thereby avoiding habituation [36–37]. MRI studies have previously described the involvement of the

Table 1. Demographic and clinical characteristics of the study participants.

		TI	Controls
Gender	**Male**	**06**	**06**
	Female	14	11
Age (Mean+SD)		42.95 (9.03)	41.41 (9.98)
Years of education (Mean+SD)		11.2 (3.87)	11.41 (3.78)
Pure-tone average (0.25–8 kHz)			
Mean right (+SD)		13.4 (5.65)	10.63 (4.28)
Mean left (+SD)		14.24 (4.92)	10.53 (3.86)
THI total (Mean+SD)		50.8 (18.2)	N/A
THI emotional (Mean+SD)		18.2 (7.9)	N/A
THI physical (Mean+SD)		20.4 (9.39)	N/A
THI catastrophic (Mean+SD)		12.2 (3.94)	N/A
TI laterality	Right	01	N/A
	Left	03	N/A
	Bilateral	13	N/A
	Head	03	N/A

THI, Tinnitus Handicap Inventory; TI, Tinnitus.

Table 2. Regional cerebral blood flow increase in tinnitus patients compared with control subjects.

Brain regions	MNI Coordinates of the peak voxel			Cluster size		pFWE after SVC
Increase	x	y	z	K$_E$	t	
Parahippocampal_L	−26	−2	−30	1322	5.02	0.021

FWE, Family-wise error; KE, number of voxels per cluster;

parahippocampal region in the judgment of inharmonious and unpleasant music, showing the activation of this region in response to aversive stimuli [38]. It has been postulated that due to the strong reciprocal connection between the parahippocampal gyrus and amygdala, these structures function as components of the neural system that help the body to cautiously explore and protect itself from harmful experiences [39]. Joos et al (2012) concluded that due to parahippocampal connectivity with the anterior cingulate and orbitofrontal cortices, the parahippocampal gyrus could be the decisive link between the network associated with tinnitus and attentional-emotional neural circuitry, underlying emotional disturbances associated with the symptoms [35].

Other structures of the paralimbic network associated with the amygdala, such as the nucleus accumbens of ventral striatum (NAc) and prefrontal cortex ventromedial (vmPFC) have been implicated in the assessment of emotional sound content. Rauschecker et al (2010) recently proposed a model of tinnitus pathophysiology, which suggests that efferents are involved in the cancellation of the tinnitus signal in the thalamus, and although tinnitus signals might initially be generated in parts of the auditory system, the limbic structures are compromised, the cancellation of tinnitus signals in the thalamus is disrupted and does not prevent the tinnitus signal from reaching the auditory cortex, leading to ongoing reorganization and chronic tinnitus [40]. Recent evidence that the NAc and vmPFC do indeed differ in the brains of individuals with tinnitus support the current hypothesis [8].

We speculate that the failure to detect significant differences in the cerebral perfusion of the superior and medial temporal gyrus and frontal areas, as demonstrated in previous studies [4;14;28], might reflect the observation of clinically normal audiograms. Although there might be bias towards the periphery auditory fibers in the presence of normal audiograms, this unbalance may not be sufficient to produce a significant change in cerebral blood flow in these regions, consistent with the view that the cortical network is involved in the conscious perception of tinnitus and the emotional symptoms that accompany this condition.

In the present study, we identified a change in cerebral perfusion, which was not specific to the auditory pathway in patients with tinnitus and normal hearing, suggesting the involvement of central mechanisms in the pathophysiology of symptoms, even in the presence of clinically normal hearing.

Acknowledgments

The authors would like to thank the patients and health volunteers for participating in this study.

Author Contributions

Conceived and designed the experiments: MRL ETO RAB RRDA APJ. Performed the experiments: MRL ETO. Analyzed the data: MRL GJG APJ. Contributed reagents/materials/analysis tools: MRL MLVC IRB MAR MVG ANDA GJG APJ. Wrote the paper: MRL IRB GJG APJ.

References

1. Eggermont JJ, Roberts LE (2004) The neuroscience of tinnitus. TRENDS in Neurosciences 27(11): 676–682.
2. Jastreboff PJ (1990) Phantom auditory perception (tinnitus): mechanisms of generation and perception. Neurosci Res 8: 221–254.
3. Gardner A, Pagani M, Jacobsson H, Lindberg G, Larsson SA, et al. (2002) Differences in resting state regional cerebral blood flow assessed with 99mTc-HMPAO SPECT and brain atlas matching between depressed patients with and without tinnitus. Nuclear Medicine Communications 23: 429–439.
4. Vanneste S, De Ridder D (2012) The auditory and non-auditory brain areas involved in tinnitus. An emergent property of multiple parallel overlapping subnetworks. Front Syst Neurosci 6: 31.
5. Noreña AJ, Farley BJ (2013) Tinnitus-related neural activity: theories of generation, propagation, and centralization. Hear Res 295: 161–171.
6. Balkenhol T, Wallhäusser-Franke E, Delb W (2013) Psychoacoustic tinnitus loudness and tinnitus-related distress show different associations with oscillatory brain activity. PLoS One 8(1): e53180.
7. Eggermont JJ (2006) Cortical tonotopic map reorganization and its implications for treatment of tinnitus. Acta Otolaryngol Suppl 556: 9–12. Review.
8. Baizer JS, Lobarinas E, Salvi R, Allman BL (2012) Brain Research special issue: advances in the neuroscience of tinnitus. Brain Res 1485: 1–2.
9. Leaver AM, Renier L, Chevillet MA, Morgan S, Kim HJ, et al. (2011) Dysregulation of limbic and auditory networks in tinnitus. Neuron 69(1): 33–43.
10. Maudoux A, Lefebvre P, Cabay JE, Demertzi A, Vanhaudenhuyse A, et al. (2012) Auditory resting-state network connectivity in tinnitus: a functional MRI study. PLoS One7(5): e36222.
11. Schlee W, Weisz N, Bertrand O, Hartmann T, Elbert T (2008) Using auditory steady state responses to outline the functional connectivity in the tinnitus brain. PLoS One 3(11): e3720.
12. De Ridder D, Vanneste S, Weisz N, Londero A, Schlee W, et al. (2013) An integrative model of auditory phantom perception: Tinnitus as a unified percept of interacting separable subnetworks. Neurosci Biobehav Rev. pii: S0149-7634 (13) 00081-X.
13. Langguth B, Schecklmann M, Lehner A, Landgrebe M, Poeppl TB, et al. (2012) Neuroimaging and neuromodulation: complementary approaches for identifying the neuronal correlates of tinnitus. Front Syst Neurosci 6: 15.
14. Farhadi M, Mahmoudian S, Saddadi F, Karimian AR, Mirzaee M, et al. (2010) Functional brain abnormalities localized in 55 chronic tinnitus patients: fusion of SPECT coincidence imaging and MRI. Journal of Cerebral Blood Flow & Metabolism 30: 864–870.
15. Schaette R, McAlpine D (2011) Tinnitus with a Normal Audiogram: Physiological Evidence for Hidden Hearing Loss and Computational Model. The Journal of Neuroscience 31(38): 13452–13457.
16. Sataloff RT, Mandel S, Muscal E, Park CH, Rosen DC, et al. (1996) Single-photon-emission computed tomography (SPECT) in neurotologic assessment: a preliminary report. Am J Otol 17(6): 909–916.
17. Ferreira PA, Cunha F, Onishi ET, Branco-Barreiro FCA, Ganança FF (2005) Tinnitus handicap inventory: adaptação cultural para o Português brasileiro. Pró-Fono R Atual Cient 17: 277–280.
18. Newman CW, Jacobson GP, Spitzer JB (1996) Development of the tinnitus handicap inventory. Arch Otolaryngol Head Neck Surg 122: 143–148.
19. McCombe A, Bagueley D, Coles R, McKenna L, McKinney C, et al. (2001) Guidelines for the grading of tinnitus severity : the results of a working group commissioned by the British Association of Otolaryngologists, Head and Neck Surgeons, 1999. Clin Otolaryngol 26: 388–393.
20. Ashburner J, Friston KJ (2005) Unified segmentation. Neuroimage 26: 839–851.
21. Morbelli S, Rodriguez G, Mignone A, Altrinetti V, Brugnolo A, et al The need of appropriate brain SPECT templates for SPM comparisons. (2008) Q J Nucl Med Mol Imaging 52(1): 89–98.
22. Tzourio-Mazoyer N, Landeau B, Papathanassiou D, Crivello F, Etard O, et al. (2002) Automated Anatomical Labeling of activations in SPM using a Macroscopic Anatomical Parcellation of the MNI MRI single-subject brain. NeuroImage 15(1): 273–289.

23. Shulman A, Strashun AM, Afriyie M, Aronson F, Abel W, et al. (1995) SPECT Imaging of Brain and Tinnitus-Neurotologic/Neurologic Implications. Int Tinnitus J 1(1): 13–29.

24. Staffen W, Biesinger E, Trinka E, Ladurner G (1999) The effect of lidocaine on chronic tinnitus: a quantitative cerebral perfusion study. Audiology 38(1): 53–57.

25. Shulman A, Strashun AM, Seibyl JP, Daftary A, Goldstein B (2000) Benzodiazepine receptor deficiency and tinnitus. Int Tinnitus J 6(2): 98–111.

26. Shulman A, Strashun AM, Goldstein BA (2002) GABAA-benzodiazepine-chloride receptor-targeted therapy for tinnitus control: preliminary report. Int Tinnitus J 8(1): 30–36.

27. Shulman A, Goldstein B (2006) Brain and inner-ear fluid homeostasis, cochleovestibular-type tinnitus, and secondary endolymphatic hydrops. Int Tinnitus J 12(1): 75–81.

28. Shulman A, Goldstein B, Strashun AM (2007) Central nervous system neurodegeneration and tinnitus: a clinical experience. Part I: Diagnosis. Int Tinnitus J 13(2): 118–131.

29. Marcondes RA, Sanchez TG, Kii MA, Ono CR, Buchpiguel CA, et al. (2010) Repetitive transcranial magnetic stimulation improve tinnitus in normal hearing patients: a double-blind controlled, clinical and neuroimaging outcome study. Eur J Neurol 17(1): 38–44.

30. Mahmoudian S, Farhadi M, Gholami S, Saddadi F, Karimian AR, et al. (2012) Pattern of brain blood perfusion in tinnitus patients using technetium-99m SPECT imaging. J Res Med Sci 17(3): 242–247.

31. Weisz N, Dohrmann K, Elbert T (2007) The relevance of spontaneous activity for the coding of the tinnitus sensation. Prog Brain Res 166: 61–70.

32. Adjamian P, Sereda M, Zobay O, Hall DA, Palmer AR (2012) Neuromagnetic indicators of tinnitus and tinnitus masking in patients with and without hearing loss. J Assoc Res Otolaryngol 13(5): 715–731.

33. Lockwood AH, Salvi RJ, Coad ML, Towsley ML, Wack DS, et al. (1998) The functional neuroanatomy of tinnitus: evidence for limbic system links and neural plasticity. Neurology 50(1): 114–20.

34. Jastreboff PJ, Jastreboff MM (2000) Tinnitus Retraining Therapy (TRT) as a method for treatment of tinnitus and hyperacusis patients. J Am Acad Audiol 11(3): 162–77.

35. Joos K, Vanneste S, De Ridder D (2012) Disentangling depression and distress networks in the tinnitus brain. PLoS One 7(7): e40544.

36. De Ridder D, Fransen H, Francois O, Sunaert S, Kovacs S, et al. (2006) Amygdalohippocampal involvement in tinnitus and auditory memory. Acta OtoLaryngologica 126: 50–53.

37. De Ridder D, Elgoyhen AB, Romo R, Langguth B (2011) Phantom percepts: tinnitus and pain as persisting aversive memory networks. Proc.Natl.Acad.Sci 108: 8075–8080.

38. Gosselin N, Samson S, Adolphs R, Noulhiane M, Roy M, et al. (2006) Emotional responses to unpleasant music correlates with damage to the parahippocampal cortex. Brain 129(Pt 10): 2585–2592.

39. McNaughton N, Corr PJ (2004) A two-dimensional neuropsychology of defense: fear/anxiety and defensive distance. Neurosci Biobehav Rev 28: 282–305.

40. Rauschecker JP, Leaver AM, Mühlau M (2010) Tuning out the noise: limbic-auditory interactions in tinnitus. Neuron 66(6): 819–26.

21

Neuronal Correlates of Maladaptive Coping: An EEG-Study in Tinnitus Patients

Sven Vanneste[1,2]*, Kathleen Joos[1], Berthold Langguth[3], Wing Ting To[4], Dirk De Ridder[5,6]

1 Department of Translational Neuroscience, Faculty of Medicine, University of Antwerp, Antwerp, Belgium, **2** School of Behavioral and Brain Sciences, The University of Texas at Dallas, Richardson, Texas, United States of America, **3** Department of Psychiatry and Psychotherapy, University Regensburg, Regensburg, Germany, **4** Faculty of Social Work and Welfare Studies, University College Ghent, Ghent, Belgium, **5** Department of Surgical Sciences, Dunedin School of Medicine, University of Otago, Dunedin, New Zealand, **6** BRAI²N, Sint Augustinus Hospital, Antwerp, Belgium

Abstract

Here we aimed to investigate the neuronal correlates of different coping styles in patients suffering from chronic tinnitus. Adaptive and maladaptive coping styles were determined in 85 tinnitus patients. Based on resting state EEG recordings, coping related differences in brain activity and connectivity were found. Maladaptive coping behavior was related to increases in subjective tinnitus loudness and distress, higher tinnitus severity and higher depression scores. EEG recordings demonstrated increased alpha activity over the left dorsolateral prefrontal cortex (DLPFC) and subgenual anterior cingulate cortex (sgACC) as well as increased connectivity in the default (i.e. resting state) network in tinnitus patients with a maladaptive coping style. Correlation analysis revealed that the changes in the DLPFC correlate primarily with maladaptive coping behavior, whereas the changes in the sgACC correlate with tinnitus severity and depression. Our findings are in line with previous research in the field of depression that during resting state a alpha band hyperconnectivity exists within the default network for patients who use a maladaptive coping style, with the sgACC as the dysfunctional node and that the strength of the connectivity is related to focusing on negative mood and catastrophizing about the consequences of tinnitus.

Editor: Manuel S. Malmierca, University of Salamanca- Institute for Neuroscience of Castille and Leon and Medical School, Spain

Funding: No current external funding sources for this study.

Competing Interests: The authors have declared that no competing interests exist.

* E-mail: sven.vanneste@utdallas.edu

Introduction

It is well established chronic medical conditions can cause a high amount of burden in some patients, whereas other patients can tolerate the same medical condition much easier. Adaptively coping with chronic health impairment is a self-regulatory challenge. Failing to meet this challenge has serious consequences, as intrusive and emotionally charged thoughts about the disorder contribute decisively to the health related burden.

One chronic medical condition is tinnitus, a subjective auditory phantom phenomenon in which patients perceive an internal sound in the absence of an external sound source, which can be very distressing [1,2]. Whereas more people who experience tinnitus can perfectly well live with it, 1 in 5 is emotionally affected by it [3], with 2.4% of the population suffering in the worst degree [4]. In those patients tinnitus is frequently accompanied by annoyance, concentration problems, depression, anxiety, irritability, sleep disturbances and intense worrying [5,6]. Even if these symptoms have been traditionally considered as a learned reaction to tinnitus [1] their exact relationship to tinnitus is still a matter of debate [5]. Theoretically, it is also conceivable that these symptoms may be preceding the tinnitus onset and predispose for it or they may represent non-auditory symptoms resulting from the same pathophysiological changes that are involved in tinnitus generation [7]. One approach to answer this question is the investigation of the relationship between tinnitus related handicap and coping behavior, since coping is assumed to mediate the relationship between disease symptoms and the related handicap or distress [8,9]. Previous research on tinnitus has already shown that the emotion regulation or coping style that tinnitus patients engage in is influencing tinnitus related stress [8,9]. However, no study addressed the neural bases of successful and non-successful coping styles in tinnitus.

Functional imaging studies suggest that the subgenual anterior cingulate cortex (sgACC) plays an important role in adaptive versus maladaptive regulation of negative autobiographical memories [10]. The sgACC has been shown to be critically implicated in major depressive disorders (MDD) [11–14] and also in poor emotion regulation [15]. Recent structural and functional imaging studies suggest the involvement of the sgACC in tinnitus [16–18] and source localized EEG studies demonstrated an important role for this area in the amount of distress perceived by tinnitus patients [19,20] and depressive feelings [21].

With respect to the neural bases of coping behavior it has been demonstrated that mind-wandering about the severity of a medical condition appears to engage regions of the default network, a set of brain areas that are active during rest periods, which include the posterior cingulate cortex, portions of lateral parietal cortex as well as the medial temporal lobe and medial prefrontal cortex [22–24]. It has recently been shown that MDD is characterized by increased default network connectivity and sgACC activity [25]. A seed-based connectivity approach further revealed that MDDs show more neural functional connectivity between the posterior cingulate cortex, which is part of the default network and the sgACC, than healthy individuals during rest periods [11].

In the present study we aimed to identify the neural bases of differences in coping behavior among tinnitus patients by using resting state electroencephalography (EEG). The study focuses on the cortical source differences in resting-state eyes closed EEG activity and connectivity between tinnitus patients who use different forms of coping. We differentiate between maladaptive, active and passive coping behavior. While maladaptive coping behavior involves focusing on negative mood, venting feelings and catastrophizing about the consequences of tinnitus, active coping behavior involves the use of a broad range of adaptive coping mechanisms. Active coping strategies are either behavioral or psychological responses designed to change the nature of the stressor itself or how one thinks about it. Passive coping behavior involves attempts to avoid tinnitus by masking the noises using background sounds and tinnitus maskers. It is further known that active styles are considered to be leading to improved psychosocial functioning, whilst maladaptive coping styles such as rumination about negative states are linked to increased depression. We hypothesize that a maladaptive coping style would be reflected in the default-mode network in tinnitus patients analogous to what is seen in depressed patients, generating increased activity of the sgACC and increased communication between the sgACC and the default network during resting state. We hypothesize that alpha activity might play an important role, as increased alpha activity has already been related to tinnitus related distress in previous EEG studies [19,20].

Methods

Patients

Eighty-five tinnitus patients (57 males and 28 females) with a mean age of 48.20 years (Sd = 14.53 years) and a mean tinnitus duration of 6.02 years (Sd = 7.54 years) were selected from the multidisciplinary Tinnitus Research Initiative (TRI) Clinic of the University Hospital of Antwerp, Belgium. For the clinical and demographic characterization of the sample see Table 1. Individuals with pulsatile tinnitus, Ménière disease, otosclerosis, chronic headache, neurological disorders such as brain tumors, and individuals being treated for mental disorders were not included in the study in order to obtain a homogeneous sample. All patients were investigated for the extent of hearing loss using audiograms. Tinnitus matching was performed looking for tinnitus pitch (frequency) and tinnitus intensity.

Antwerp University Ethics Committee reviewed and approved the study and all applicable documents prior to study initiation. All patients signed an approved informed consent in order to enroll into the study.

Questionnaires

TCSQ. A Dutch translation was made from the Tinnitus Coping Style Questionnaire (TCSQ). This questionnaire assesses the frequency in which sufferers use a broad range of tinnitus-specific coping actions to manage the intrusiveness of the tinnitus sound. The questionnaire identifies three tinnitus coping behaviors, namely maladaptive coping, effective or active coping, and passive coping [8,26]. One item was excluded from the questionnaire ('Using a pillow speaker to help you sleep') as most tinnitus patients are not familiar with this product. As such, the translated TCSQ consisted of 39 items measured on a 7-point scale, ranging from 'never' (scored as 1) to 'always' (scored as 7). This questionnaire was used as the primary outcome measure as

Table 1. Population statistics.

| | | Coping style | | Total |
		adaptive	maladapative	
Gender	Male	35	22	57
	Female	14	14	28
Age	Mean	49.04	47.06	48.20
	Sd	13.56	14.78	14.53
Tinnitus type	Pure tone	22	15	37
	Narrow Band Noise	27	21	48
Tinnitus lateralization	Unilateral	24	16	40
	Bilateral	25	20	45
Tinnitus Duration	Mean	5.78	6.34	6.02
	Sd	5.79	9.24	7.54
Hearing loss (dB HL)	Mean	27.18	32.05	29.24
	SD	14.59	16.43	15.03

this questionnaire was specifically developed to measure coping behavior in tinnitus.

To validate the TCSQ in Dutch the COPE, Beck Depression Scale (BDI), the Tinnitus Questionnaire (TQ), Visual Analogue Scale (VAS) for tinnitus loudness were measured.

COPE. A Dutch translation of the COPE [27] was used, a coping inventory that includes 53 items and exist out of 13 subscales: Active coping, Planning, Suppression of competing activities, Restraint coping, Seeking social support for instrumental reasons, Seeking social support for emotional reason, Positive reinterpretation & growths, Acceptance, Turning to Religion, Focus on & venting of emotions, Denial, Behavioral disengagement, Mental disengagement, Alcohol-drug disengagement [28].

VAS. A visual analogue scale for loudness ('How loud is your tinnitus?') was assessed.

TQ. We used the Dutch translation of the Tinnitus Questionnaire validated by Meeus et al. [29]. This scale comprised of 52 items and is a well-established measure for the assessment of a broad spectrum of tinnitus-related psychological complaints. The TQ measures emotional and cognitive distress, intrusiveness, auditory perceptual difficulties, sleep disturbances, and somatic complaints. As previously mentioned, the global TQ score can be computed to measure the general level of psychological and psychosomatic distress. A 3-point scale is given for all items, ranging from 'true' (2 points) to 'partly true' (1 point) and 'not true' (0 points). The total score (from 0–84) was computed according to standard criteria published in previous work [29,30].

BDI. Beck Depression Inventory is a depression test to measure the severity and depth of depression symptoms. Each of the inventory items corresponds to a specific category of depressive symptom and/or attitude according to DSM-IV. This questionnaire was validated in Dutch [31].

EEG data collection

EEG recordings (Mitsar-201, NovaTech http://www.novatecheeg.com/) were obtained in a quiet and dimly lighted room with each participant sitting upright on a small but comfortable chair. Participants were requested to abstain from alcohol consumption 24 hours prior to recording, and from caffeinated beverages consumption on the day of recording. The actual recording lasted approximately 5 min. The EEG was sampled with 19 electrodes in the standard 10–20 International placement referenced to linked ears and impedances were checked to remain below 5 $k\Omega$. Data were collected eyes-closed (sampling rate = 1024 Hz, band passed 0.15–200 Hz). Data were resampled to 128 Hz, band-pass filtered (fast Fourier transform filter) to 2–44 Hz and subsequently transposed into Eureka! Software [32], plotted and carefully inspected for manual artifact-rejection (i.e. eye blinks, eye movements, teeth clenching, body movement, or ECG artifact) and removed. Average Fourier cross-spectral matrices were computed for bands delta (2–3.5 Hz), theta (4–7.5 Hz), alpha1 (8–10 Hz), alpha2 (10–12 Hz), beta1 (13–18 Hz), beta2 (18.5–21 Hz), beta3 (21.5–30 Hz) and gamma (30.5–44 Hz).

Source localization

Standardized low-resolution brain electromagnetic tomography (sLORETA) was used to estimate the intracerebral electrical sources that generated the scalp-recorded activity in each of the eight frequency bands [33]. sLORETA computes electric neuronal activity as current density (A/m^2) without assuming a predefined number of active sources. The sLORETA solution space consists of 6,239 voxels (voxel size: 5×5×5 mm), computations were made in a realistic head model, and is restricted to cortical gray matter and hippocampi, as defined by digitized MNI152 template [34]. Scalp electrode coordinates on the MNI brain are derived from the international 5% system [35].

Lagged phase coherence (connectivity)

Lagged phase coherence between two sources can be interpreted as the amount of cross-talk between the regions contributing to the source activity [36]. Since the two brain areas oscillate coherently with a phase lag, the cross-talk can be interpreted as information sharing by axonal transmission. More precisely, the discrete Fourier transform decomposes the signal in a finite series of cosine and sine waves (in-phase and out-of-phase carrier waves, forming the real and imaginary part of the Fourier decomposition) at the Fourier frequencies. The lag of the cosine waves with respect to their sine counterparts is inversely proportional to their frequency and amounts to a quarter of the period; The threshold of significance for a given lagged phase coherence value according to asymptotic results can be found as described by Pascual-Marqui [37,38], where the definition of lagged phase coherence can be found as well.

Time-series of current density were extracted for different regions of interest using sLORETA. Power in all 6,239 voxels was normalized to a power of 1 and log transformed at each time point. Region of interest values thus reflect the log transformed fraction of total power across all voxels, separately for specific frequencies. Regions of interest were defined based on previous brain research on default network by Fox et al. [39] as well as the findings based on source localization (BA25, BA9/46) on tinnitus (Table 2).

Table 2. Default network [39].

Common names	Brodmann's areas
Posterior cingulate cortex	BA 31
Retro-splenial cortex	BA 30
Lateral parietal cortex	BA 39
Medial prefrontal cortex	BA 32/10
Superior frontal cortex	BA 8
Inferior temporal cortex	BA 20/21
Parahippocampal gyrus	BA 35

Region of interest analysis

The log-transformed electric current density was averaged across all voxels belonging to the region of interest, respectively BA25 left and right, BA9/46 left and BA9/46 right separately across all frequency bands.

Statistical analyses

The methodology used is non-parametric. It is based on estimating, via randomization, the empirical probability distribution for the max-statistic, under the null hypothesis comparisons [40]. This methodology corrects for multiple testing (i.e., for the collection of tests performed for all voxels and for all frequency bands). Due to the non-parametric nature of the method, its validity does not rely on any assumption of Gaussianity [40]. Statistical contrast maps were calculated through multiple voxel-by-voxel comparisons in a logarithm of F-ratio. The significance threshold was based on a permutation test with 5000 permutations. A comparison was made between tinnitus patients using an adaptive coping style in comparison to tinnitus patients using a maladaptive coping style as well as correlation were calculated with different questionnaires.

Factor analysis using principal component extraction was performed on the TCSQ. Based on the scree test plot the number of components is determined. Internal consistency for the different components was calculated using Cronbach Alpha. To verify the construct validity the components were correlated with different subscales of the COPE questionnaire using Pearson correlations. To further verify the convergent validity the different components of the TCSQ were correlated with the BDI, the subscales of the TQ, the total score of the TQ, and the VAS loudness.

In order to differentiate the sample in groups, a hierarchical cluster analysis based on the squared Euclidean distance was conducted on the 39 coping items of the TCSQ. A multivariate ANOVA with the 3 components as dependent variables and the cluster groups as an independent variable was conducted to further explore these different clusters. In addition, a multivariate analysis was conducted with the clusters as independent variable and VAS loudness, BDI, and the TQ subscales (emotional aspects, cognitive aspects, intrusiveness, perceptual differences, sleep disturbance, and somatic problems) as dependent variables.

To compare sample correlation coefficients drawn from the same sample we rely on a formula described in Cohen and Cohen [41]. The formula yields in a t-statistic with n-3 degrees of freedom. The formula tests for a significant difference in the correlation between variables X & Y and V & Y.

Results

Coping behavior and coping style

Factor analysis using principal component extraction was performed on the TCSQ. A scree plot indicates that three factors would be ideal (Figure 1). The first factor explained 20.75% of the total variance (eigenvalue = 8.09), a second factor explained 12.95% of the total variance (eigenvalue = 5.05) and a third factor 6.58% of the total variance (eigenvalue = 2.57). Table 3 presents the factor pattern matrix after oblique rotation. Similar to previous research using the same questionnaire [8,26], factor 1 corroborates with *maladaptive coping behavior*, factor 2 with *active coping behavior*, and factor 3 with *passive coping behavior*. These three factors show a good internal consistency measured with Cronbach α coefficient: maladaptive coping behavior (α = .88), active coping behavior (α = .76), and passive coping behavior (α = .69).

To verify the construct validity of the TCSQ we correlated the different subscales with the 13 subscales of COPE. Correlation analyses revealed for *maladaptive coping behavior as measured by the TCSQ* a positive correlation with the following items of COPE: *suppression of competing activities, seeking social support for emotional reasons, focus on and venting of emotions, behavioral disengagement, mental disengagement* and a negative correlation with *positive reinterpretation and growth* (Table 4). The subscale *active coping behavior* of the TCSQ correlated positively with *active coping, positive reinterpretation and growth*, and *mental disengagement of the COPE questionnaire*. The TCSQ subscale *passive coping behavior* correlated positively with COPE's *restraint coping*, and *focus on and venting of emotions*.

Convergent validity was found by correlating the TCSQ with typical measures used in tinnitus research indicating that tinnitus loudness, tinnitus distress, BDI, the different subscales of the TQ and the total score of the TQ correlated positively with maladaptive coping behavior, but not with active and passive coping (Table 4).

In order to differentiate the sample in groups that differ in their general coping behavior a hierarchical cluster analysis based on the squared Euclidean distance was conducted on the 39 coping items. This analysis revealed that 2 clusters (i.e. 2 groups) give a reliable solution. A multivariate ANOVA with the 3 TCSQ coping

dimensions as dependent variables and the 2 cluster groups as an independent variable indicates a significant effect, $F = 61.32$, $p < .001$. Univariate analysis indicates that the effect can mainly be explained by a significant effect of factor 1 *maladaptive coping behavior*, but not by factor 2 *active coping behavior* and factor 3 *passive coping behavior* of the TCSQ (Table 5). For maladaptive behavior it was shown that the second cluster had a higher score on this dimension in comparison to the first cluster. As such, one can interpret cluster 1 as patients making use of adaptive coping styles, while the second group uses maladaptive coping styles.

A multivariate analysis with groups *adaptive coping style* versus *maladaptive coping style* as independent variable and VAS loudness, BDI and the TQ subscales (emotional aspects, cognitive aspects, intrusiveness, perceptual differences, sleep disturbance and somatic problems) as dependent variables revealed a significant effect, $F = 8.42$, $p < .001$. Univariate analysis revealed that the maladaptive group has higher scores on the different dependent variables in comparison to the adaptive group (Table 6).

Neural correlates of the 2 clusters: maladaptive vs. adaptive coping styles

For the alpha 1 and alpha2 band sLORETA revealed a higher current source density for the maladaptive coping style as compared to the adaptive coping style over the left dorsolateral prefrontal cortex (DLFPC) (Figure 2A) and sgACC (BA25) (Figure 2C&D). In the other frequency bands (delta, theta, beta 1, beta 2, beta 3 and gamma) there were no statistically significant differences between the two groups.

To confirm these results and based on previous research a ROI analysis of these two regions was conducted. An ANOVA with coping style (maladaptive versus adaptive coping) as independent variable and log-transformed current density for respectively the left DLPFC and sgACC revealed a significant effect for coping style, demonstrating that the maladaptive coping style had a higher log-transformed current density in comparison to the adaptive coping style for respectively the left DLPFC ($F = 4.83$, $p < .05$; Figure 2B) and sgACC ($F = 4.30$, $p < .05$; Figure 2E).

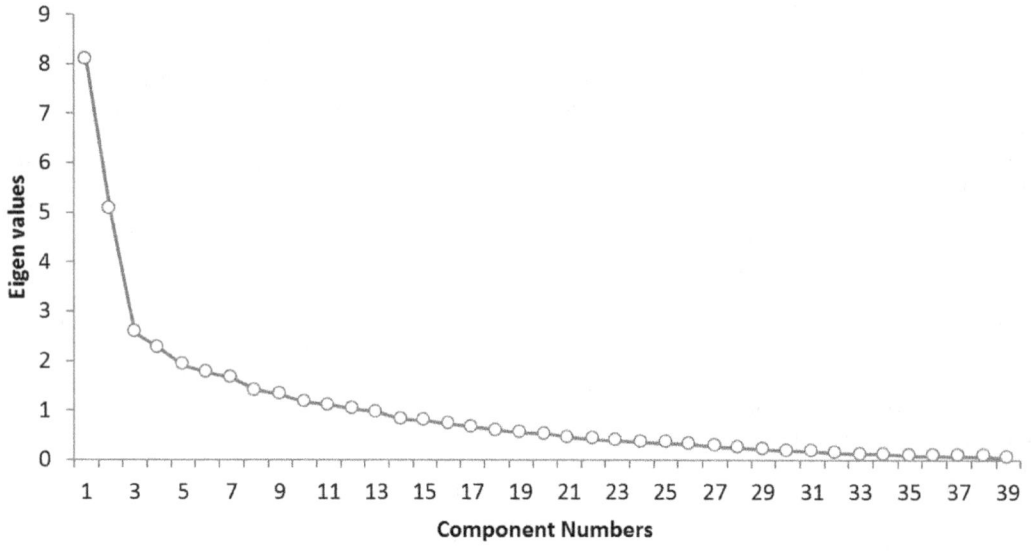

Figure 1. Scree plot for the THQ shows the number of components and the corresponding eigenvalues (see Figure 1). When the drop ceases and the curve makes an elbow toward less steep decline, all further components after the one starting the elbow can be dropped. The scree plot indicates that three factors would be ideal.

Table 3. The items for the TCSQ. Results from the factor analysis using principal component extraction.

	Component		
	Factor 1	Factor 2	Factor 3
	maladaptive	active	passive
1. Ik gebruik bepaalde middelen om mijn tinnitus te maskeren.	.12	.00	**.49**
Using a masker for tinnitus			
2. Ik probeer aan plezante dingen te denken, in plaats van me op mijn tinnitus te concentreren.	.09	**.71**	.06
Thinking of something pleasant rather than concentrating on your tinnitus			
3. Ik denk erover om het op te geven.	**.44**	−.13	.29
Thinking of giving up			
4. Ik probeer mezelf eraan te herinneren dat mijn leven over het algemeen voldoening geeft en bevredigend is.	−.08	**.57**	.00
Reminding yourself that your life is generally fulfilling and satisfying			
5. Nadenken hoe erg en onplezierig dit geluid is.	**.70**	.11	−.03
Thinking about how awful and unpleasant the noises sound			
6. Gebruik maken van achtergrondlawaai om te helpen slapen.	.02	.04	**.74**
Using background noise mask your tinnitus			
7. Bidden helpt om mijn tinnitus te doen verminderen of te laten verdwijnen.	.13	.08	**.32**
Praying yours tinnitus will suddenly diminish or stop			
8. Ik doe bewust moeite om mijn tinnitus weg te denken.	.30	**.60**	.11
Making a conscious effort to think your tinnitus away			
9. Ik vertel andere hoe erg mijn tinnitus is.	**.79**	.17	−.12
Telling others how awful your tinnitus is			
10. Ik dagdroom over hoe mijn leven zou zijn zonder tinnitus.	**.78**	.15	.14
Daydreaming about what life would be like without tinnitus			
11. Ik vraag mij af waaraan ik mijn tinnitus verdiend heb.	**.68**	.14	.17
Asking what you have done to deserve your tinnitus			
12. Luisteren naar de radio, muziek of TV kijken maskeert mijn tinnitus.	−.14	.26	**.59**
Listening to the radio, music, or watching TV to mask your tinnitus			
13. Ik bekijk tinnitus als een deel van het alledaagse achtergrond lawaai.	−.19	**.64**	.05
Thinking of your tinnitus as part of everyday background noise			
14. Ik doe alsof mijn tinnitus er niet is.	−.24	**.58**	.22
Pretending your tinnitus is not there			
15. Ik vermijd sociale situaties als gevolg van mijn tinnitus.	**.56**	−.12	.00
Avoiding social situations because of your tinnitus			
16. Ik focus mij volledig op de dingen waar ik mee bezig ben, of op dingen die gebeuren rondom mij.	−.04	**.38**	−.15
Focusing your attention fully on what you are doing, or on the things that are happening around you			
17. Ik kruip in mijn bed en/of slaap tijdens de dag om van mijn tinnitus af te zijn.	.28	−.27	**.35**
Going to bed and/or sleeping during the day to get away from your tinnitus			
18. Ik verzeker mezelf ervan dat ik mijn tinnitus kan tolereren/negeren.	**−.45**	.30	.12
Reassuring yourself that you can learn to tolerate/ignore your tinnitus			
19. Ik probeer niet aan mijn tinnitus te denken.	−.39	**.59**	.17
Trying not to think about your tinnitus			
20. Ik consulteer een therapeut of psycholoog om nieuwe manieren te leren om met mijn tinnitus om te gaan.	.03	−.18	**.64**
Consulting a professional counselor, or psychologist, to learn new ways of coping with tinnitus			
21. Ik neem hobby's en passies op om mezelf af te leiden van mijn tinnitus.	.27	**.36**	.28
Taking up hobbies and interests to distract yourself from your tinnitus			
22. Ik denk dat tinnitus mijn levenskwaliteit heeft geruïneerd.	**.72**	−.19	.30

Table 3. Cont.

	Component		
	Factor 1	**Factor 2**	**Factor 3**
	maladaptive	active	passive
Thinking that your tinnitus has ruined the quality of your life			
23. Ik verzeker mezelf ervan dat ik kan omgaan met mijn tinnitus, aangezien dat ik in het verleden ook heb gedaan.	**−.53**	.18	.38
Reassuring yourself that you can cope with your tinnitus now because you have coped in the past			
24. Ik luister vaak naar mijn tinnitus.	**.68**	−.01	−.03
Listening to your tinnitus			
25. Ik denk aan dingen om te doen om mijzelf van mij tinnitus af te leiden.	.31	**.59**	.02
Thinking of things to do to distract yourself from your tinnitus			
26. Ik probeer mij eraan te herinneren dat ik nog altijd van het leven kan genieten.	−.03	**.73**	−.06
Reminding yourself that you can still enjoy life despite your tinnitus			
27. Ik hoop dat er binnenkort een oplossing kan gevonden worden voor tinnitus.	**.32**	.22	−.02
Hoping that a cure for tinnitus will be found soon			
28. Ik zeg tegen mijzelf dat tinnitus gewoon één van de uitdagingen in het leven is.	−.35	**.50**	.19
Saying to yourself that tinnitus is just one of life's many challenges			
29. Ik neem voorgeschreven medicatie om mij te helpen slapen.	**.40**	−.19	.30
Taking prescribed medication to help your tinnitus			
30. Ik kijk naar mensen rondom mij die in een ergere situatie zitten dan ik.	**.37**	.27	.04
Looking at others around you who are in a worse situation than yourself			
31. Ik denk vaak aan vroegere tijden waar ik geen tinnitus had.	**.67**	−.01	.07
Thinking of times in the past when you did not have tinnitus			
32. Ik probeer bezig te blijven of actief te zijn om mijzelf af te leiden van mijn tinnitus.	.34	**.50**	−.14
Staying busy or active to distract yourself from your tinnitus			
33. Ik denk dat ik niets kan doen om te leren omgaan met mijn tinnitus.	**.51**	−.28	.25
Thinking that you cannot do anything to cope with your tinnitus			
34. Ik laat tinnitus niet mijn leven beheersen.	**−.39**	.06	.26
Thinking that you won't let your tinnitus get the better of you			
35. Ik verzeker mezelf ervan dat ik toegang heb tot professioneel advies en ondersteuning.	.11	−.07	**.30**
Reassuring yourself that you have access to professional advice and support			
36. Ik lees om mij af te leiden van mijn tinnitus.	.06	**.33**	−.02
Reading in order to distract yourself from your tinnitus			
37. Ik ben bang dat het geluid mij een zenuwinzinking zal bezorgen.	**.54**	−.05	.32
Worrying that the noises will give you a nervous breakdown			
38. Ik leer en gebruik relaxtatie technieken	−.25	.21	**.52**
Learning and practicing relaxation techniques			
39. Ik denk dat ik niet instaat ben om, om te gaan met mijn tinnitus.	**.70**	−.18	.27
Thinking about not being able to put up with tinnitus			

	Correlation		
	Factor 1	**Factor 2**	**Factor 3**
	maladaptive	active	passive
Factor 1 maldaptive	-	−.07	.16
Factor 2 active	-	-	.08
Factor 3 passive	-	-	-

The communality is the sum of the squared correlations between a variable and each of the three factors.
Extraction Method: Principal Component Analysis.
Rotation Method: Oblique with Kaiser Normalization.
a. Rotation converged in 7 iterations.

Table 4. Correlation analysis between the TCSQ and respectively COPE, Tinnitus loudness, Tinnitus distress, BDI, the different subscales of the TQ and the total score of the TQ.

	TCSQ Coping behavior		
	maladaptive	active	passive
COPE scale			
Active coping	.18	.31**	.07
Planning	.20†	−.08	.19†
Suppression of competing activities	.29**	−.14	.15
Restraint coping	.14	−.05	.21*
Seeking social support for instrumental reasons	.14	−.08	.00
Seeking social support for emotional reasons	.23*	.03	.12
Positive reinterpretation & growth	−.50***	.24*	.00
Acceptance	−.59***	.24*	−.08
Turning to Religion	.13	.20	−.07
Focus on & venting of emotions	.54***	.01	.30**
Denial	.17	.02	.02
Behavioral disengagement	.40**	−.03	.05
Mental disengagement	.28**	.33**	.15
Alcohol-drug disengagement	.07	.11	.03
Tinnitus loudness	.38***	.01	.04
BDI	.65***	.00	.21
TQ			
distress (emotional)	.59***	−.02	.21
distress (cognitive)	.68***	−.05	.00
intruisiveness	.66***	−.16	.01
perceptual difficulties	.45***	−.15	−.05
sleep distubance	.41***	.07	.05
somatic problems	.46***	.12	.11
total	.77***	−.05	.09

†*p*<.10;
* *p*<.05;
** *p*<.01;
*** *p*<.001.

Table 5. A comparison of the mean score on the three factors for the two cluster groups.

	Coping style		
	adaptive	maladaptive	*F*-value
TCSQ maladaptive coping behavior	2.72	4.39	188.37***
TCSQ active coping behavior	3.96	3.74	1.52
TCSQ passive coping behavior	2.64	2.95	1.40

* *p*<.05;
** *p*<.01;
*** *p*<.001.

n.s.), and VAS loudness. To compare sample correlation coefficients between the left DLPFC and respectively the maladaptive coping behavior and BDI an additional analysis was conducted revealing that the correlation was marginally significantly; stronger for maladaptive coping behavior than for the BDI (t = 1.37, *p* = .09). A similar analysis for active coping behavior and passive coping behavior groups did not yield in significant effects.

Maladaptive coping behavior and the subgenual Anterior Cingulate Cortex

To further evaluate the involvement of the sgACC in *maladaptive coping behavior, TQ, BDI, and VAS loudness*, a region of interest of the sgACC was extracted for alpha2 activity and correlated to each of these characteristics (maladaptive coping behavior, TQ, BDI, VAS loudness). A significant correlation was found for sgACC alpha2 activity and the TQ (r = .34, *p*<.01) as well as the BDI (r = .24, *p*<.05), but not for maladaptive coping behavior (r = .08, *n.s.*) and VAS loudness (r = −.08, *n.s.*).

Table 6. Tinnitus loudness, Tinnitus annoyance, BDI, subscale of TQ (emotional distress, cognitive distress, intrusiveness, perceptual differences, sleep disturbance, somatic problems) & Total score on the TQ.

	Coping style		
	adaptive	maladaptive	
Tinnitus loudness	5.21	6.60	23.35***
Tinnitus annoyance	4.06	6.91	5.11*
BDI	7.20	19.20	39.07***
TQ			
distress (emotional)	4.91	11.57	55.34***
distress (cognitive)	5.13	8.05	28.04***
intruisiveness	9.88	13.66	31.51***
perceptual difficulties	4.56	6.98	17.79***
sleep distubance	2.28	4.18	5.14*
somatic problems	2.72	4.77	15.87**
Total	29.47	49.20	8.42***

* *p*<.05;
** *p*<.01;
*** *p*<.001.

Maladaptive coping behavior and the left dorsolateral prefrontal cortex

A correlation analysis on the whole brain with maladaptive coping behavior indicates a significant positive correlation between the left dorsolateral prefrontal cortex (DLPFC) and maladaptive coping behavior for the alpha 1 band (Figure 3A,B). No significant effects were obtained for delta, theta, alpha2, beta 1, beta 2, beta 3 and gamma frequency band. Similar analyses with respectively the active coping behavior and passive coping behavior yielded no significant effects.

To further confirm this finding and based on previous research, a ROI analysis was conducted correlating respectively the left and right DLPFC with the maladaptive coping behavior. This analysis revealed a significant positive correlation between the left DLPFC and maladaptive coping behavior (r = .40, *p*<.001; Figure 3B), but not with the right DLPFC (r = .17, *p* = .14). To further explore this latter effect, alpha 1 activity within the left DLPFC was also correlated with respectively the BDI (r = .27, *p*<.05), TQ (r = .14,

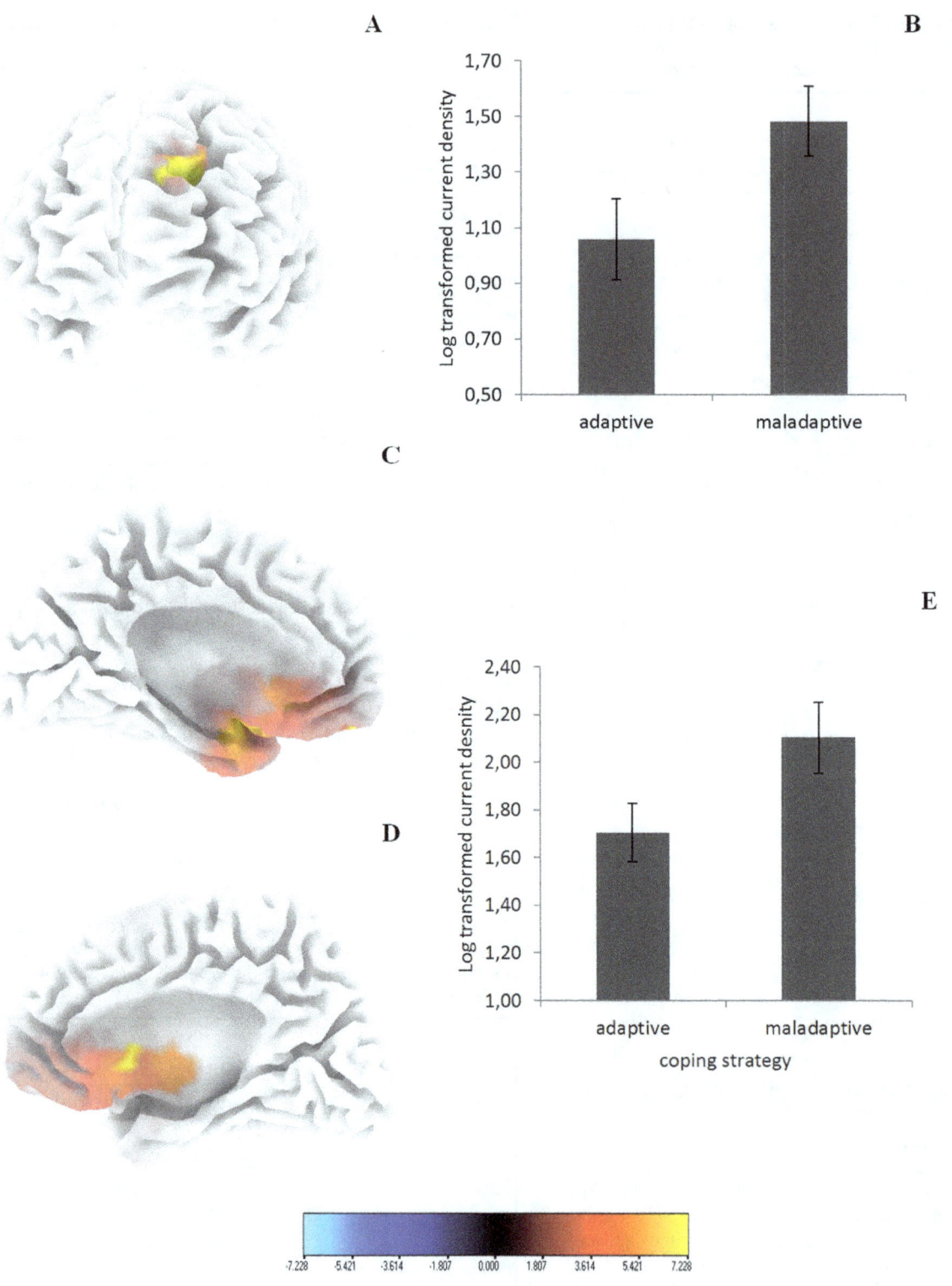

Figure 2. (A) Increased activity in the left dorsolateral prefrontal cortex (BA9) for tinnitus patients using a maladaptive coping style in comparison to tinnitus patients using an adaptive coping style for the frequency band Alpha1. (B) Region of interest analysis shows increased activity in the left dorsolateral prefrontal cortex (BA9) for tinnitus patients using a maladaptive coping style in comparison to tinnitus patients using an adaptive coping style for Alpha1. (C & D) Increased activity in the subgenual anterior cingulate cortex (BA25) for tinnitus patients using a maladaptive coping style in comparison to tinnitus patients using an adaptive coping style for the frequency band Alpha2. (E) Region of interest analysis shows increased activity in the subgenual anterior cingulate cortex (BA25) for tinnitus patients using a maladaptive coping style in comparison to tinnitus patients using an adaptive coping style for Alpha2.

A   **B**

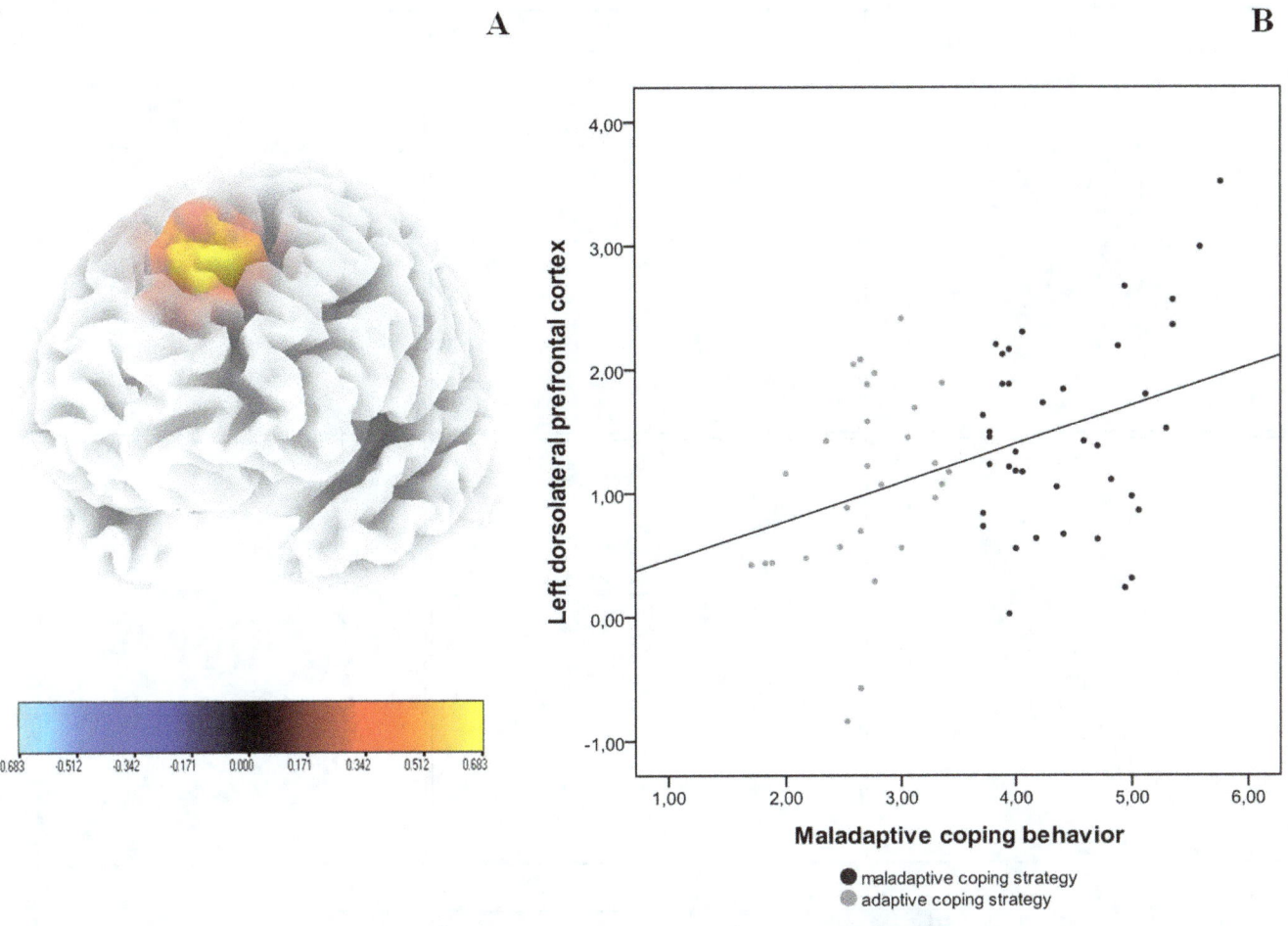

Figure 3. (A) A significant positive correlation between maladaptive coping behavior and alpha1 activity in the left dorsolateral prefrontal cortex on whole brain analysis. (B) A significant positive correlation after a ROI analysis between the left DLPFC (BA9/46) and maladaptive coping behavior.

Differences within the default network between tinnitus patients groups with maladaptive vs. adaptive coping styles

Connectivity analysis yielded in a significant difference ($p<.05$) between maladaptive and adaptive tinnitus patients for the alpha2 frequency band (Figure 4). Increased lagged phase coherence could be found in general for tinnitus patients using a maladaptive coping style in comparison to tinnitus patients using an adaptive coping style in default network extending to the sgACC. No significant effects were obtained for delta, theta, alpha1, beta1, beta2, beta3 and gamma.

Correlation analysis: Default network of maladaptive coping behavior

A correlation analysis between lagged phase coherence and maladaptive coping behavior revealed significant effects for the alpha 1 and alpha2 default network (Figure 5 A & B) which also includes the sgACC. No significant effects were obtained for the other frequency bands (delta, theta, beta1, beta2, beta3 and gamma). Similar analyses were conducted between lagged phase coherence and BDI, TQ, VAS loudness, Age for alpha 1 and alpha2. These additional analyses revealed no significant effects.

Discussion

In the present study, we examined cortical differences in resting-state EEG activity between tinnitus patients who use an adaptive coping style versus those who use a maladaptive coping style.

Coping behavior and style

We demonstrated that the Tinnitus Coping Style Questionnaire is a reliable and valid questionnaire measuring coping behavior on three dimensions, namely *maladaptive*, *active* and *passive* coping behavior. These three factors are similar to previous research on tinnitus coping [8] or coping with general life stress [42]. Furthermore, we found that tinnitus loudness, tinnitus distress, BDI, the different subscales of the TQ, and the total score of the TQ correlated positively with maladaptive coping behavior, but not with active and passive coping. This finding is in line with earlier studies investigating the relationship between TCSQ results and tinnitus related handicap [26].

Based on these three coping behaviors a cluster analysis indicated that some tinnitus patients apply an adaptive coping style, while others apply a maladaptive coping style. The latter group had higher scores on maladaptive coping behavior, but not on active and passive coping behavior. The tinnitus patients using a maladaptive coping style are characterized by increased scores

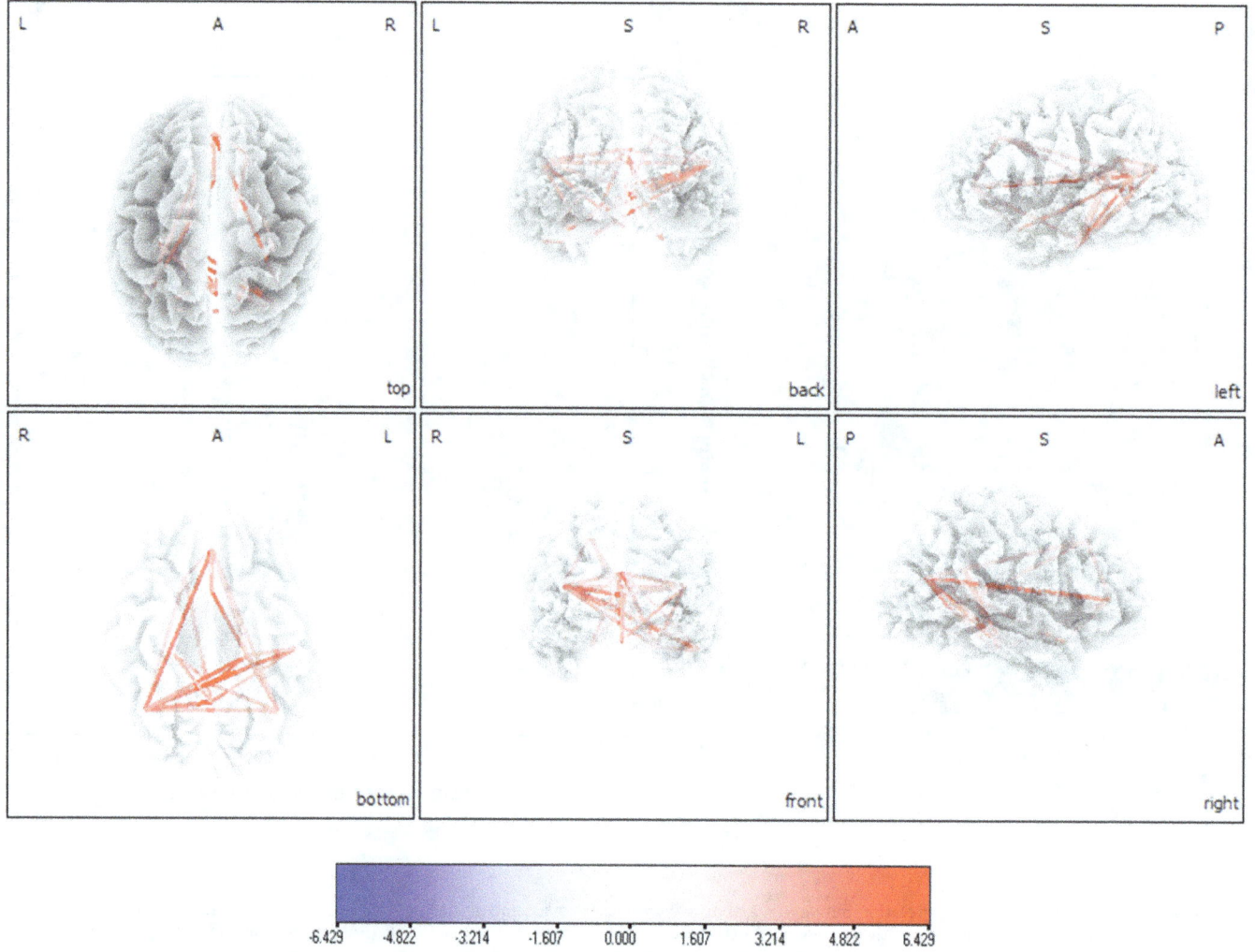

Figure 4. Connectivity analysis (lagged phase synchronization) yielded in a significant difference (*p*<.05) between maladaptive and adaptive tinnitus patients for the alpha2 frequency band. Increased lagged phase coherence could be found in general for tinnitus patients using a maladaptive coping style in comparison to tinnitus patients using an adaptive coping style in default network extending to the sgACC.

on the depression scale, tinnitus questionnaire, and experienced their tinnitus as louder and more distressing in comparison to tinnitus patients using an adaptive coping style. This fits with previous results that showed that a maladaptive coping style is linked with increased depression [43]. It is possible that tinnitus patients suffering from depression are not able to use adaptive coping styles or, vice versa, the inability to use adaptive coping could lead to depression. It is known that depressive patients use maladaptive coping styles more frequently in comparison to healthy subjects [44]. These encompass rumination about negative affect, catastrophizing and self-blame in response to negative events. However, further longitudinal research is needed to have a better understanding on how coping styles relate to coping with tinnitus and its relationship with depression.

Coping behavior, style, and the neural correlates

Activity changes were obtained in the left DLPFC and sgACC alpha 1 and alpha 2 frequency band. Our results indicated increased activity when patients applied a maladaptive coping strategy in comparison to adaptive coping strategy. A positive association was found between increased alpha1 activity in the left DLPFC with maladaptive coping behavior and a positive

association was found between alpha2 activity in the sgACC and tinnitus related distress and depressive feelings. Furthermore increased lagged phased synchronization was noted between the default network and sgACC for the alpha2 frequency band for patients using a maladaptive coping style, and the higher the lagged phased synchronization was between different parts of the default network and the sgACC the higher the tinnitus patients scored on maladaptive coping behavior for respectively alpha1 and alpha2 frequency bands.

The involvement of the DLPFC and sgACC in tinnitus is not that rare. Both areas are already discussed in previous studies on tinnitus [19,21]. It is known that the DLPFC plays an important role in anxiety [45], the unpleasantness related to pain [46] and in aversive auditory stimuli [47]. Further support for the involvement of the DLPFC in tinnitus stems from studies using brain stimulation. High frequency rTMS and tDCS of the left DLPFC is capable of reducing tinnitus severity [48–54] as well as enhancing effects of temporal cortex rTMS [55]. In addition, previous research has demonstrated that the distress network in tinnitus is characterized by increased alpha activity in the sgACC [16,19,20]. Highly distressed tinnitus patients have increased alpha activity within the sgACC in comparison to tinnitus patients with

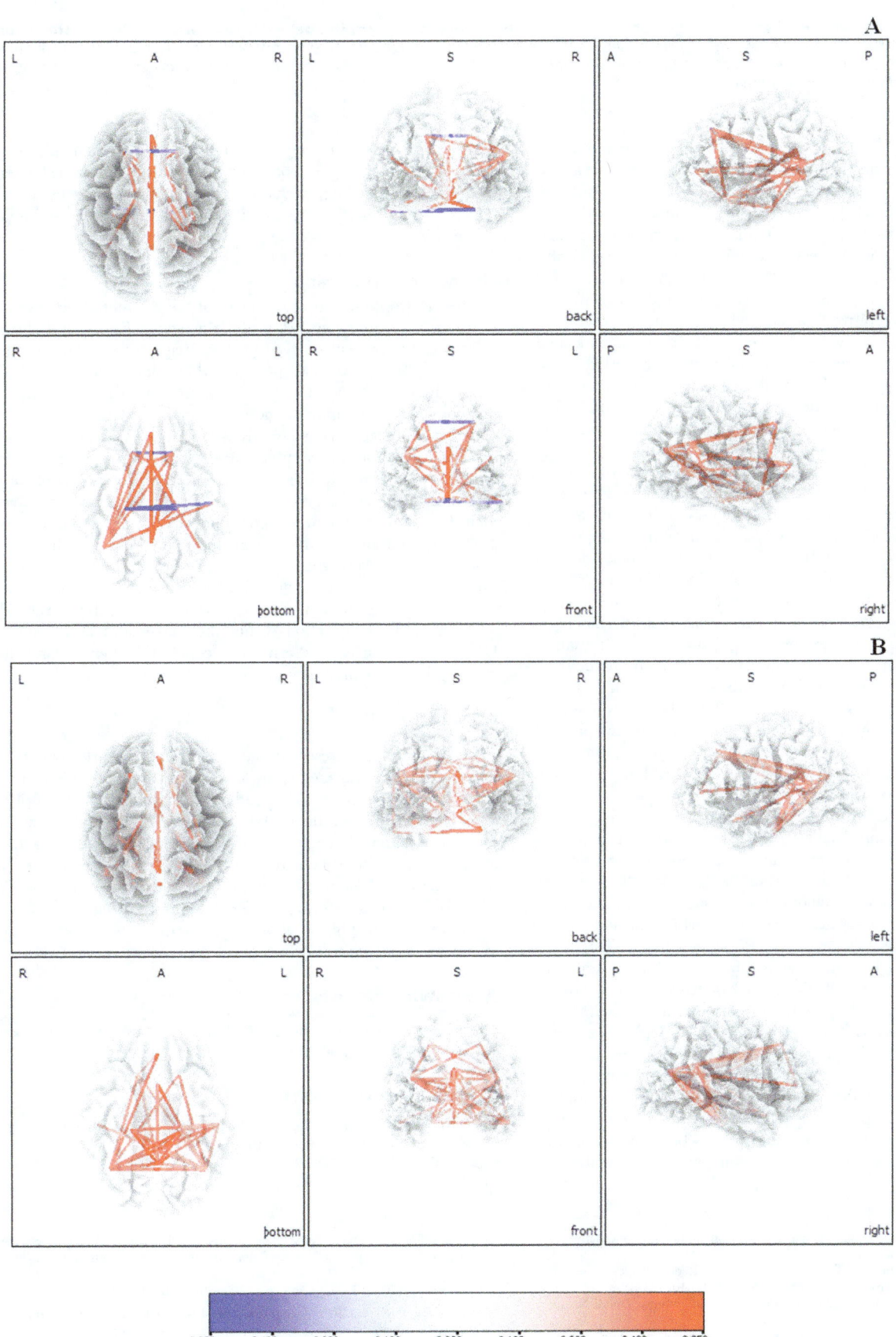

Figure 5. A correlation analysis between lagged phase coherence and maladaptive coping behavior revealed significant effects for the alpha 1 and alpha2 default network. (A) Increased functional connectivity (lagged phase synchronization) correlated with maladaptive behavior for the default network in Alpha1. (B) Increased functional connectivity (lagged phase synchronization) correlated with maladaptive behavior for the default network in Alpha2.

low distress [16,19,20]. Furthermore there is an increased functional connectivity between the parahippocampal area and the sgACC at 10 Hz and 11.5 Hz in grade III and grade IV distress respectively [16]. The sgACC has gained considerable attention both for its putative role in a mood-regulation circuit and for its specific role in depression [25,56], pain distress [57,58], distress in asthmatic dyspnea [59,60], and distress in functional somatic syndromes such as electro-sensitivity for mobile phones [61], social rejection distress [10], as well as tinnitus [19,62]. In the depression literature activation of the sgACC has been associated with autonomic responses of emotional processing during rumination and brooding [11]. Our findings are in agreement with this previous research and add the important role of these brain areas in tinnitus specifically when patients apply a maladaptive coping style.

Our findings indicate that increased maladaptive coping behavior is associated with an increased resting state functional connectivity in the default network in tinnitus patients and is connected to sgACC. The sgACC is considered an important dysfunctional node in MDD [25,56,63] and associated with functional connectivity increases with increasing length of depressive episode. A 'hyper'-connectivity in the default system extending to the sgACC during resting state in MDD has been associated to depressive rumination [25,56,63] or rumination during idle moments [11]. This corroborates with our findings and suggests that the resting-state signal in the sgACC region may be a marker for refractoriness to treatment [25]. The involvement of the sgACC is in agreement with the recent tinnitus model introduced by Rauschecker et al. [62] suggesting that the sgACC/ventromedial prefrontal cortex might be a central hub in tinnitus and that this limbic structure shows a stronger hyperactivity and structural differences in tinnitus patients than the auditory cortex in comparison to control subjects [17]. It is known that subgenual region is extremely rich in serotonin transporters and is considered as a governor for a vast network. Rauschecker and colleagues [62] reinvoked the serotonin hypothesis that suggested that tinnitus goes together with a serotonin depletion [64,65] in addition to hypersensitivity to noise reduced REM sleep and depression [66,67]. Interestingly, recent research revealed that serotonin depletion in animals within the medial prefrontal cortex induces stress and passive coping [68]. Furthermore the default mode network is involved in self-referential processing [69], mind-wandering [70], thinking about the future [71] and the past [72], as well as in goal directed cognition, coping and goal directed behavior [73]. When the sgACC, which is involved in tinnitus loudness and distress processing [16,17,19–21,62], becomes tightly coupled to this default network, the tinnitus becomes coupled to the mind-wandering and self-referential processing resulting in

tinnitus related ruminating [74]. This coupling potentially also explains why maladaptive coopers perceive their tinnitus as louder as the noise cancelling mechanism is possibly inhibited by alpha activity, which can have an inhibitory function in the auditory system [75].

The role of alpha band

The electrophysiological correlate of self-referential processing in the default mode network is alpha activity [76–78], and alpha activity correlates with fMRI BOLD activity in the default mode network [79,80]. During periods when attention is focused internally (mind wandering) there is more neural phase synchronization between brain regions associated with the default network, whereas during periods when subjects are focused on performing a more neural phase synchrony within a task-specific brain network is noted [81]. As in maladaptive coping people are constantly ruminating about their tinnitus, it seems logical that their default mode system is hyper-connected in the default mode's physiological frequency and that the more they ruminate the more alpha synchronization they have in the DMN. If this is corrected it can be predicted that in a study that looks at the percentage of the time that patients focus on their tinnitus in a day will be correlated with alpha synchronization within the DMN and between the DMN and the sgACC. We need to conduct further research to explore this latter proposition.

Conclusion

In summary, the present findings add to prior work suggesting that the DLPFC and sgACC are involved in tinnitus patients who use a maladaptive coping style leading to the probability to display more distressed and depressed behavior. Our results extend previous research in the field of depression by demonstrating that maladaptive coping style is related to alpha "hyper"-connectivity within the default network during rest as well as with the sgACC. The strength of the connectivity is related to focusing on negative mood and catastrophizing about the consequences of tinnitus (i.e. maladaptive coping behavior).

Acknowledgments

The authors thank Jan Ost, Bram Van Achteren, Bjorn Devree and Pieter van Looy for their help in preparing this manuscript.

Author Contributions

Conceived and designed the experiments: SV DDR. Performed the experiments: SV DDR. Analyzed the data: SV WTT DDR. Wrote the paper: SV KJ BL WTT DDR.

References

1. Jastreboff PJ (1990) Phantom auditory perception (tinnitus): mechanisms of generation and perception. Neurosci Res 8: 221–254.
2. Muhlnickel W, Elbert T, Taub E, Flor H (1998) Reorganization of auditory cortex in tinnitus. Proc Natl Acad Sci U S A 95: 10340–10343.
3. Eggermont JJ, Roberts LE (2004) The neuroscience of tinnitus. Trends Neurosci 27: 676–682.
4. Axelsson A, Ringdahl A (1989) Tinnitus–a study of its prevalence and characteristics. Br J Audiol 23: 53–62.
5. Langguth B, Landgrebe M, Kleinjung T, Sand GP, Hajak G (2011) Tinnitus and depression. World J Biol Psychiatry 12: 489–500.

6. Scott B, Lindberg P (2000) Psychological profile and somatic complaints between help-seeking and non-help-seeking tinnitus subjects. Psychosomatics 41: 347–352.
7. Moller AR (2007) Tinnitus and pain. Prog Brain Res 166: 47–53.
8. Budd RJ, Pugh R (1995) The relationship between locus of control, tinnitus severity, and emotional distress in a group of tinnitus sufferers. J Psychosom Res 39: 1015–1018.
9. Vanneste S, De Ridder D (2012) The use of alcohol as a moderator for tinnitus-related distress. Brain Topogr 25: 97–105.

10. Kross E, Davidson M, Weber J, Ochsner K (2009) Coping with emotions past: the neural bases of regulating affect associated with negative autobiographical memories. Biol Psychiatry 65: 361–366.

11. Berman MG, Peltier S, Nee DE, Kross E, Deldin PJ, et al. (2010) Depression, rumination and the default network. Soc Cogn Affect Neurosci.

12. Drevets WC, Price JL, Furey ML (2008) Brain structural and functional abnormalities in mood disorders: implications for neurocircuitry models of depression. Brain Struct Funct 213: 93–118.

13. Mayberg HS (1997) Limbic-cortical dysregulation: a proposed model of depression. J Neuropsychiatry Clin Neurosci 9: 471–481.

14. Sheline YI, Barch DM, Price JL, Rundle MM, Vaishnavi SN, et al. (2009) The default mode network and self-referential processes in depression. Proc Natl Acad Sci U S A 106: 1942–1947.

15. Abler B, Hofer C, Viviani R (2008) Habitual emotion regulation strategies and baseline brain perfusion. Neuroreport 19: 21–24.

16. Vanneste S, Congedo M, De Ridder D (2013) Pinpointing a Highly Specific Pathological Functional Connection That Turns Phantom Sound into Distress. Cereb Cortex.

17. Leaver AM, Renier L, Chevillet MA, Morgan S, Kim HJ, et al. (2011) Dysregulation of limbic and auditory networks in tinnitus. Neuron 69: 33–43.

18. Muhlau M, Rauschecker JP, Oestreicher E, Gaser C, Rottinger M, et al. (2006) Structural brain changes in tinnitus. Cereb Cortex 16: 1283–1288.

19. Vanneste S, Plazier M, der Loo E, de Heyning PV, Congedo M, et al. (2010) The neural correlates of tinnitus-related distress. Neuroimage 52: 470–480.

20. De Ridder D, Vanneste S, Congedo M (2011) The distressed brain: a group blind source separation analysis on tinnitus. PLoS One 6: e24273.

21. Joos K, Vanneste S, De Ridder D (2012) Disentangling depression and distress networks in the tinnitus brain. PLoS One 7: e40544.

22. Baliki MN, Geha PY, Apkarian AV, Chialvo DR (2008) Beyond feeling: chronic pain hurts the brain, disrupting the default-mode network dynamics. J Neurosci 28: 1398–1403.

23. Christoff K, Gordon AM, Smallwood J, Smith R, Schooler JW (2009) Experience sampling during fMRI reveals default network and executive system contributions to mind wandering. Proc Natl Acad Sci U S A 106: 8719–8724.

24. Hamilton JP, Furman DJ, Chang C, Thomason ME, Dennis E, et al. (2011) Default-Mode and Task-Positive Network Activity in Major Depressive Disorder: Implications for Adaptive and Maladaptive Rumination. Biol Psychiatry.

25. Greicius MD, Flores BH, Menon V, Glover GH, Solvason HB, et al. (2007) Resting-state functional connectivity in major depression: abnormally increased contributions from subgenual cingulate cortex and thalamus. Biol Psychiatry 62: 429–437.

26. Budd RJ, Pugh R (1996) Tinnitus coping style and its relationship to tinnitus severity and emotional distress. J Psychosom Res 41: 327–335.

27. Bijttebier P, Vertommen H (1997) Psychometric properties of the Coping Strategy Indicator in a Flemish sample. Personality and Individual Differences 23: 157–160.

28. Carver CS, Scheier MF, Weintraub JK (1989) Assessing coping strategies: a theoretically based approach. J Pers Soc Psychol 56: 267–283.

29. Meeus O, Blaivie C, Van de Heyning P (2007) Validation of the Dutch and the French version of the Tinnitus Questionnaire. B-ENT 3 Suppl 7: 11–17.

30. Goebel G, Hiller W (1994) [The tinnitus questionnaire. A standard instrument for grading the degree of tinnitus. Results of a multicenter study with the tinnitus questionnaire]. HNO 42: 166–172.

31. Bouman T, Luteijn F, Albersnagel FA, van der Ploeg FAE (1985) Enige ervaringen met de Beck Depression Inventory. Gedrag – Tijdschrift voor psychologie 13: 13–24.

32. Congedo M (2002) EureKa! (Version 3.0) [Computer Software]. Knoxville, TN: NovaTech EEG Inc. Available: www.NovaTechEEG.

33. Pascual-Marqui RD (2002) Standardized low-resolution brain electromagnetic tomography (sLORETA): technical details. Methods Find Exp Clin Pharmacol 24 Suppl D: 5–12.

34. Fuchs M, Kastner J, Wagner M, Hawes S, Ebersole JS (2002) A standardized boundary element method volume conductor model. Clin Neurophysiol 113: 702–712.

35. Jurcak V, Tsuzuki D, Dan I (2007) 10/20, 10/10, and 10/5 systems revisited: their validity as relative head-surface-based positioning systems. Neuroimage 34: 1600–1611.

36. Congedo M, John RE, De Ridder D, Prichep L, Isenhart R (2010) On the "dependence" of "independent" group EEG sources; an EEG study on two large databases. Brain Topogr 23: 134–138.

37. Pascual-Marqui R (2007) Instantaneous and lagged measurements of linear and nonlinear dependence between groups of multivariate time series: frequency decomposition. Available: http://arxiv.org/abs/0711.1455.

38. Pascual-Marqui RD, Lehmann D, Koukkou M, Kochi K, Anderer P, et al. (2011) Assessing interactions in the brain with exact low-resolution electromagnetic tomography. Philos Transact A Math Phys Eng Sci 369: 3768–3784.

39. Fox MD, Snyder AZ, Vincent JL, Corbetta M, Van Essen DC, et al. (2005) The human brain is intrinsically organized into dynamic, anticorrelated functional networks. Proc Natl Acad Sci U S A 102: 9673–9678.

40. Nichols TE, Holmes AP (2002) Nonparametric permutation tests for functional neuroimaging: a primer with examples. Hum Brain Mapp 15: 1–25.

41. Cohen J, Cohen P, West SG, Aiken LS (2003) Applied Multiple Regression/Correlation Analysis for the Behavioral Sciences (3rd edition). Mahwah, NJ.: Lawrence Earlbaum Associates.

42. Schwarzer R, Schwarzer C (1995) A critical survey on coping instruments. In: Zeidner M, Endler NS, editors. Handbook of coping: theory, research, applications. New York: John Wiley & Sons.

43. Fletcher K, Parker GB, Manicavasagar V (2013) Coping profiles in bipolar disorder. Compr Psychiatry.

44. Green MJ, Lino BJ, Hwang EJ, Sparks A, James C, et al. (2011) Cognitive regulation of emotion in bipolar I disorder and unaffected biological relatives. Acta Psychiatr Scand 124: 307–316.

45. Fregni F, Marcondes R, Boggio PS, Marcolin MA, Rigonatti SP, et al. (2006) Transient tinnitus suppression induced by repetitive transcranial magnetic stimulation and transcranial direct current stimulation. Eur J Neurol 13: 996–1001.

46. Freund W, Stuber G, Wunderlich AP, Schmitz B (2007) Cortical correlates of perception and suppression of electrically induced pain. Somatosens Mot Res 24: 203–212.

47. Mirz F, Gjedde A, Ishizu K, Pedersen CB (2000) Cortical networks subserving the perception of tinnitus–a PET study. Acta Otolaryngol Suppl 543: 241–243.

48. Piccirillo JF, Kallogjeri D, Nicklaus J, Wineland A, Spitznagel EL, Jr., et al. (2013) Low-frequency repetitive transcranial magnetic stimulation to the temporoparietal junction for tinnitus: four-week stimulation trial. JAMA Otolaryngol Head Neck Surg 139: 388–395.

49. Frank E, Schecklmann M, Landgrebe M, Burger J, Kreuzer P, et al. (2011) Treatment of chronic tinnitus with repeated sessions of prefrontal transcranial direct current stimulation: outcomes from an open-label pilot study. J Neurol.

50. Faber M, Vanneste S, Fregni F, De Ridder D (2011) Top down prefrontal affective modulation of tinnitus with multiple sessions of tDCS of dorsolateral prefrontal cortex. Brain Stimul.

51. Plazier M, Joos K, Vanneste S, Ost J, De Ridder D (2011) Bifrontal and biooccipital transcranial direct current stimulation (tDCS) does not induce mood changes in healthy volunteers: a placebo controlled study. Brain Stimul.

52. Vanneste S, Focquaert F, Van de Heyning P, De Ridder D (2011) Different resting state brain activity and functional connectivity in patients who respond and not respond to bifrontal tDCS for tinnitus suppression. Exp Brain Res 210: 217–227.

53. Vanneste S, Langguth B, De Ridder D (2011) Do tDCS and TMS influence tinnitus transiently via a direct cortical and indirect somatosensory modulating effect? A combined TMS-tDCS and TENS study. Brain Stimul 4: 242–252.

54. Vanneste S, Plazier M, Ost J, van der Loo E, Van de Heyning P, et al. (2010) Bilateral dorsolateral prefrontal cortex modulation for tinnitus by transcranial direct current stimulation: a preliminary clinical study. Exp Brain Res 202: 779–785.

55. Kleinjung T, Eichhammer P, Landgrebe M, Sand P, Hajak G, et al. (2008) Combined temporal and prefrontal transcranial magnetic stimulation for tinnitus treatment: a pilot study. Otolaryngol Head Neck Surg 138: 497–501.

56. Cooney RE, Joormann J, Eugene F, Dennis EL, Gotlib IH (2010) Neural correlates of rumination in depression. Cogn Affect Behav Neurosci 10: 470–478.

57. Price DD (2000) Psychological and neural mechanisms of the affective dimension of pain. Science 288: 1769–1772.

58. Moisset X, Bouhassira D (2007) Brain imaging of neuropathic pain. Neuroimage 37 Suppl 1: S80–88.

59. von Leupoldt A, Sommer T, Kegat S, Eippert F, Baumann HJ, et al. (2009) Down-regulation of insular cortex responses to dyspnea and pain in asthma. Am J Respir Crit Care Med 180: 232–238.

60. von Leupoldt A, Sommer T, Kegat S, Baumann HJ, Klose H, et al. (2009) Dyspnea and pain share emotion-related brain network. Neuroimage 48: 200–206.

61. Landgrebe M, Frick U, Hauser S, Hajak G, Langguth B (2009) Association of tinnitus and electromagnetic hypersensitivity: hints for a shared pathophysiology? PLoS One 4: e5026.

62. Rauschecker JP, Leaver AM, Muhlau M (2010) Tuning out the noise: limbic-auditory interactions in tinnitus. Neuron 66: 819–826.

63. Botteron KN, Raichle ME, Drevets WC, Heath AC, Todd RD (2002) Volumetric reduction in left subgenual prefrontal cortex in early onset depression. Biol Psychiatry 51: 342–344.

64. Dobie RA (2003) Depression and tinnitus. Otolaryngol Clin North Am 36: 383–388.

65. Simpson JJ, Davies WE (2000) A review of evidence in support of a role for 5-HT in the perception of tinnitus. Hear Res 145: 1–7.

66. Geyer MA, Vollenweider FX (2008) Serotonin research: contributions to understanding psychoses. Trends Pharmacol Sci 29: 445–453.

67. Marriage J, Barnes NM (1995) Is central hyperacusis a symptom of 5-hydroxytryptamine (5-HT) dysfunction? J Laryngol Otol 109: 915–921.

68. Andolina D, Maran D, Valzania A, Conversi D, Puglisi-Allegra S (2013) Prefrontal/amygdalar system determines stress coping behavior through 5-HT/GABA connection. Neuropsychopharmacology 38: 2057–2067.

69. Gusnard DA, Akbudak E, Shulman GL, Raichle ME (2001) Medial prefrontal cortex and self-referential mental activity: relation to a default mode of brain function. Proc Natl Acad Sci U S A 98: 4259–4264.

70. Mason MF, Norton MI, Van Horn JD, Wegner DM, Grafton ST, et al. (2007) Wandering minds: the default network and stimulus-independent thought. Science 315: 393–395.

71. Buckner RL, Andrews-Hanna JR, Schacter DL (2008) The brain's default network: anatomy, function, and relevance to disease. Ann N Y Acad Sci 1124: 1–38.

72. Schacter DL (2012) Constructive memory: past and future. Dialogues Clin Neurosci 14: 7–18.

73. Schacter DL, Addis DR, Hassabis D, Martin VC, Spreng RN, et al. (2012) The future of memory: remembering, imagining, and the brain. Neuron 76: 677–694.

74. Nejad AB, Fossati P, Lemogne C (2013) Self-Referential Processing, Rumination, and Cortical Midline Structures in Major Depression. Front Hum Neurosci 7: 666.

75. Weisz N, Hartmann T, Muller N, Lorenz I, Obleser J (2011) Alpha rhythms in audition: cognitive and clinical perspectives. Front Psychol 2: 73.

76. Knyazev GG (2012) Extraversion and anterior vs. posterior DMN activity during self-referential thoughts. Front Hum Neurosci 6: 348.

77. Knyazev GG (2012) EEG delta oscillations as a correlate of basic homeostatic and motivational processes. Neurosci Biobehav Rev 36: 677–695.

78. Knyazev GG, Slobodskoj-Plusnin JY, Bocharov AV, Pylkova LV (2011) The default mode network and EEG alpha oscillations: an independent component analysis. Brain Res 1402: 67–79.

79. Jann K, Dierks T, Boesch C, Kottlow M, Strik W, et al. (2009) BOLD correlates of EEG alpha phase-locking and the fMRI default mode network. Neuroimage 45: 903–916.

80. Mo J, Liu Y, Huang H, Ding M (2013) Coupling between visual alpha oscillations and default mode activity. Neuroimage 68: 112–118.

81. Kirschner A, Kam JW, Handy TC, Ward LM (2012) Differential synchronization in default and task-specific networks of the human brain. Front Hum Neurosci 6: 139.

22

Brain Areas Controlling Heart Rate Variability in Tinnitus and Tinnitus-Related Distress

Sven Vanneste[1,2]*, Dirk De Ridder[1]

1 Brai²n, Tinnitus Research Initiative Clinic Antwerp & Department of Neurosurgery, University Hospital Antwerp, Antwerp, Belgium, **2** Department of Translational Neuroscience, Faculty of Medicine, University of Antwerp, Antwerp, Belgium

Abstract

Background: Tinnitus is defined as an intrinsic sound perception that cannot be attributed to an external sound source. Distress in tinnitus patients is related to increased beta activity in the dorsal part of the anterior cingulate and the amount of distress correlates with network activity consisting of the amygdala-anterior cingulate cortex-insula-parahippocampus. Previous research also revealed that distress is associated to a higher sympathetic (OS) tone in tinnitus patients and tinnitus suppression to increased parasympathetic (PS) tone.

Methodology: The aim of the present study is to investigate the relationship between tinnitus distress and the autonomic nervous system and find out which cortical areas are involved in the autonomic nervous system influences in tinnitus distress by the use of source localized resting state electroencephalogram (EEG) recordings and electrocardiogram (ECG). Twenty-one tinnitus patients were included in this study.

Conclusions: The results indicate that the dorsal and subgenual anterior cingulate, as well as the left and right insula are important in the central control of heart rate variability in tinnitus patients. Whereas the sympathovagal balance is controlled by the subgenual and pregenual anterior cingulate cortex, the right insula controls sympathetic activity and the left insula the parasympathetic activity. The perceived distress in tinnitus patients seems to be sympathetically mediated.

Editor: Mathias Baumert, University of Adelaide, Australia

Funding: This work was supported by Research Foundation Flanders (FWO). The funders had no role in study design, data collection and analysis, decision to publish, or preparation of the manuscript.

Competing Interests: The authors have declared that no competing interests exist.

* E-mail: sven.vanneste@ua.ac.be

Introduction

Tinnitus is defined as an intrinsic sound perception that cannot be attributed to an external sound source. This phantom perception is a common disorder. The American Tinnitus Association estimates that 50 million Americans are affected by it, and that 12 million of these people seek medical attention because of their tinnitus [1]. In about 6 to 25% of the affected people tinnitus causes a considerable amount of distress [2–4], resulting in about 2–4% of the population who are severely impaired in their quality of life [5]. Tinnitus can interfere with sleep and concentration, social interaction and work [6]. Increased prevalence rates of anxiety and depression are reported among tinnitus patients [7,8].

Distress in tinnitus patients is related to increased beta activity in the dorsal part of the anterior cingulate and the amount of distress correlates with an EEG alpha network activity consisting of the amygdala-anterior cingulate cortex-insula-parahippocampus as demonstrated both by source analysis of Fourier based data [9] and independent component analysis [10]. Using MEG, long-range coupling between frontal, parietal and cingulate brain areas in alpha and gamma phase synchronization has been shown to be related to tinnitus distress [11]. The distress in tinnitus patients also correlates with an increase in incoming and outgoing connections

in the gamma band in the prefrontal cortex and the parieto-occipital region [12].

Adaptation under conditions of stress is a priority for all organisms. Stress can be broadly defined as an actual or anticipated disruption of homeostasis or an anticipated threat to well-being [13]. Stressor-related information from all major sensory systems is conveyed to the brain, which recruits neural and neuroendocrine systems (effectors) to minimize the net cost to the animal. The physiological response to stress involves an efficient and highly conserved set of interlocking systems and aims to maintain physiological integrity even in the most demanding of circumstances [13].

The autonomic nervous system provides the most immediate response to stressor exposure - through its sympathetic and parasympathetic arms, which provoke rapid alterations in physiological states through neural innervation of end organs. The autonomic nervous system is a collection of afferent and efferent neurons that link the central nervous system with visceral effectors. The two efferent arms of the autonomic nervous system - the sympathetic and parasympathetic arms - consist of parallel and differentially regulated pathways made up of cholinergic neurons (preganglionic neurons) located within the central nervous system that innervate ganglia (for example, para- or pre-vertebral sympathetic ganglia), glands (adrenal glands) or neural networks of varying complexity (enteric or cardiac ganglionic networks). These peripheral ganglia and networks contain the motor neurons (ganglionic neurons) that control smooth muscles and other visceral targets. The sympathetic ganglionic neurons that control cardiovascular targets are primarily noradrenergic [14]. The sympatho-adrenomedullary arm can rapidly (in seconds) increase heart rate and blood pressure by exciting the cardiovascular system. Importantly, excitation of the autonomic nervous system wanes quickly - owing to reflex parasympathetic activation - resulting in short-lived responses [13]. Previous research also revealed that distress is associated to a higher sympathetic (OS) tone in tinnitus patients [15] and tinnitus suppression to increased parasympathetic (PS) tone [16]. The heart is dually innervated by the autonomic nervous system such that relative increases in sympathetic activity are associated with heart rate increases and relative increases in parasympathetic activity are associated with heart rate decreases. In addition, human lesion and electrical stimulation studies have revealed that the right insula controls cardiac sympathetic activity whereas the left insula is predominantly associated to parasympathetic activity [17–19].

Heart rate variability (HRV) is a physiological phenomenon where the time interval between heart beats varies. It is measured by the variation in the beat-to-beat interval. HRV is a simple and non-invasive quantitative marker of autonomic function. As a result of continuous variations of the balance between OS and PS neural activity influencing heart rate, intervals between consecutive heartbeats (RR intervals) show spontaneously occurring oscillations. For HRV analysis, a Fourier-based spectral analysis is performed of the beat to beat intervals, yielding two main frequencies: a low frequency range (LF: 0.05–0.15 Hz) and a high frequency range (HF 0.15–0.4 Hz) [20]. The high frequency component of HRV is believed to be influenced by vagal activity and is also related to the frequency of respiration [21]. Low-frequency (LF) power is modulated by baroreceptor activities and fluctuations in heart rate in the LF range reflect OS as well as PS influences. Low-frequency power, therefore, cannot be considered to reflect selective OS activity. However if normalized units of LF and HF are considered, the OS and PS influences respectively are emphasized [20]. In HRV frequency domain, normalized units of LF and HF components therefore reflect OS and PS influences respectively.

In two recent PET studies it was demonstrated that inducing a certain amount of stress, HRV correlates positively with activity in the anterior cingulate cortex, caudate nucleus, insula, medial prefrontal cortex extending into the dorsal prefrontal cortex [22,23]. These areas are also involved in tinnitus related distress [9]. Using similar PET studies, the neural correlates of the HF component (PS) have been delineated as the caudate nucleus, periaqueductal gray and left mid-insula [23], while in fMRI the HF component correlates positively with activity in the hypothalamus, amygdala and anterior hippocampal area, dorsomedial/dorsolateral prefrontal cortex and negatively with the cerebellum, parabrachial nucleus/locus coeruleus, periaqueductal gray, posterior parahippocampal area, thalamus, posterior insular and middle temporal cortices [24]. The left inferior part of the pregenual anterior cingulate cortex also correlates with the HF component of the HRV [25]. The increased LF/HF-ratio (in rectal distension) is correlated with activity in the bilateral insula, putamen, thalamus, midbrain, pons, and cerebellum [26].

The aim of the present study is to investigate the relationship between tinnitus distress and the autonomic nervous system and find out which cortical areas are involved in the autonomic nervous system influences in tinnitus distress by the use of source

localized resting state electroencephalogram (EEG) recordings and electrocardiogram (ECG).

Quantitative analysis of EEG is a low-cost and useful neurophysiological approach to study the brain physiology and pathology [27]. Cortical sources of the EEG rhythms were estimated by standardized low-resolution brain electromagnetic tomography (sLORETA) [28]. sLORETA is a functional imaging technique estimating maximally smoothed linear inverse solutions accounting for distributed EEG sources within Montreal Neurological Institute (MNI) space [28]. This feature is of special importance for the comparison of EEG results with those of most structural and functional neuroimaging studies. sLORETA has been successfully used in recent EEG studies on tinnitus [29]. In this study we investigate which brain areas are involved in tinnitus distress and in the autonomic nervous system control of the distress.

Materials and Methods

Participants

Twenty-one patients (N = 21; 15 males and 6 females) with a mean age of 47.44 (Sd = 12.72 were selected from the multidisciplinary Tinnitus Research Initiative (TRI) Clinic of the University Hospital of Antwerp, Belgium. Tinnitus lateralization and tinnitus type was verified by asking the patient in which ear they perceived the tinnitus and whether they perceived a tone or a noise-like sound. Six patients presented with unilateral tinnitus and 15 patients with bilateral tinnitus. Nine patients perceived a pure tone phantom sound and 16 patients a narrow band noise (hearing a noise-like tone within a certain frequency range). No patients included in the study perceived their tinnitus centrally in the head. Individuals with pulsatile tinnitus, Ménière's disease, otosclerosis, chronic headache, neurological disorders such as brain tumors, and individuals being treated for mental disorders were not included in the study.

Participants were requested to refrain from alcohol consumption 24 hours prior to recording, and from caffeinated beverages consumption on the day of recording. Patients were also given the validated Dutch version of the Tinnitus Questionnaire [30] originally published by Goebel and Hiller [31]. Goebel and Hiller described this TQ as a global index of distress and the Dutch version was further confirmed as a reliable measure for tinnitus-related distress [30,32]. At the moment of the study patients did not take any pharmacological agent.

This study was approved by the local ethical committee (Antwerp University Hospital) and was in accordance with the declaration of Helsinki. Written informed consent was obtained from all patients.

EEG/ECG Data Collection

Recordings (Mitsar-201, NovaTech http://www.novatecheeg.com/) were obtained in a fully lighted room with each participant sitting upright on a small but comfortable chair. The actual recording lasted approximately 5 min. The EEG was sampled with 19 electrodes (Fp1, Fp2, F7, F3, Fz, F4, F8, T7, C3, Cz, C4, T8, P7, P3, Pz, P4, P8, O1 O2) in the standard 10–20 International placement referenced to linked ears and impedances were checked to remain below 5 kΩ. Two ECG electrodes were place on the heart axis. EEG and ECG were measured for 5 minutes. Data were collected eyes-closed (sampling rate = 1024 Hz, band passed 0.15–200 Hz). To minimize respiratory influences on HRV, respiration is controlled at 12 beats per minute using auditory cues (i.e. tone 1000 Hz). We selected auditory cues as this is the standard method when collecting ECG data during eyes closed EEG [33]. No patients indicate that this auditory cue interfered with the tinnitus perception or auditory attention to the tinnitus.

EEG Analysis

Data were resampled to 128 Hz, band-pass filtered (fast Fourier transform filter) to 2–44 Hz and subsequently transposed into Eureka! Software [34], plotted and carefully inspected for manual artifact-rejection. All episodic artifacts including eye blinks, eye movements, teeth clenching, or body movement were removed from the stream of the EEG. Average Fourier cross-spectral matrices were computed for bands delta (2–3.5 Hz), theta (4–7.5 Hz), alpha (8–12 Hz), low beta (13–21 Hz), high beta (21.5–30 Hz) and gamma (30.5–44 Hz) [28,35].

ECG Analysis

ECG signals are processed by frequency domain methods as recommended by the Task force [20]: QRS complexes are recognized from the short-term artifact-free ECG recordings from which peaks (R-waves) are detected and from which intervals between two consecutive peaks (RR intervals) are calculated. Once HRV time series are extracted they are analyzed in frequency domain using HRV Analysis Software 1.1 for windows developed by The Biomedical Signal Analysis Group, Department of Applied Physics, University of Kuopio, Finland (see http://kubios.uku.fi/) and generating low frequency (LF: 05–.15 Hz) and high frequency (HF:.15–.40 Hz). Also the LF/HF-ratio was calculated.

Source Localization

Standardized low-resolution brain electromagnetic tomography (sLORETA) was used to estimate the intracerebral electrical sources that generated the scalp-recorded activity in each of the eight frequency bands [28]. sLORETA computes electric neuronal activity as current density (A/m^2) without assuming a predefined number of active sources. The sLORETA solution space consists of 6239 voxels (voxel size: 5×5×5 mm) and is restricted to cortical gray matter and hippocampi, as defined by digitized MNI152 template [36].

The tomography sLORETA has received considerable validation from studies combining LORETA with other more established localization methods, such as functional Magnetic Resonance Imaging (fMRI) [37,38], structural MRI [39], Positron Emission Tomography (PET) [40–42]. Further sLORETA validation has been based on accepting as ground truth the localization findings obtained from invasive, implanted depth electrodes, in which case there are several studies in epilepsy [43,44] and cognitive ERPs [45]. It is worth emphasizing those deep structures such as the anterior cingulate cortex [46], and mesial temporal lobes [47] can be correctly localized with these methods.

Region of Interest Analysis

The log-transformed electric current density was averaged across all voxels belonging to the region of interest. Regions of interest were defined based on previous brain research on HRV as well as tinnitus related distress. Regions of interest were respectively the left insula (LI) and right insula (RI)(BA13) [9], dorsal anterior cingulate cortex (BA24 left and right) [9] and subgenual anterior cingulate cortex (BA25 left and right) [9], primary (BA41) and secondary (BA21) auditory cortex [48] and the orbitofrontal cortex (BA10) [12]. Region of interest analyses were computed for the different frequency bands separately.

A lateralization index for the insula was calculated for each frequency band,

$$\text{Lateralization index} = \frac{(LI - RI)}{(LI + RI)}$$

where LI and RI are the log-transformed electrical current density in the left and right insula, respectively. This method is similar to Weisz et al. [49]. Pearson Correlations were calculated and corrections for multiple comparisons for the frequency bands (i.e. Bonferroni) were applied.

Statistical Analyses

We conducted a whole brain analysis and region of interest (ROI) analyses. Whole-brain analysis is automated and un-biased, making no assumptions about any regions of particular interest. However, this technique requires a great number of subjects to achieve statistical significance and it is possible that smaller changes may not be easily identified. This is one of the reasons why it is common practice to conduct a secondary ROI analysis, testing for statistically significant differences only in the voxels that are deemed of interest by an *a priori* hypothesis. An ROI analysis

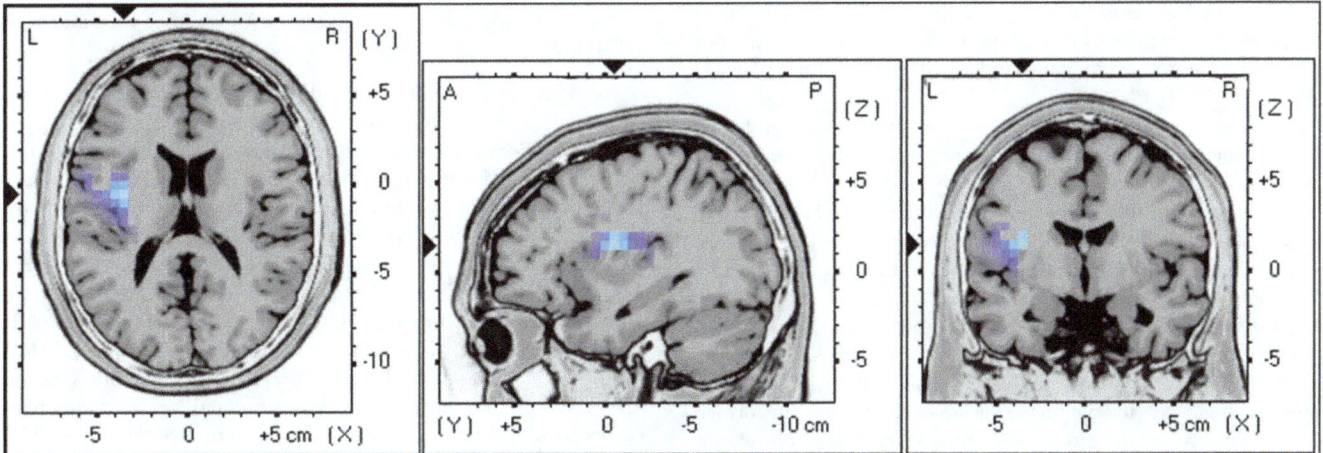

Figure 1. Negative correlation between LF (sympathetic+parasympathetic) HRV and Alpha activity in the left insula (BA13), indicating that decreased alpha activity in the left insula goes together with increased LF-HRV.

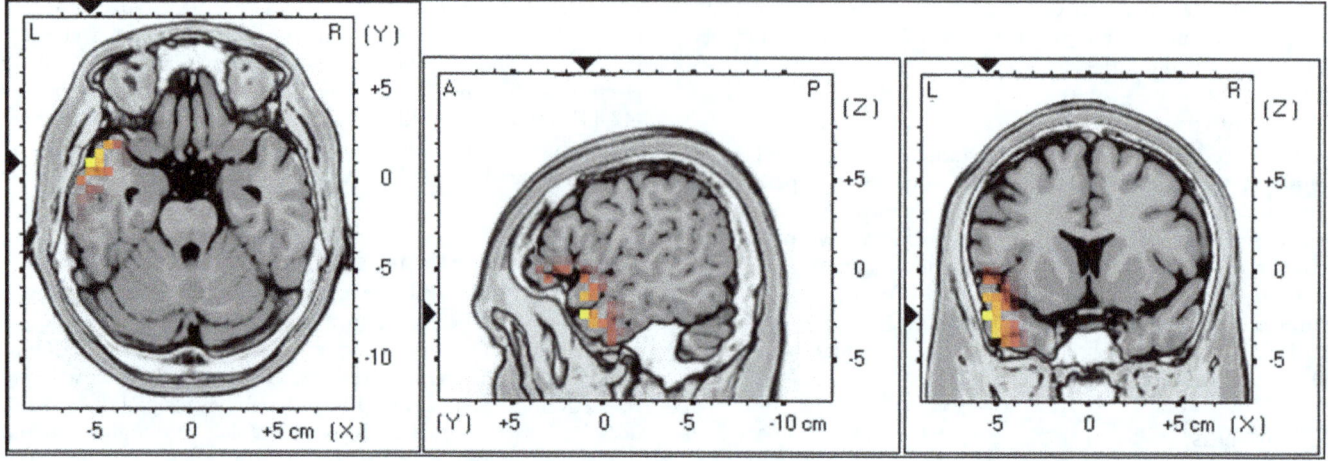

Figure 2. Positive correlation between HF (parasympathetic) HRV and Alpha activity in the rostral portions of the superior temporal gyrus and the middle temporal gyrus (BA21/38). That is increased activity in the rostral portions of the superior temporal gyrus and the middle temporal gyrus goes together with increased HF-HRV.

can be used to corroborate the findings of previous studies, or those obtained during the whole-brain analysis. This is of special importance in studies with a small sample size.

First, correlations are calculated between respectively LF, HF, LF/HF and distress with brain activity (whole brain analysis). The methodology used for the sLORETA correlations is non-parametric. It is based on estimating, via randomization, the empirical probability distribution for the max-statistic, under the null hypothesis comparisons [50]. This methodology corrects for multiple testing (i.e., for the collection of tests performed for all voxels, and for all frequency bands). Due to the non-parametric nature of the method, its validity does not rely on any assumption of Gaussianity [50]. sLORETA statistical contrast maps were calculated through multiple voxel-by-voxel comparisons in a logarithm of F-ratio. The significance threshold was based on a permutation test with 5000 permutations.

Secondly, Pearson correlations are calculated between the lateralization index of the insula and LF/HF-ratio. Based on these findings we conducted a third step, a multivariate ANOVA with LF/HF-ratio and TQ as dependent variables and the lateralization index of the insula in both the alpha and gamma band as independent variables. The reason to include these frequency bands was that both frequency bands correlated with the LF/HF-ratio.

In addition a Pearson correlation analysis was conducted between the dorsal, subgenual and pregenual anterior cingulate cortex, primary and secondary auditory cortex and the orbito-frontal cortex with the respectively the LF, HF, LF/HF-ratio and the TQ, to validate previously obtained results [9,10].

Lastly, we applied a median-split on both the TQ and the LF/HF-ratio. A median split [51] is a data driven post-hoc stratification that allows us to test the group difference between a low versus high TQ (i.e. distress) and low and high LF/HF-ratio. We applied an ANOVA with TQ (low vs. high) and LF/HF-ration (low vs. high) as independent variables and log-transformed current density at the pregenual anterior cingulate cortex for respectively the high beta and gamma band as dependent variable. We opt to do this analysis for the pregenual anterior cingulate cortex as region of interest for these specific frequency bands, as both frequencies correlated with the TQ and LF/HF ratio.

Results

Tinnitus Questionnaire

The mean TQ was 39.22 (Sd = 15.13). No correlation could be found between the TQ and respectively LF, HF and LF/HF-ratio HRV.

Whole Brain and HRV

1. LF-HRV. Analysis of LF-HRV (a combination of sympathetic and parasympathetic activity) and the left insula (BA13) for alpha activity revealed a significant negative correlation (r = −.42, p<.05) indicating that decreased alpha activity in the left insula goes together with increased LF-HRV (see Figure 1).

No significant correlation could be retrieved in delta, theta, low beta, high beta and gamma frequency bands.

2. HF-HRV. Results yielded as a significant positive correlation (r = .68, p<.05) between HF-HRV (i.e. sympathetic activity) and rostral portions of the superior temporal gyrus and the middle temporal gyrus (BA21/38) for alpha activity (see Figure 2). That is increased activity in the rostral portions of the superior temporal gyrus and the middle temporal gyrus goes together with increased HF-HRV.

No significant correlation could be retrieved in delta, theta, low beta, high beta and gamma frequency bands.

3. LF/HF-ratio. Analysis demonstrated a positive correlation between LF/HF-ratio (i.e. high numbers mean dominance of sympathetic activity while low numbers mean dominance of the para-sympathetic activity) and Theta activity (r = .43, p<.05) in the subgenual anterior cingulate cortex (BA25) (see Figure 3a). This correlation indicates that increased activity in the subgenual anterior cingulate cortex goes together with increased LF/HF-ratio. Also a negative correlation was revealed between LF/HF-ratio HRV and high Beta (r = −.45, p<.05) and Gamma (r = −.46, p<.05) activity in the pregenual anterior cingulate cortex (BA24) extending into dorsal lateral prefrontal cortex (BA9) (see Figure 3b&c). This latter correlation shows that decreased activity in the pregenual anterior cingulate cortex goes together with increased LF/HF-ratio. No significant correlation could be retrieved in delta, theta and low beta frequency bands.

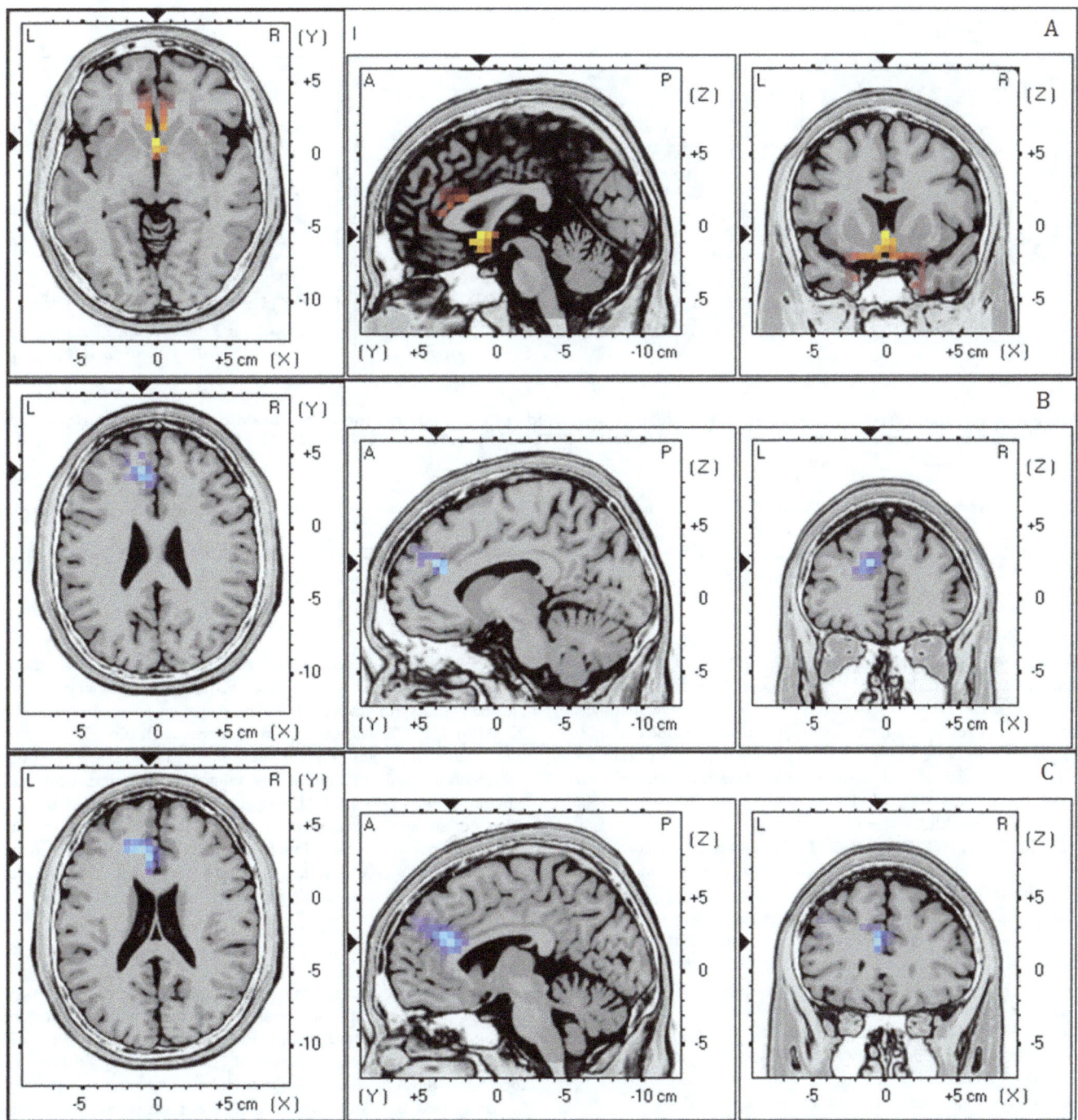

Figure 3. (a) Positive correlation between LF/HF-ratio (sympathetic/parasympathetic ratio) HRV and theta activity in the subgenual anterior cingulate cortex (BA25) (r = .43, *p*<.05); (b) & (c) Negative correlation between LF/HF-ratio HRV and High Beta (r = −.45, *p*<.05) and Gamma activity (r = −.46, *p*<.05) in the left pregenual anterior cingulate cortex (BA24) extending into dorsal lateral prefrontal cortex (BA9).

Whole Brain and Distress

A correlation analysis between the distress as measured with the TQ and the whole brain demonstrated a significant effect for the pregenual/subgenual anterior cingulate cortex (r = .42, *p*<.05 (see Figure 4) for the alpha frequency band. This correlation indicates that increased activity in the anterior cingulate cortex goes together with increased distress. No significant correlation could be retrieved in delta, theta, low and high beta and gamma frequency bands.

Region of Interest Analysis

1. Lateralisation index. Significant negative correlations were found between lateralization index of the insula for Alpha activity and LF/HF-ratio (r = −.45, *p*<.05) and Gamma activity

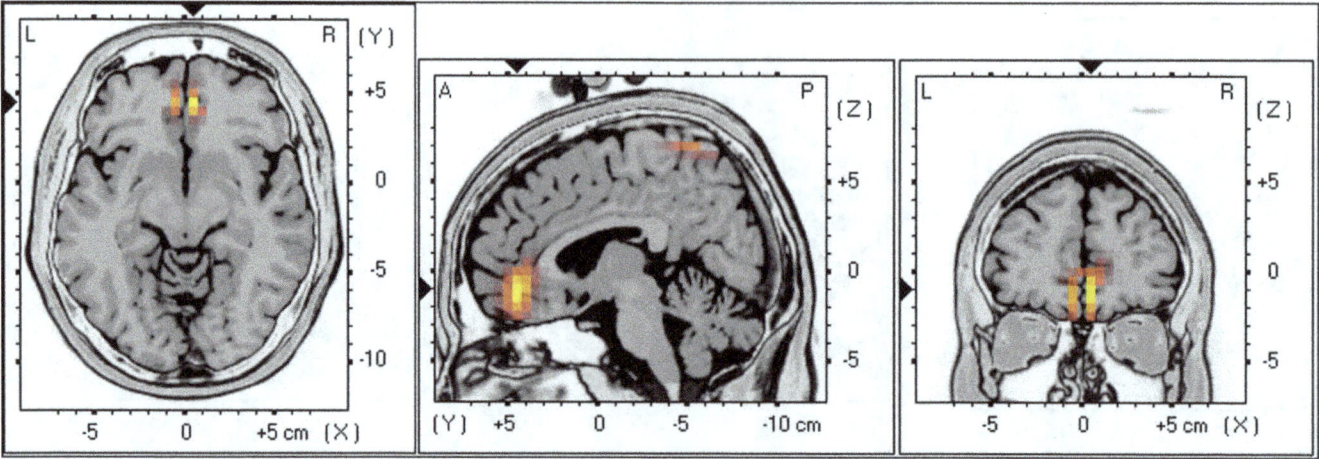

Figure 4. A positive correlation between the distress as measured with the TQ and the whole brain demonstrated a significant effect for the pregenual/subgenual anterior cingulate cortex (BA24/25) (r = .42, p<.05) for the alpha frequency band.

and LF/HF-ratio (r = −.43, p<.05) (see figure 5). In addition, a significant negative correlation was found between lateralization index of the insula for Alpha activity with TQ (r = −.48, p<.05). No significant effects were obtained for the delta, theta, low and high beta frequency bands.

A multivariate ANOVA revealed that both for the lateralization index of the insula for alpha activity (F(2,17) = 11.48, p<.001) and gamma activity (F(2,17) = 4.11, p<.05) could be associated with the TQ and LF/HF–ratio (see figure 5). A test of between-subjects effects further revealed that the alpha lateralisation index could be associated with both TQ (F(1,20) = 5.69, p<.05) and LF/HF-ratio (F(1,20) = 6.01, p<.05), while the gamma lateralisation index could be associated only with LF/HF-ratio (F(1,20) = 3.82, p<.05) and no TQ (F(1,20) = .52, p = .45).

2. LF-HRV, HF-HRV and LF/HR-ratio. A correlation between the LF-HRV, HF-HRV and LF/HR-ratio and respectively the dorsal, pregunal and subgenual anterior cingulate cortex, primary and secondary auditory cortex and the orbitofrontal cortex was computed. This analysis revealed as significant effect for LF/HF with respectively the subgenual anterior cingulate (r = .43, p<.05) for the theta frequency band, the pregenual anterior cingulate cortex for the high beta (r = −.45, p<.05) and gamma (r = −.46, p<.05) frequency band. No significant effects were obtained for primary and secondary auditory cortex and the orbitofrontal cortex.

3. TQ. A significant correlation was obtained for the dorsal anterior cingulate cortex and the TQ for High Beta activity (r = .34, p<.05), while the subgenual anterior cingulate cortex was correlated with Alpha activity (r = .34, p<.01). No significant effects where obtained for the other frequency bands.

No significant effects could be obtained for the orbitofrontal cortex and the primary and secondary auditory cortex.

4. Interaction between HRV and TQ. A marginal significant interaction effect (see figure 6), was obtained between distress (low vs. high) and LF/HF-ratio (low vs. high) for the pregenual anterior cingulate cortex in the high beta (F = 2.93, p = .10) and gamma (F = 3.27, p = .09) frequency band. A detailed analysis demonstrates that patients with a low LF/HF ratio and high distress have a lower current density with these specific frequency bands in the pregenual anterior cingulate cortex in comparison to patients with a low LF/HF ratio and high distress. No difference

was found in comparison to patients with high LF/HF ratio irrespective of low or high distress.

No significant effects were obtained for the delta, theta, alpha and low beta frequency bands.

Discussion

The autonomic nervous system is controlled by the sympathetic and parasympathetic system. The cardiac sympathetic/parasympathetic or sympathovagal balance is reflected by the LF (OS+PS)/HF (PS) ratio [52]. Previous research already revealed the relationship between the autonomic nervous system and specific brain regions such as the subgenual and dorsal anterior cingulate cortex and insula. Interestingly, these brain areas are also involved in tinnitus related distress [9]. The aim of the present study is to investigate the relationship between tinnitus distress and the autonomic nervous system and find out which cortical areas are involved in the autonomic nervous system influences in tinnitus distress.

Heart Rate Variability and the Brain

A negative correlation was demonstrated between LF/HF-ratio and the pregenual anterior cingulate cortex extending into the dorsal lateral prefrontal cortex for respectively high beta and gamma activity. That is, decreased LF and/or increased HF goes together with an intensification of high beta and gamma activity in the pregenual anterior cingulate cortex. A positive correlation has previously been found between neural activity in the pregenual anterior cingulate cortex and the parasympathetically linked HF component of heart rate variability in an anxious population [22] and when performing a Stroop task [25]. Together with the pregenual anterior cingulate also the dorsal lateral prefrontal cortex was involved with regulating LF/HF-ratio. This was similarly to previous research indicating that during social threat the dorsal lateral prefrontal cortex activity appears reduced in social phobia compared to controls [53]. The pregenual anterior cingulate cortex extending into the ventro-medial prefrontal cortex predominantly mediates parasympathetic control [54–56], and the ventromedial prefrontal cortex inactivates sympathetic activity [57], suggesting that the ventromedial prefrontal cortex exerts an predominantly parasympathetic modulation of the sympathovagal balance. This is in accordance with the positive correlation found

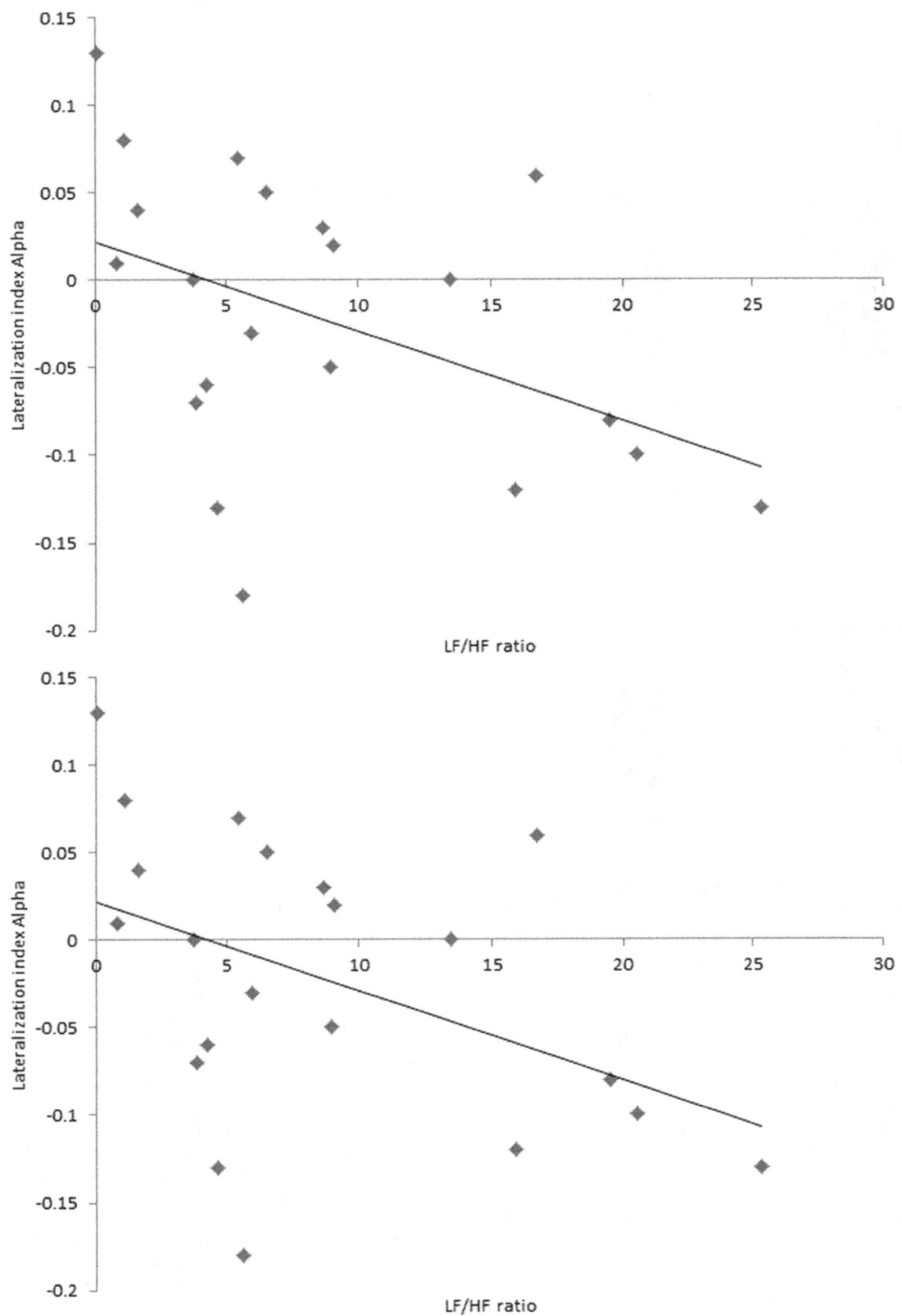

Figure 5. Scatterplots and regression lines for respectively the lateralization index of the insula for Alpha and LF/HF-ratio. Significant negative correlation were found between lateralization tinnitex of the insula for Alpha activity and LF/HF-ratio ($r = -.45$, $p < .05$) and Gamma activity and LF/HF-ratio ($r = -.43$, $p < .05$).

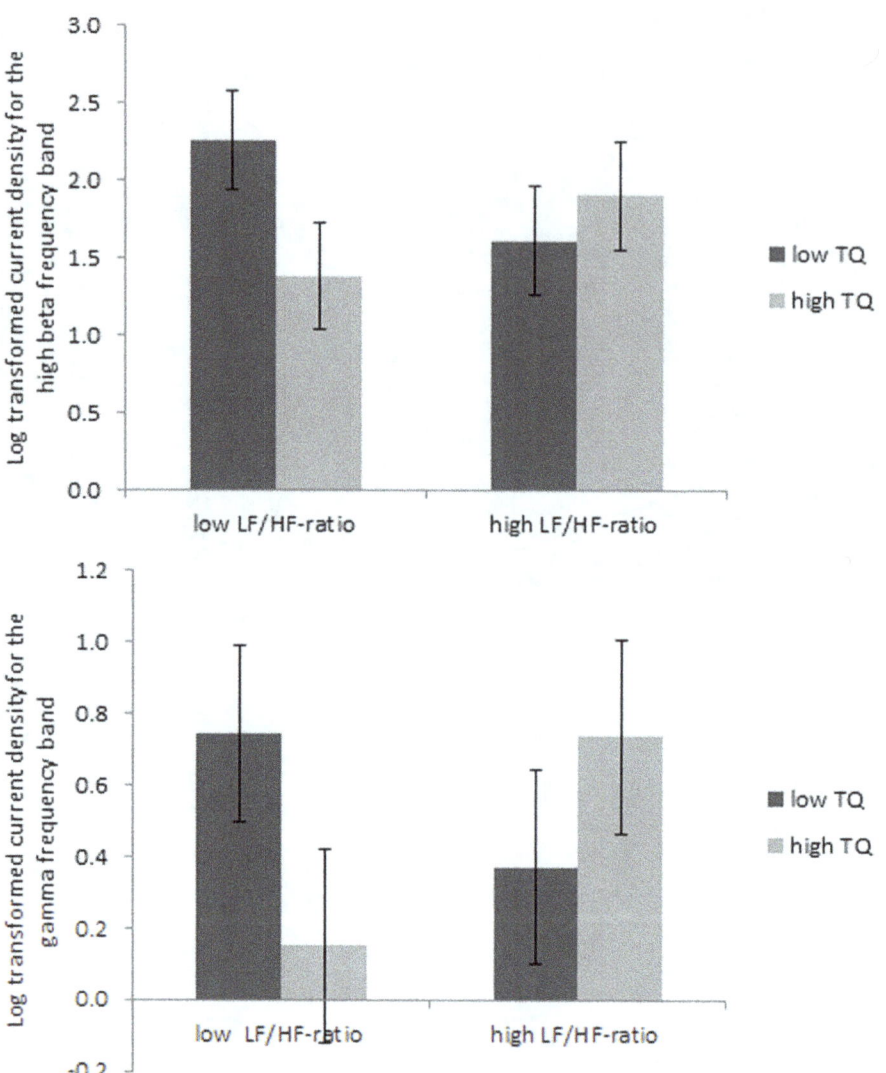

Figure 6. A marginal significant interaction effect between distress (low vs. high) and LF/HF-ratio (low vs. high) for the pregenual anterior cingulate cortex in the high beta ($F=2.93$, $p=.10$) and gamma ($F=3.27$, $p=.09$) frequency band.

between LF/HF-ratio and the subgenual anterior cingulate cortex for theta activity, revealing that increased LF and decrease HF goes together with an increase of theta activity in the subgenual anterior cingulate cortex. A fMRI study also related HRV and sympathetic cardiac influence with the subgenual anterior cingulate cortex [58]. It has also been shown that increased activity in posterior subgenual anterior cingulate cortex extending into nucleus accumbens-ventral tegmental area is involved in processing of aversive sounds [59] and unpleasant music [60] and this area has been implicated in mediating limbic-autonomic interactions in tinnitus as well [61,62]. This area in animals has been considered a visceromotor cortex, due to its connections with the parasympathetic nucleus tractus solitarius [63] and the sympathetic areas in the periaquaductal grey [64]. Furthermore it is functionally connected to the insula and anticorrelated to the dorsal anterior cingulate cortex [65–67]. Dorsal anterior cingulate activity covaries with blood pressure, emotional heart rate changes, cardiac sympathetic tone and pupillary changes [68].

Our results further revealed that increased LF goes together with a decrease in activity in the left insula. Furthermore tinnitus distress correlates negatively with the lateralization index of the

insula for alpha, revealing that increased tinnitus distress is associated with a decrease in the lateralization index in the insula. These findings are in accordance with previous research revealing that increased insular activity is associated with subjective emotional and bodily awareness, as well as interoception [69]. The insula has been implicated in autonomic nervous system control [20,68,70,71] and might therefore be related to the autonomic components involved in distress [72,73], induced by the phantom sound. In a recent study it was further revealed that the insula is involved in pain sensitivity [74]. In addition, a region of interest analysis revealed that LF/HF-ratio correlates negatively with the lateralization index for alpha and gamma activity in the insula. This latter result demonstrates that increased LF and(or) decreased HF goes together with a decrease of activity in the left insula and an increase of activity in the right insula.

Distress and the Brain

Tinnitus distress, as reflected by the TQ, correlates positively with the lateralization index of the insula in alpha, indicating that an increase in right insula and/or a decrease in left insula go together with an increase in tinnitus related distress. It has already been shown that alpha activity in both the left and right insula correlates with the severity of tinnitus-related distress [9]. In addition also a correlation was found between TQ and the dorsal anterior cingulate cortex for high beta frequency band and the TQ and subgenual anterior cingulate cortex for alpha frequency band [9].

Heart Rate Variability and Distress

No correlation could be found between the TQ and respectively LF, HF and LF/HF-ratio HRV. This is similar to previous research demonstrating no correlation between trait anxiety and LF, HF and LF/HF-ratio HRV [75]. However research further revealed that the lateralisation index for alpha activity can be associated with both TQ and LF/HF-ratio, while the lateralisation index for gamma could only be associated to the LF/HF-ratio. Taking these findings together this would suggest that the left and right insula in alpha activity influence the TQ and LF/HF-ratio.

Heart Rate Variability, Distress and the Brain

Our results seem to indicate that the sympathovagal balance is controlled by subgenual and pregenual anterior cingulate cortex, whereas the left and right insula control parasympathetic and sympathetic activity respectively. Interestingly, the tinnitus distress correlates positively with the lateralization index of the insula, indicating that distress seems to be sympathetically mediated, as has been demonstrated previously [76]. In addition we found an interaction effect between the LF/HF ratio and distress for the pregenual anterior cingulate cortex within high beta and gamma frequency band. It has been proposed [77] and shown [81] that the pregenual anterior cingulate cortex mediates a the top-down inhibitory effect on tinnitus [78], analogous to what has been shown for pain [79–81]. This top-down, descending pain inhibitory system involves the anterior insula, pregenual anterior cingulate cortex, and periaqueductal gray [81]. In the auditory system it involves the subgenual and pregenual anterior cingulate cortex [62,78,82], and could also involve the anterior insula and the longitudinal tectal column, a recently discovered structure, adjacent to the periaqueductal gray, the auditory analogue of the somatosensory periaqueductal gray [77]. In pain, fluctuations of activity in the dorsal anterior cingulate cortex and anterior insula determine whether a near threshold pain stimulus is consciously perceived or not [83], and the same holds for an auditory stimulus [84]. Thus by decreasing the anterior cingulate and anterior

insular activity painful and auditory stimuli can be processed without the stimuli reaching awareness, linked to the anterior insula [85–87].

Limitations of the Study

One major limitation of this and any EEG based approach is that no subcortical activity can be analyzed, limiting network description to cortical sources. The data presented should therefore be viewed acknowledging this limitation. Another limitation of the present study is that no control group was included in the study. However, our analysis shows that within tinnitus patients certain brain areas play an important role in the central control of HRV and that these brain areas are also correlated to tinnitus related distress. This does not exclude that for control subjects this could also be the matter. Yet previous research has shown that dorsal anterior cingulate cortex and the subgenual anterior cingulate cortex show increased activity in respectively the Beta and Alpha activity in comparison to a control group [9,10]. Hence, we think that the results obtained in our study might be reliable and valid, but it should be stressed that further research confirming and extending these results is needed, e.g. by using a control group.

Conclusion

In conclusion our data suggest that the dorsal and subgenual anterior cingulate cortex, as well as the left and right insula are important in the central control of heart rate variability in tinnitus patients. Whereas the sympathovagal balance is controlled by the subgenual and pregenual anterior cingulate cortex, the right insula controls sympathetic activity and the left insula the parasympathetic activity. The perceived distress in tinnitus patients seems to be sympathetically mediated.

Acknowledgments

The authors thank Jan Ost, Bram Van Achteren, Bjorn Devree and Pieter van Looy for their help in preparing this manuscript.

Author Contributions

Conceived and designed the experiments: SV DD. Performed the experiments: SV DD. Analyzed the data: SV DD. Contributed reagents/materials/analysis tools: SV DD. Wrote the paper: SV DD.

References

1. Moller AR (2007) Tinnitus: presence and future. Prog Brain Res 166: 3–16.
2. Baguley DM (2002) Mechanisms of tinnitus. Br Med Bull 63: 195–212.
3. Eggermont JJ, Roberts LE (2004) The neuroscience of tinnitus. Trends Neurosci 27: 676–682.
4. Heller AJ (2003) Classification and epidemiology of tinnitus. Otolaryngol Clin North Am 36: 239–248.
5. Axelsson A, Ringdahl A (1989) Tinnitus–a study of its prevalence and characteristics. Br J Audiol 23: 53–62.
6. Cronlein T, Langguth B, Geisler P, Hajak G (2007) Tinnitus and insomnia. Prog Brain Res 166: 227–233.
7. Scott B, Lindberg P (2000) Psychological profile and somatic complaints between help-seeking and non-help-seeking tinnitus subjects. Psychosomatics 41: 347–352.
8. Erlandsson SI, Holgers KM (2001) The impact of perceived tinnitus severity on health-related quality of life with aspects of gender. Noise Health 3: 39–51.
9. Vanneste S, Plazier M, der Loo E, de Heyning PV, Congedo M, et al. (2010) The neural correlates of tinnitus-related distress. Neuroimage 52: 470–480.
10. De Ridder D, Vanneste S, Congedo M (2011) The distressed brain: a group blind source separation analysis on tinnitus. PLoS One 6: e24273.
11. Schlee W, Weisz N, Bertrand O, Hartmann T, Elbert T (2008) Using auditory steady state responses to outline the functional connectivity in the tinnitus brain. PLoS ONE 3: e3720.
12. Schlee W, Mueller N, Hartmann T, Keil J, Lorenz I, et al. (2009) Mapping cortical hubs in tinnitus. BMC Biol 7: 80.

13. Ulrich-Lai YM, Herman JP (2009) Neural regulation of endocrine and autonomic stress responses. Nat Rev Neurosci 10: 397–409.
14. Guyenet PG (2006) The sympathetic control of blood pressure. Nat Rev Neurosci 7: 335–346.
15. Datzov E, Danev S, Haralanov H, Naidenova V, Sachanska T, et al. (1999) Tinnitus, heart rate variability, and some biochemical indicators. Int Tinnitus J 5: 20–23.
16. Matsushima JI, Kamada T, Sakai N, Miyoshi S, Uemi N, et al. (1996) Increased Parasympathetic Nerve Tone in Tinnitus Patients Following Electrical Promontory Stimulation. Int Tinnitus J 2: 67–71.
17. Oppenheimer SM, Kedem G, Martin WM (1996) Left-insular cortex lesions perturb cardiac autonomic tone in humans. Clin Auton Res 6: 131–140.
18. Oppenheimer S (2006) Cerebrogenic cardiac arrhythmias: cortical lateralization and clinical significance. Clin Auton Res 16: 6–11.
19. Craig AD (2005) Forebrain emotional asymmetry: a neuroanatomical basis? Trends Cogn Sci 9: 566–571.
20. Oppenheimer S (1993) The anatomy and physiology of cortical mechanisms of cardiac control. Stroke 24: 13–5.
21. Yasuma F, Hayano J (2004) Respiratory sinus arrhythmia: why does the heartbeat synchronize with respiratory rhythm? Chest 125: 683–690.
22. Ahs F, Sollers JJ, 3rd, Furmark T, Fredrikson M, Thayer JF (2009) High-frequency heart rate variability and cortico-striatal activity in men and women with social phobia. Neuroimage 47: 815–820.

23. Lane RD, McRae K, Reiman EM, Chen K, Ahern GL, et al. (2009) Neural correlates of heart rate variability during emotion. Neuroimage 44: 213–222.

24. Napadow V, Dhond R, Conti G, Makris N, Brown EN, et al. (2008) Brain correlates of autonomic modulation: combining heart rate variability with fMRI. Neuroimage 42: 169–177.

25. Matthews SC, Paulus MP, Simmons AN, Nelesen RA, Dimsdale JE (2004) Functional subdivisions within anterior cingulate cortex and their relationship to autonomic nervous system function. Neuroimage 22: 1151–1156.

26. Suzuki H, Watanabe S, Hamaguchi T, Mine H, Terui T, et al. (2009) Brain activation associated with changes in heart rate, heart rate variability, and plasma catecholamines during rectal distention. Psychosom Med 71: 619–626.

27. Babiloni C, Binetti G, Cassarino A, Dal Forno G, Del Percio C, et al. (2006) Sources of cortical rhythms in adults during physiological aging: a multicentric EEG study. Hum Brain Mapp 27: 162–172.

28. Pascual-Marqui RD (2002) Standardized low-resolution brain electromagnetic tomography (sLORETA): technical details. Methods Find Exp Clin Pharmacol 24 Suppl D: 5–12.

29. Moazami-Goudarzi M, Michels L, Weisz N, Jeanmonod D (2010) Temporo-insular enhancement of EEG low and high frequencies in patients with chronic tinnitus. QEEG study of chronic tinnitus patients. BMC Neurosci 11: 40.

30. Meeus O, Blaivie C, Van de Heyning P (2007) Validation of the Dutch and the French version of the Tinnitus Questionnaire. B-ENT 3 Suppl 7: 11–17.

31. Goebel G, Hiller W (1994) [The tinnitus questionnaire. A standard instrument for grading the degree of tinnitus. Results of a multicenter study with the tinnitus questionnaire]. HNO 42: 166–172.

32. Vanneste S, Plazier M, van der Loo E, Ost J, Meeus O, et al. (2010) Validation of the Mini-TQ in a Dutch-speaking population. A rapid assessment for tinnitus-related distress. B-ENT.

33. van der Loo E, Congedo M, Vanneste S, De Heyning PV, De Ridder D (2011) Insular lateralization in tinnitus distress. Auton Neurosci.

34. Congedo M (2002) EureKa! (Version 3.0) [Computer Software]. Knoxville, TN: NovaTech EEG Inc. Freeware available at www.NovaTechEEG. Accessed 2013 Feb 26.

35. Pascual-Marqui RD, Esslen M, Kochi K, Lehmann D (2002) Functional imaging with low-resolution brain electromagnetic tomography (LORETA): a review. Methods Find Exp Clin Pharmacol 24 Suppl C: 91–95.

36. Fuchs M, Kastner J, Wagner M, Hawes S, Ebersole JS (2002) A standardized boundary element method volume conductor model. Clin Neurophysiol 113: 702–712.

37. Mulert C, Jager L, Schmitt R, Bussfeld P, Pogarell O, et al. (2004) Integration of fMRI and simultaneous EEG: towards a comprehensive understanding of localization and time-course of brain activity in target detection. Neuroimage 22: 83–94.

38. Vitacco D, Brandeis D, Pascual-Marqui R, Martin E (2002) Correspondence of event-related potential tomography and functional magnetic resonance imaging during language processing. Hum Brain Mapp 17: 4–12.

39. Worrell GA, Lagerlund TD, Sharbrough FW, Brinkmann BH, Busacker NE, et al. (2000) Localization of the epileptic focus by low-resolution electromagnetic tomography in patients with a lesion demonstrated by MRI. Brain Topogr 12: 273–282.

40. Dierks T, Jelic V, Pascual-Marqui RD, Wahlund L, Julin P, et al. (2000) Spatial pattern of cerebral glucose metabolism (PET) correlates with localization of intracerebral EEG-generators in Alzheimer's disease. Clin Neurophysiol 111: 1817–1824.

41. Pizzagalli DA, Oakes TR, Fox AS, Chung MK, Larson CL, et al. (2004) Functional but not structural subgenual prefrontal cortex abnormalities in melancholia. Mol Psychiatry 9: 325, 393–405.

42. Zumsteg D, Wennberg RA, Treyer V, Buck A, Wieser HG (2005) H2(15)O or 13NH3 PET and electromagnetic tomography (LORETA) during partial status epilepticus. Neurology 65: 1657–1660.

43. Zumsteg D, Lozano AM, Wennberg RA (2006) Depth electrode recorded cerebral responses with deep brain stimulation of the anterior thalamus for epilepsy. Clin Neurophysiol 117: 1602–1609.

44. Zumsteg D, Lozano AM, Wieser HG, Wennberg RA (2006) Cortical activation with deep brain stimulation of the anterior thalamus for epilepsy. Clin Neurophysiol 117: 192–207.

45. Volpe U, Mucci A, Bucci P, Merlotti E, Galderisi S, et al. (2007) The cortical generators of P3a and P3b: a LORETA study. Brain Res Bull 73: 220–230.

46. Pizzagalli D, Pascual-Marqui RD, Nitschke JB, Oakes TR, Larson CL, et al. (2001) Anterior cingulate activity as a predictor of degree of treatment response in major depression: evidence from brain electrical tomography analysis. Am J Psychiatry 158: 405–415.

47. Zumsteg D, Lozano AM, Wennberg RA (2006) Mesial temporal inhibition in a patient with deep brain stimulation of the anterior thalamus for epilepsy. Epilepsia 47: 1958–1962.

48. Weisz N, Moratti S, Meinzer M, Dohrmann K, Elbert T (2005) Tinnitus perception and distress is related to abnormal spontaneous brain activity as measured by magnetoencephalography. PLoS Med 2: e153.

49. Weisz N, Muller S, Schlee W, Dohrmann K, Hartmann T, et al. (2007) The neural code of auditory phantom perception. J Neurosci 27: 1479–1484.

50. Nichols TE, Holmes AP (2002) Nonparametric permutation tests for functional neuroimaging: a primer with examples. Hum Brain Mapp 15: 1–25.

51. Schlee W, Leirer V, Kolassa IT, Weisz N, Elbert T (2012) Age-related changes in neural functional connectivity and its behavioral relevance. BMC Neurosci 13: 16.

52. Kamath MV, Fallen EL (1993) Power spectral analysis of heart rate variability: a noninvasive signature of cardiac autonomic function. Crit Rev Biomed Eng 21: 245–311.

53. Goldin PR, Manber T, Hakimi S, Canli T, Gross JJ (2009) Neural bases of social anxiety disorder: emotional reactivity and cognitive regulation during social and physical threat. Arch Gen Psychiatry 66: 170–180.

54. Wong SW, Masse N, Kimmerly DS, Menon RS, Shoemaker JK (2007) Ventral medial prefrontal cortex and cardiovagal control in conscious humans. Neuroimage 35: 698–708.

55. Hansel A, von Kanel R (2008) The ventro-medial prefrontal cortex: a major link between the autonomic nervous system, regulation of emotion, and stress reactivity? Biopsychosoc Med 2: 21.

56. Nicotra A, Critchley HD, Mathias CJ, Dolan RJ (2006) Emotional and autonomic consequences of spinal cord injury explored using functional brain imaging. Brain 129: 718–728.

57. Verberne AJ, Owens NC (1998) Cortical modulation of the cardiovascular system. Prog Neurobiol 54: 149–168.

58. Critchley HD, Mathias CJ, Josephs O, O'Doherty J, Zanini S, et al. (2003) Human cingulate cortex and autonomic control: converging neuroimaging and clinical evidence. Brain 126: 2139–2152.

59. Zald DH, Pardo JV (2002) The neural correlates of aversive auditory stimulation. Neuroimage 16: 746–753.

60. Blood AJ, Zatorre RJ, Bermudez P, Evans AC (1999) Emotional responses to pleasant and unpleasant music correlate with activity in paralimbic brain regions. Nat Neurosci 2: 382–387.

61. Muhlau M, Rauschecker JP, Oestreicher E, Gaser C, Rottinger M, et al. (2006) Structural brain changes in tinnitus. Cereb Cortex 16: 1283–1288.

62. Rauschecker JP, leaver AM, Muhlau M (2010) Tuning Out the Noise: Limbic-Auditory Interactions in Tinnitus. Neuron 66: 819–826.

63. Frysztak RJ, Neafsey EJ (1994) The effect of medial frontal cortex lesions on cardiovascular conditioned emotional responses in the rat. Brain Res 643: 181–193.

64. Ongur D, Price JL (2000) The organization of networks within the orbital and medial prefrontal cortex of rats, monkeys and humans. Cereb Cortex 10: 206–219.

65. Stein JL, Wiedholz LM, Bassett DS, Weinberger DR, Zink CF, et al. (2007) A validated network of effective amygdala connectivity. Neuroimage 36: 736–745.

66. Margulies DS, Kelly AM, Uddin LQ, Biswal BB, Castellanos FX, et al. (2007) Mapping the functional connectivity of anterior cingulate cortex. Neuroimage 37: 579–588.

67. Kahn I, Andrews-Hanna JR, Vincent JL, Snyder AZ, Buckner RL (2008) Distinct cortical anatomy linked to subregions of the medial temporal lobe revealed by intrinsic functional connectivity. J Neurophysiol 100: 129–139.

68. Critchley HD (2005) Neural mechanisms of autonomic, affective, and cognitive integration. J Comp Neurol 493: 154–166.

69. Craig AD (2003) Interoception: the sense of the physiological condition of the body. Curr Opin Neurobiol 13: 500–505.

70. Oppenheimer SM, Gelb A, Girvin JP, Hachinski VC (1992) Cardiovascular effects of human insular cortex stimulation. Neurology 42: 1727–1732.

71. Critchley HD, Wiens S, Rotshtein P, Ohman A, Dolan RJ (2004) Neural systems supporting interoceptive awareness. Nat Neurosci 7: 189–195.

72. Wang J, Rao H, Wetmore GS, Furlan PM, Korczykowski M, et al. (2005) Perfusion functional MRI reveals cerebral blood flow pattern under psychological stress. Proc Natl Acad Sci U S A 102: 17804–17809.

73. Critchley HD, Corfield DR, Chandler MP, Mathias CJ, Dolan RJ (2000) Cerebral correlates of autonomic cardiovascular arousal: a functional neuroimaging investigation in humans. J Physiol 523 Pt 1: 259–270.

74. Baliki MN, Geha PY, Apkarian AV (2009) Parsing pain perception between nociceptive representation and magnitude estimation. J Neurophysiol 101: 875–887.

75. Tolkunov D, Rubin D, Mujica-Parodi L (2010) Power spectrum scale invariance quantifies limbic dysregulation in trait anxious adults using fMRI: adapting methods optimized for characterizing autonomic dysregulation to neural dynamic time series. Neuroimage 50: 72–80.

76. van der Loo E, Congedo M, Vanneste S, De Heyning PV, De Ridder D (2011) Insular lateralization in tinnitus distress. Auton Neurosci 165: 191–194.

77. De Ridder D, Vanneste S, Menovsky T, Langguth B (2012) Surgical brain modulation for tinnitus: the past, present and future. J Neurosurg Sci 56: 323–340.

78. Vanneste S, De Ridder D (2011) Bifrontal transcranial direct current stimulation modulates tinnitus intensity and tinnitus-distress-related brain activity. Eur J Neurosci 34: 605–614.

79. Kong J, Loggia ML, Zyloney C, Tu P, Laviolette P, et al. (2010) Exploring the brain in pain: activations, deactivations and their relation. Pain 148: 257–267.

80. Bingel U, Tracey I (2008) Imaging CNS modulation of pain in humans. Physiology (Bethesda) 23: 371–380.

81. Fields H (2004) State-dependent opioid control of pain. Nat Rev Neurosci 5: 565–575.

82. Leaver AM, Renier L, Chevillet MA, Morgan S, Kim HJ, et al. (2011) Dysregulation of limbic and auditory networks in tinnitus. Neuron 69: 33–43.

83. Boly M, Balteau E, Schnakers C, Degueldre C, Moonen G, et al. (2007) Baseline brain activity fluctuations predict somatosensory perception in humans. Proc Natl Acad Sci U S A 104: 12187–12192.

84. Sadaghiani S, Hesselmann G, Kleinschmidt A (2009) Distributed and antagonistic contributions of ongoing activity fluctuations to auditory stimulus detection. J Neurosci 29: 13410–13417.

85. Craig AD (2002) How do you feel? Interoception: the sense of the physiological condition of the body. Nat Rev Neurosci 3: 655–666.

86. Bamiou DE, Musiek FE, Luxon LM (2003) The insula (Island of Reil) and its role in auditory processing. Literature review. Brain Res Brain Res Rev 42: 143–154.

87. Fifer RC (1993) Insular stroke causing unilateral auditory processing disorder: case report. J Am Acad Audiol 4: 364–369.

Permissions

The contributors of this book come from diverse backgrounds, making this book a truly international effort. This book will bring forth new frontiers with its revolutionizing research information and detailed analysis of the nascent developments around the world.

We would like to thank all the contributing authors for lending their expertise to make the book truly unique. They have played a crucial role in the development of this book. Without their invaluable contributions this book wouldn't have been possible. They have made vital efforts to compile up to date information on the varied aspects of this subject to make this book a valuable addition to the collection of many professionals and students.

This book was conceptualized with the vision of imparting up-to-date information and advanced data in this field. To ensure the same, a matchless editorial board was set up. Every individual on the board went through rigorous rounds of assessment to prove their worth. After which they invested a large part of their time researching and compiling the most relevant data for our readers.

The editorial board has been involved in producing this book since its inception. They have spent rigorous hours researching and exploring the diverse topics which have resulted in the successful publishing of this book. They have passed on their knowledge of decades through this book. To expedite this challenging task, the publisher supported the team at every step. A small team of assistant editors was also appointed to further simplify the editing procedure and attain best results for the readers.

Apart from the editorial board, the designing team has also invested a significant amount of their time in understanding the subject and creating the most relevant covers. They scrutinized every image to scout for the most suitable representation of the subject and create an appropriate cover for the book.

The publishing team has been an ardent support to the editorial, designing and production team. Their endless efforts to recruit the best for this project, has resulted in the accomplishment of this book. They are a veteran in the field of academics and their pool of knowledge is as vast as their experience in printing. Their expertise and guidance has proved useful at every step. Their uncompromising quality standards have made this book an exceptional effort. Their encouragement from time to time has been an inspiration for everyone.

The publisher and the editorial board hope that this book will prove to be a valuable piece of knowledge for researchers, students, practitioners and scholars across the globe.

List of Contributors

Avril Genene Holt, David Bissig, Najab Mirza and Gary Rajah
Department of Anatomy and Cell Biology, Wayne State University School of Medicine, Detroit, Michigan, United States of America

Bruce Berkowitz
Department of Anatomy and Cell Biology, Wayne State University School of Medicine, Detroit, Michigan, United States of America
Department of Ophthalmology, Wayne State University School of Medicine, Detroit, Michigan, United States of America

Elisabeth Peltier, Cedric Peltier, Stephanie Tahar and Evelyne Alliot-Lugaz
Laboratoire Chelles surdité, Chelles, France

Yves Cazals
Laboratoire de Neurosciences Intégratives et Adaptatives, Aix-Marseille Université, CNRS UMR 7260, Féderation de Recherche 3C (Cerveau, Comportement, Cognition), Marseille, France

Elisabeth Wallhäusser-Franke, Tobias Balkenhol, Andrea Seegmüller and Wolfgang Delb
Department of Phoniatrics and Audiology, Medical Faculty Mannheim, Heidelberg University, Mannheim, Germany

Roberto D'Amelio
Department of Phoniatrics and Audiology, Medical Faculty Mannheim, Heidelberg University, Mannheim, Germany
Department of Internal Medicine IV and Neurocenter, University Clinic, Saarland University, Homburg/Saar, Germany

Joachim Brade
Department of Medical Statistics and Biomathematics, Medical Faculty Mannheim, Heidelberg University, Mannheim, Germany

Veronika Vielsmeier and Jürgen Strutz
Department of Otorhinolaryngology, University of Regensburg, Regensburg, Germany

Tobias Kleinjung
Department of Otorhinolaryngology, University of Zurich, Zurich, Switzerland

Martin Schecklmann, Peter Michael Kreuzer, Michael Landgrebe and Berthold Langguth
Department of Psychiatry and Psychotherapy, University of Regensburg, Regensburg, Germany

Sönke Ahlf, Konstantin Tziridis, Sabine Korn, Ilona Strohmeyer and Holger Schulze
Experimental Otolaryngology, University of Erlangen-Nuremberg, Erlangen, Germany

Henning Teismann and Christo Pantev
Institute for Biomagnetism and Biosignalanalysis, University of Muenster, Muenster, Germany

Hidehiko Okamoto
Institute for Biomagnetism and Biosignalanalysis, University of Muenster, Muenster, Germany
Department of Integrative Physiology, National Institute for Physiological Sciences, Okazaki, Japan

Tobias Balkenhol, Elisabeth Wallhäusser-Franke and Wolfgang Delb
Department of Phoniatrics and Audiology, Medical Faculty Mannheim, Heidelberg University, Mannheim, Germany

Kathleen Joos, Sven Vanneste and Dirk De Ridder
Brai^{2}n, Tinnitus Research Initiative Clinic Antwerp, Department of Neurosurgery, University Hospital Antwerp, Belgium

Nadia Müller
Università degli Studi di Trento, Center for Mind/Brain Sciences, Mattarello, Italy

Nathan Weisz
Università degli Studi di Trento, Center for Mind/Brain Sciences, Mattarello, Italy
Zukunftskolleg, University of Konstanz, Konstanz, Germany

Isabel Lorenz
University of Konstanz, Department of Psychology, Konstanz, Germany

Berthold Langguth
University Hospital Regensburg, Department of Psychiatry and Psychotherapy, Regensburg, Germany

Athena Demertzi, Audrey Vanhaudenhuyse and Andrea Soddu
Coma Science Group, Cyclotron Research Centre, University of Liège, Liège, Belgium

Audrey Maudoux
Coma Science Group, Cyclotron Research Centre, University of Liège, Liège, Belgium
OtoRhinoLaryngology Head and Neck Surgery Department, University of Liège, Liège, Belgium

Steven Laureys
Coma Science Group, Cyclotron Research Centre, University of Liège, Liège, Belgium
Neurology Department, CHU Sart Tilman Hospital, University of Liège, Liège, Belgium

Philippe Lefebvre
OtoRhinoLaryngology Head and Neck Surgery Department, University of Liège, Liège, Belgium

Jean-Evrard Cabay
Radiology Department, CHU Sart Tilman Hospital, University of Liège, Liège, Belgium

Dirk De Ridder and Sven Vanneste
Brain, TRI & Department of Neurosurgery, Antwerp University Hospital, Antwerp, Belgium,

Marco Congedo
Team ViBS (Vision and Brain Signal Processing), GIPSA-lab, National Center for Scientific Research, Grenoble University, Grenoble, France

Lukas Rüttiger., Wibke Singer., Rama Panford-Walsh., Masahiro Matsumoto, Sze Chim Lee, Annalisa Zuccotti, Ulrike Zimmermann, Mirko Jaumann, Karin Rohbock, Hao Xiong and Marlies Knipper
Department of Otolaryngology, Hearing Research Centre Tübingen (THRC), Molecular Physiology of Hearing, University of Tübingen, Tübingen, Germany

Sylvie Hébert
É cole d'orthophonie et d'audiologie, Faculté de médecine, Université de Montréal, BRAMS, International Laboratory for Brain, Music, and Sound Research, and Centre de recherche de l'Institut universitaire de gériatrie de Montréal, Montréal, Québec, Canada

Linda L. Magnusson Hanson and Hugo Westerlund
Stress Research Institute, Stockholm University, Stockholm, Sweden

Töres Theorell
Stress Research Institute, Stockholm University, Stockholm, Sweden
Department of Public Health, Karolinska Institute, Stockholm, Sweden

Dan Hasson
Stress Research Institute, Stockholm University, Stockholm, Sweden

Department of Physiology and Pharmacology, Karolinska Institute, Stockholm, Sweden

Barbara Canlon
Department of Physiology and Pharmacology, Karolinska Institute, Stockholm, Sweden

Winfried Schlee and Iris-Tatjana Kolassa
Department of Clinical and Biological Psychology, University of Ulm, Ulm, Germany

Tobias Kleinjung
Department of Otorhinolaryngology, University of Zurich, Zurich, Switzerland
Interdisciplinary Tinnitus Clinic, University of Regensburg, Regensburg, Germany

Berthold Langguth
Interdisciplinary Tinnitus Clinic, University of Regensburg, Regensburg, Germany
Department of Psychiatry and Psychotherapy, University of Regensburg, Regensburg, Germany

Wolfgang Hiller
Department of Clinical Psychology, University of Mainz, Regensburg, Germany

Gerhard Goebel
Medical-Psychomatic Hospital, Schoen Clinic Roseneck, Prien, Germany

Yan-Yan Su, Bin Luo, Yan Jin and Lin Chen
CAS Key Laboratory of Brain Function and Disease, School of Life Sciences, University of Science and Technology of China, Hefei, China
Auditory Research Laboratory, University of Science and Technology of China, Hefei, China

Shu-Hui Wu
Department of Neuroscience, Carleton University, Ottawa, Ontario, Canada

Edward Lobarinas and Richard J. Salvi
Center for Hearing and Deafness, State University of New York at Buffalo, Buffalo, New York, United States of America

Sven Vanneste, Kathleen Joos and Dirk De Ridder
Brai^{2}n, TRI & Department of Neurosurgery, University Hospital Antwerp, Belgium

Juen-Haur Hwang
Department of Otolaryngology, Buddhist Dalin Tzu-Chi General Hospital, Dalin, Chiayi, Taiwan
School of Medicine, Tzu Chi University, Hualien, Taiwan

Jin-Cherng Chen
School of Medicine, Tzu Chi University, Hualien, Taiwan
Department of Neurosurgery, Buddhist Dalin Tzu-Chi
General Hospital, Dalin, Chiayi, Taiwan

Yin-Ching Chan
Department of Food and Nutrition, Providence
University, Shalu, Taichung, Taiwan

Andreas Wollbrink and Christo Pantev
Institute for Biomagnetism and Biosignalanalysis,
University Hospital, Münster, Germany

Henning Teismann
Institute for Biomagnetism and Biosignalanalysis,
University Hospital, Münster, Germany
Institute for Epidemiology and Social Medicine,
University Hospital, Münster, Germany

Hidehiko Okamoto
Department of Integrative Physiology, National
Institute for Physiological Sciences, Okazaki, Japan

Gottfried Schlaug
Department of Neurology, Beth Israel Deaconess
Medical Center and Harvard Medical School, Boston,
Massachusetts, United States of America

Claudia Rudack
Department of Otorhinolaryngology, University
Hospital, Münster, Germany

Hugo Hesser and Peter Molander
Department of Behavioural Sciences and Learning,
Swedish Institute for Disability Research, Linkö ping
University, Linköping, Sweden

Gerhard Andersson
Department of Behavioural Sciences and Learning,
Swedish Institute for Disability Research, Linkö ping
University, Linköping, Sweden
Psychiatry Section, Department of Clinical Neuroscience,
Karolinska Institutet, Stockholm, Sweden

Mikael Jungermann
Department of Behavioural Sciences and Learning,
Linkö ping University, Linköping, Sweden

**Maura Regina Laureano, Roberta Ribeiro de Almeida
and Andrea Parolin Jackowski**
Laboratório Interdisciplinar de Neurociências Clínicas
(LiNC), Departamento de Psiquiatria, Universidade
Federal de São Paulo, São Paulo, Brasil

**Rodrigo Affonseca Bressan, Ilza Rosa Batista and
Marilia Alves Reis**
Laboratório Interdisciplinar de Neurociências Clínicas
(LiNC), Departamento de Psiquiatria, Universidade
Federal de São Paulo, São Paulo, Brasil
Instituto do Cérebro – Hospital Israelita Albert
Einstein, São Paulo, Brasil

Ektor Tsuneo Onishi
Departamento de Otorrinolaringologia e Cirurgia de
Cabeça e Pescoço, Universidade Federal de São Paulo,
São Paulo, Brasil

Mario Luiz Vieira Castiglioni
Seção de Medicina Nuclear, Departamento de
Radiologia, Universidade Federal de São Paulo, São
Paulo, Brasil

**Michele Vargas Garcia and Adriana Neves de
Andrade**
Departamento de Fonoaudiologia, Universidade
Federal de São Paulo, São Paulo, Brasil

Griselda J. Garrido
Western Australian Centre for Health and Ageing,
Centre for Medical Research, University of Western
Australia, Perth, Australia

Kathleen Joos
Department of Translational Neuroscience, Faculty of
Medicine, University of Antwerp, Antwerp, Belgium

Sven Vanneste
Department of Translational Neuroscience, Faculty of
Medicine, University of Antwerp, Antwerp, Belgium
School of Behavioral and Brain Sciences, The University
of Texas at Dallas, Richardson, Texas, United States of
America

Index